Nerves: Anatomy, Exposures, and Techniques

Amgad S. Hanna
Editor

Nerves: Anatomy, Exposures, and Techniques

Second Edition

Springer

Editor
Amgad S. Hanna
Department of Neurosurgery
University of Wisconsin School
of Medicine and Public Health
Madison, WI, USA

ISBN 978-3-031-73930-9 ISBN 978-3-031-73931-6 (eBook)
https://doi.org/10.1007/978-3-031-73931-6

This Springer imprint is published by the registered company Springer Nature Switzerland AG
The registered company address is: Gewerbestrasse 11, 6330 Cham, Switzerland

To all students, residents, and fellows seeking a career in Nerve Surgery

To my family

In memory of our colleague and friend Dr. Lynda J-S Yang

Foreword to First Edition

Most physicians' understanding of the anatomy of the spinal nerves is limited throughout the fields of medicine, in spite of that system's exquisite importance to normal function. Often this is the result of a lack of experience with the pathology involved or impractical training methods. The functionality of these nerves for qualities of occupation, ambulation, and eye-hand coordination to name but a few, deserves better. Traditional teaching techniques lack the organization that would enhance understanding and familiarity.

In this volume, Hanna and Ehlers provide a straightforward approach to the surgical anatomy of the spinal nerves by emphasizing the steps of surgery and the actual structures that are seen. Their approach is concise and practical. It emphasizes a surgeon's view of the anatomy in a step-by-step pattern that facilitates understanding of the surrounding musculature, vasculature, and their location and importance. By working through each of the major surgical nerves they cover most clinical scenarios. This makes the book invaluable for students attempting to understand the practical implications of this system or surgeons efficiently studying their work and building on this platform to improve surgical techniques. The practicality of this book is obvious in that it serves the surgeons in an anatomically based fashion through a practical rather than cadaveric approach. It is a welcome addition to literature, and in a concise fashion, thoroughly covers the topic. The authors are to be congratulated for this contribution.

Department of Neurological Surgery
University of Wisconsin School
of Medicine and Public Health
Madison, WI, USA

Robert J. Dempsey

Foreword to First Edition

Nerve anatomy is often a stumbling block for neurosurgeons preparing for board examinations or contemplating unusual cases. Outside of academic centers, limited volume and sub-specialization in other fields limits the exposure of neurosurgeons to these types of cases. Traditional resources for trainees and those wishing to "brush up" on nerve cases consist of anatomic textbooks, which largely rely on traditional anatomic exposures to illustrate the structures of interest. These "anatomical" exposures are not always directly relevant to surgical exposures, which in general are less extensile in order to minimize morbidity.

Hanna and Ehlers have provided a concise and useful text for the study of practical nerve anatomy. This work differs from traditional texts in that the approach is surgically based. The chapters are geared towards answering two or three questions per topic: What anatomy do you see? When do you see it? How do you get there? The text is limited to stripped-down bullet points, which makes it an efficient way to review for board examinations or bone up on a case the night before. Ample illustrations and supplemental videos aid the learner by providing the same information in multiple formats. This work will be a useful addition to the library of neurosurgeons who perform nerve cases on occasion and for trainees who are preparing for upcoming cases or for board examination.

Daniel K. Resnick

Department of Neurological Surgery
University of Wisconsin School
of Medicine and Public Health
Madison, WI, USA

Foreword to Second Edition

Dr. Hanna has provided here a timely update to his very successful first edition, *Anatomy and Exposures of Spinal Nerves*. As we pleasantly discovered in his first edition, learning nerve anatomy and surgical exposures does not have to be difficult or drudgery. His approach is very practical and simplistic; he understands very well that our lives are busy, and we do not have the time or inclination to pore for hours over detailed descriptions of anatomical minutiae. As surgeons we tend to be goal-directed, visual learners, and thus his emphasis on clear intraoperative photos and cadaver dissections provides us with a prompt understanding of the essentials of each procedure. The step-by-step illustrations allow both the novice and the experienced surgeon to learn or review the essential surgical anatomy, identify the important landmarks, appreciate the potential hazards to avoid, and focus the exposure on the pathology to be encountered. Most major clinical scenarios are addressed, and now in this second edition he has added new chapters on more recently developed nerve procedures, including corneal neurotization, lower extremity nerve transfers, surgery for spasticity, spinal cord injury, and torticollis. The text is clear and concise, and the illustrations are accurate and well-labelled. The supplementary material with operative videos is clearly presented and very useful. We are indebted to Dr. Hanna for his meticulous presentation of this important material in a very user-friendly fashion.

Eric L. Zager

Department of Neurosurgery
University of Pennsylvania
Philadelphia, PA, USA

Foreword to Second Edition

This is a follow-up second edition to the initial publication of *Anatomy and Exposure of Spinal Nerves* by Hanna and Ehlers, published in 2015, which in a concise and beautifully illustrated way, provided exposure and relevant surgical anatomical detail for spinal nerves. In this highly anticipated second edition, Hanna has now expanded the format and changed the title to *Nerves: Anatomy, Exposures, and Techniques*. In this new edition, additional chapters on basic neuroanatomy and neurophysiology of nerves, and specialized techniques such as corneal neurotization, facial palsy, lower extremity nerve transfers, surgeries for spasticity, and others have been added. What is retained and the best aspect of this book are the excellent point by point and bulleted concise notes on key anatomical details which allow the practitioner as well as student interested in nerve anatomy and surgery great clarity. The illustrations particularly are fabulous and together with the videos provided allow within only a few and at the most up to 15 min the surgeon to hone up on the surgical anatomy of nerves and techniques to guide surgical exploration. The reader will appreciate immediately the straightforward approach outlined including the several key steps required to expose nerves at surgery. This book will be useful to all students who are interested in nerve anatomy and surgery. It will also be a handy reference to faculty and all surgeons who are encountering nerve conditions in various parts of the body and are planning an operative procedure. By bringing a handy yet masterful approach to the exposure of nerves as well as some important nerve operations, the authors have done a tremendous service to the overall academic as well as clinical community, which will serve to advance the care of patients with surgical nerve disorders. Dr Hanna and his team are to be congratulated for this effort.

Rajiv Midha

Department of Clinical Neurosciences
Hotchkiss Brain Institute,
Cumming School of Medicine
University of Calgary
Calgary, AB, Canada

Preface to First Edition

This book was mainly inspired by deficiencies in most neurosurgery training programs in the field of nerves. I prefer the term spinal nerves as they contrast to cranial nerves. There is a huge gap between the knowledge requirements and what we actually teach. Simplicity was key in writing this book. I intended to avoid the sophistication of textbooks, and burdening you with lots of references. Each chapter is 1–2 pages of text and plenty of figures. There are video recordings for each described approach. Most of the videos are less than 5 min long. The goal is to be able to review each topic in less than 10 min. Whether you are a resident studying for written boards, a junior faculty studying for oral boards, or getting ready for a case that you haven't seen for years, this book should provide you with easy information, and ample illustrations, concise enough to match your busy schedule. The axial cuts and their MRI correlates are unique and will be extremely helpful not only to the nerve surgeon but also to radiologists. I hope you will enjoy going through the material of this book.

Madison, WI, USA | Amgad S. Hanna

Preface to Second Edition

Since its publication in 2015, *Anatomy and Exposures of Spinal Nerves* has had a huge success with over 80,000-chapter downloads and translations to Chinese and Russian. Since then, there have been numerous advances in the nerve world, with newer techniques that should help the field progress forward and improve patient outcomes. We felt compelled to publish a second edition under the title *Nerves: Anatomy, Exposures, and Techniques*. This project is no more a monograph; we have asked the experts in each field to write about their favorite technique. Techniques, such as corneal neurotization, facial reanimation, and penile reinnervation, have been added. Surgeries for torticollis, spasticity, spinal cord injury, and pain are also included. We have also added a whole section on nerve fundamentals including histology, electrodiagnostics, and imaging. This update will significantly enrich the knowledge in the book.

Each author can express her/his own opinion, at times based on evidence and others based on experience, which the reader should be critical of. While some topics could be controversial, the book intends to focus on surgical techniques rather than management debates.

With more than double the number of chapters compared to the first edition, we are sure the reader will savor the beauty of Nerve Surgery, in a more comprehensive yet still concise format. We have intentionally left out the term "peripheral" nerves, since it's a misnomer and does not exist in recently published anatomical nomenclature (Terminologia Anatomica).

Madison, WI, USA

Amgad S. Hanna

Acknowledgments

The authors would like to thank those who donated their bodies for education and science, and their families. Our sincere gratitude to our patients as well.

Contents

Part V Surgical Techniques

Contributors

Amruth K. V. Addanki Doris Duke Clinical Research Continuum, Duke University, Durham, NC, USA
University of Wisconsin–Madison, Madison, WI, USA

Ahmed M. Afifi Division of Plastic and Reconstructive Surgery, Department of Surgery, University of Wisconsin-Madison, Madison, WI, USA

Abdulaziz F. Ahmed Missouri Orthopaedic Institute, Department of Orthopaedic Surgery, University of Missouri School of Medicine, Columbia, MO, USA

Maya Alexis Perelman School of Medicine, University of Pennsylvania, Philadelphia, PA, USA

Asim Ali Department of Ophthalmology and Vision Sciences, University of Toronto and The Hospital for Sick Children, Toronto, ON, Canada

Zarina S. Ali Department of Neurosurgery, Penn Presbyterian Medical Center, University of Pennsylvania, Philadelphia, PA, USA

Simon G. Ammanuel Department of Neurological Surgery, University of Wisconsin Hospitals and Clinics, Madison, WI, USA

Oskar C. Aszmann Clinical Laboratory for Bionic Extremity Reconstruction, Department of Plastic, Reconstructive and Aesthetic Surgery, Medical University of Vienna, Vienna, Austria

Pradeep K. Attaluri Division of Plastic Surgery, Department of Surgery, University of Wisconsin-Madison, Madison, WI, USA

Christopher D. Baggott Department of Neurosurgery, SSM Health—Dean Medical Group, Madison, WI, USA

Niles J. Batdorf Plastic and Reconstructive Surgery Department, The Ohio State University, Columbus, OH, USA

Stanley F. Bazarek Department of Neurological Surgery, Case Western Reserve University School of Medicine, Cleveland, OH, USA

Michael L. Bentz Division of Plastic and Reconstructive Surgery, Department of Surgery, University of Wisconsin-Madison, Madison, WI, USA

Sandip Biswal Department of Radiology, University of Wisconsin-Madison, Madison, WI, USA

Gregory H. Borschel Division of Plastic Surgery, Riley Hospital for Children, Indianapolis, IN, USA

Kelsey M. Bowman Deparment of Neurosurgery, University of Wisconsin School of Medicine and Public Health, Madison, WI, USA

Justin M. Brown Department of Neurosurgery, Massachusetts General Hospital, Harvard Medical School, Boston, MA, USA

Daniel J. Burkett Department of Neurosurgery, SSM Health—Dean Medical Group, Madison, WI, USA

Joaquim Casañas-Sintes Teknon Hospital, Barcelona, Spain
Orthopaedic Surgery and Traumatology, Bellvitge Hospital, Barcelona, Spain

Liann C. Casey University of Cincinnati, Cincinnati, OH, USA

Tak Ho Chu Department of Clinical Neurosciences, University of Calgary, Calgary, AB, Canada

Eric J. Cotter Department of Orthopedics and Rehabilitation, University of Wisconsin School of Medicine and Public Health, Madison, WI, USA

Simeon C. Daeschler Department of Hand, Plastic and Reconstructive Surgery, Burn Center, BG-Trauma Center, University of Heidelberg, Ludwigshafen/Rhine, Germany

Nora F. Dengler Fakultät für Gesundheitswissenschaften Brandenburg, Medizinische Hochschule Brandenburg Theodor Fontane, Bad Saarow Klinik für Neurochirurgie, HELIOS Klinik Bad Saarow Charité – Universitaetsmedizin, Berlin, Germany

Karan Dua Department of Orthopaedic Surgery, New York-Presbytarian/Columbia University Irving Medical Center, New York, NY, USA

Armin Edalatpour Division of Plastic and Reconstructive Surgery, Department of Surgery, University of Wisconsin Hospitals and Clinics, Madison, WI, USA

Mark E. Ehlers Urology, Aurora Health Care Medical Group, Milwaukee, WI, USA

Bassem T. Elhassan Department of Orthopaedic Surgery, Harvard Medical School, Massachusetts General Hospital, Boston, MA, USA

Shady Elmaraghi Department of Plastic Surgery, Vanderbilt Health, Nashville, TN, USA

Akram M. Eraky Department of Neurosurgery, University of Wisconsin School of Medicine and Public Health, Madison, WI, USA

Asma Eslami Department of Neurosurgery, University of Wisconsin School of Medicine and Public Health, Madison, WI, USA

Gustavo L. Fernandes Department of Gynecologic Oncology at Santa Casa, São Paulo, Brazil

Aaron G. Filler Institute for Nerve Medicine, Santa Monica, CA, USA

Júlia Flores-Benítez Department of Human Anatomy, University of Barcelona Medical School, Barcelona, Spain
Orthopaedic Surgery and Traumatology, Bellvitge Hospital, Barcelona, Spain

Anton Fornieles-Espinel Department of Human Anatomy, University of Barcelona Medical School, Barcelona, Spain
Department of Orthopaedic Surgery and Traumatology Department, Vall d'Hebron Hospital, Barcelona, Spain

Rebecca D. Funk Department of Orthopedics and Rehabilitation, University of Wisconsin, Madison, WI, USA

Brian H. Gander Division of Plastic and Reconstructive Surgery, Department of Surgery, University of Wisconsin Hospitals and Clinics, Madison, WI, USA

Robert E. George Division of Plastic and Reconstructive Surgery, Department of Surgery, University of Wisconsin-Madison, Madison, WI, USA

Allison M. Grayev Department of Radiology, University of Wisconsin School of Medicine and Public Health, Madison, WI, USA

Natalia Guevara-Moriones Faculty of Medicine, Universidad Juan N. Corpas, Bogotá, Colombia

Benjamin K. Gundlach Boston Children's Hospital, Harvard Medical School, Department of Orthopedics, Boston, MA, USA

Forrest A. Hamrick School of Medicine, University of Utah, Salt Lake City, UT, USA

Amgad S. Hanna Department of Neurosurgery, University of Wisconsin School of Medicine and Public Health, Madison, WI, USA

Barbara A. Hanna Mayo Clinic Alix School of Medicine, Rochester, MN, USA

Michael J. Hansen Department of Neurology, University of Wisconsin School of Medicine and Public Health, Madison, WI, USA

Christian Heinen Department Neuro-, Spine- and Nerve Surgery, Christliches Krankenhaus, Quakenbrück, Germany

Bermans J. Iskandar Department of Neurosurgery, University of Wisconsin Hospitals and Clinics, Madison, WI, USA

Jacqueline S. Israel Division of Plastic and Reconstructive Surgery, Department of Surgery, University of Wisconsin Hospitals and Clinics, Madison, WI, USA

Benjamin R. Johnston Department of Neurological Surgery, Brigham and Women's, Boston Children's Hospital, Harvard Medical School, Boston, MA, USA

Luke T. Juckett Department of Plastic and Reconstructive Surgery, Maxillofacial and Oral Health, University of Virginia, Charlottesville, VA, USA

Thomas G. Knoedler Department of Orthopaedic Surgery, Lewis Katz School of Medicine at Temple University, Philadelphia, PA, USA

Joyce A. Koueik Department of Neurological Surgery, University of Wisconsin Hospitals and Clinics, Madison, Wisconsin, USA

Scott H. Kozin Lewis Katz School of Medicine at Temple University, Sidney Kimmel Medical College at Thomas Jefferson University, Philadelphia, PA, USA
Shriners Hopsital for Children, Philadelphia, PA, USA

Thomas Kretschmer Department of Neurosurgery and Neurorestoration, Federal State Hospital Klinikum, Klagenfurt, Austria

Nucelio Lemos Temerty Faculty of Medicine, University of Toronto, Toronto, ON, Canada

Kevin J. Little Cincinnati Children's Hospital Medical Center, Cincinnati, OH, USA

Manuel Llusa-Pérez Department of Human Anatomy, University of Barcelona Medical School, Barcelona, Spain
Department of Orthopaedic Surgery and Traumatology, Vall d'Hebron Hospital, Barcelona, Spain

Ryan Lohre Department of Orthopaedic Surgery, Harvard Medical School, Massachusetts General Hospital, Boston, MA, USA

Lucas V. Magnani School of Medicine of Botucatu, São Paulo State University, UNESP, São Paulo, Brazil

Mark A. Mahan Division of Nerve and Pain Surgery, Department of Neurosurgery, University of Utah, Salt Lake City, UT, USA

Udo Maierhofer Clinical Laboratory for Bionic Extremity Reconstruction, Department of Plastic, Reconstructive and Aesthetic Surgery, Medical University of Vienna, Vienna, Austria

Pablo Martínez-Collado Department of Human Anatomy, University of Barcelona Medical School, Barcelona, Spain
Department of Orthopaedic Surgery and Traumatology Department, Vall d'Hebron Hospital, Barcelona, Spain

Lars W. Meisner Department of Neurological Surgery, University of Wisconsin Hospitals and Clinics, Madison, Wisconsin, USA

Rajiv Midha Department of Clinical Neurosciences, Hotchkiss Brain Institute, Cumming School of Medicine, University of Calgary, Calgary, AB, Canada

Stephen P. Miranda Neurosurgery Department, University of Pennsylvania, Philadelphia, PA, USA

Amy M. Moore Plastic and Reconstructive Surgery Department, The Ohio State University Wexner Medical Center, Columbus, OH, USA

Augusta Morgado-Ribeiro Neuropelveology at UNIFESP, São Paulo, Brazil

M. Rosa Morro-Martí Department of Human Anatomy, University of Barcelona Medical School, Barcelona, Spain
Department of Orthopaedic Surgery and Traumatology, Vall d'Hebron Hospital, Barcelona, Spain

Luis Rafael Moscote-Salazar Department of Neurosurgery, University of Wisconsin School of Medicine and Public Health, Madison, WI, USA

Amer Mustafa-Gondolbeu Department of Human Anatomy, University of Lleida Medical School, Lleida, Spain
Department of Orthopaedic Surgery and Traumatology, Arnau de Vilanova Hospital, Lleida, Spain

Balduino F. M. Neto Botucatu School of Medicine, HC-FMB, UNESP, São Paulo, Brazil

Denise Ng Department of Laboratory Medicine, University of Calgary, Calgary, AB, Canada

Ahmed H. Omar Department of Neurosurgery, University of Wisconsin School of Medicine and Public Health, Madison, WI, USA
Department of Neurosurgery, Cairo University, Giza, Egypt

Paul S. Page Department of Neurological Surgery, University of Wisconsin School of Medicine and Public Health, Madison, WI, USA
Goodman Campbell Brain and Spine, Carmel, IN, USA

Eugene Park Sidney Kimmel Medical College of Thomas Jefferson University, Shriners Hospital for Children, Philadelphia, PA, USA

Rajesh K. Pathiyil Department of Clinical Neurosciences, University of Calgary, Calgary, AB, Canada

Maria T. Pedro Sektion Periphere Nerven, Klinik für Neurochirurgie, Universitaetsklinik Ulm am Bezirkskrankenhaus, Günzburg, Germany

Marta Pérez-Montoya Department of Human Anatomy, University of Barcelona Medical School, Barcelona, Spain
Orthopaedic Surgery and Traumatology, Asepeyo Hospital, Sant Cugat del Vallès, Spain

Elise B. Raney Department of Orthopedics and Rehabilitation, University of Wisconsin School of Medicine and Public Health, Madison, WI, USA

Shai M. Rozen Department of Plastic and Reconstructive Surgery, University of Texas Southwestern Medical Center, Dallas, TX, USA

A. Neil Salyapongse Madison Surgery Center, Department of Orthopedics, University of Wisconsin School of Medicine and Public Health, Madison, WI, USA

Ann R. Schwentker University of Cincinnati, Cincinnati Children's Hospital Medical Center, Cincinnati, OH, USA

Allison J. Seitz Division of Plastic and Reconstructive Surgery, Department of Surgery, University of Wisconsin Hospitals and Clinics, Madison, WI, USA

Ellen C. Shaffrey Division of Plastic Surgery, Department of Surgery, University of Wisconsin-Madison, Madison, WI, USA

Alexander Y. Shin Mayo Clinic, Division of Hand Surgery, Department of Orthopaedic Surgery, Rochester, MN, USA

Brandon W. Smith Cone Health Neurosurgery, Burlington, NC, USA

David A. Spinner Department of Rehabilitation and Human Performance, Mount Sinai Hospital, New York, NY, USA

Robert J. Spinner Department of Neurologic Surgery, Mayo Clinic, Rochester, MN, USA

Thomas M. Staniszewski Department of Neurological Surgery, University of Wisconsin School of Medicine and Public Health, Madison, WI, USA

Margaret S. Sten Georgetown University School of Medicine, Washington, DC, USA

Jacob W. Sveum Department of Neurosurgery, University of Wisconsin School of Medicine and Public Health, Madison, WI, USA

John S. Symanski Department of Radiology, University of Wisconsin School of Medicine and Public Health, Madison, WI, USA

Guillermo Tarnawski-Español Department of Human Anatomy, University of Barcelona Medical School, Barcelona, Spain
Department of Orthopaedic Surgery and Traumatology Department, Fraternidad Muprespa Habana Hospital, Madrid, Spain

Jasmine A. Thum Department of Neurosurgery, Massachusetts General Hospital, Harvard Medical School, Boston, MA, USA
Department of Neurosurgery, University of Alabama at Brimingham, Birmingham, AL, USA

Caroline A. Varlotta Department of Rehabilitation and Human Performance, Mount Sinai Hospital, New York, NY, USA

Fausto Viterbo Plastic Surgery, University of the State of São Paulo (UNESP), São Paulo, Brazil
Fausto Viterbo's Plastic Clinic, School of Medicine of Botucatu, São Paulo, Brazil

Y. Edward Wen Department of Plastic and Reconstructive Surgery, University of Texas Southwestern Medical Center, Dallas, TX, USA

Kathryn L. Williams Foot and Ankle Division, Department of Orthopedics and Rehabilitation, University of Wisconsin School of Medicine and Public Health, Madison, WI, USA

Emily Xu Perelman School of Medicine, University of Pennsylvania, Philadelphia, PA, USA

Adolfo Zamora-Madrazo Department of General Surgery, Hospital General de México Dr. Eduardo Liceaga, Ciudad de méxico, Mexico
Department of Plastic and Reconstructive Surgery, University of Texas Southwestern Medical Center, Dallas, TX, USA

Nicole A. Zelenski Department of Orthopaedics, Emory University School of Medicine, Atlanta, GA, USA

Dan A. Zlotolow Sidney Kimmel Medical College of Thomas Jefferson University, Shriners Hospital for Children, Philadelphia, PA, USA
The Hospital for Special Surgery, New York, NY, USA

Part I

Introduction

Anatomization: The History of a Uniquely Human Art

1

Christopher D. Baggott

The opportunity to "anatomize" the human body: The introduction to a modern gross anatomy class inevitably reminds those newly initiated dissectors of a certain *gravitas* that comes with this opportunity. To introduce this atlas, created with such respect for its object, appreciation for the generosity of those who proffered their body after death for the betterment of our science is almost certainly implicit.

However, there exists a trail through human history, which when followed from its origin in prescientific anatomic exploration through its modern course reminds me of an appreciation that I owe to the anatomists as much as to the anatomized. What started as a search for divinity progressed to a discovery of humanity. What started with *careful observations* by dissectors with *prepared minds* was passed forward as truth. The accumulated truths of human experience define our collective history. We continue this work of discovery, of teaching, and of healing.

While creation stories staunchly carry the Neolithic human's anatomic understanding to us nearly unblemished, as in the story of Adam's rib, the careful observations of many knowledgeable anatomists over centuries have been manipulated, distorted, and overlooked by history [1]. Out of respect, I offer a brief account of what we know about the people who helped humanity see what is on the other side of the skin.

Almost a millennium before the birth of Christ, the Hellenistic Greeks flow into the Aegean Peninsula as Minoan culture ebbs. Collecting and synthesizing the anatomic knowledge of the Mediterranean region, the Greek travelers and traders bring Egyptian and Mesopotamian anatomic experience home with them. While anatomic knowledge manifests in these other Mediterranean cultures by way of spiritual or mystical embarkations, the Greeks' *Canon of Proportion* elegantly incorporates anatomic truths with the meticulous artistic tradition of their Minoan predecessors.

Greece is the *patria* of our modern anatomic state. The crude descriptions of the wounds of war brought to us through the Greek poet historians, most notably Homer in his *Iliad*, quickly gain sophistication as sculptors demonstrate anatomic understanding at a level that overwhelms language.

While art, philosophy, and medicine flourish as Greece flourishes, a stronghold of knowledge develops across the Mediterranean. Alexandria emerges as a city empowered not by armies or industry but by knowledge. The Alexandrian Library is adorned with the greatest texts of the known world. The halls of the library accommodate the first known scientific dissectors of the human body, Herophilus and Erasistratus, in the fifth century BC [2].

The contribution of Herophilus, the Father of Anatomy, to neuroanatomy is preserved in the names of the *torcular* and the *calmus scriptorius*, both attributed to Herophilus [3]. Erasistratus, the Father of Physiology, described the passage of *animal spirit* from the cerebral ventricles through the intangible lumina of the nerves, engorging and distending muscles to cause contraction. I am unaware of any eponym commemorating Erasistratus.

Though Fathers of Anatomy and Physiology, respectively, the works of these two men are cloaked in mystery and rumor. Their work is known to us secondhand, primarily through the writings of Galen of Pergamon, as the primary texts are burned in two great fires at the Alexandrian Library.

Galen comments on the texts of Herophilus and Erasistratus critically, reworking the understanding of anatomy and physiology with the knowledge he gathers from his own human dissections. Galen described the vertebral column including the most "sacred" bone *sacrum*, described seven cranial nerves, and even described the differences in spinal cord injury based on the injury level with good accuracy [2]. The great cerebral vein is attributed to a worthy Greek.

The contribution of Galen to medicine, anatomy, and philosophy should not be understated. However, he does seem particularly prominent in the history of medicine. His writing

C. D. Baggott (✉)
Department of Neurosurgery, SSM Health—Dean Medical Group, Madison, WI, USA
e-mail: Christopher.Baggott@SSMHealth.com

A. S. Hanna (ed.), *Nerves: Anatomy, Exposures, and Techniques*, https://doi.org/10.1007/978-3-031-73931-6_1

is unusually well preserved. His work appealed broadly to pagan and Christian alike; Stoic philosophy infused his writing, his dissection, and his understanding of the world he explored so carefully [3]. His popularity was also aided by his status as the physician to Marcus Aurelius, Commodus, and the gladiators.

Despite his prominence in history, not to mention in Rome itself, Galen does not inspire any notable disciples. The status of physicians in Rome is that of a *respected outsider*. The stench of mystery and rumor that surrounds the dissectors in Alexandria follows the early physicians. Stories of death by "anatomization," vivisection, and the like make the field of medicine, rather ironically, the work of those undeserving of Roman citizenry [1, 2].

As the dark ages begin, the Roman Empire is crumbling, the Alexandrian library has suffered two great fires, and the mass of accumulated knowledge of the pagan world is consumed or forgotten. The mob of fanatic Christians awaiting the day of reckoning, the day of salvation, and the day of fire and brimstone see plague and pestilence as a sign of apocalyptic imminence. Every day is a reminder that the flesh is of no importance compared to the soul. Anatomic inquiry is of no use and falls by the wayside.

In the ninth century, during the heart of darkness, the seat of human intellect moves East. Arabic translations and commentaries of the great Galenic and Hippocratic works arm the Persian physicians with the tools to advance diagnosis and treatment to a degree that cannot be understated.

Though the neoclassicism of the Renaissance scrubs much of the Arabic dialect from our modern anatomic and medical nomenclature, the names of Rhazes, Hali Abbas, and the great Avicenna are as critical to the story of medicine as Galen, Hippocrates, and Vesalius. However, the care of the body after death in Islamic religion precludes dissection, inhibiting real progress in anatomic discovery during this period. The contribution of Persian physicians is really that of preservation when looking purely at the field of anatomy independent of medicine.

Back in the West, a zeal for scholasticism, particularly in the monasteries of Northern Italy, inspires the collection and translation of the Greco-Arabic and original Greek texts. This establishes a foundation upon which the first universities are built. At Salerno and Bologna, universities are no more than direct secular extensions of monastic scholasticism.

It is at the University of Bologna that our story accelerates. At the beginning of the fourteenth century, there emerge three students of the University that possess real experience in human dissection, knowledge that does not come from the preserved texts of Greeks or Persians.

The common thread is a mysterious professor, *Thaddeus of Florence*. The work of Thaddeus is largely unknown, but unpublished documents regarding this man are rumored to exist in the Vatican Library [2]. Among his students, *Bartolomeo da Varignama* performs the first documented postmortem examination (which he conducts for forensic purposes at the order of the "jurists" of Bologna's prominent law school), *Henri de Mondeville* brings academic human dissection to the great medical schools that develop in France at Paris and Montpellier, and *Mondino de' Luzzi* pens *Anathomia*, a dissection manual so revolutionary that history labels him as the "Great Restorer of Anatomy" [3].

While there is little more than recapitulation of the Bolognese experience of Mondino and the others for the remainder of the fourteenth century, dissection gains traction in medical school curricula and gains acceptance in popular culture. Even the omnipresent Catholic Church accepts this new mode in the exploration of humanity, owing in large part to Pope Sixtus IV, an alumnus from the University of Bologna. Pope Alexander V, in fact, is examined postmortem prior to his burial at the Church of San Francesco in Bologna, of all places.

Now, the artistic, scientific, and philosophical tides of the time are soon to swell into a great wave of human achievement, the Renaissance.

Here, we must acknowledge a great anachronism: Leonardo da Vinci. Although da Vinci's legacy is that of an intellectual superhero, his works do not contribute to the linear advancement of human understanding. When his partner, Anatomy Professor Marc Antonio della Torre, dies in the midst of their creation of an anatomic text, his 700+ anatomic illustrations are shelved. The sketches, though brilliant, are unpublished until 1784.

We return, then, to the work of mere mortals. In the early Renaissance, anatomic knowledge is disseminated in printed versions of Mondino's *Anathomia*, along with illustrated commentaries on Mondino. Anatomy gains popularity in both scientific and lay communities. Anatomic illustrations take on a certain showmanship that suggests a dual purpose: education and entertainment [3].

With the texts of Galen, Mondino, and Mondino's commentators now printed, distributed, and accessible, we have the dénouement of anatomy's modernization. A man not yet 30 years of age named Andreas Vesalius publishes *De humani corporis fabrica,* translated *On the Fabric of the Human Body* (Fig. 1.1). This text has the greatest influence on the course of anatomic science. The *Fabrica,* as it is known, and its sequel *Epitome,* are masterpieces that showcase the knowledge, the skill, and the passion of Vesalius [1–3].

It was the accuracy, artistry, and draftsmanship of *Fabrica* that captured the attention and imagination of academics, royalty, and the common person alike (Fig. 1.2). The great anatomic dissection and illustration of Vesalius not only conveyed the facts hidden under the skin but also evoked the response that all great art evokes [4–6]. A dramatized and

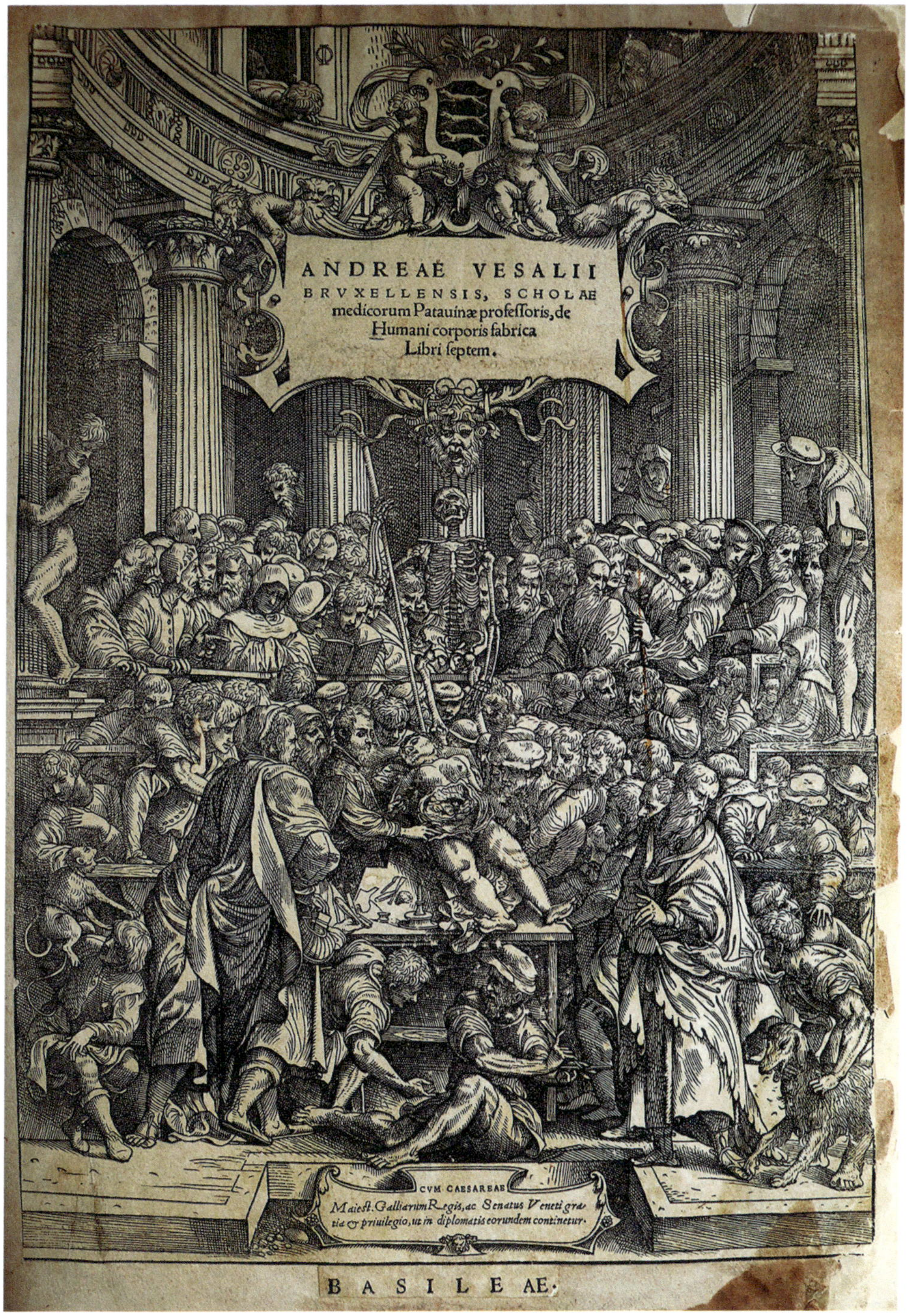

Fig. 1.1 Frontispiece from Vesalius' masterpiece *On the Fabric of the Human Body*, 1543, known fondly as *Fabrica*. Vesalius is the young, bearded man boldly instructing the clamoring crowd, not from the professor's chair as was tradition but from the work itself, the careful anatomization of the human body [5]. (*Courtesy of Ebling Library, Rare Books and Special Collections, University of Wisconsin-Madison*)

artistic presentation of anatomy persisted despite evolution in the processes of dissection, illustration, and publication. A plate from the seventeenth century *Anatomia humani corporis* by the Dutch anatomist Govard Bidloo (Fig. 1.3) demonstrates the artistic and dramatic presentation of anatomy, with a prosected arm dangling from the dissection table, muscles pinned back as the figure was sketched [4, 7].

Like da Vinci, like Galen, and like Herophilus, Vesalius was not divine. These men might not have thought that what they were doing would change the world like it has. The greatness of their work can be explained without mysticism, divine intervention, or even luck. It was by the power of *careful observation* and a *prepared mind* that these anatomists changed the collective understanding of the human body.

We are learning about the nervous system now like centuries past have learned about the rest of the body. Remember the work of the functional anatomists of the nineteenth century: Charcot, Bell, and Magendie. Remember the work of the surgical anatomists of the twentieth century: Cushing,

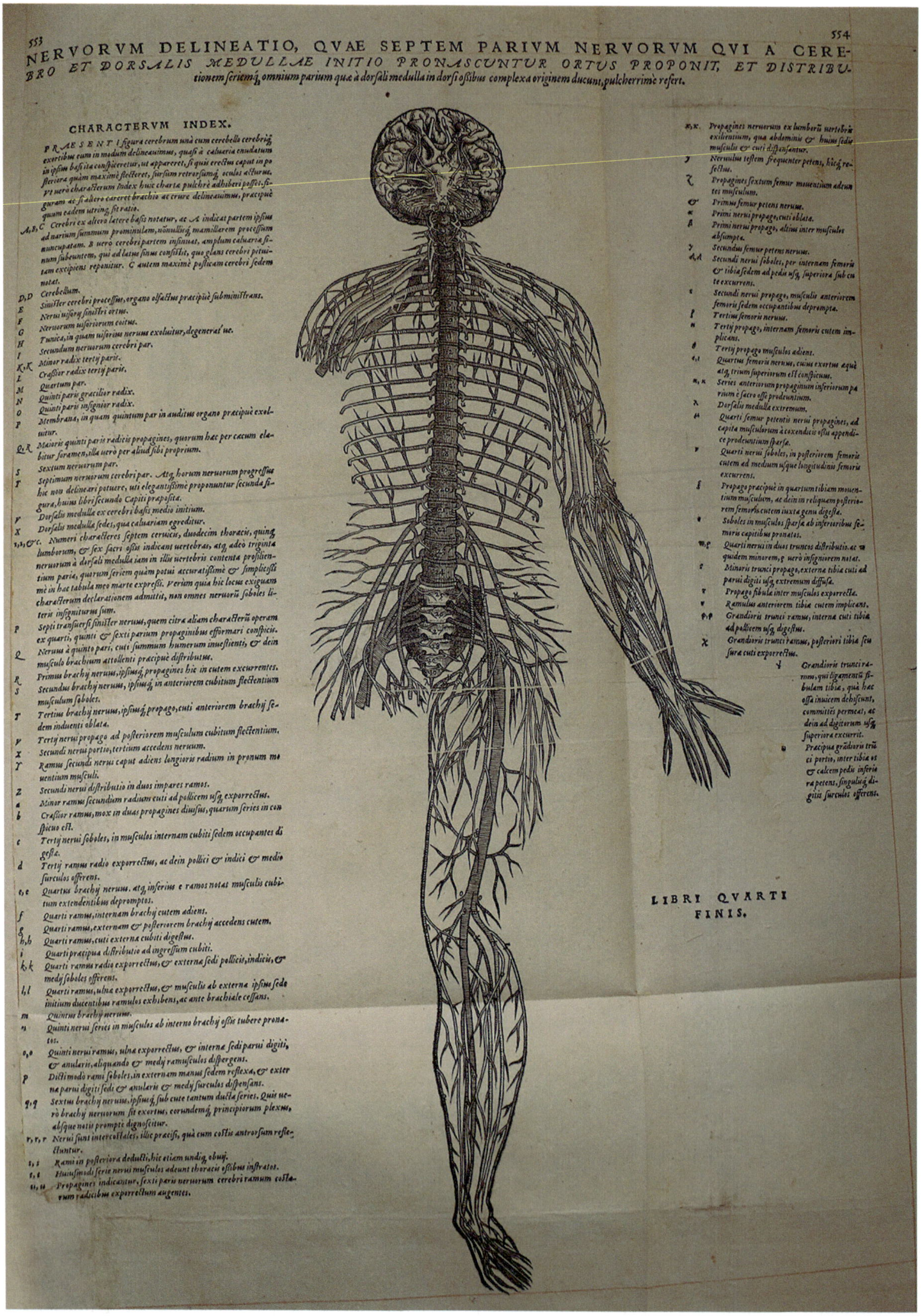

Fig. 1.2 In this fold-out figure from the 1555 edition of *Fabrica*, Vesalius delineates the nervous system impressively. Although dissections and sketches had to be carried out hastily in the absence of tissue fixation techniques, the accuracy of Vesalius' work set him apart from his contemporaries. The brachial plexus and lumbosacral plexus, despite some errors, are fairly represented [6]. (*Courtesy of Ebling Library, Rare Books and Special Collections, University of Wisconsin-Madison*)

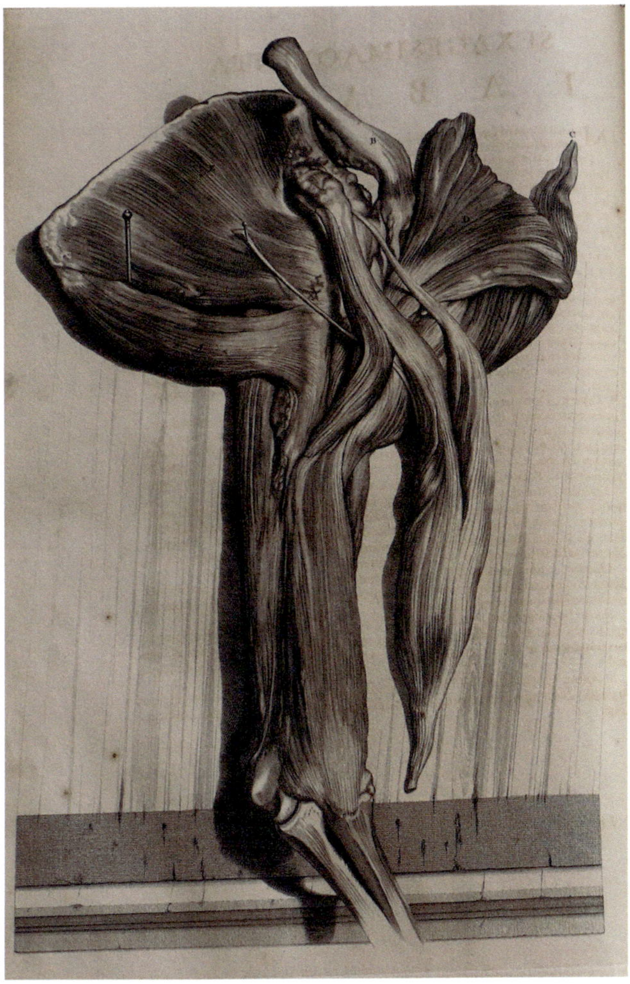

Fig. 1.3 The musculocutaneous nerve piercing the coracobrachialis in Bidloo, 1685. Anatomic dissection and illustration proceeded in the traditions of Vesalius for centuries. Although printing techniques and anatomic knowledge pressed forward, the stylized and dramatized artistic presentation of anatomic dissection was preserved. Vesalius' work was printed with wooden plates, which were carved by hand as a "negative" image, then inked and pressed. The plate shown here from Bidloo's text was etched in copper plates, allowing the texture and lines of the anatomy to be printed in more fine detail. The craftsmanship required to print these Renaissance texts remains impressive today [4, 7]. *(Courtesy of Ebling Library, Rare Books and Special Collections, University of Wisconsin-Madison)*

Penfield, and Rhoton. How will the twenty-first century anatomist be remembered? Our work is influenced by our heritage, our environment, our way of thinking, our educational background, our rivals, and our collaborators.

By looking at the accumulated achievements of the past, perhaps it is easy to say that everything that can be discovered has already been discovered. But I argue that this well will not run dry. The accumulated knowledge of humanity is moving from the monotonous shelves of the world's libraries to the phone in my back pocket. The time for discovery is now.

With careful observation, this atlas has been compiled. It has been created so that you might draw forth from the well of knowledge merely one pail among all that you will ever learn. When you imbibe, the knowledge will manifest uniquely. No student will have the same preface, and no teacher will have the same conclusion.

With this collection of anatomic truths drawn forth from under the skin of the laudable dissected, prepare your mind *to discover*, *to teach*, and *to heal* as no one has done before you.

References

1. Hurren ET (2014) Personal communication (C. D. Baggott, Interviewer)
2. Singer C (1957) A short history of anatomy from the Greeks to Harvey. Dover Publications, New York
3. Singer C (1926) Evolution of anatomy : a short history of anatomical and physiological discovery to Harvey: being the substance of the Fitzpatrick lectures delivered at the Royal College of Physicians of London in the years 1923 and 1924. Alfred A. Knopf, New York. Reprint, Hertford: Stephen Austin & Sons; 1982
4. Fowler-Sullivan M (2014) Personal Communication (C. D. Baggott, Interviewer)
5. Vesalius A, van Calcar JS (1543) De humani corporis fabrica libri septem. ex officina Joannis Oporini, Basileae (Basel)
6. Vesalius A, Oporinus J (1555) De humani corporis fabrica libri septem. Per Ioannem Oporinum, Basileae [Basel]
7. Bidloo, Govard, Gérard de Lairesse (1685) Anatomia Hvmani Corporis, Centum & Quinque Tabvlis, Per Artificiosiss. Amsteledami: sumptibus viduae Joannis à Someren [etc.] (Amsterdam: for the widow of Joannes van Someren, the heirs of Joannes van Dyk, Henry Boom and widow of Theodore Boom)

2 This Body of Literature: Classical Influences on Human Neuroanatomy

Barbara A. Hanna

Introduction

The human body contains many scientific allures, from the atomic level to the anatomic level. Beyond science, though, the study of the human body cannot be separated from its historical, literary, and etymological influences. The way these disciplines collide is especially apparent in researching the reference points for anatomic nomenclature. Greek and Roman languages and mythology were heavily used as source materials in the formation of anatomical terms. These connections are often referenced in the literature to enliven the process of learning and studying anatomy. Visual art can be utilized as a tool to further enrich the communication of anatomical origin stories. Each of the following pieces visualizes an aspect of neuroanatomy as related to its origin within the context of Greek and Roman mythology. These drawings take artistic liberties with less emphasis on anatomical accuracy.

Narcissus (Fig. 2.1)

Ovid, an ancient Roman writer, writes the story of Narcissus in his *Metamorphoses*. Narcissus, a very attractive young man, gains the attention of Echo, a nymph, as he walks through the woods one day. Having fallen in love with Narcissus, Echo approaches him to act on her feelings. Narcissus rejects Echo with no trace of sympathy and runs away, gaining the attention of Nemesis, the goddess of revenge. Nemesis curses Narcissus, declaring that he would fall in love with someone he would never be able to court. After running from Echo, Narcissus stops to rest by a spring of water. Leaning over the pool, Narcissus is mesmerized by the person he sees. Per the curse of Nemesis, Narcissus falls in love with his own reflection [1]. Anatomists and surgeons are mesmerized by the self but not for its exterior. In Fig. 2.1, Narcissus is shown falling in love not with his own beauty but with his own anatomy.

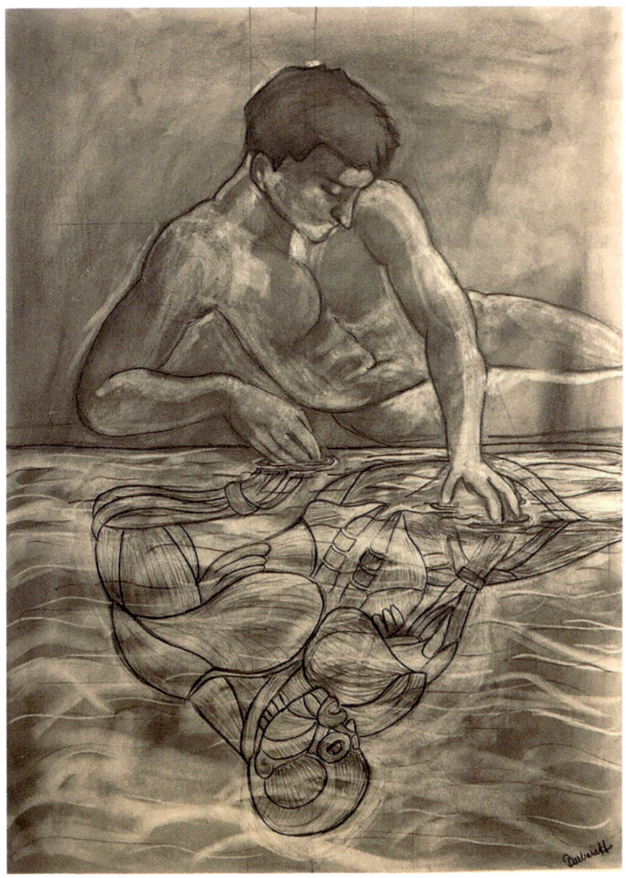

Fig. 2.1 The myth of Narcissus from Ovid's *Metamorphoses*. Narcissus is not mesmerized by his physical reflection but by his anatomy. Copyright Barbara Hanna, published with permission [1]

B. A. Hanna (✉)
Mayo Clinic Alix School of Medicine, Rochester, MN, USA
e-mail: hanna.barbara@mayo.edu

A. S. Hanna (ed.), *Nerves: Anatomy, Exposures, and Techniques*, https://doi.org/10.1007/978-3-031-73931-6_2

Homunculus (Fig. 2.2)

The homunculus is used by physiologists, neurologists, and neurosurgeons to help understand and summarize the functions of the primary motor and somatosensory cortices [2]. The homunculus has its roots in Latin. *Homo, hominis* translates to "man" [3]. The suffix *ulus* indicates what linguists call the diminutive form of a word, telling the reader that this word is "little." Thus, *homunculus* literally translates to "little man." Figure 2.2 shows the homunculus through the Greek myth of Athena's birth from the head of Zeus. Zeus and his wife, Metis, conceive a daughter, but Zeus is warned that his unborn daughter will one day threaten his sovereignty. Terrified of this outcome and seeking to change fate, Zeus swallows his wife whole. After some time, though, Zeus suffers a terrible headache. Athena then bursts from his headache, victoriously defeating her father's attempts to destroy her [4]. In this piece, Athena is positioned as the homunculus of the primary somatosensory cortex on the postcentral gyrus of Zeus' brain.

Axilla (Fig. 2.3)

The armpit region of the human body is known anatomically as the axillary area. *Axilla* is another anatomic term of Latin origin, coming from the root *ala, alae*, translating to "wing" [3] The suffix *illa* is another Latin diminutive suffix [5], so *axilla* literally translates to "little wing." Another story Ovid tells in his *Metamorphoses* is that of Daedalus and his son, Icarus. Daedalus angers King Minos, the ruler of the land, and Daedalus must use his innovative mind to devise a way for him and Icarus to escape. Daedalus crafts wings, one set for himself and one for Icarus, to fly them away to safety. Icarus flies higher and higher, despite his father's caution, and ends up too close to the sun. His wings melt, and Icarus fatally descends into the sea below [1]. In Fig. 2.3, Icarus is shown with little wings, too fragile to support his proximity to the sun. The veins of the wings are designed to reflect the organization of the brachial plexus, the major neuroanatomy of the axillary area.

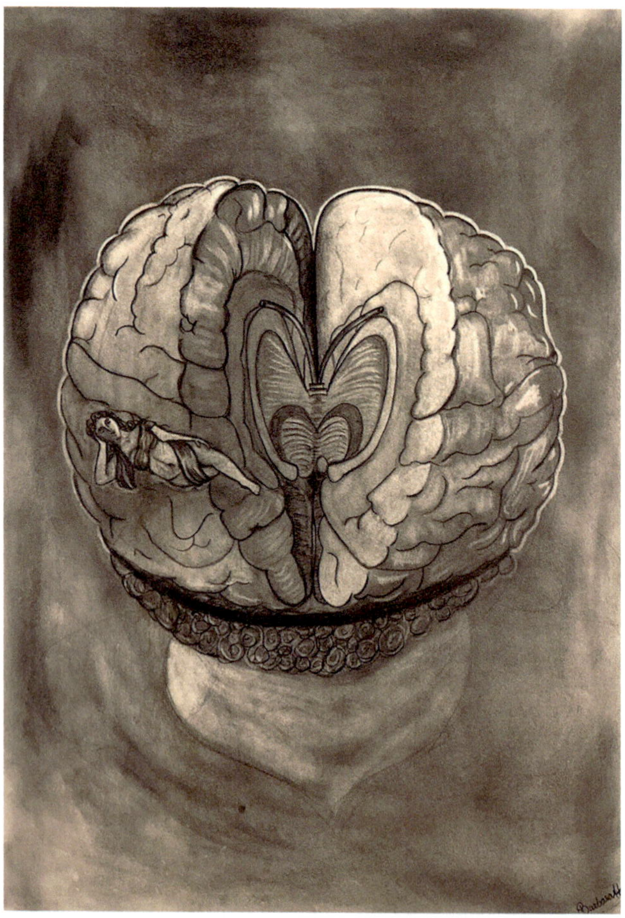

Fig. 2.2 Athena as the homunculus of the primary somatosensory cortex on the postcentral gyrus of Zeus' brain. Copyright Barbara Hanna, published with permission [1]

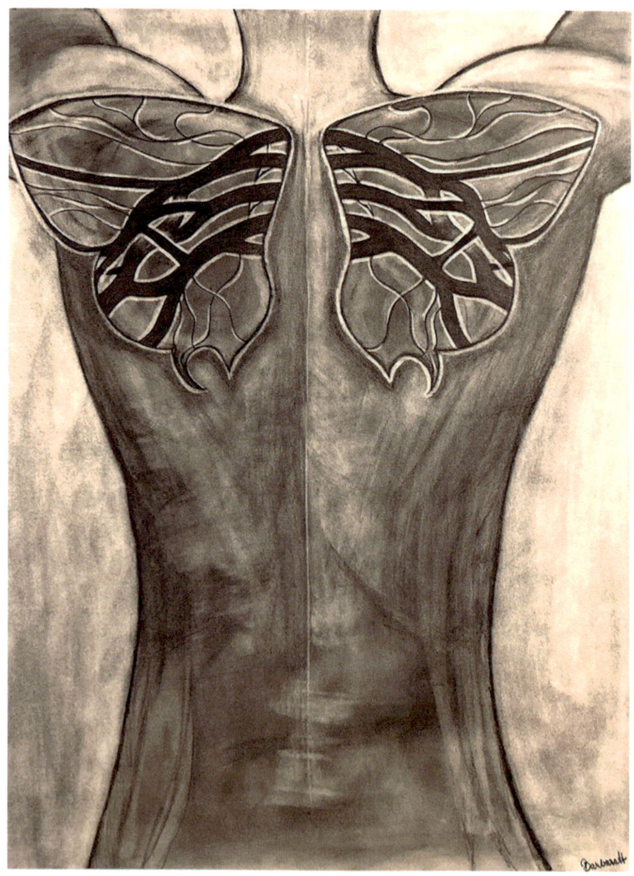

Fig. 2.3 The little wings of Icarus drawn with the major neuroanatomy of the axilla, the brachial plexus, to represent the etymological origin of axilla. Copyright Barbara Hanna, published with permission [1]

Achilles Tendon (Fig. 2.4)

The Achilles tendon, also known as the calcaneal tendon, connects the gastrocnemius and soleus muscles to the calcaneus [6]. In Greek mythology, Achilles' mother takes her young child to the River Styx to give him the immortality of the gods that comes from bathing in its waters. Dipping Achilles in water, she covers his body. Holding his heel too tightly, though, the Stygian waters never contact Achilles' ankle. Growing to be a powerful man and a Trojan war hero, Achilles fights in great battles and remains triumphant throughout; that is, until Paris, the Prince of Troy, shoots an arrow into Achilles' heel. Achilles dies immediately [7]. In Fig. 2.4, the Trojan hero has been drawn in as the calcaneal tendon, made vulnerable by the muscles tying him up. The sural nerve has been drawn lateral to Achilles.

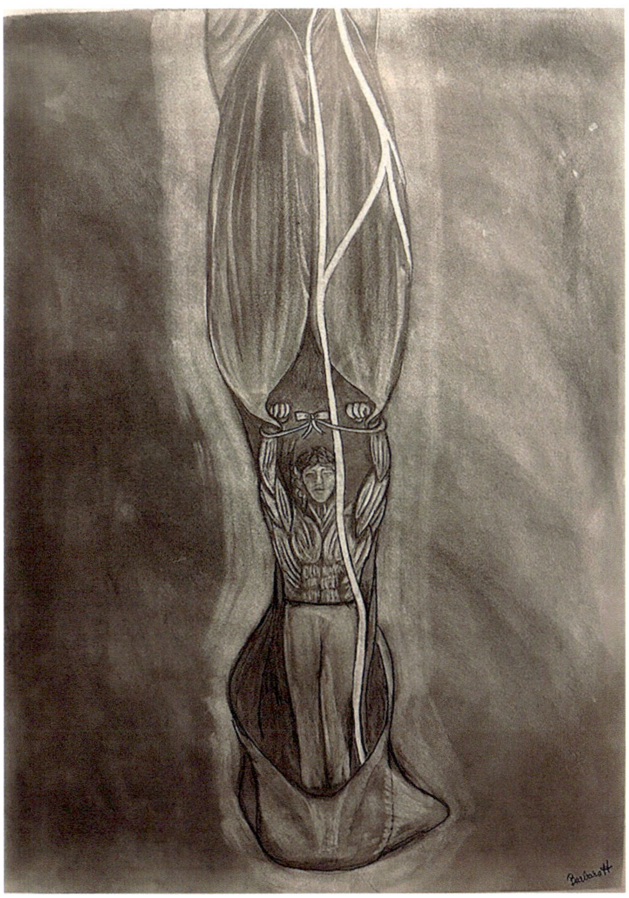

Fig. 2.4 Achilles, the Trojan war hero, tied up by the soleus and gastrocnemius and standing on the calcaneus. The sural nerve is visualized lateral to Achilles. Copyright Barbara Hanna, published with permission [1]

Atlas (Fig. 2.5)

The first cervical vertebra is also known as the atlas, and it contacts the skull at the occipital condyles, carrying the weight of the head. The atlas gets its name from a titan, Atlas, who leads a battle against Zeus in Greek mythology. Atlas is defeated. As punishment, Atlas is condemned to carry the heavens on his shoulders for eternity [7]. Figure 2.5 is an image of Atlas the Titan bearing the skull above him.

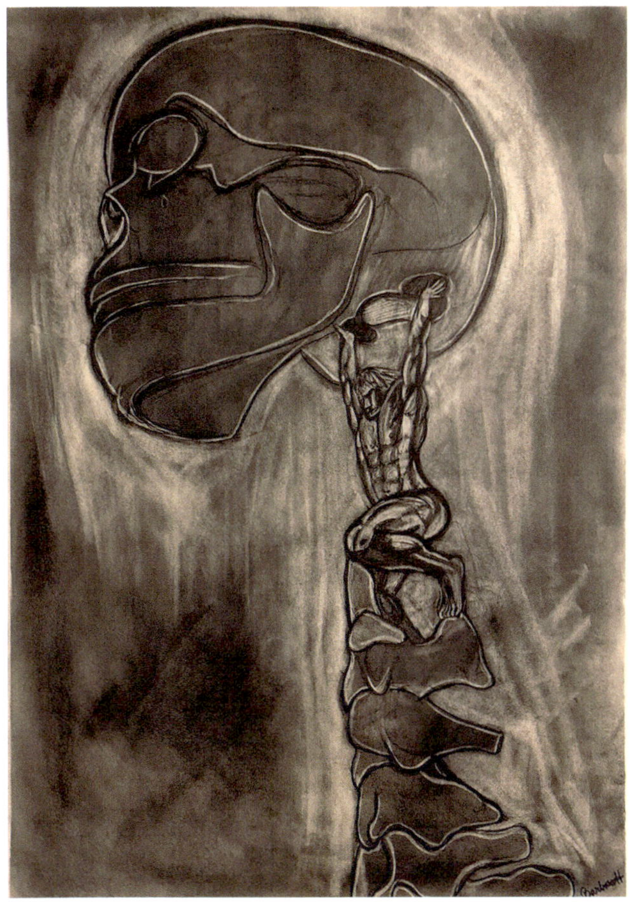

Fig. 2.5 The first cervical vertebra drawn as Atlas the Titan, bearing the skull above him and kneeling on the axis below. Copyright Barbara Hanna, published with permission [1]

Conclusion

Medicine cannot be separated from the history, culture, language, and literature that has shaped its conception. In recognizing these intersections that anatomy can have with the literature and art, the subject becomes even more engrossing, not just as a physical science but as a human one, tracing the story of the body all the way back to the start of civilization.

References

1. Hanna BA (2021) In the eyes of Herophilus: a Greco-Roman design of human neuroanatomy. J Neurosurg 136(3):927–930. https://doi.org/10.3171/2021.6.JNS211464
2. Jones P (2007) Reading Ovid: stories from the metamorphoses. Cambridge University Press
3. Roux FE, Djidjeli I, Durand JB (2018) Functional architecture of the somatosensory homunculus detected by electrostimulation. J Physiol 596(5):941–956. https://doi.org/10.1113/JP275243
4. Julius D (2006) Latin made simple: a complete introductory course in classical Latin. Crown Publishing Group, New York
5. Strodach GK (1933) Latin diminutives in-Ello/A-and-Illo/A-A study in diminutive formation. Language dissertations. Linguistic Society of America, Philadelphia, pp 7–98
6. Neri B, Sonnet I, Sonnet II OF (2005) Elizabeth Barrett browning's sonnets from the Portuguese: setting the stage for divine reunification. Studies Browning His Circle 26:41–53. Armstrong Browning Library, Baylor University
7. Dayton P (2017) Anatomic, vascular, and mechanical overview of the Achilles tendon. Clin Podiatr Med Surg 34(2):107–113. https://doi.org/10.1016/j.cpm.2016.10.002

Part II

Fundamentals of Nerve Surgery

Nerve Histology and Physiology in Health and Disease

3

Rajesh K. Pathiyil, Denise Ng, Tak Ho Chu, and Rajiv Midha

Nerve Microstructure

A nerve is an organ consisting of bundles of neuronal axons arranged in an orderly fashion within a connective tissue stroma, supported by a blood supply. It relays communication between the central nervous system and the end organs. This includes axons which are involved in general somatosensory (afferent), general motor (efferent) and autonomic (sympathetic and parasympathetic) functions. The nerve cell bodies are absent in most parts of the nerves except in areas where they form ganglia.

Nerve Axons

The axons are peripheral extensions of neuronal cell bodies which are situated within the central nervous system or peripheral ganglia. Axons contain axoplasm and a few organelles. The structural support of the axon is provided by neurofilaments, whereas microtubules aid in axoplasmic transport. The axoplasm has vesicles containing neurotransmitter chemicals which are transported to and concentrated at the tip of the axons (synaptic knobs or terminal buttons). Abundant mitochondria within the axoplasm provide energy for all these processes.

Nerve Fascicle

A group of axons forming a small bundle is called a nerve fascicle. Most nerves are comprised of multiple fascicles.

Myelin Sheath

The axons in a nerve may be myelinated or nonmyelinated depending on the presence or absence of myelin sheath, respectively. Myelin is a protein–lipid complex, resulting from many layers (up to a 100) of the Schwann cell plasma membrane. During the wrapping of the axon by the membrane, Schwann cell cytoplasm is lost as the membrane layers get tightly compacted around the axon by the interlocking of a membrane protein called protein zero (P_0) [1].

Initial Segment

Also called axon hillock, this is the unmyelinated segment located at the proximal axon in myelinated fibers. It is the site of action potential initiation.

Nodes of Ranvier

In between the areas of myelin sheath, there are small spaces (1 μm spaces about 1 mm apart) devoid of myelin, which are known as nodes of Ranvier. Their exposed axonal membranes have a higher concentration of sodium channels which helps in rapid transmission of impulses along the myelinated axons (saltatory conduction). Juxtaparanode region, which is endowed with a higher concentration of potassium channels, is situated next to the nodes of Ranvier.

Clefts (Incisures) of Schmidt–Lantermann

These are "interruptions" in the internodal region of myelin sheath. They consist of angular spiral of Schwann cell cytoplasm between myelin lamellae. They don't have any effect on nerve conduction.

R. K. Pathiyil · T. H. Chu
Department of Clinical Neurosciences, University of Calgary, Calgary, AB, Canada
e-mail: thchu@ucalgary.ca

D. Ng
Department of Laboratory Medicine, University of Calgary, Calgary, AB, Canada
e-mail: denise.ng@albertaprecisionlabs.ca

R. Midha (✉)
Department of Clinical Neurosciences, University of Calgary, Calgary, AB, Canada

Hotchkiss Brain Institute, Cumming School of Medicine, University of Calgary, Calgary, AB, Canada
e-mail: rajmidha@ucalgary.ca; rajiv.midha@ahs.ca

A. S. Hanna (ed.), *Nerves: Anatomy, Exposures, and Techniques*, https://doi.org/10.1007/978-3-031-73931-6_3

Connective Tissue

The connective tissue within and around the nerve is organized into the following layers (Figs. 3.1 and 3.2).

Paraneurium (Circumneurium)

This is the loose connective tissue around the nerve which connects the nerve to the surrounding structures and holds the nerve in its normal anatomical position while acting as a gliding layer. This layer of collagen is more evident outside complex nerves such as sciatic and femoral nerves. This collagen layer has interconnections which extend to the adventitia and epimysium of neighboring vessels and muscles, respectively. It is the structure that the surgeon can "handle" while doing circumferential nerve dissection during what's commonly called *external neurolysis*.

Epineurium

Epineurium is made up of loose connective tissue and fat. It has an inner and an outer layer. Epineurial vessels are present in the inner layer. Fascicles are embedded within the inner epineurium. Internal epineurium has variable thickness, being much more robust in larger diameter nerves as well as adjacent to joints to provide greater protection to the nerve. *Internal neurolysis*, as frequently called, entails an epineurotomy, followed by micro-dissection within the internal epineurium to separate fascicles from each other.

Perineurium

Perineurium surrounds each nerve fascicle. It is comprised of multiple layers of flattened perineurial cells joined by tight gap junctions, which form one of the sites contributing to the blood–nerve barrier. This structure provides considerable internal strength to the nerve, and it is the smallest structure in the nerve that can be repaired using microsutures.

Endoneurium

Endoneurium surrounds individual axons and consists of fibroblasts with an extracellular matrix containing collagen. Schwann cells reside with this layer and are invested in basal lamina, rich in extracellular proteins, laminin, and fibronectin. The basal laminae are the microstructure counterparts of endoneurial tubes which guide nerve fibers as they regenerate following injury.

Blood Supply of Nerves

The nerves are supplied by longitudinal vessels running with the endoneurium and epineurium, which are connected by small bridging vessels. They derive their segmental feeders at the levels of joints in the extremities. The endothelial tight junctions in the capillaries and microvessels within the endoneurium are less permeable than the epineurial vessels and form the second site of blood–nerve barrier, along with the tight cell junctions of the perineurium.

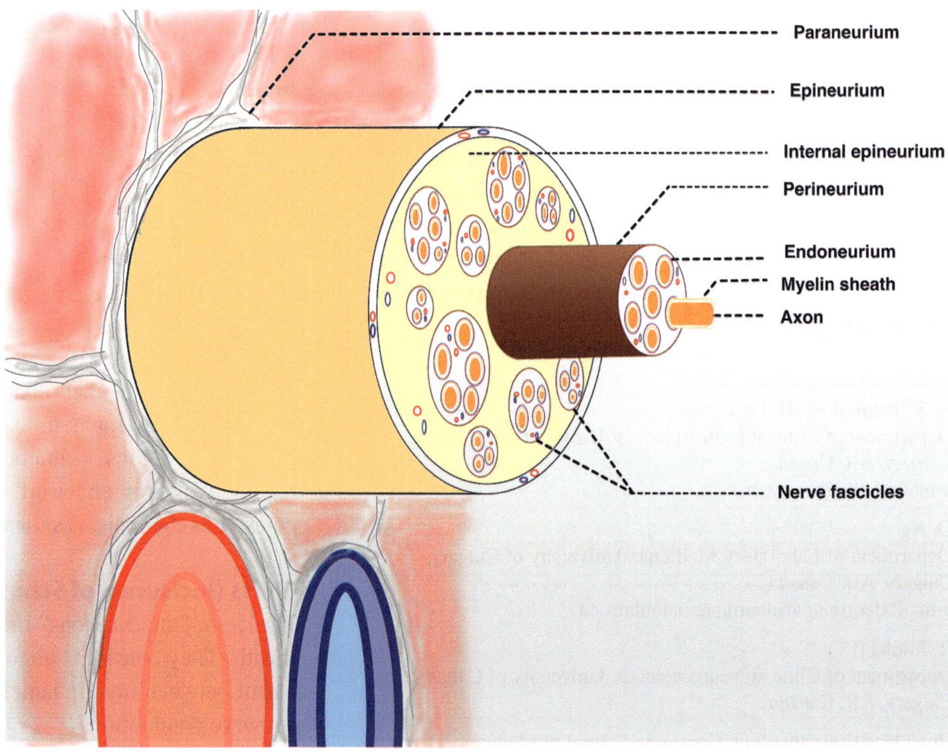

Fig. 3.1 Schematic representation of nerve microstructure

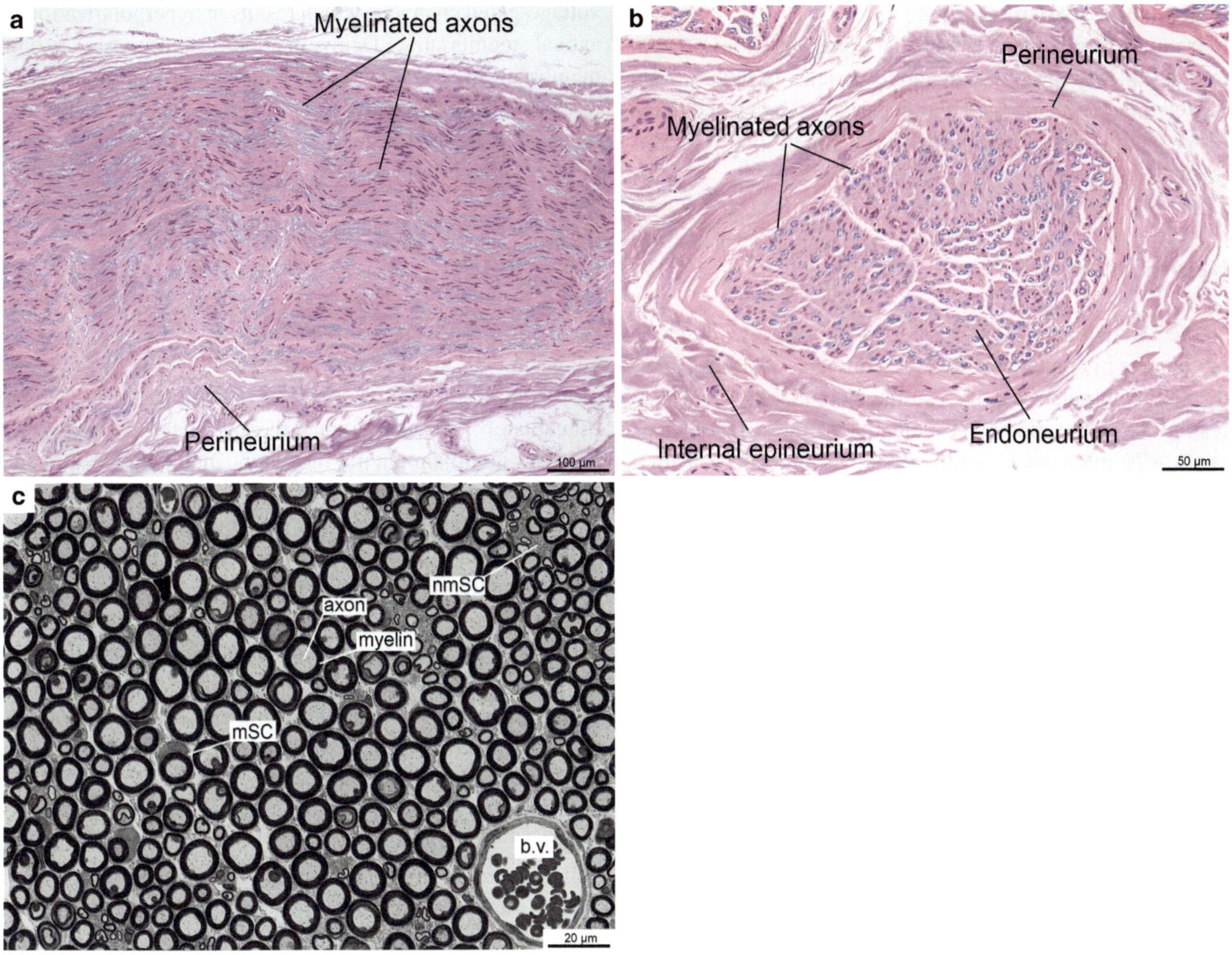

Fig. 3.2 Low- and high-power histomicrographs showing normal nerve microstructure in longitudinal and cross sections. (**a&b**) Hematoxylin and eosin (H&E) and Luxol fast blue (LFB), (**c**) Osmium fixed and toluidine blue stained semithin sections. (**a**) Normal human nerve longitudinal section. (**b**) Normal human nerve cross section. (**c**) High-power cross section of rodent nerve to demonstrate endoneurial contents of nerve. *mSC* myelinating Schwann cells, *nmSC* nonmyelinating Schwann cells, *b.v.* blood vessel

Decellularized Nerve Allografts

Nerve allografts were used for nerve reconstruction as early as the nineteenth century but were met with the problem of immune rejection and the need for host immunosuppression. Decellularized nerve allografts (DCAs) were developed to eliminate the need for immunosuppression while providing a readily available tissue source for nerve reconstruction. The cellular components of the nerve are eliminated by the processing steps, and the graft is rendered nonimmunogenic by appropriate treatment while preserving its microstructure and connective scaffold. DCAs contain endoneurium, perineurium, and epineurium but lack axons and cells. The DCAs get revascularized and repopulated with host Schwann cells, which provide the microenvironment conducive for nerve regeneration. The endoneurial tubes in the DCA serve as a conduit for regenerating axons.

Nerve Physiology

Axonal Transport

Axoplasmic flow, which is aided by microtubules, helps to transport proteins and polypeptides along the length of the axons.

Orthograde (Anterograde) Transport

This involves transport from the cell body toward the terminal buttons. It has both fast (100–400 mm/day) and slow (0.5–10 mm/day) components [1]. The phase of slow axonal transport of 1–2 mm/day transports cell membrane components to the nerve and thus is the limiting factor determining the rate of nerve regeneration.

Retrograde Transport

It occurs toward the cell body, fast only, at about 50–200 mm/day [1]. Some of the synaptic vesicles (which are not recycled in the membrane) and materials endocytosed at the nerve endings are transported to the cell body in this manner.

Nerve Conduction

Nerve excitation and transmission of impulses is a function of changes in conduction of electrically charged ions across the cell membranes and the resulting potential difference. At resting state, the membrane potential of the nerve fiber is about −70 mV (inside negative relative to outside), with a higher concentration of K^+ inside and Na^+ outside the axonal membrane. This electrochemical gradient is maintained by Na^+-K^+ ATPase. Simply stated, the nerve action potential in response to a depolarizing stimulus is generated by the influx of Na^+ which overwhelms K^+ ion channels early on, followed by late opening of K^+ ion channels and efflux of K^+ ions which bring the membrane potential toward a hyperpolarized state.

Voltage-gated Na^+ channels which play a very important role in the generation and conduction of action potentials are highly concentrated in the initial segment (350–500 per μm^2) and nodes of Ranvier (2000–12,000 per μm^2), as compared to myelinated areas (<25 per μm^2) and to the axonal membranes of unmyelinated nerves (110 per μm^2) [1].

When membrane polarity gets reversed during action potential, it generates a current sink which causes a flow of positive ions from the nearby axonal membrane into the depolarized segment. This reduces the membrane potential of the membrane ahead, and when the firing potential is reached, it leads to the propagation of action potential. As the membrane on one side of the current sink is in a refractory period, the propagation of impulses usually occurs only in one direction (orthodromic) under physiological conditions.

In myelinated nerves, myelin acts as an insulator and also covers areas of axonal membrane largely devoid of ion channels, and as a result, the impulses "jump" from one node of Ranvier to the next. This is called saltatory conduction and is up to 50 times faster than the conduction in unmyelinated axons [1].

Pathological States

Demyelination

Conditions causing demyelination include hereditary, inflammatory, compressive, toxic, and metabolic insults. Segmental loss of myelin causes leakage of K^+ ions through voltage-gated channels, which results in hyperpolarization of axonal membranes. Demyelination also exposes axonal membranes that are devoid of ion channels and hence relatively incapable of propagating an action potential. The combination of these changes slows down or completely blocks nerve conduction.

Nerve Injury

Histological Changes (Fig. 3.3)

Schwann cells are the "first responders" to a nerve injury as they significantly outnumber the macrophages in nerves. Immediately after nerve injury, there is an abrupt rise (within 5–24 h) in inflammatory mediators including TNF-α and IL-1β in the local environment. This is followed by microstructural changes within the cell body, proximal stump, interstump gap, and in the distal stump. Hematogenous-derived macrophages infiltrate the nerve in response to chemokines and other mediators released by denervated Schwann cells. The macrophages and Schwann cells clear the debris. The inflammatory mediators and the debris cleanup create a permissive environment which allows axons regenerating from the proximal nerve stump to elongate in the distal nerve [2].

Cell Body

Following nerve injury, there occurs a metabolic switch from "maintenance mode" to "regenerative mode" with an increased synthesis of proteins and other molecules required for nerve repair. This is associated with a set of morphological changes in the cell body known as chromatolysis, where the cell body swells up with the displacement of the nucleus to the periphery and profound disorganization of the basophilic granules (Nissl bodies). The intrinsic growth capacity of the neuronal cell is activated, which involves c-AMP-mediated pathways, and there occurs a shift of metabolism from neurotransmission to membrane synthesis in order to aid axonal regeneration.

Proximal Stump

After injury, the axon in the proximal stump usually degenerates up to the nearest node of Ranvier. Axonal sprouts come out of the proximal stump 2–3 days following injury. Schwann cells provide the growth factors required for the process of regeneration, which occurs via a vascularized bridge in the interstump gap within the proximal and distal stumps [3].

Distal Stump

After injury, the distal stump is cut off from the supply of endogenous survival factors produced by the cell body. It undergoes a process called Wallerian degeneration (named

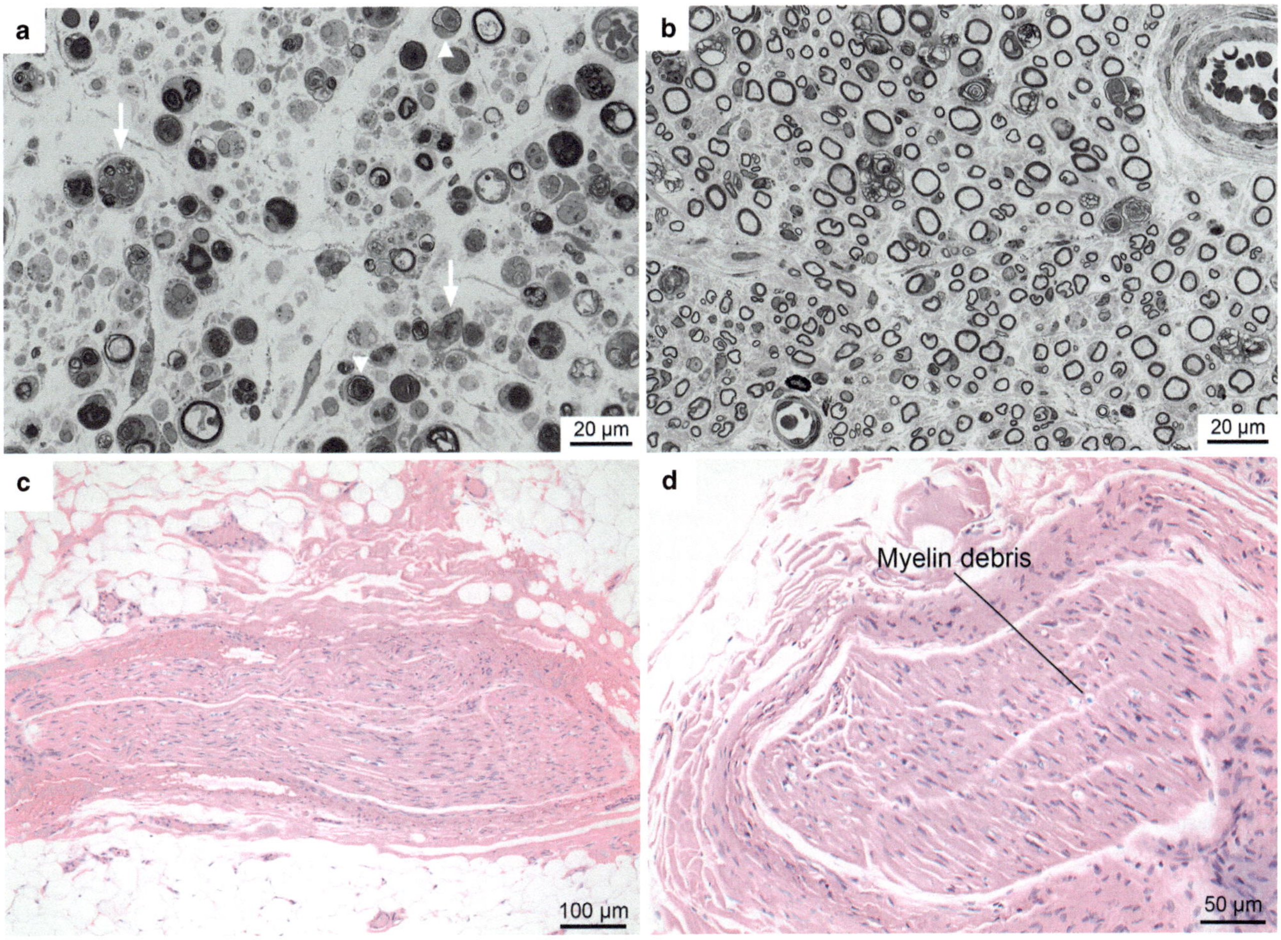

Fig. 3.3 Response of nerve to injury. (**a**) Early (within days) response with Wallerian degeneration, myelin phagocytosis, and inflammatory cell infiltrate. Macrophages with phagocytosed debris (*arrows*) and disintegrating myelin associated with Schwann cells (*arrow heads*) are seen. (**b**) Few weeks after injury with regeneration response, note the overall decrease and variability in the size of myelinated axon profiles and decreased myelination as compared to normal nerve (in Fig. 3.2c) (Panels **a** and **b** are experimental examples from rodents, Osmium fixed and toluidine blue stained semithin sections). (**c**, **d**) Histopathology of human neuropathy demonstrating axonal dropout and decreased myelin content, Hematoxylin and eosin (H&E) and Luxol fast blue (LFB)

after Augustus Waller who first described the process), which starts 24–48 h after the injury (Fig. 3.3a). The process is initiated by the entry of calcium into the axons and subsequent activation of proteases and axonal dissolution. Schwann cells and macrophages subsequently clear the axon and myelin debris; this occurs over days to weeks in nerves (Fig. 3.3a). Clearance of myelin is very important for axonal regeneration, as myelin contains axonal growth inhibitory factors. The Schwann cells switch their gene expression to a "repair" mode expressing neurotrophic factors required for regeneration [4]. They also proliferate to form cell columns contained within the basal lamina-lined endoneurial tubes which act as "lane markers" for regenerating axons from the proximal stump. The regenerating axons are initially small and mature over time with increasing diameter and myelination (Fig. 3.3b). The axonal regeneration typically occurs at a rate of 1 mm/day or 3 cm/month.

Table 3.1 Seddon's classification of nerve injuries

Type of injury	Description of injury
Neurapraxia	Transient block—nerve conduction is temporarily impaired without any structural damage to the axons
Axonotmesis	Lesion in continuity—This involves degeneration of the axons, but the connective tissue structure of the nerve is not completely divided. The nerve as a mass is still in continuity
Neurotmesis	Complete division of a nerve

Classification of Nerve Injuries

In 1942, Sir Herbert Seddon classified nerve injuries into three types [5] (Table 3.1). Each of Seddon's class contained heterogeneous injury patterns. In 1951, Sydney Sunderland proposed a grading system of nerve injury based on the extent of axonal and connective tissue damage [6] (Table 3.2). He described five grades of injury based on increasing injury

Table 3.2 Sunderland's classification of nerve injuries

Grade	Seddon's class	Description of injury	Electrophysiology	MRN	Treatment
I	Neurapraxia	Focal segmental demyelination; connective tissues and axons in continuity; autonomic function usually spared	NCS—Partial/complete conduction block at the level of injury; preserved conduction distally, even after 2 weeks. EMG—Normal morphology and poor MUAP recruitment	Nerve—Increased T2 SI Muscle—normal	Medical; spontaneous recovery (weeks–few months)
II	Axonotmesis	Damaged axon with intact endoneurium	NCS—Partial/complete conduction block at the level of injury; distal conduction normal till Wallerian degeneration sets in (few days), then lost	Nerve—diffuse enlargement; increased T2 SI. Fascicles—enlarged or effaced due to edema Muscles—denervation	Medical; spontaneous recovery expected and occurs in target end-organ based on rate of regeneration.
III		Damaged axon and endoneurium with intact perineurium	EMG—Abnormal activity and denervation changes in 2 weeks		Surgical intervention may be required
IV		Damaged axon, endoneurium, and perineurium, with intact external epineurium		Nerve—focally enlarged, heterogeneous SI. Fascicles—disrupted, heterogeneous SI Neuroma in continuity Muscles—denervation	Surgical intervention necessary
V	Neurotmesis	Complete nerve transection	NCS—Complete conduction block proximally and distally EMG—Abnormal activity; denervation	Nerve—complete nerve discontinuity; possible hemorrhage and fibrosis in the nerve gap; end-bulb neuroma proximally; epineurial thickening. Muscles—denervation	

MRN magnetic resonance neurography, *NCS* nerve conduction study, *EMG* electromyography, *MUAP* motor unit action potential, *SI* signal intensity

Table 3.3 Common mechanisms of nerve injury

Mechanism	Description of injury	Likely Sunderland's grade	Treatment
Compression (pressure)	• Produces mechanical as well as ischemic injury, along with the breakdown of blood nerve barrier • Can result in focal demyelination and transient conduction block, or axonal damage in severe cases, e.g., entrapment neuropathies	I–II	Release the compressing factor and wait for recovery. Management is elective unless sudden severe compression from compartment syndrome, expanding hematoma, etc., where emergency decompression warranted to prevent irreversible nerve damage
Stretch (traction)	• Usually results in axonal discontinuity • Epineurium allows stretch up to 15–20% of its length • Severity of damage depends on the rate and duration of stretch, as well as on the total increase in length of the nerve	I–IV (Grade V in cases of nerve root avulsion)	Conservative measures initially; allow Grade 1–2 injury elements to recover; surgical measures (grafts/transfers) if there is no improvement and/or for higher grade elements, usually delayed (3–6 months)
Crush	• Results in axonal discontinuity	II–IV	Conservative measures initially; surgical measures (grafts/transfers) if there is no improvement
Laceration	• Results in discontinuity of the nerve • Both proximal and distal stumps form neuromas and retract	V	Requires surgical repair. Immediate to early if sharp, delayed (3–4 weeks) for blunt
Injection palsy	• Not necessarily by direct needle trauma • Toxicity of injected substance can cause local inflammatory reaction, scarring, and necrosis	II–III; rarely Grade IV	Conservative measures initially. Surgical intervention (nerve release [also called neurolysis] or rarely repair) if there is no improvement

severity. Electrophysiological studies, nerve conduction studies (NCS), electromyographic (EMG) tests, and magnetic resonance neurography (MRN) can help distinguish between grades to a certain extent.

Mechanisms of Nerve Injury

Table 3.3 summarizes the common mechanisms of nerve injury encountered in clinical practice.

References

1. Barret KE, Barman SM, Brooks HL, Yuan J (eds) (2019) Excitable tissue: nerve. Ganong's review of medical physiology, 26th edn. McGraw Hill, New York
2. Umansky D, Midha R (2022) Peripheral nerve injury. In: Steinmetz MP, Berven SH, Benzel Edward C (eds) Benzel's spine surgery: techniques, complication avoidance, and management, 5th edn. Elsevier Inc., Philadelphia, pp 356–370
3. Cattin AL, Burden JJ, Van Emmenis L et al (2015) Macrophage-induced blood vessels guide Schwann cell-mediated regeneration of peripheral nerves. Cell 162:1127–1139. https://doi.org/10.1016/j.cell.2015.07.021
4. Jessen KR, Mirsky R (2016) The repair Schwann cell and its function in regenerating nerves. J Physiol 594:3521–3531. https://doi.org/10.1113/JP270874
5. Seddon HJ (1942) A classification of nerve injuries. Br Med J 2:237–239. https://doi.org/10.1136/bmj.2.4260.237
6. Sunderland S (1951) A classification of peripheral nerve injuries producing loss of function. Brain 74:491–516. https://doi.org/10.1093/brain/74.4.491

Electrodiagnosis of the Peripheral Nervous System

4

Michael J. Hansen

Anatomy

The peripheral nervous system (PNS) consists of both motor and sensory components. The cell bodies of the sensory neurons are located within the dorsal root ganglia (DRG) which are outside of the spinal cord. The cells within the DRG are bipolar, with one axonal projection forming the sensory nerve root (projecting centrally) and the other forming the sensory fibers of the nerves (projecting peripherally). This contrasts with the cell body of the motor neurons which are located within the spinal cord (anterior horn cells). These cell bodies are technically within the central nervous system and are also referred to as lower motor neurons. Their projections exit the spinal cord as the motor roots. The PNS includes the nerve roots, the nerves, and the neuromuscular junction (NMJ), while the muscles are the end-organs supplied by the PNS. Fundamentally, these are the systems studied when employing nerve conduction studies (NCS) and needle electromyography (EMG).

Ordering NCS/EMG

The ability for a patient to tolerate a study will vary greatly, even if the patient has a good understanding of why the study is being performed. At times, a more focused study is pursued due to poor toleration. Performing NCS/EMG in uncooperative patients is extremely challenging, and often incomplete or no meaningful information can be obtained. The setting of the study is also important and is ideally performed on an outpatient basis in properly engineered examination rooms. Inpatient rooms have environmental factors that can lead to a significant artifact and can result in nondiagnostic studies. The prior medical history of a patient is vital. Prior history of neuropathy-causing conditions such as diabetes can reduce the ability to obtain sensory responses which are essential in proving if a lesion is truly distal to the DRG. Certain muscles such as paraspinal muscles and those near blood vessels may not be able to be sampled if the patient is on antiplatelet medications or anticoagulants.

When placing an order for electrodiagnostic studies, it is important to provide relevant history, important neurological examination findings, and the differential diagnosis in question. Writing requests such as "update EMG," "hand numbness," or "weakness" are not focused, and one may not get the answer that is clinically helpful. If the request is vague, the patient may give history that is not relevant to the question, and a wrong study may be performed. Instead, it is wise to provide the person performing the EMG more guidance such as "evaluate for right median neuropathy at the wrist vs. C7 radiculopathy," "S1 radiculopathy vs. length-dependent peripheral neuropathy," or "upper trunk brachial plexopathy vs C5/C6 radiculopathy."

Nerve Conduction Studies [1]

The most studied nerves in routine practice include the median, radial, and ulnar nerves in the upper extremities and the peroneal, sural, and tibial nerves in the lower extremities. There are techniques to study other nerves; however, many are more technically demanding, prone to artifact, and/or poorly tolerated by the patient and thus are not employed routinely. The selection of what nerves to study depends on the history and physical examination of the patient, as well as the clinical question to be answered. Unfortunately, not all nerve fibers can be studied with routine NCS. In fact, only the largest, myelinated fibers can be tested in the EMG laboratory. This excludes smaller or unmyelinated fibers.

M. J. Hansen (✉)
Department of Neurology, University of Wisconsin School of Medicine and Public Health, Madison, WI, USA
e-mail: hansen@neurology.wisc.edu

A. S. Hanna (ed.), *Nerves: Anatomy, Exposures, and Techniques*, https://doi.org/10.1007/978-3-031-73931-6_4

Compound Muscle Action Potential (CMAP)

Motor conduction studies typically employ what is referred to as the belly-tendon montage, where an active recording electrode is placed over the muscle belly, and a reference electrode is placed distally on the tendon of the muscle. The nerve that supplies the muscle is then stimulated proximal to the recording site, and a response is recorded, typically in the range of millivolts (mV). As an example, the setup for recording the median motor response would have the recording electrode on the muscle belly of the abductor pollicis brevis, the reference electrode on the first metacarpophalangeal joint and the stimulator slightly lateral to the midwrist. Additional, more proximal stimulation sites can be studied through the course of the median nerve, most commonly in the antecubital fossa. These are performed by moving the stimulation site, while the recording electrodes remain in place. The waveform that is recorded is typically biphasic, with the first phase occurring above the baseline and the second phase below the baseline. This is referred to as a compound muscle action potential (CMAP). An initial positive (below baseline) deflection can indicate that the recording electrode is not properly placed over the motor endplate and should be moved before the study is continued.

At each stimulation site, the current starts at 0, and the intensity of the stimulation at each site is gradually increased until the waveform no longer grows in amplitude. This technique ensures what is referred to as supramaximal stimulation, which means that all nerve fibers in the studied nerve are being stimulated. However, it is equally important to stop increasing the current once the waveform no longer grows to avoid co-stimulation of nearby nerves. For instance, in the wrist, the median and ulnar nerves are in relatively close proximity. If enough current is used, both the median and ulnar nerves can be stimulated and recorded, even if the stimulator is immediately over the median nerve in the wrist, and the recording electrodes are placed properly over the muscle belly of the abductor pollicis brevis (there are adjacent ulnar innervated muscles).

Several aspects of the CMAP are analyzed (Fig. 4.1). The *amplitude* is typically measured from the baseline to the negative (above baseline) peak and represents the number of depolarized muscle fibers. Several neuropathological processes can lower the CMAP amplitude, including axonal loss, conduction block, muscle loss, or failure of the NMJ. The *latency* is a measure of the time that elapses between the stimulation of the nerve and the beginning of the CMAP waveform. Because it is recording the beginning of the deflection, this represents the fastest (most heavily myelinated) fibers and also includes the time of NMJ transmission. The CMAP *area* is measured from the baseline to the negative peak and can be used to help determine if conduction block is present. The CMAP *duration* is commonly measured from the initial negative deflection to the next crossing of the baseline and is a measure of synchrony of the motor fibers. The duration will typically increase in demyelinating lesions when some fibers are slowed more than others. Motor *conduction velocity* measurements require at least two sites of stimulation and measure the speed of the fastest fibers along a motor nerve. For example, the median nerve can be stimulated in the antecubital fossa and at the wrist, and the conduction velocity of the forearm segment can be calculated. This measure does not include the time of neuromuscular transmission or time for muscle depolarization and is typically reduced in demyelinating lesions, although it can be affected by axonal lesions if the fastest fibers are affected.

Sensory Nerve Action Potentials (SNAPs)

Sensory nerve conduction studies are typically performed using either ring electrodes (a small wire that wraps around a finger) with a second reference electrode placed ~3 cm away or a bar electrode that contains both a recording electrode and a reference electrode. SNAPs are small in comparison to CMAPs and are measured in μV (Fig. 4.2). The waveforms are of much shorter duration, which is one clue that can be utilized in determining the source of an unknown waveform. Due to their small nature, they are much more susceptible to artifacts, injury, or various technical difficulties. Similar aspects of SNAPs are analyzed when compared to CMAPs

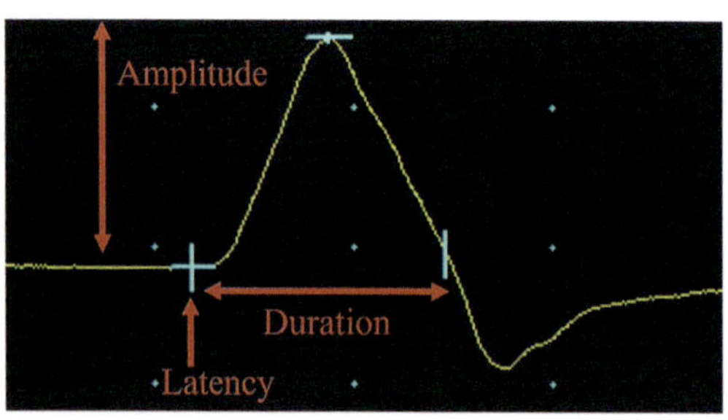

Fig. 4.1 Compound muscle action potential (CMAP)

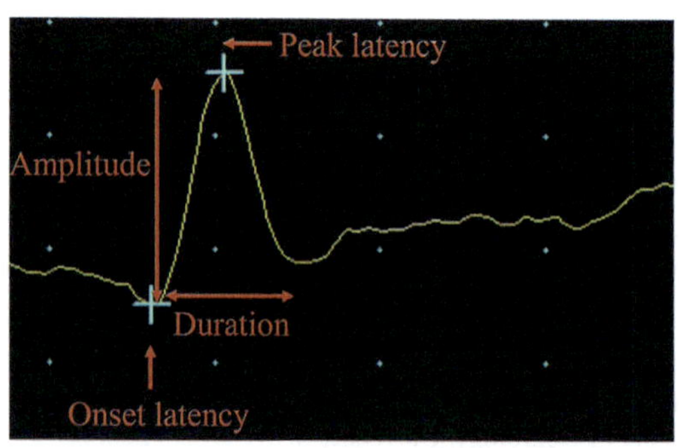

Fig. 4.2 Sensory nerve action potential (SNAP)

with some important distinctions. *Amplitude* is measured from the baseline to the negative peak and indicates nerve pathology when decreased. In contrast to CMAPs, two measures of latency are commonly used when evaluating SNAPs. *Peak latency* measures the time to the first negative peak. The benefits of this measure include higher reliability (it is easy to place a marker on the peak of a waveform); however, the exact population of sensory neurons that are studied is uncertain. This is in contrast with the *onset latency* which is measured at the initial deflection from the baseline. The onset latency measures the fastest fibers but can be obscured by artifacts which lead to less precise measurement in some situations. A *conduction velocity* can be determined distally, with one stimulation site, as there is no neuromuscular transmission or muscle depolarization time to consider. This is essentially the same measure as the onset latency, except that the distance traveled is considered in the calculation. More proximal conduction velocity on SNAPs can also be measured in a similar fashion to CMAPs with two sites of stimulation. However, these can often be difficult to obtain due to the small nature of SNAPs and phase cancelation, which is a phenomenon where the sensory response waveforms are of significantly lower amplitude and increased duration, the further away the stimulation is from the recording site. SNAPs can be recorded using both an antidromic (proximal stimulation with distal recording) and orthodromic (distal stimulation with proximal recording) technique. Antidromic recording, which is more commonly utilized, will record a larger amplitude SNAP but can be susceptible to muscle artifact. An orthodromic technique will eliminate many artifacts, but the recorded SNAP will be smaller.

Interpretation of NCS

One of the most important aspects to understand with NCS is that damage must affect the nerve cell body or occur between the nerve cell body and the recording site in order to be detected. For a CMAP, the cell body is in the anterior horn cells in the spinal cord, so a lesion in any part of that circuit can affect the CMAP. This is not the case when interpreting SNAPs, as the sensory cell body is in the DRG. *If the lesion is proximal to the DRG, the SNAP will remain normal.* This fact cannot be repeated enough as it is one of the most frequently misunderstood concepts in electrodiagnostics and leads to countless clinical errors. If an isolated lesion is in the nerve root (radiculopathy, avulsion), spinal cord, or brain, the SNAP will remain normal with only extremely rare exceptions.

Late responses include the *F response* (also referred to as an F-wave), which is a late motor response obtained with distal motor stimulation, antidromic signal to the anterior horn cells, and orthodromic response back to the muscle belly. These are sensitive (though nonspecific) studies as they test the entire nerve circuit and thus will have prolonged latency if there is damage anywhere along the motor pathway. The F-wave studies are especially helpful in the assessment of proximal nerve segments, which are not accessible for direct nerve stimulation.

Timing of NCS

Wallerian (axonal) degeneration generally takes 3–5 days for motor fibers and 6–10 days for sensory fibers. In general, this process should be complete prior to obtaining a study, otherwise false normal results can occur. If nerve conduction testing is performed prior to the completion of Wallerian degeneration, a phenomenon called *pseudoconduction block* can occur in which it can appear that a conduction block is present (evidence of demyelination), while the true pathology is axonal and the pattern will only manifest after Wallerian degeneration is complete.

Basic Nerve Conduction Patterns

Neuropathic lesions have two main patterns, axonal and demyelinating. In axonal lesions, the most common finding is a reduced amplitude of the motor and/or sensory responses. Other findings such as mildly prolonged latency and mildly slowed conduction velocity may be present (likely related, in part, to pathology of the fastest nerve fibers). In demyelinating lesions, the amplitude can be normal or reduced if conduction block or temporal dispersion is present. Temporal dispersion represents desynchronization of components of a CMAP due to different rates of conduction among the individual axons secondary to varying degrees of demyelination. The waveform will be wider (increased duration) and have less amplitude. Conduction block refers to a decrease in amplitude when comparing a distal CMAP amplitude to a proximal CMAP amplitude. Although different definitions exist, a *20% drop in amplitude* in most nerves is a concern for a possible conduction block. Supramaximal stimulation proximal to the conduction block needs to be obtained to ensure proper interpretation of findings. This makes finding a direct evidence to support very proximal (brachial plexus/root) conduction blocks challenging as supramaximal stimulation of proximal nerves is quite painful and technically challenging. *Latency needs to be >130%* of normal and conduction *velocity needs to be <75%* of normal to state that findings are unequivocally related to underlying demyelination. Often, neuropathic lesions will have mixed findings with evidence of both axonal loss and demyelination.

Electromyography [1]

Needle EMG employs the use of a concentric needle electrode. The tip of this needle has a beveled surface with both an active (small wire in the center of the needle) and a reference electrode (shaft). Electrical activity is recorded from muscle fibers immediately adjacent (~1 mm) to the beveled surface. The needle is first inserted into a target muscle to assess for spontaneous activity. At rest, the muscle is normally quiet, with brief bursts of potentials when the needle is moved. Normal insertional activity should last no longer than 300 ms (when the needle is moved), with abnormal spontaneous activity being any activity persisting longer than 3 s when at rest. Techniques vary, but generally several quadrants at different depths should be sampled in every muscle to assess for abnormal spontaneous activity. Some spontaneous activity is nonspecific, whereas others can be associated with certain disorders. Analysis of spontaneous activity involves evaluation of the waveform morphology, stability, and firing characteristics, which requires both visual and audio representations to properly identify waveforms.

Fibrillation potentials and *positive sharp* waves are both generated by the muscle fiber and represent active denervation. If these are present, it can be assumed there is damage to the circuit. This can be in the cell body, axon, NMJ, or muscle fiber itself and thus can be caused by a variety of conditions. They are generally graded on a 4-point scale, with 0 representing nonpresent, up to 4 which is essentially a full interference pattern of potentials. Fibrillation potentials and positive sharp waves are not observed if there is only isolated demyelination of the nerve fiber. Proper timing of the study is important to find these potentials, as the appearance depends on the distance between the lesion site and the muscle being sampled. *If a lesion is at the root level in the lumbar spine, it can take 10–14 days for fibrillation potentials/positive sharp waves to appear in the paraspinal muscles, 2–3 weeks in the proximal thigh, 3–4 weeks in the leg, and 5–6 weeks in the distal foot. Conversely, if the lesion is at the site of the muscle such as a necrotizing myopathy or botulism, these potentials can appear within the first few days.* Thinking through the potential site of the lesion in question will help determine the proper time to perform the study.

There are several other spontaneous discharges that can also be observed. *Complex repetitive discharges* (CRDs) require chronically denervated muscle fibers and can be seen in chronic denervation followed by reinnervation or myopathic disorders that lead to denervation of muscle fibers in the course of muscle degeneration. *Myotonic discharges* are waxing/waning discharges observed most often in myotonia congenita or myotonic dystrophies. *Fasciculation potentials* are generated from the motor neuron/axon and are notoriously associated with motor neuron disease. However, they can be observed in many other conditions including neuropathies and radiculopathies and can often be benign. There is no reliable way to distinguish "benign" (fasciculations that occur without other evidence of injury to the lower motor neurons) from "malignant" fasciculations in isolation, and the rest of the history, examination, and NCS/EMG must be considered. *Myokymia* is also generated from the motor neuron/axon. They are often associated with prior radiation therapies and can be helpful, if present, to distinguish a radiation plexopathy from malignant infiltration of nerves, e.g., the brachial plexus in cases of breast cancer. They can also be observed (although less frequently) in other conditions such as immune-mediated neuropathies, entrapment neuropathies, or radiculopathies. *Cramps* can be observed on needle EMG and are not generated in the muscle, but instead are generated from rapid discharges of motor axons. *Neuromyotonia* is a rare, high-frequency discharge and is associated with its own set of neuromyotonic syndromes.

Next, the motor unit action potential (MUAP) or voluntary motor activity is analyzed (Table 4.1). Each motor unit represents a single anterior horn cell, axon, NMJ, and the individual muscle fibers it innervates. MUAPs are generally triphasic, and there are three main morphological features that are assessed. *Duration* is a measure of the initial deflection from baseline to the final return to baseline and reflects both the number of fibers in a motor unit and how they depolarize over time. *Polyphasia* describes the number of phases of a motor unit and is a measure of how synchronous muscle fibers are firing. *Amplitude* is the peak-to-peak measurement of the waveform. Its measure is highly dependent on the distance of the needle tip to the muscle fibers and thus is generally less reliable than the duration and polyphasia in determining the underlying pathology. Changes to the MUAP morphology evolve over several months and thus may not be observed if the EMG is performed too early after the onset of a nerve injury or other axonal neuropathic processes.

MUAPs can also be evaluated for their firing pattern. *Recruitment* describes the firing rate compared to the number of distinct MUAPs observed. There are only two ways to increase strength, by firing motor units faster or by firing more motor units. Reduced recruitment is seen when there are too few distinct motor units firing at too high frequency. Reduced recruitment is the earliest finding in most neuropathic lesions, even before changes in the NCS. Early or increased recruitment refers to many motor units firing despite the minimal force exerted by the muscle. This generally requires opposition of the patient's movement by the person performing the EMG as well as significant experience with "normal" recruitment and the force generated. Early

Table 4.1 Outline of common patterns in MUAP morphology and the firing pattern (however, this list is not comprehensive, and exceptions may be encountered)

Lesion	MUAP morphology	MUAP firing pattern
Acute neuropathic (axonal) if axon is in continuity	Normal	Reduced recruitment
Chronic neuropathic (axonal)	Increased duration, large amplitude, increased phases	Reduced recruitment
Demyelinating	Normal	Normal
Demyelinating with conduction block	Normal	Reduced recruitment
Acute myopathy	Short duration, low amplitude, increased phases	Early recruitment
Chronic myopathy	Variable	Early recruitment

recruitment is most often observed in myopathic conditions where abnormal muscle fibers require significant MUAP recruitment to generate a muscle force. If a MUAP is observed, this is evidence of axonal continuity between the anterior horn cells and the muscle being sampled.

Activation, when used in an electrophysiological context, is a measure of the ability to increase the rate in which one fires a MUAP. Poor activation occurs when the patient cannot adequately move a muscle and can be related to a disorder in the central nervous system, pain, effort, or functional neurologic disorder. It is important to note that if a patient is unable to activate a muscle, the information gathered from the EMG will be limited to spontaneous activity which can limit the overall interpretation of the study. Some muscles require activation to ensure that the needle is in the correct location. The needle may pass through the muscle, especially if atrophic, and may sample MUAPs from adjacent muscles which may have different innervations. This can lead to misinterpretation and improper localization of the lesion.

Nerve Regeneration

NCS/EMG can be very helpful tools in determining if there is evidence of nerve regeneration. Regeneration occurs when there is an injury to the anterior horn cell, its axon, the NMJ, or the muscle fiber it innervates. It does not occur in lesions that are exclusively demyelinating, although many primarily demyelinating conditions also have secondary axonal damage. Without intervention, there are typically two main mechanisms of regeneration. The most common type of nerve regeneration is from *collateral sprouting* of surviving motor neurons. In severe nerve injuries where there are no surviving motor neurons to provide collateral sprouting, the mechanism of nerve regeneration is *axonal regrowth* from the site of the injury. This process is slow and can take many months to years.

In general, NCS can be used to measure the overall signal that is being carried by the axons of a nerve. The amplitude of a CMAP represents the number of muscle fibers that are being depolarized. In an axonal nerve injury, the amplitude will be decreased, although it is important to note that there are many other pathologies that can result in a reduction in amplitude as previously discussed. Improvement in CMAP amplitude over time following a nerve injury represents the overall nerve regeneration. For example, a distal median motor CMAP amplitude of 1 mV following a gunshot wound to the median nerve in the forearm, if at 1 year CMAP amplitude is 5 mV, represents axonal regrowth as long as the coexisting conduction block/demyelination were properly ruled out.

Needle EMG is a more sensitive measure of nerve regeneration. If voluntary motor units are observed in a muscle, it can be assumed that there is some degree of axonal continuity to that muscle. Following an axonal injury, the axon regrows and begins to reinnervate some of the denervated muscle fibers. *Polyphasia* of voluntary motor units is an early sign of reinnervation and represents the dyssynchronous firing of the individual muscle fibers of one motor unit. Over many months, this will synchronize, resulting in large-amplitude, long-duration units that are associated with chronic reinnervation. At times, *nascent motor units* can be observed following severe denervation and are a sign of early reinnervation These are short, narrow, polyphasic units that can resemble myopathic motor units. Nascent motor units can be differentiated from myopathic units as they have reduced recruitment compared to the normal to early recruitment observed in myopathic motor units.

Radiculopathy [2]

One of the most common conditions evaluated in the EMG laboratory is radiculopathy. Ultimately, it is a clinical diagnosis; however, correlation between imaging, clinical examination, and EMG findings can increase the certainty of the correct diagnosis. A myotome refers to all the muscles that are innervated by a single spinal segment, and a dermatome refers to the cutaneous sensory distribution innervated by a single spinal segment. There is significant overlap in both of these distributions, with muscles often innervated by several adjacent spinal segments (i.e., triceps innervated by C6/C7/C8) and sensory overlap in dermatomal segments. Although the dermatomes are often depicted as distinct barriers, the reality is there is a tremendous amount of variability and dual innervation by adjacent levels; thus, these should be used as a rough guideline. Both paralysis of a muscle and severe sensory loss are unusual to be caused by radiculopathy, although not impossible, and may suggest root avulsion, a more distal nerve lesion, or a central lesion depending on the clinical circumstance.

NCS are typically normal in radiculopathy, but severe and/or multilevel involvement can cause low CMAPs. *SNAPs are normal as the lesion is proximal to the DRG*. Therefore, the diagnosis is typically established with the needle EMG. Muscles are sampled that are innervated by different nerves but the same myotome to help exclude a mononeuropathy. Both proximal and distal muscles should be sampled to exclude a length-dependent peripheral neuropathy (which would preferentially affect the distal muscles).

There are several limitations to needle EMG. The yield of EMG is higher if there is clinical weakness. Time course is also important as it can take time for denervation potentials to develop (up to 6 weeks) and longer for chronic reinnervation changes. At times, the level cannot be determined with exact certainty given the tendency of muscles to be innervated by multiple adjacent spinal segments. Paraspinal muscles are helpful if they are abnormal but are only found in ~50% of radiculopathies. Thus, *the absence of paraspinal abnormalities should never exclude a radiculopathy*. Paraspinal muscles can only identify that the lesion is at or above the root level but cannot be used to localize the root level. Furthermore, there are several situations where paraspinal muscles may be abnormal, including diabetes or in a prior surgical site, and thus may not be sampled as they do not add relevant information. If the lesion is purely demyelinating or if there is only sensory involvement, the needle EMG will be normal. Similarly, if the lesion affects only certain fascicles, these may not be sampled in a routine study. Lumbosacral spinal stenosis can often have normal EMG findings, especially as neurogenic claudication is intermittent compression, and thus may not cause the axonal damage.

Plexus Lesions (Table 4.2)

The brachial plexus and lumbosacral plexus are both complicated anatomical structures. Evaluating these lesions with NCS/EMG is demanding and relies primarily on the SNAPs as well as extensive needle EMG study. Abnormal SNAPs are often the most useful piece of information in a properly diagnosed plexus lesion. Normal SNAPs indicate that the lesion is preganglionic. Contralateral studies should be performed as a control, as the side of the lesion may have "normal" SNAP amplitude, but it is considered abnormal if it is <50% of the healthy side.

Table 4.2 In the brachial plexus, there are many sensory potentials that can be used to localize the site of the lesion

Brachial plexus structure	Corresponding sensory potential
Upper trunk	Lateral antebrachial cutaneous, radial (thumb, snuffbox), median (thumb and index finger)
Middle trunk	Median (middle and ring finger)
Lower trunk	Median (ring finger), ulnar (ring and little fingers), dorsal ulnar cutaneous, medial antebrachial cutaneous
Lateral cord	Lateral antebrachial cutaneous, median (thumb, index, and middle finger)
Posterior cord	Radial (thumb, snuffbox)
Medial cord	Median (ring finger), ulnar (ring, little fingers), dorsal ulnar cutaneous, medial antebrachial cutaneous

Needle EMG should be performed to evaluate all relevant trunks, cords, and nerve branches if tolerated by the patient. Muscles that are innervated directly from the nerve roots (rhomboids, serratus anterior, paraspinal muscles) will be normal in a brachial plexus lesion but can be abnormal if there is an accompanied root avulsion. EMG findings can often be identical in both radiculopathies and plexus injuries (such as a C5/C6 radiculopathy vs upper trunk plexopathy); therefore, it is essential to demonstrate SNAP abnormalities before one is confident the pathology is distal to the DRG and in the plexus.

The approach to the lumbosacral plexus is similar in principle; however, there are more limited options for sensory studies (superficial peroneal, sural, and saphenous nerves). Thus, it can often be more difficult to confidently differentiate a multilevel lumbosacral radiculopathy from plexopathy on the basis of NCS/EMG alone.

Nerve Entrapments [2] (Tables 4.3, 4.4, and 4.5)

There are several areas in the body where nerves are commonly entrapped/impinged such as the median nerve at the wrist, ulnar nerve at the elbow, and peroneal nerve at the fibular head. The sensory disturbance is often more concentrated, especially in severe lesions. They are more likely to result in anesthesia in contrast to radicular lesions which tend to have more altered or diminished sensation. NCS and EMG can be used to confirm an entrapment, but this does not absolve the clinician from taking a history and performing an appropriate clinical examination. For example, a report may indicate a median neuropathy across the wrist; however, this could be an incidental finding in the absence of an appropriate clinical scenario. This principle is especially relevant in diabetics where evidence of entrapment is common, although the patient may be asymptomatic.

Table 4.3 Demonstration of common patterns of median neuropathy at the wrist, recording the abductor pollicis brevis

Nerve/site	Latency	Amplitude	Conduction velocity
(A) Median (motor)	(≤4.5)	(≥4.0)	(≥48.0)
Wrist	3	10	
Elbow		9.6	60
Median (sensory)	(≤3.6)	(≥15.0)	(≥51.0)
Wrist	**4.0**	20	51
(B) Median (motor)	(≤4.5)	(≥4.0)	(≥48.0)
Wrist	**5.0**	6	
Elbow		5.7	54
Median (sensory)	(≤3.6)	(≥15.0)	(≥51.0)
Wrist	**6.2**	**6.0**	**35**
(C) Median (motor)	(≤4.5)	(≥4.0)	(≥48.0)
Wrist	**7.2**	**2.0**	
Elbow		1.5	48
Median (sensory)	(≤3.6)	(≥15.0)	(≥51.0)
Wrist	**NR**	**NR**	**NR**

(A) A mild median neuropathy across the wrist. Note the normal motor study, with only mild prolongation of the median nerve sensory latency. If the above testing is normal yet median neuropathy at the wrist is suspected, additional comparison studies such as comparing the latency of the palmar mixed fibers of the median and ulnar nerves (not pictured), can be pursued
(B) A moderate median neuropathy across the wrist. Note the motor latency is now prolonged, with a lower amplitude (although still may be normal). The sensory amplitude is now diminished with a prolonged latency and slowed conduction velocity
(C) A severe median neuropathy across the wrist. Note the significant reduction in the motor amplitude with prolonged latency. The sensory study is now absent. Motor reference values are in mV and sensory reference values are in μV. *NR* no response, **Bold** abnormal finding

Table 4.4 Demonstration of common patterns in entrapment neuropathies using the ulnar nerve recording the adductor digiti minimi as an example

Nerve/site	Latency	Amplitude	Conduction velocity
(A) Ulnar (motor)	(≤3.6)	(≥6.0)	(≥51.0)
Wrist	3	8	
Below elbow		7.8	60
Above elbow		7.7	**45**
Ulnar (sensory)	(≤3.1)	(≥10)	(≥51.0)
Wrist	**3.2**	12	52
(B) Ulnar (motor)	(≤3.6)	(≥6.0)	(≥51.0)
Wrist	3.6	7	
Below elbow		6.9	60
Above elbow		**4.0**	**30**
Ulnar (sensory)	(≤3.1)	(≥10)	(≥51.0)
Wrist	**3.7**	**4**	**45**
(C) Ulnar (motor)	(≤3.6)	(≥6.0)	(≥51.0)
Wrist	**4.2**	**2**	
Below elbow		**1.7**	**45**
Above elbow		**NR**	
Ulnar (sensory)	(≤3.1)	(≥10)	(≥51.0)
Wrist	**NR**	**NR**	**NR**

(A) A mild ulnar neuropathy across the elbow. Note the normal motor amplitudes, slowing of conduction velocity across the elbow, indicating focal demyelination, and borderline normal sensory amplitude with mildly prolonged latency
(B) A moderate ulnar neuropathy across the elbow. Note the drop in amplitude from the below to above elbow stimulation indicating conduction block and reduced amplitude on the sensory response
(C) A severe ulnar neuropathy across the elbow. Note the significant reduction in all motor amplitudes, which suggests axonal loss, and conduction block across the elbow, as well as absent sensory responses. Motor reference values are in mV and sensory reference values are in μV and may vary among labs. *NR* no response, **Bold** abnormal finding

Table 4.5 Demonstration of common patterns of peroneal neuropathy

Nerve/site	Latency	Amplitude	Conduction velocity
(A) Peroneal (motor) EDB	(≤6.0)	(≥2.0)	(≥41.0)
Ankle	4.6	10	
Below fibular neck		9.7	45
Knee		**4.0**	**20**
Peroneal (motor) TA	(≤4.0)	(≥5.0)	(≥41.0)
Below fibular neck	3.6	7.0	
Knee		**2.7**	**24**
Peroneal (sensory)	(≤4.5)	(≥5.0)	(≥40.0)
Ankle	4.2	**4.0**	41
(B) Peroneal (motor) EDB	(≤6.0)	(≥2.0)	(≥41.0)
Ankle	4.6	**1.8**	
Below fibular neck		**1.6**	45
Knee		**1.5**	42
Peroneal (motor) TA	(≤4.0)	(≥5.0)	(≥41.0)
Below fibular neck	3.6	**3.0**	
Knee		**2.7**	43
Peroneal (sensory)	(≤4.5)	(≥5.0)	(≥40.0)
Ankle	**NR**	**NR**	**NR**

(**A**) Common peroneal neuropathy across the fibular head. Note the slowing of velocity and conduction block in both motor studies. The sensory amplitude is low which supports involvement in the common peroneal nerve. Often, due to significant variability of "normal" values obtained in the lower extremities, contralateral studies may need to be performed to increase the sensitivity of testing

(**B**) A nonlocalizable peroneal neuropathy vs sciatic neuropathy. Note the reduction in motor amplitudes without focal slowing or conduction block. The absent peroneal sensory response indicates a lesion distal to the DRG. Further localization would be found on needle EMG, with the lesion located "at or above the takeoff" to the most proximal, abnormal muscle. Sampling tibial-innervated muscles as well as the short head of biceps femoris, which is the last muscle supplied by peroneal nerve in the thigh, is important for localization. Peroneal fibers are preferentially affected in most sciatic nerve lesions; thus, there can be a significant crossover between the findings observed in the electromyography laboratory. Motor reference values are in mV, and sensory reference values are in μV and may vary among labs. *EDB* extensor digitorum brevis, *TA* tibialis anterior, *NR* no response, **Bold** abnormal finding

In nerve entrapment, changes in SNAPs are typically more sensitive and found earlier than changes in CMAPs. SNAPs cannot be used to localize the exact site of the lesion. Some entrapments, such as median neuropathy at the wrist, have several comparison studies such as comparing the latency of the palmar mixed fibers of the median and ulnar nerves, among several others, that can increase the overall sensitivity of testing and aid in localization. On the motor studies, focal slowing of conduction velocity and/or conduction block can be used to localize the site of the lesion. For example, slowing of conduction velocity between the below-elbow and above-elbow stimulation sites with conduction block can diagnose ulnar neuropathy across the elbow.

Needle EMG is also used for localization purposes but not in isolation. If there are changes on the needle examination, one can assume that there is damage, at some place, to the motor unit (presumably the axon if related to a nerve entrapment) and that the area of damage is at or above the takeoff point of the nerve branch to the target muscle. At times, electromyographers will try to localize a nerve lesion based on the needle examination alone which can result in diagnostic errors. For example, if the needle examination for the first dorsal interosseous is abnormal but is normal for the abductor digiti minimi, one may propose that the lesion is somewhere in the ulnar nerve in the hand. However, another possibility is a more proximal lesion preferentially affecting the fascicle destined for the first dorsal interosseous in the ulnar nerve at the elbow. This is why it is critical to use both the NCS and EMG data to localize a lesion and why certain studies may be reported as "nonlocalizable" lesion- or clinical correlation-recommended.

Polyneuropathy

Polyneuropathy is a general term meaning dysfunction of multiple nerves. It describes a diverse set of conditions that can be divided by several different factors including temporal course, pattern of involvement, fiber type involved, and underlying pathology, among others.

The most common pattern is a *length-dependent peripheral polyneuropathy*. Symptoms develop in the feet first and ascend, with hand involvement beginning typically when symptoms reach the knees, or the so-called "stocking-glove" pattern. NCS and EMG can be very useful in the diagnosis. Typically, these are primarily axonal neuropathies but can have a coexisting demyelinating component. If they involve both the motor and sensory fibers, mildly symptomatic patients will typically have low-amplitude sensory responses in the legs. As symptoms progress, distal motor nerve conduction studies in the legs will begin to reveal different degrees of CMAP amplitude decreases. In severe cases, the sensory and motor responses are unobtainable in the lower extremities, with significant reduction in amplitudes in both sensory and motor studies in the upper extremities. Similarly, needle EMG abnormalities are often limited to the most distal muscles but will advance proximally as the polyneuropathy progresses. As NCS only study the large fibers, neuropathies isolated to the small nerve fibers typically have normal NCS and EMG studies.

Demyelinating neuropathies are diagnosed by finding evidence of diffuse demyelination or focal conduction blocks at non-entrapment sites. If the demyelination is severe enough, there can be secondary axonal loss as well. If the pathology is predominantly in the nerve roots (such as in many cases of the Guillain-Barré syndrome), conduction block, temporal dispersion, or other evidence of demyelination may be difficult to observe as there is no practical way to stimulate the nerves proximally. In those polyneuropathic processes, the F-wave may be most helpful.

Indications for Nerve Biopsy

Nerve biopsy is often utilized to help provide additional information on the underlying pathology of nerve injury or disease. Due to the invasive nature of the procedure, this is typically reserved for situations where additional knowledge of the underlying pathology would change management. Vasculitis affecting the PNS is one of the more common indications for nerve biopsy. Obtaining a muscle biopsy in addition to the nerve biopsy is generally recommended to increase yield when vasculitis is on differential diagnosis. The sural nerve is a common target for biopsy due to the minimal neurological deficit that results after the biopsy; alternatively, the superficial radial nerve can be used for upper limb involvement. Traditionally, nerve biopsy was used to identify both genetic and acquired demyelinating neuropathies. However, due to the advancements in both genetic testing and nerve ultrasound, these can often be differentiated non-invasively. A fascicular biopsy can be pursued if there is a focal involvement of pathology, especially when nerves exhibit an increase in size and/or signal changes on magnetic resonance neurography (MRN), in order to detect focal chronic immune-mediated polyradiculoneuropathy, benign tumors such as perineurioma, or malignant tumors like lymphoma. Nerve biopsy is typically not helpful in most axonal neuropathies unless there is concern for amyloidosis. Other targets such as a fat pad biopsy or cardiac tissue biopsy are commonly pursued first; however, if amyloid is primarily involving nerves, a nerve biopsy can be useful.

Motor Neuron Disease

The most common motor neuron disease in adults is amyotrophic lateral sclerosis (ALS). This disorder only involves the motor neurons; therefore, sensory studies should be normal. Ultimately, ALS is a clinical diagnosis; however, EMG is essential to confirm the diagnosis. Typically, there is significant and widespread active and chronic denervation on needle EMG, with widespread fasciculation potentials. These changes should be seen in multiple myotomes, as well as multiple segments of the nervous system in order to differentiate motor neuron disease from other conditions such as multilevel radiculopathies. One challenge, especially in early disease affecting one body segment, is that the needle EMG findings can be identical to those in radiculopathy; thus, strong clinical correlation is required, and a repeat study may need to be performed in 3–6 months to assess for progression that would support a more widespread degenerative process affecting the anterior horn cells.

References

1. Preston D, Shapiro B (2020) Electromyography and neuromuscular disorders: clinical-electrophysiologic-ultrasound correlations. Elsevier, Philadelphia
2. Bashar K (2018) Electromyography in clinical practice: a case study approach. Oxford University Press, New York, NY

Diagnostic Ultrasound of Nerves and Ultrasound-Guided Procedures

5

John S. Symanski

Indications

- Diagnosis and localization of neuropathy, trauma, and nerve sheath tumors
- Imaging nerves around metal implants and shrapnel or in patients with MRI contraindications such as pacemakers
- Dynamic evaluation of nerve subluxation
- Image guidance for nerve blocks, wire localizations, and nerve ablation (radiofrequency, alcohol, microwave, and cryoablation)

Equipment

Superficial nerves should be imaged with a high-frequency probe (10–24 MHz) to maximize spatial resolution. Imaging deeper nerves may necessitate the use of a lower frequency probe (6–10 MHz), which will produce images with a lower spatial and contrast resolution.

Ultrasound Appearance of Normal Nerves (Fig. 5.1)

In short axis, most large- and medium-sized nerves have a characteristic honeycomb appearance with a hyperechoic outer epineurium surrounding hypoechoic nerve fascicular bundles, which are invested by a hyperechoic inner epineurium [1, 2]. Smaller nerves may only have one hypoechoic fascicular bundle. The hyperechoic epineurium of some nerves may not be apparent if surrounded by similarly hyperechoic connective tissues. In the long axis, the hyperechoic epineurium parallels the hypoechoic nerve fascicular bundles. In contrast, tendons have a finer, more fibrillar architecture.

Supplementary Information The online version contains supplementary material available at https://doi.org/10.1007/978-3-031-73931-6_5.

J. S. Symanski (✉)
Department of Radiology, University of Wisconsin School of Medicine and Public Health, Madison, WI, USA
e-mail: JSymanski@uwhealth.org

A. S. Hanna (ed.), *Nerves: Anatomy, Exposures, and Techniques*, https://doi.org/10.1007/978-3-031-73931-6_5

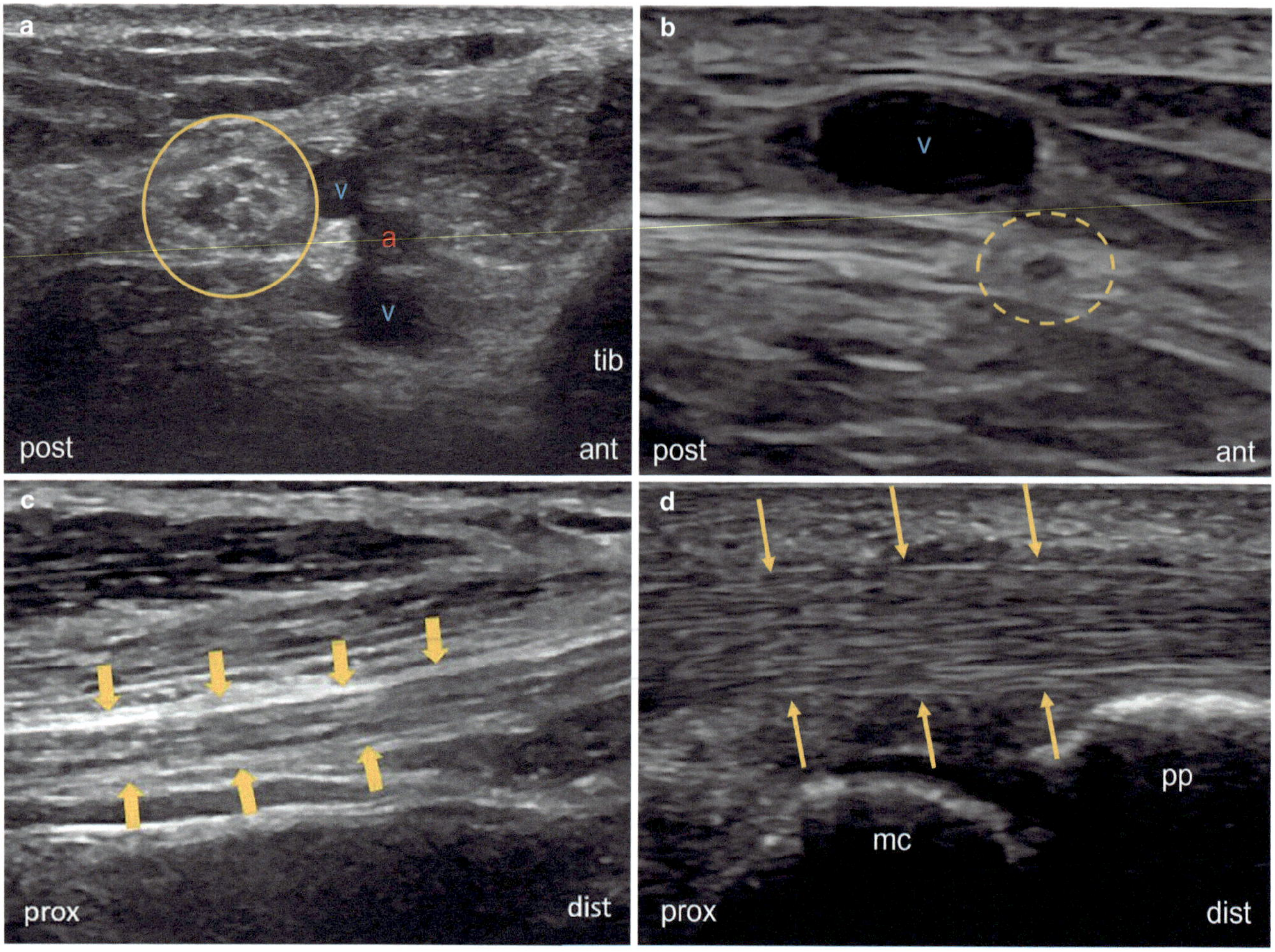

Fig. 5.1 Normal US appearance of nerves. (**a**) The tibial nerve (*gold circle*) imaged in short axis in the tarsal tunnel with a characteristic honeycomb appearance; *a* posterior tibial artery, *tib* tibia, *v* posterior tibial veins. (**b**) The saphenous nerve (*dashed gold circle*) imaged in short axis in the leg with only a single visible hypoechoic fascicular bundle; *v* great saphenous vein. (**c**) The ulnar nerve (*thick gold arrows*) imaged in long axis near the elbow with a characteristic fascicular appearance. (**d**) Unlike nerves, tendons have a finer more fibrillar appearance, as seen with the flexor tendons in the hand (*thin gold arrows*); *mc* metacarpal head, *pp* proximal phalanx

Ultrasound Appearance of Neuropathy (Figs. 5.2 and 5.3)

Hallmarks of low-grade nerve injuries and entrapment neuropathy are generalized nerve enlargement, increase in size of one or all of the hypoechoic fascicular bundles, and decreased nerve echogenicity, which may impart a coalesced appearance to the hypoechoic fascicular bundles [1, 2]. Nerve enlargement may occur at or adjacent to the site of compression. The diagnosis of nerve enlargement may be made by comparison to the presumable normal contralateral nerve, established normative cross-sectional area measurements, or changes in nerve cross-sectional area along its longitudinal course. For example, threshold cross-sectional area measurements and threshold caliber changes have been established for the median nerve at the carpal tunnel, with a median nerve cross-sectional area of > 14 mm^2 in the carpal tunnel essentially diagnostic of entrapment neuropathy [3]. A cross-sectional area of 10–14 mm^2 at the carpal tunnel or a change in median nerve cross-sectional area of >2 mm^2 at the carpal tunnel compared to the distal forearm at the level of the pronator quadratus muscle is equivocal for neuropathy [3]. Ultrasound may also establish nerve subluxation or dislocation as a cause for neuropathy, which is commonly seen with the ulnar nerve at the elbow (Video 5.1).

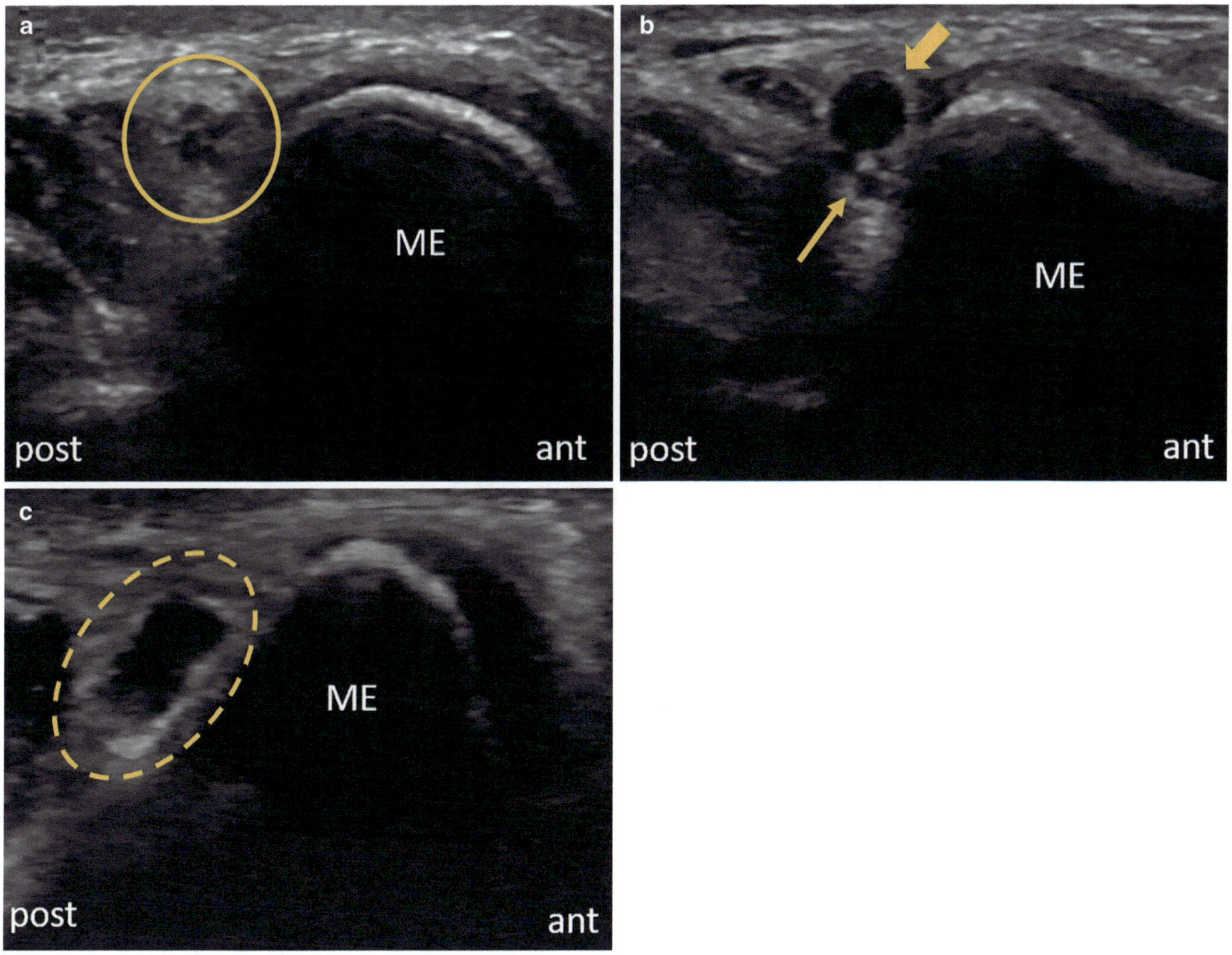

Fig. 5.2 Spectrum of neuropathy. (**a**) For reference, a normal ulnar nerve (*gold circle*) in short axis posterior to the medial epicondyle (*ME*) at the elbow. (**b**) Enlargement of one of the ulnar nerve fascicles (*thick gold arrow*) in contrast to the other normal fascicles (*thin gold arrow*). (**c**) Diffuse ulnar nerve enlargement with coalesced fascicles (*dashed gold oval*). The cause for this ulnar neuropathy was hypermobility with dynamic dislocation over the medial epicondyle with flexion (see Video 5.1)

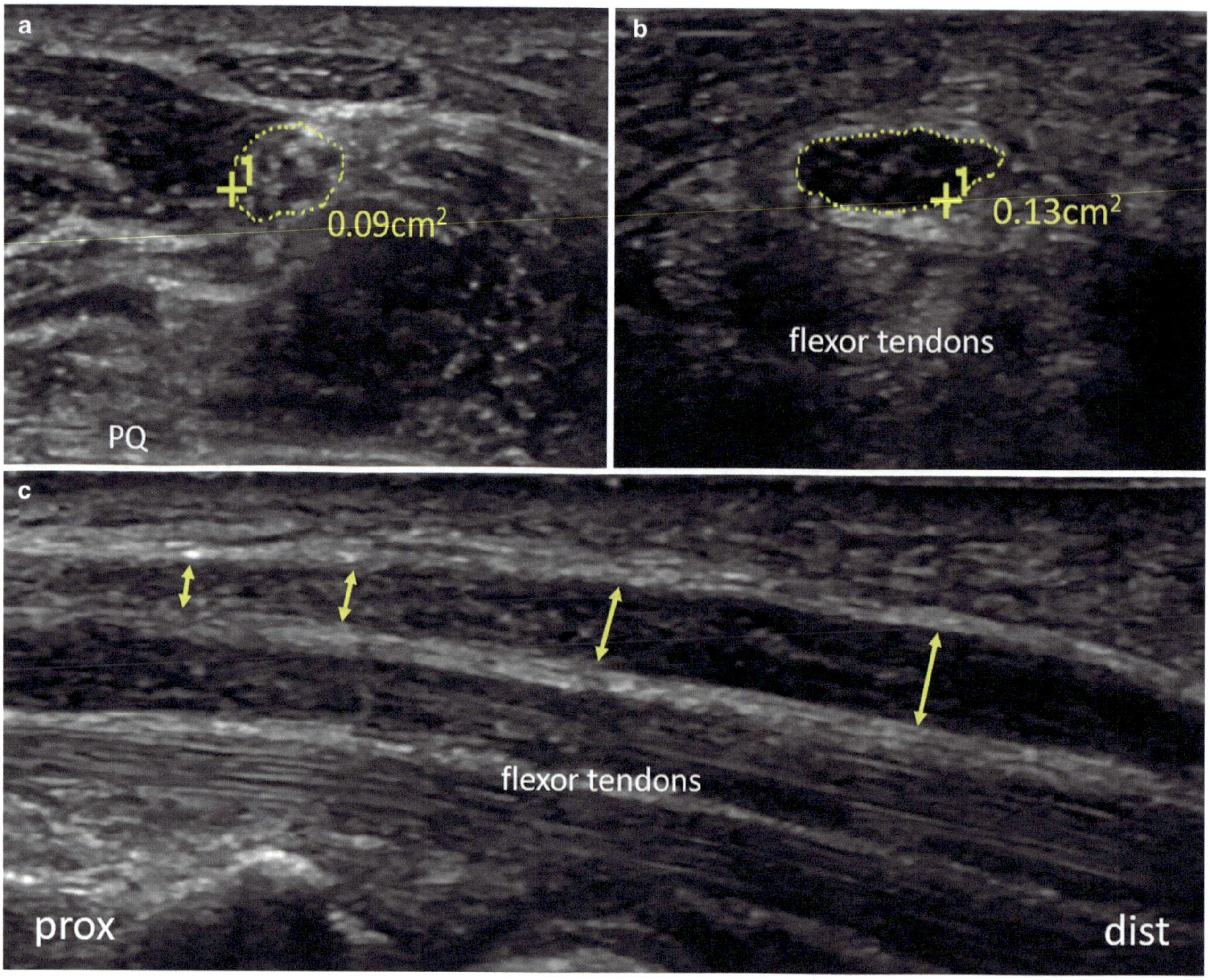

Fig. 5.3 (**a**) Normal appearance and cross-sectional area of the median nerve (*dashed yellow circle*) in the distal forearm at the level of the pronator quadratus muscle (*PQ*). (**b**) Median nerve enlarges in the carpal tunnel with increased cross-sectional area and overall decreased nerve echogenicity. (**c**) Same median nerve in long axis demonstrates progressive thickening (*double yellow arrows*) as it courses from the forearm to the carpal tunnel

Ultrasound Appearance of Nerve Trauma (Figs. 5.4 and 5.5)

In high-grade nerve injuries, a neuroma will form, which is recognized by focal hypoechoic enlargement of the nerve without any recognizable nerve architecture [1]. A neuroma can be further characterized as a neuroma-in-continuity with intact epineurium (Sunderland Grave IV) or a stump neuroma with disrupted epineurium (Sunderland Grade V).

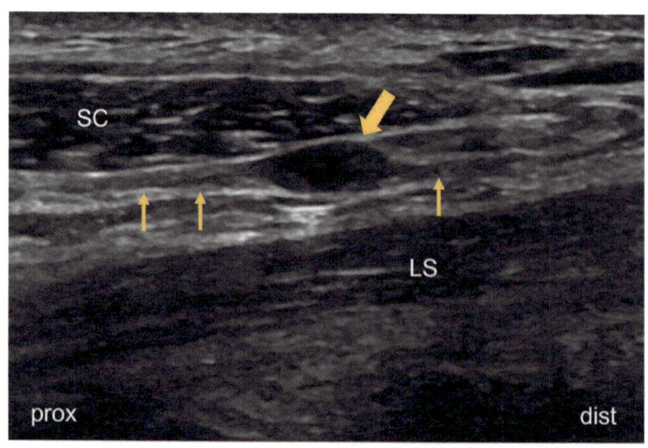

Fig. 5.4 Sagittal image of the lateral neck at the posterior cervical triangle producing a long-axis image of the spinal accessory nerve (*thin gold arrows*) and neuroma-in-continuity (*thick gold arrow*) between the sternocleidomastoid muscle (SC) and the levator scapulae muscle (LS) after lipoma resection. This neuroma-in-continuity is hypoechoic and has no organized internal architecture, but the hyperechoic epineurium is preserved

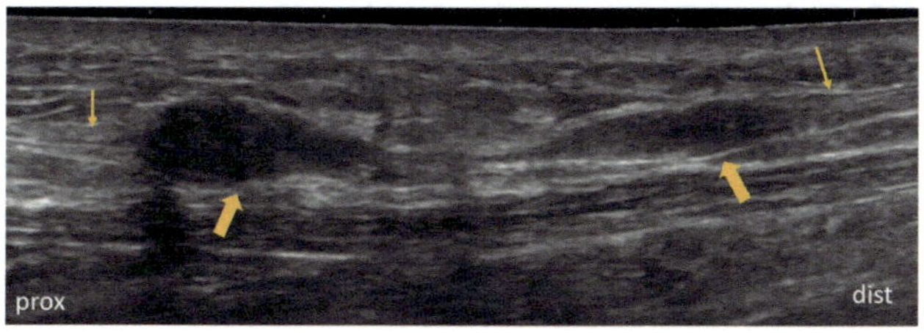

Fig. 5.5 Sagittal image of the leg producing a long-axis image of the sural nerve (*thin gold arrows*) after iatrogenic injury and subsequent neurectomy. Stump neuromas (*thick gold arrows*) have formed at the proximal and distal cut ends of the sural nerve. A stump neuroma is hypoechoic and contains no organized neural architecture, but unlike neuroma-in-continuity, the echogenic epineurium is disrupted, and a gap exists between the nerve's cut ends

Ultrasound Appearance of Nerve Sheath Tumors (Figs. 5.6 and 5.7)

The most specific imaging feature of a nerve sheath tumor is identification of the entering and exiting nerve [4]. Characteristic sonographic findings also include relatively homogeneous hypoechogenicity, posterior acoustic enhancement, and pain with targeted nerve compression. Imaging, especially ultrasound, cannot reliably distinguish schwannoma from neurofibroma or benign from malignant tumors [4]. A greater body of literature exists for using FDG-PET and MRI for benign versus malignant characterization, but some features are likely transferrable to US. Intratumoral

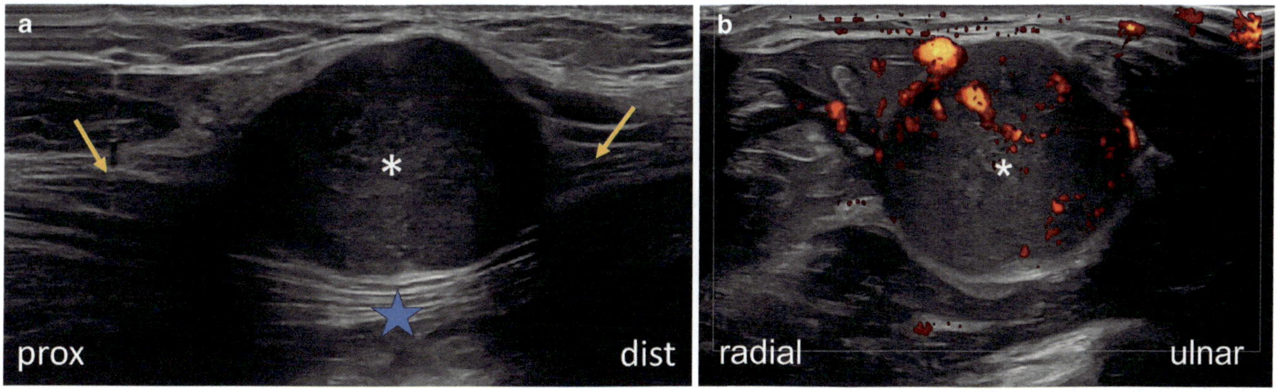

Fig. 5.6 Ulnar nerve schwannoma (*) in the forearm. (**a**) Long-axis US image demonstrating entering and exiting ulnar nerve fascicles (*gold arrows*). The high cellularity of the schwannoma causes posterior acoustic enhancement (*blue star*). (**b**) Short-axis image with power Doppler demonstrating increased internal blood flow

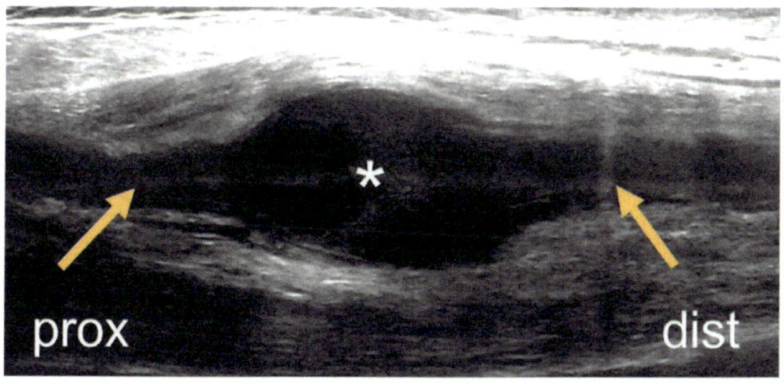

Fig. 5.7 Long-axis US image of a malignant nerve sheath tumor (MPNST) (*) arising from the tibial nerve (*gold arrows*), which is diffusely thickened secondary to plexiform neurofibroma in a patient with neurofibromatosis type 1 (NF1)

necrosis with cystic-like change occurs more frequently with malignant tumors, but degeneration may also occur in benign nerve sheath tumors, e.g., "ancient schwannoma." Additionally, a size greater than 5 cm favors malignant rather than benign tumor. Increased color Doppler blood flow should be observed in non-necrotic portions of malignant tumors but is also commonly observed with benign tumors.

US-Guided Perineural Injection (Nerve Block) (Figs. 5.8, 5.9 and 5.10)

1. May be performed for diagnostic and/or therapeutic intent.
2. Nerve is first visualized in short axis, and an appropriate needle entry site is marked on the skin.

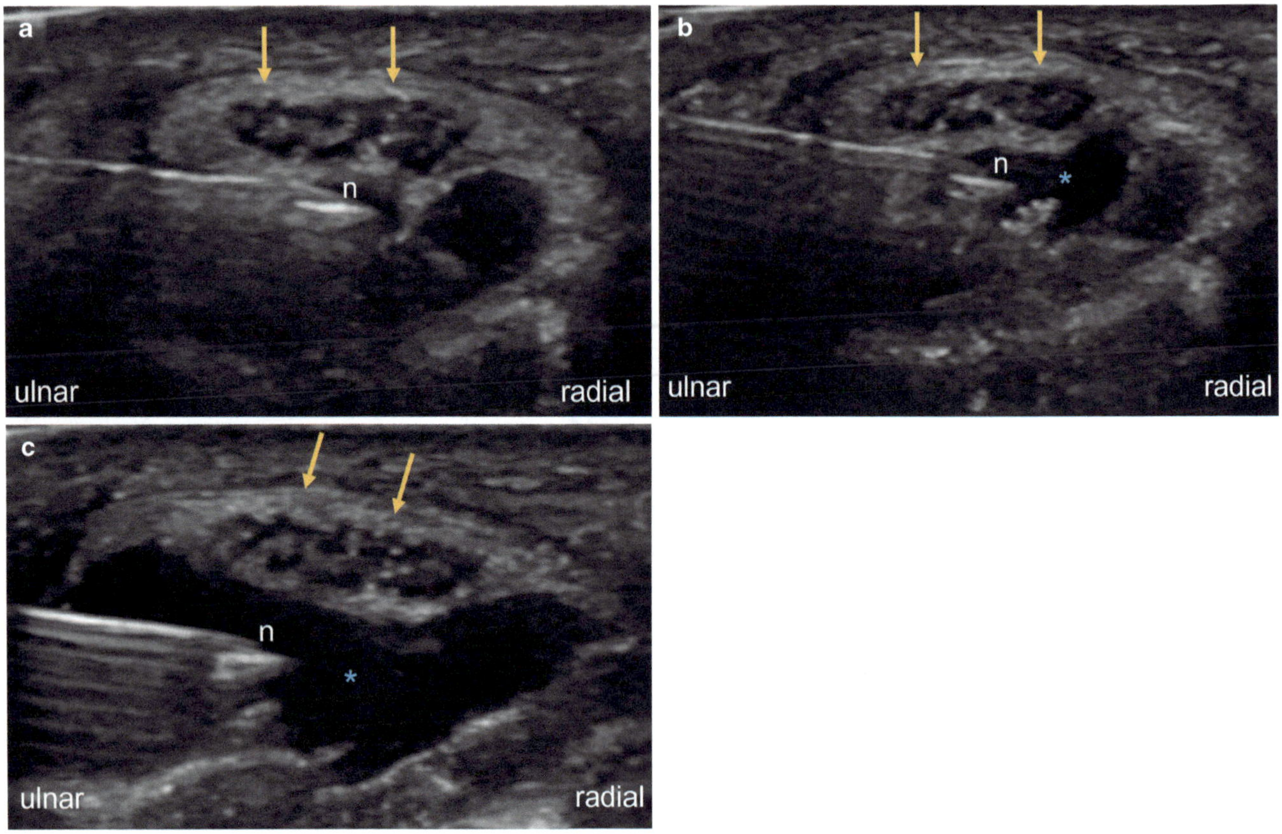

Fig. 5.8 Short-axis images of the median nerve (*gold arrows*) at the carpal tunnel for nerve block with noncircumferential hydrodissection. (**a**) Needle advanced in short axis from an ulnar-sided approach to the margin of the hyperechoic epineurium with the needle bevel (*n*) facing the nerve. (**b**) Epineurium hydrodissected from the adventitial glide layer with injection (*) of a short-acting anesthetic (lidocaine). (**c**) After partial hydrodissection of the epineurium from surrounding soft tissue, a therapeutic mixture of a longer acting anesthetic and a corticosteroid is injected

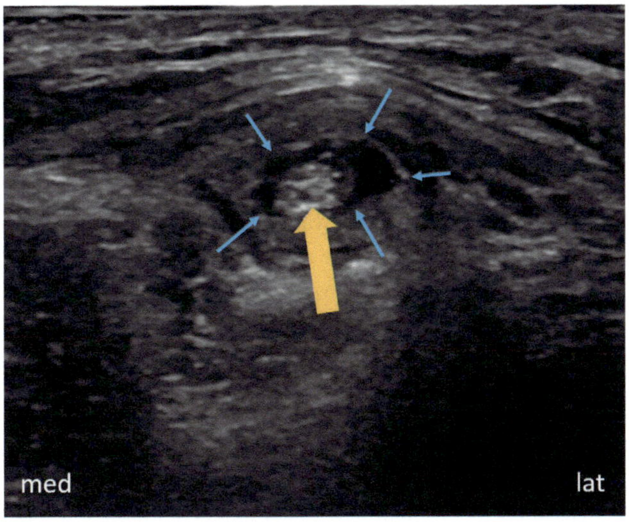

Fig. 5.9 Circumferential spread of injectate (*thin blue arrows*) around the lateral femoral cutaneous nerve (*gold yellow arrow*) after block (needle removed) in the proximal thigh just distal to the level of the anterior superior iliac spine (ASIS)

3. Standard sterile techniques are used including a sterile US probe cover.
4. Needle is advanced in-plane to the outer edge of the epineurium. Needle visualization is improved when the needle is parallel to the ultrasound transducer.
5. Hydrodissection of the epineurium from the surrounding adventitial glide layer is performed with a small volume of short-acting anesthetic such as lidocaine [1].
6. Repositioning the needle tip to achieve circumferential hydrodissection may maximize the therapeutic benefit of nerve block but is not required and sometimes precluded by adjacent vascular structures and the lack of a robust adventitial gliding layer with small nerves [5]. For nerves located in a well-defined fascial plane, injecting the fascial plane adjacent to the nerve is effective such as with the ilioinguinal nerve in the lower abdominal wall [1]. *Intraneural injection should be avoided.*
7. After satisfactory hydrodissection, a longer acting anesthetic and/or steroid is injected into the fluid surrounding the nerve.

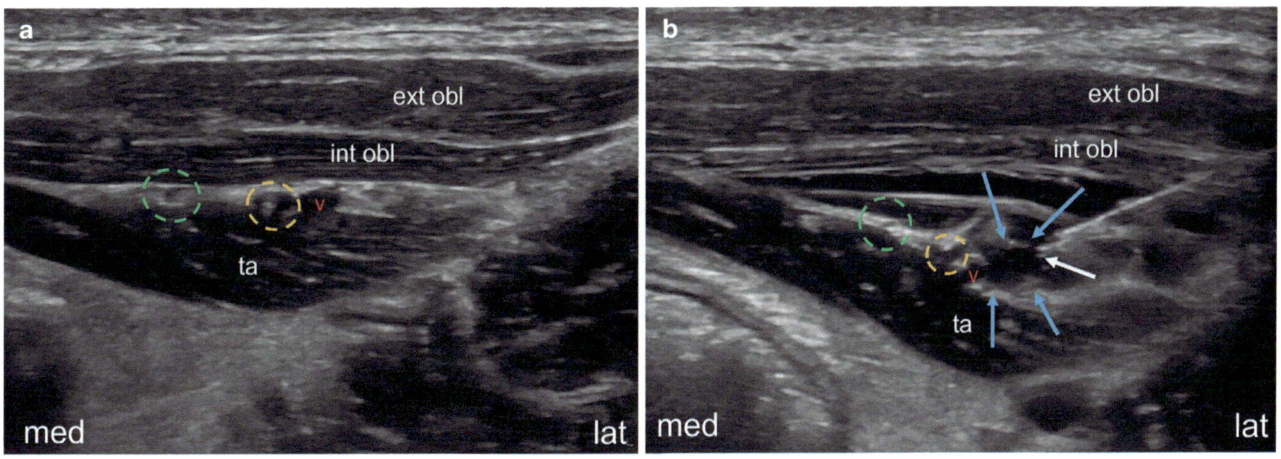

Fig. 5.10 Ultrasound-guided ilioinguinal nerve block performed in the lower abdominal wall. (**a**) Ilioinguinal nerve (*dashed gold circle*) located in the fascial plane between the internal oblique (*int obl*) and transversus abdominis (*ta*) muscles. External oblique muscle (*ext obl*), deep circumflex iliac vessel (*v*), and iliohypogastric nerve (*dashed green circle*) are shown for reference. (**b**) Needle (*white arrow*) visualized in-plane with injectate (*blue arrows*) flooding the fascial plane between the internal oblique and the transversus abdominus muscles. Off-target fluid was also injected into more superficial fascial layers

Nerve Block Medication Selection

A longer acting anesthetic such as ropivacaine or bupivacaine may be used after injection to prolong the anesthetic effect. For nerves, bupivacaine is often favored over ropivacaine, which is more expensive, a vasoconstrictor and may form crystal aggregates when combined with a water-soluble steroid such as dexamethasone [6]. Steroids are frequently combined with the anesthetic mixture to potentiate the anesthetic effect and provide a longer lasting benefit. Particulate steroids such as triamcinolone have a theoretically longer duration of action but come with a risk of local skin depigmentation if injected superficially. While the safety profile of particulate steroids is high for perineural injections, rare microvascular embolization events have been reported, particularly when injected adjacent to blood vessels such as in the spine and at the stellate ganglion. Nonparticulate, fully water-soluble steroids such as dexamethasone minimize the risk of embolic events. No published studies definitively demonstrate the superiority of particulate steroids over water-soluble steroids for perineural injections.

Nerve Hydrodissection

The hydrostatic pressure achieved with a high-volume perineural injection theoretically may more robustly release adhesions that exert direct pressure on the nerve and restrict normal gliding. Most nerve hydrodissection clinical trials have studied the median nerve at the carpal tunnel and have compared different solutions including dextrose 5% in water (D5W), normal saline (NS), and NS + hyaluronidase, with D5W and NS + hyaluronidase, each demonstrating superiority to NS alone [7].

Preoperative Wire Localization (Fig. 5.11)

1. Decreases "skin-to-nerve time" for nerves that are difficult to identify intraoperatively, due to small size and/or variable anatomy such as the lateral femoral cutaneous nerve (LFCN) [8].
2. Target nerve and any relevant branches are mapped with US and are marked on the patient's skin.
3. Target location of the nerve is identified in short axis, and the skin entry site for wire localization needle is marked.
4. Standard sterile techniques are used including a sterile US probe cover.
5. After injection of a local anesthetic, a straight needle containing a curved-tip retractable wire is advanced in plane until the tip is just subjacent to the nerve [8].
6. The wire is deployed/advanced under the nerve, and the needle is retracted over the wire, which stays in place. A wire without substantial soft tissue purchase may back out, so it's important to pick a skin entry point and a wire trajectory that provides enough soft tissue to stabilize the wire.
7. Depth of the nerve from the skin surface and the horizontal distance from the wire entry site to the nerve projection on the skin are measured; the latter guides the surgeon to where the skin incision should be made [8].
8. Protective dressing is applied over the exposed wire. Care should be taken to avoid excessive movement of the limb to prevent wire dislodgement.

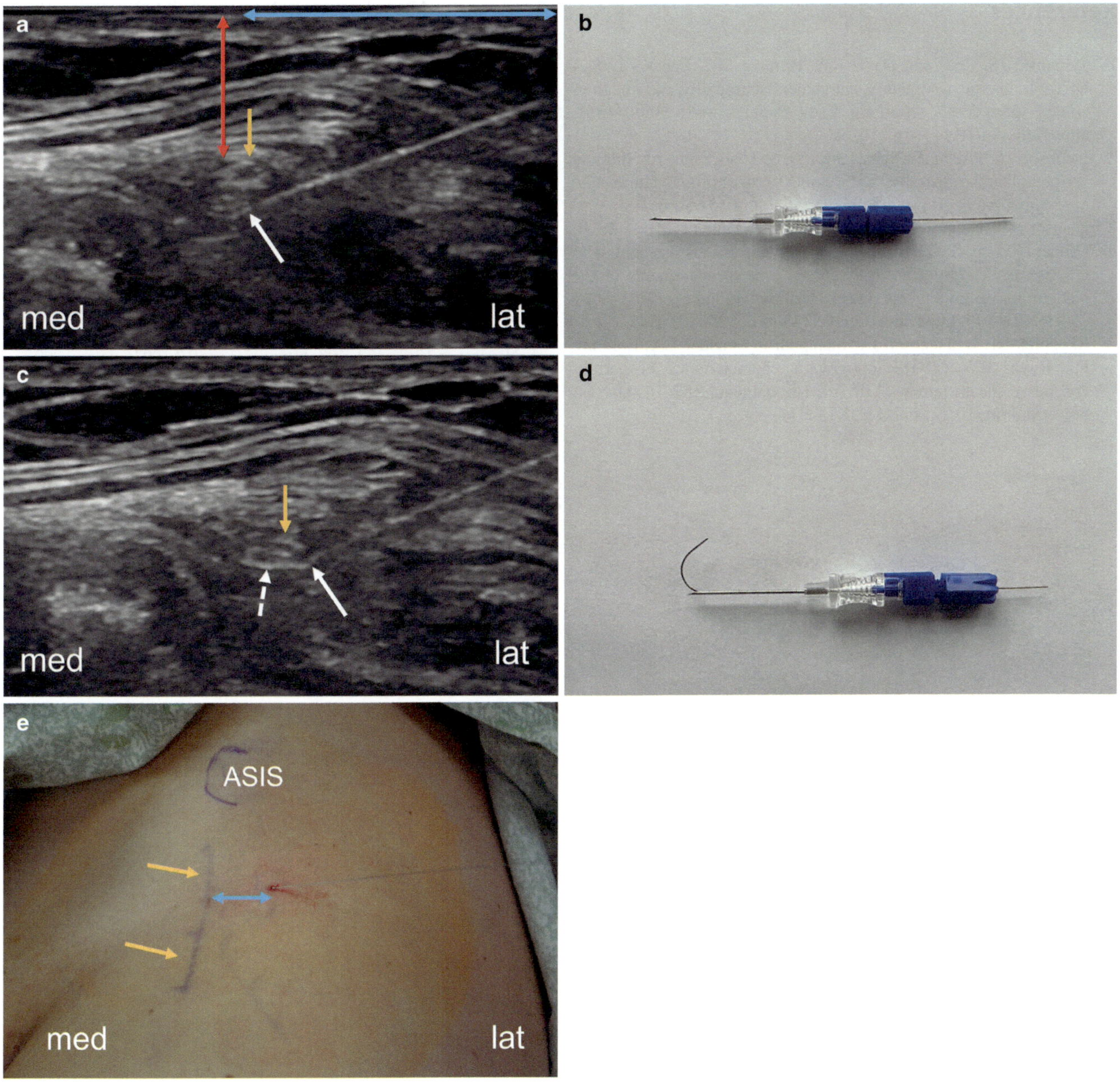

Fig. 5.11 Ultrasound-guided lateral femoral cutaneous nerve (LFCN) wire localization. (**a**) LFCN (*gold arrow*) is visualized in short axis, and wire localization needle (*white arrow*) tip is advanced just deep to the LFCN. Depth of the nerve from the skin surface (*red double arrow heads*) is measured. *Blue double arrow heads* show the measured horizontal distance from the wire skin entry site to the point on the skin directly overlying the target nerve. (**b**) Homer needle-wire system (Argon Medical, Plano TX) with undeployed wire. (**c**) Wire is advanced through needle with the curved tip (*dashed arrows*) just deep to the LFCN (*gold arrow*). (**d**) Wire advanced through the needle showing the J-curve tip. (**e**) Photograph with localization wire in place after the introducer needle removal. The course of the LFCN (*golden arrows*) and the anterior superior iliac spine (*ASIS*) are marked on the skin. As shown in (**a**), the *blue double arrow heads* are the measured horizontal distance from the wire skin entry site to the point on the skin directly over the target nerve. *Med* medial, *lat* lateral

References

1. Symanski JS, Ross AB, Davis KW, Brunner MC, Lee KS (2022) US for traumatic nerve injury, entrapment neuropathy, and imaging-guided perineural injection. Radiographics 42(5):1546–1561. https://doi.org/10.1148/rg.210152
2. Jacobson JA, Wilson TJ, Yang LJ-S (2016) Sonography of common peripheral nerve disorders with clinical correlation. J Ultrasound Med 35:683–693. https://doi.org/10.7863/ultra.15.05061
3. Klauser AS, Halpern EJ, De Zordo T, Feuchtner GM, Arora R, Gruber J et al (2009) Carpal tunnel syndrome assessment with US: value of additional crosssectional area measurements of the median nerve in patients versus healthy volunteers. Radiology 250(1):171–177. https://doi.org/10.1148/radiol.2501080397
4. Reynolds DL Jr, Jacobson JA, Inampudi P, Jamadar DA, Ebrahim FS, Hayes CW (2004) Sonographic characteristics of peripheral nerve sheath tumors. AJR Am J Roentgenol 182(3):741–744. https://doi.org/10.2214/ajr.182.3.1820741
5. Choquet O, Morau D, Biboulet P, Capdevila X (2012) Where should the tip of the needle be located in ultrasound-guided peripheral nerve blocks? Curr Opin Anaesthesiol 25(5):596–602. https://doi.org/10.1097/ACO.0b013e328356bb40
6. Watkins TW, Dupre S, Coucher JR (2015) Ropivacaine and dexamethasone: a potentially dangerous combination for therapeutic pain injections. J Med Imaging Radiat Oncol 59(5):571–577. https://doi.org/10.1111/1754-9485.12333
7. Lam KHS, Hung CY, Chiang YP, Onishi K, Su DCJ, Clark TB et al (2020) Ultrasound-guided nerve hydrodissection for pain management: rationale, methods, current literature and theoretical mechanisms. J Pain Res 13:1957–1968. https://doi.org/10.2147/JPR.S247208
8. Hanna AS, Ehlers ME, Lee KS (2017) Preoperative ultrasound-guided wire localization of the lateral femoral cutaneous nerve. Oper Neurosurg 13(3):402–408. https://doi.org/10.1093/ons/opw009

Magnetic Resonance Neurography: MR Imaging of Nerves

6

Sandip Biswal

Magnetic Resonance Neurography (MRN): Definition and Background

In the past 20 years, there has been a concerted effort to provide high-quality, high-resolution imaging of the brachial/lumbar plexuses and the nerves. Referred to as magnetic resonance neurography (MRN), the technical improvements in MRI during this same period, which include increased field strength, better coils, faster gradients, diffusion-weighted imaging, 3D imaging, etc., have made the visualization of nerves clearer and more detailed than ever, allowing for the noninvasive, more comprehensive evaluation of nerves [1–3]. This enhanced assessment afforded by MRN (especially when compared to more conventional MR techniques) includes not only its ability to identify, localize, visualize, and determine the integrity and intrinsic quality of individual "named" nerves but is also utilized to characterize sites of constriction/entrapment, determine the size of individual fascicles within a nerve, the condition of epineurium in large- to medium-sized nerves, and, perhaps most importantly, the degree of edema/swelling in the nerve and/or individual fascicles. It also allows for the visualization of the nerves and surrounding structures in great detail, including the nerve fibers and surrounding tissue, and, perhaps most importantly, facilitates the discrimination between nerve and vessel, which are usually immediately adjacent to each other and often indistinguishable on more conventional MR sequences such as T1-weighted or fat-saturated T2-weighted fast spin echo. By utilizing a combination of pulse sequences, MRN has become an important opportunity to observe nerves with greater clarity and accuracy with regards to its signal intensity and morphology and has facilitated changes in diagnosis and management.

S. Biswal (✉)
Department of Radiology, University of Wisconsin-Madison, Madison, WI, USA
e-mail: biswal3@wisc.edu

Patient Selection and Preparation

The technique is used in patients with different pain syndromes, such as peripheral neuropathies, radiculopathies, and plexopathies, and it can be used to help diagnose conditions such as nerve entrapment, nerve compression, and nerve injury. Referring physicians have been increasingly sending patients for evaluation of possible entrapment of specific nerves in the extremities, trunk, and pelvis (as described in the following sections). Some common requests include brachial plexus and cervical nerves in patients with neck and shoulder pain, imaging of the lumbosacral plexus and lumbar nerves in patients with low back pain, and imaging of nerves in the upper and lower extremities in patients with neuropathic pain. MRN can also be used to help plan and monitor treatment for these conditions. One of the main advantages of MRN is that it is noninvasive and does not use ionizing radiation. This makes it safe and effective for patients, particularly those who may not be able to undergo other imaging modalities.

Is MRN Impactful?

MRN has the potential to be an important tool for improving clinical outcomes in patients with pain. By identifying areas of nerve impingement or other pathologies, MRN can help guide the selection of appropriate treatment options. For example, if a herniated disc is found to be compressing a nerve, the patient may be a candidate for surgical intervention, such as a discectomy. Alternatively, if nerve thickening is detected, this may suggest that the patient has a chronic inflammatory condition, and treatment with anti-inflammatory medications may be warranted. MRN can also be useful for monitoring the effectiveness of treatment. Follow-up MRN studies can be performed to assess whether the nerve impingement or inflammation has improved and to determine whether further intervention is necessary. In addition to its diagnostic and monitoring capabilities, MRN can

A. S. Hanna (ed.), *Nerves: Anatomy, Exposures, and Techniques*, https://doi.org/10.1007/978-3-031-73931-6_6

also have a positive impact on patient outcomes by providing reassurance and reducing anxiety. Patients with chronic pain often experience significant psychological distress, and having a clear diagnosis and treatment plan can help reduce the anxiety and improve the overall quality of life.

That said, has MRN made a difference? Whether MRN has had a positive effect on patient outcomes remains to be formally determined. MRN has influenced changes in patient diagnosis and their management in cases of complex limb pain, for example. In a preliminary case series of 58 patients with previously difficult-to-diagnose limb pain, MRN and electrodiagnostic studies were used to identify injured nerves [4]. Abnormal findings from these diagnostics were compared to the patient's reported outcome after ultrasound-guided nerve block. The most identified abnormality on MRN was nerve signal alteration on fluid-sensitive sequences, followed by caliber change and impingement. Comparing the outcome of diagnostic nerve blocks with abnormal nerve findings on MRN or electrodiagnostics, the investigators found that MRN had a sensitivity of 67% and specificity of 100%, while for electrodiagnostic studies, they were 45% and 0%, respectively. Reviewing the imaging findings before a multidisciplinary group of specialists in pain medicine/anesthesia, neurology, plastic surgery, neurosurgery and radiology, a more specific diagnosis was produced in 78% of evaluated cases opening additional treatment pathways such as nerve-targeted surgery, which was performed in 36% cases. While outcomes were not monitored following these cases, this descriptive case series demonstrates the use of the moderately sensitive but highly specific MRN imaging modality that helped facilitate a change in the diagnosis for most patients with complex limb pain.

MRN has also been shown to affect patient-reported pain outcomes in 202 patients with chronic lumbosacral radiculopathy, pelvic pain, and groin pain. In a study by Dessouky et al., MRN findings were found instrumental to change the diagnosis in 92% of the subjects and change the management in 71% of the patients [5]. Changes in management included changes from narcotic to non-narcotic medications (or vice versa), medication dosage, type of treatment, or the introduction of a new treatment.

Technical Considerations

As a team, the referring clinician, protocoling radiologist, performing technologist, patient, and interpreting radiologist should all participate in a good MRN examination that adheres to the principles outlined in this section [6, 7].

To take advantage of the superior signal-to-noise ratio (SNR), imaging is best done on a 3T scanner since it allows for shorter imaging times, higher SNR, and better contrast. When compared to 1.5 T and 3 T scanners, keep slice thickness to a minimum, allowing for excellent through-plane resolution for 2D sequences and thinner isotropic resolution for 3D imaging. That said, 1.5 T scanners can be used when 3 T scanners are not available, although 1.5 T scanners have some limitations in terms of 3D imaging capability and longer examination periods. Additionally, all imaging planes can be employed, but the author typically prefers imaging orthogonal to the long axis of the nerve, e.g., axial/transverse imaging planes are applied when imaging the arms and legs. Regardless of the differences of using 1.5 T or 3.0 T magnets, optimal imaging parameters and sequences have been described for both scanners [8, 9]. Additionally, there continues to be an evolution of a variety of 3D imaging protocols for both magnetic field strengths.

The typical MR sequences employed by this author are T1-weighted fast spin echo (FSE), T2-weighted FSE with fat saturation, short tau inversion recovery (STIR) (optional, especially if the structure of interest is located off isocenter), and three-dimensional (3D) diffusion-weighted dual-echo steady state (DESS) that are all included in the protocol [7, 10]. The addition of 3D sequences with isotropic voxel sets enables multiplanar reformation, while the addition of hybrid DWI provides nerve-selective imaging and minimizes contribution from vascular structures. Of note, the administration of an intravenous gadolinium-based contrast agent is *rarely* required except in cases with suspected enhanced soft tissue mass lesions.

To obtain high-resolution imaging in the longitudinal and transverse planes, the field of view (FOV) should be chosen based on the physician's request and should be kept as small as feasible. Clinicians should therefore be as specific as they can while describing the lesion's location. However, pinpointing the exact location of a suspected lesion is typically the primary reason for the imaging, and, therefore, it is likely that multiple bed and coil positions will be needed to cover the length of the nerve in question. For example, if medial foot pain is the symptom, then imaging of the medial plantar nerve, tibial nerve, and distal sciatic nerve is needed. For the best evaluation of tiny nerves, the area around the extremity should not be more than about 20% of its diameter. But this approach might produce wraparound effects, particularly in off-center imaging. To prevent such artifacts, phase oversampling or fold-over suppression techniques may be applied.

Prior to the imaging session, patients are typically asked to refrain from eating or drinking 2–4 h before the exam. They may also be asked to wear loose-fitting clothing to avoid constriction of the nerves being imaged. Other technical considerations include the fact that patients with a tremor or an inability to hold still for several minutes at a time will likely produce lower quality images due to motion artifacts. Similarly, imaging near the heart or in the thorax, both of which contribute motion through pulsation and respiratory activity, respectively, is a significant challenge when attempting to image nerves in the anterior chest wall, lateral thorax, or upper abdomen. MR technicians should place a skin marker at the site of most pain, and the patient should be instructed to maintain stillness and normal breathing during image acquisition. To prevent movement during the examination, the extremities should be well-padded and snugly wrapped within the coil(s). To prevent a distended bladder from interfering with the images, the urine bladder should be emptied, particularly for pelvic or lumbosacral (LS) plexus imaging. As mentioned above, administration with gadolinium contrast material is not usually needed unless a tumor is in close proximity to a nerve of interest or if there is concern of perineural spread of a malignancy.

Normal Nerve MRI Characteristics (Fig. 6.1)

It is imperative to have a thorough and familiar understanding of the typical appearance of nerves, including their size, course, and signal intensity, while assessing MR images for peripheral neuropathies. To become familiar with the normal appearance of nerves on MRI, one has to repeatedly evaluate the nerves on every study, especially in patients where nerve

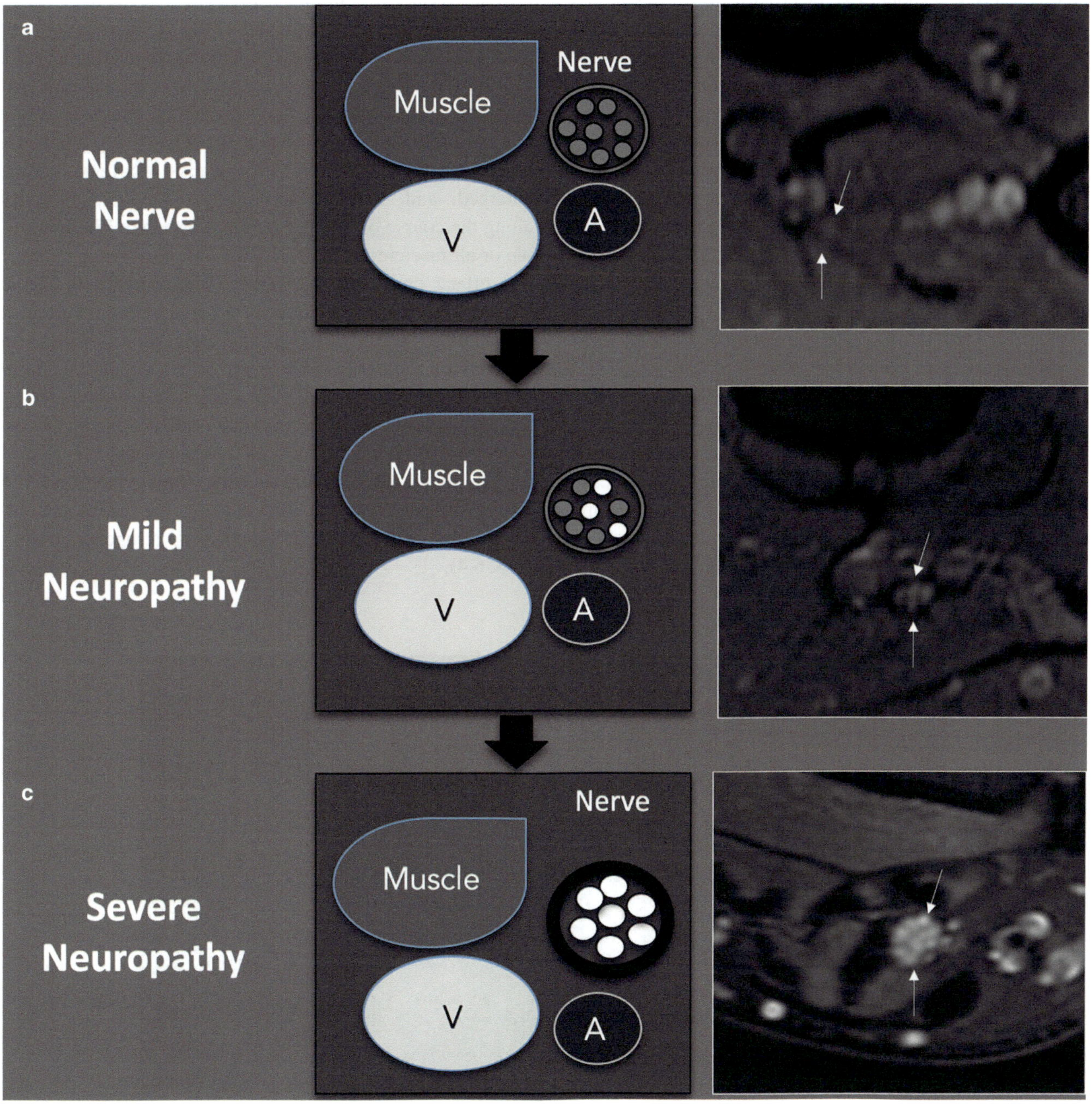

Fig. 6.1 Schematic representation of peripheral neuropathy or nerve inflammation on MR neurography (*arrows*). (**a**) In normal, medium- to small-sized nerves, the fascicular anatomy may or may not be defined in transverse (axial) MR imaging (orthogonal to the long axis of the nerve). Signal intensity of the normal nerve is isointense to the adjacent muscle on fluid-sensitive sequences and can admittedly be difficult at times to distinguish muscle from the nerve, as in this case of the tibial nerve. (**b**) In mild neuropathy, individual fascicles will be distinct, slightly enlarged, and some or all individual fascicles will be slightly elevated in signal intensity in fluid-sensitive sequences when compared to the signal intensity in adjacent muscle. (**c**) In severe neuropathy, all individual fascicles are enlarged, significantly elevated in signal intensity compared to muscle on fluid-sensitive sequences, and the entire nerve is enlarged in cross-sectional area. Severely inflamed or neuropathic nerves may or may not demonstrate the increased thickening of the epineurium (the outermost casing of the nerve), which will be low in signal intensity on multiple sequences

injury or nerve pain is not suspected. Normal nerves exhibit a fascicular appearance and may seem isointense to slightly more intense on fat-suppressed T2-weighted imaging or STIR imaging than the surrounding muscle tissue. On T1-weighted imaging, nerves are also described as being isointense to the surrounding skeletal muscle. Individual fascicles within normal nerves are relatively equal in size and homogeneous in signal intensity to each other. The entire nerve's cross-sectional area appears to be similar to that of nearby arteries. It should also be possible to see the perineural fat planes surrounding the nerve along the length of its course, especially on T1-weighted, non-fat-suppressed sequences. The course of the typical normal nerve and its branches is relatively smooth and free from abrupt changes in direction, compared to veins, which can suddenly change direction or arborize quite frequently. If intravenous contrast happens to be utilized, normal nerves are devoid of enhancement.

Abnormal MRI Features

A broad variety of pathologic conditions can give rise to abnormal MRI appearance of nerves. Direct traumatic or postsurgical injury is among the most common causes. Other possible etiologies of nerve injury or inflammation include inflammation/infection, ischemia, demyelinating diseases, and toxic exposures (e.g., radiation and chemotherapy). Physical constriction, entrapment, or impingement of the nerve can occur when a nerve passes through areas of inflammation or anatomic variants that narrow the otherwise normal aperture of a passing nerve. Alternatively, if the nerve is itself inflamed and swollen, the nerve will have to tightly course through structures that were otherwise normal in dimensions but are now too small to accommodate an engorged nerve.

Abnormal MR findings of nerves include increased signal intensity on fluid-sensitive sequences to the point that the nerve is noticeably brighter than the closely adjacent muscle tissue on fluid-sensitive MR sequences (e.g., T2-weighted Fast Spin Echo and STIR) and increased diameter (swelling) of fascicles within the nerve itself (Fig. 6.1). In mildly neuropathic cases, the finding of increased signal intensity of the individual fascicles can be relatively subtle but an important distinction to make (Figs. 6.2 and 6.3). Of note, individual, several, or all fascicles of a nerve can be enlarged, and therefore scrutiny of individual fascicles along the course of interrogation is warranted. When multiple or all fascicles are affected, the entire nerve can enlarge and efface perineural fat planes. The increase in signal intensity is thought to be attributed to the accumulation of endoneurial fluid and/or vascular congestion. Changes in the course or integrity of the nerve can especially be appreciated with a combination of imaging transverse and longitudinal to the nerve, with particular attention given to the nerve's caliber and continuity as it passes through an area of injury, inflammation, and/or scarring. Angulation or discontinuity of the nerve can be ascertained as they are more commonly associated with traumatic or iatrogenic lesions (Fig. 6.4).

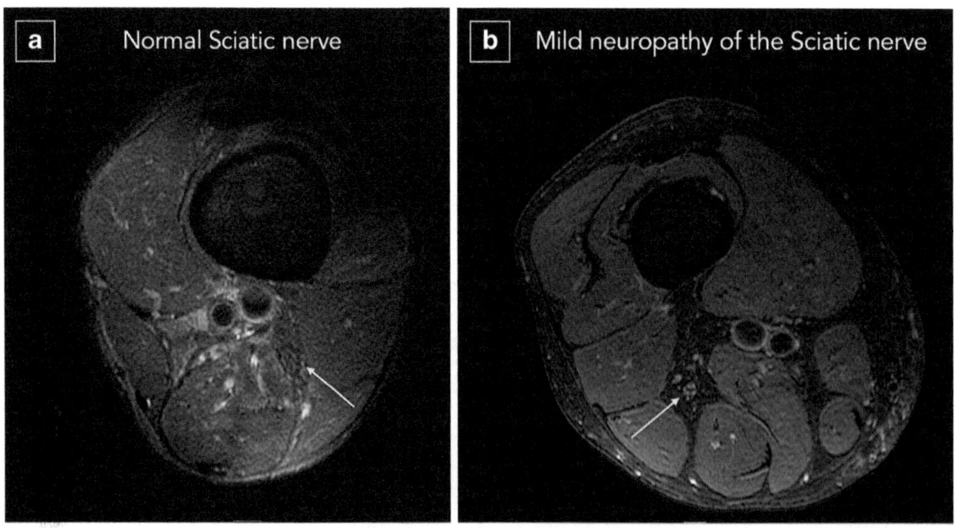

Fig. 6.2 Imaging findings in the evaluation of nerves can be subtle. (**a**) Normal appearing sciatic nerve. Transverse T2-weighted, fat-suppressed axial image through the distal sciatic nerve (*arrow*) demonstrates fascicular architecture of the nerve in which the individual fascicles demonstrate signal intensity that is isointense to the signal intensity of the surrounding musculature. The cross-sectional size of the individual fascicles and the entire nerve itself is within normal limits. (**b**) By comparison, the individual fascicles of the distal sciatic nerve (*arrow*) in another patient demonstrate increased signal intensity compared to the adjacent muscle, consistent with mild neuropathy

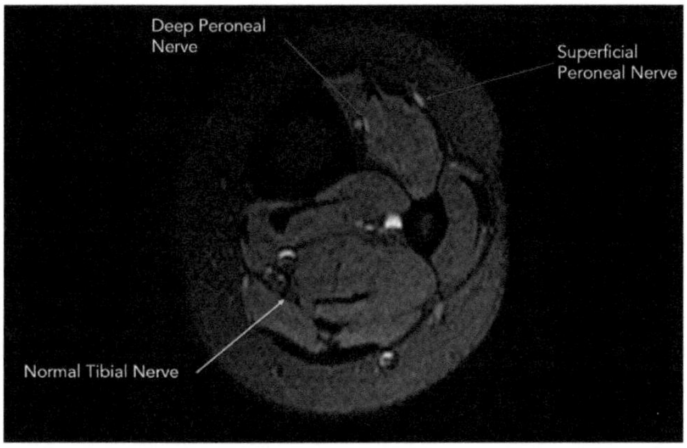

Fig. 6.3 Axial T2W fat-saturated image through the distal lower extremity shows increased signal and subtle increase in girth of the deep and superficial peroneal nerves (*red arrows*) when compared to the adjacent muscle signal intensity. Findings are consistent with neuropathy. The tibial nerve is almost indistinguishable (*green arrow*) as its signal intensity is similar to that of the adjacent muscle

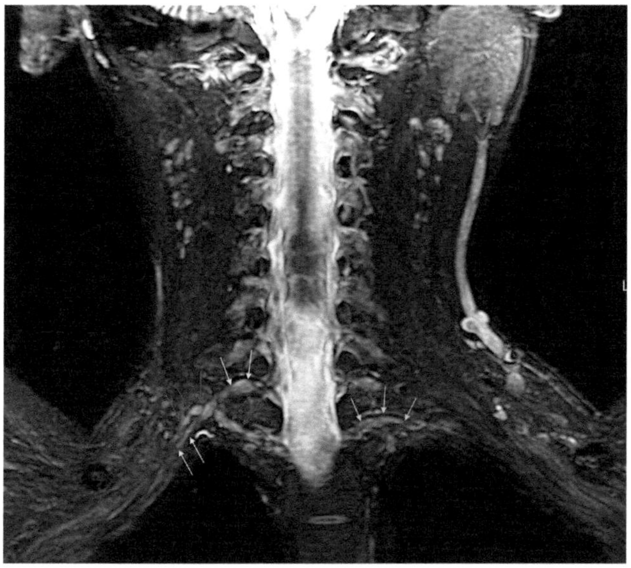

Fig. 6.4 Young adult female suffered from complex regional pain syndrome of the right upper extremity following right first rib resection for thoracic outlet syndrome. Initial workup, including conventional spinal MRI revealed no plausible explanation. MRN was ordered, and a thin slab maximum intensity projection of a 3D neurographic sequence demonstrated tethering of the *right* T1 nerve (*red arrows*) on the cut end of the resected first rib. The expected course of the T1 nerve is depicted on the *left* (*green arrows*) where it "drapes" over the apex of the left lung. *Yellow arrows* point to the right C8 nerve for reference

Familiarity with the normal anatomic course of the nerves in different planes as well as their typical spatial relationship to adjacent structures, such as muscles, tendons, ligaments, and bones, is also required. Deviation from its expected anatomic location may give rise to entrapment of the nerve. However, there are a few, relatively more common nerve–muscle anomalies that have unclear associations with pain syndromes. For example, the relationship between the anterior and middle scalene muscles with the brachial plexus is variable, and these variants are relatively prevalent. While the clinical impact of these variants remains unclear, recognition of the variants with MRN, for example, may play an important role in the stratification of patients with predominantly neurogenic thoracic outlet syndrome (nTOS), allowing for stakeholders to explore the importance of the variant anatomy with regards to specifically targeted, image-guided injections with anesthetics, botulinum toxin, or corticosteroids. Indeed, studies have shown some benefit of such injections [11], but perhaps the knowledge of the precise location of these injections with regard to variant anatomy will potentially prove a boon to outcome measures.

Traumatic, iatrogenic, entrapment, extrinsic compression, and intrinsic lesions of the nerve can also give rise to secondary signs of nerve injury or inflammation, namely, denervation edema or fatty atrophy of muscles in a distribution characteristic to the affected nerve. Signal abnormality of an affected muscle can manifest as soon as 24 h from the time of nerve injury, but it will take weeks to years after the denervating insult to demonstrate fatty replacement and volume loss/atrophy of the muscle.

Anatomic Variants of the Plexuses

In the past couple of decades, a substantial number of muscle variants and their relationship with the nerves have been increasingly realized, which is in part due to improvements in MR and ultrasound imaging technologies. The anatomic details of these variants, of which there are numerous, are beyond the scope of this article. There are a few that are occasionally encountered in an active MR neurography practice, so they are briefly summarized here to sensitize the reader of their existence and location. Of note, it remains unclear whether these variants have important clinical implications since these variants have been largely undetected and, in many cases, have not been specifically targeted therapeutically. It is the opinion of this author that many of the variants are likely clinically silent until the patient sustains an injury or inflammatory, be it traumatic, drug-induced, auto-immune insult, etc., i.e., it usually takes an additional insult for patients predisposed by such variants to manifest with nerve-related pain syndromes.

Brachial Plexus

The brachial plexus (BP) is a network of nerves that originates from the spinal nerves in the neck and upper back and provides motor and sensory innervation to the upper limb.

The brachial plexus begins in the neck region, where it is formed by the union of the anterior rami of the lower four cervical spinal nerves (C5–C8) and the first thoracic spinal nerve (T1). The roots of the plexus run between the anterior and middle scalene muscles in the neck. Nerve entrapment in the neck can occur due to conditions such as thoracic outlet syndrome (TOS), which is a group of disorders characterized by compression or irritation of nerves, arteries, and/or veins as they pass through the thoracic outlet, which is a narrow space between the clavicle, subclavius muscle, and first rib. The syndrome can cause a range of symptoms, including pain on the side of the neck and upper limb, numbness, tingling, weakness, atrophy, and/or swelling of the hand and/or arm.

With regard to TOS, there are traditionally three main types, namely, nTOS, arterial thoracic outlet syndrome (aTOS), and venous thoracic outlet syndrome (vTOS), each with its own set of causes, symptoms, and treatment options [12]. This separation is too artificial since the artery and plexus go hand-in-hand in the same tight space. This passage will focus on predominantly nTOS, which is considered the most common form of TOS [13], albeit the most challenging to diagnose. Given the overlap of clinical presentations of nTOS with other diseases and the inherent challenge in specifically diagnosing nTOS, patients are subject to a wide variety of interventions, such as cervical fusion, carpel tunnel release, cubital tunnel release, surgical treatment of the rotator cuff, or just prolonged physical therapy. Conventional MRI should theoretically reveal some kind of inflammation of the nerve or nearby soft tissue if the BP is impinged upon and plexopathy develops; however, this has not always been the case. MRN potentially offers additional sensitivity and specificity in this regard. The most common cause of nTOS is pressure on the BP from the scalene muscles in the neck, although it can also be caused by other structures, such as cervical ribs or a tight pectoralis minor muscle [12].

Once leaving the neck, the brachial plexus eventually divides into three cords—the lateral, medial, and posterior cords—in the infraclavicular region. Here, the nerves can be compressed or entrapped by various structures, including the coracoid process, the pectoralis minor muscle, and the subscapularis muscle. The cords give rise to various nerve branches that innervate the muscles of the upper limb. Nerve entrapment can occur at various sites in the arm, including the axilla (armpit), where the nerves can be compressed by structures such as the axillary vein, pectoralis minor, arterial branches, or aberrant muscles.

While the bulk of BP imaging has been in the setting of tumors in the BP itself or in the evaluation of metastatic disease and tumor spread/invasion/mass effect on the BP, MRN has been increasingly used to monitor more subtle pathologies such as the entrapment of individual components of the plexus, and MRN can be used to interrogate the common sites of nerve entrapment, including the thoracic outlet, the clavicle, the first rib, the subclavius muscle, the coracoid process, the pectoralis minor muscle, and the axilla.

MRN in conjunction with vascular imaging can be helpful in delineating which type of TOS is present and also identifying if there are any anatomic aberrations that may give rise to plexopathy. Imaging can also be performed with the arms to the side and the arms above the head, to look for dynamic compression. Among the nTOS category, a high-quality MRN can be helpful in the delineation of different subtypes; it can help delineate the relationship between a cervical rib and trunks of the BP, for example. Furthermore, MRN can potentially identify anatomic variations of the relationship between the BP and the scalene muscles, which are thought to give rise to compression of certain individual nerves in some patients. If an anatomic aberration is felt to be the cause of the symptoms, surgery may be necessary to restore a more normal course of the affected nerve or to relieve the compression or blockage and restore the normal function to the affected limb. MRN can therefore potentially aid in the design of minimally guided interventions, such as ultrasound-guided injection of anesthetic [14] or even Botox [15], or in surgical planning.

In the past several years, there has been increasing importance placed on congenital variants that alter the typical relationships between the scalene muscles, cervical ribs, and roots of the brachial plexus, and, in fact, most cases of nTOS are thought to arise from these numerous anatomical variances [16]. The existence of a cervical rib, for example, which is considered an important cause of aTOS, occurs in 1–2% of the general population and is also thought to be etiologically important in nTOS. Although the majority of people with cervical ribs are *asymptomatic*, 20% of individuals with nTOS have been found to possess a cervical rib and are at increased risk of developing the condition [16].

More recently, congenital abnormalities of the scalene muscles are being recognized as important factors in the pathogenesis of nTOS. In an excellent review by Koh [17], a number of piercing and pass-over variants of the BP upper trunk and scalene muscles have been described in which the roots of the brachial plexus pass *through* or *anterior* to the anterior scalene muscle (Fig. 6.5).

The common perception that the postganglionic C5–T1 nerve roots pass between the anterior and middle scalene muscles is actually flawed since variants of this relationship occur in up to 62.1% and have been described previously[18–20]. More specifically, aberrations in the course of the C5 and/or C6 nerve roots are common (between 25% and 60%), whereby one or both nerve roots pass through (pierce through) or pass anterior to the anterior scalene. Of note, the piercing variant tend to be more common than the variant where C5 passes anterior to the anterior scalene (~1%), as

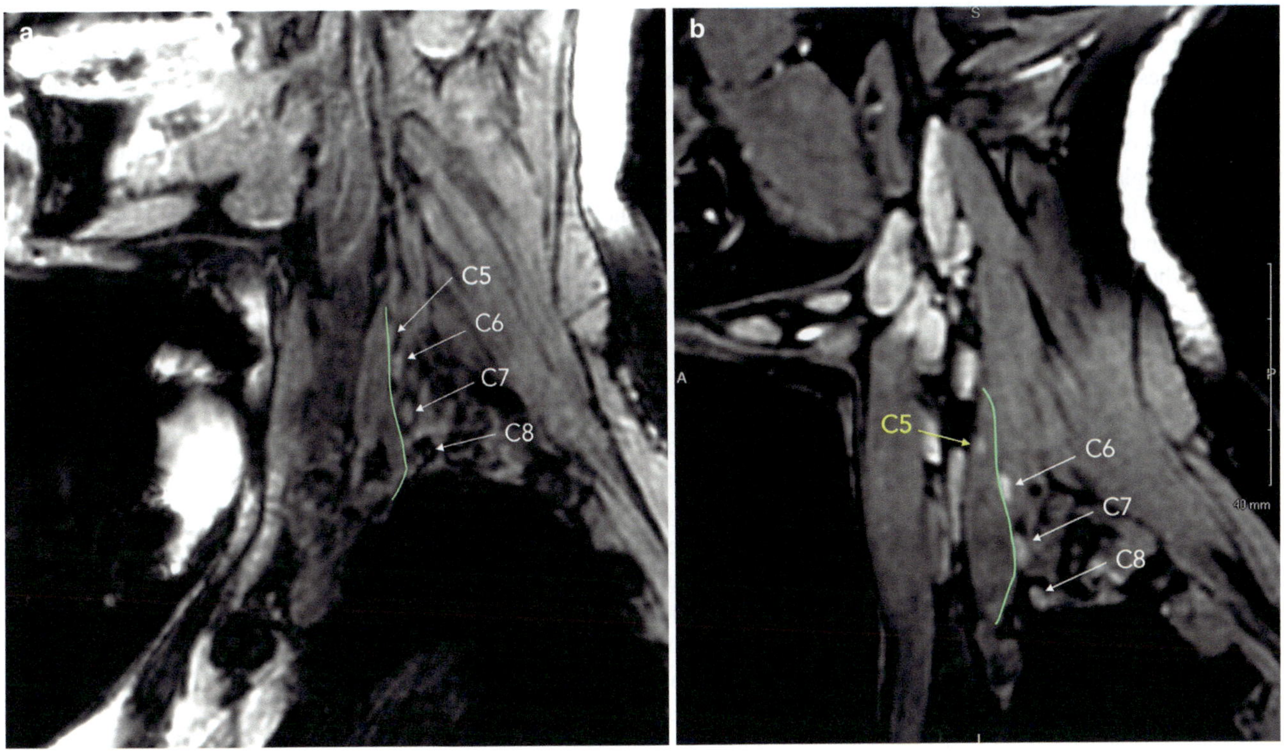

Fig. 6.5 Sagittal 3D neurographic sequence multi-echo in steady-state acquisition (MENSA) of the proximal brachial plexus; *thin green line* depicts the posterior margin of the anterior scalene. (**a**) Typical anatomy: the C5, C6, C7, and C8 nerve roots lie in their typical location within the scalene triangle (posterior to the anterior scalene and anterior to the middle scalene). (**b**) Variant anatomy: the C5 nerve root is located just anterior to or within the anterior fibers of the anterior scalene, while the C6, C7, and C8 nerve roots lie in their typical location within the scalene triangle

determined in a cadaveric study [21]. Whether these piercing or "pass-over" variants in nTOS have clinical significance remains a topic of discussion. Ultrasound-guided injections can be utilized to determine if the anatomical variant plays a contributory role in the patient's symptoms, since some of these are simply incidental findings [14].

Prefixed and postfixed plexus is yet another anatomic variant that could potentially contribute to a patient's symptoms and is amenable to interrogation with MRN. Nearly one-fifth of all BP in a cadaveric study are prefixed in which the contribution to the superior root of the BP is from C4 rather than C5, and, as a result, the plexus is positioned more cephalad than the typical position [22]. Post-fixed BP, where the most inferior root of the BP is from T2 instead of T1, occurs in less than one-tenth of cadavers and places the plexus in a more caudad position than normal. The alteration in position of the BP may create unusual stress on the nerves and result in atypical motor and/or sensory innervation patterns of the upper limb [23].

The variants listed above can potentially be seen with MRN. However, there exists anatomic variations in which MRN in its current technologic constraints will have a challenging time delineating since the variant anatomy is very small and packed into tight compartments, making the discrimination of individual cords, divisions, and their preterminal branches difficult. For example, the absence of inferior trunk (9% of all BPs) or upper trunk (1% of all BPs) will be challenging to identify with MRN [24]. Variants of the divisions are present in nearly a third of the BPs, and multiple deviations in the origin of the musculocutaneous nerve will likely be beyond the ability of MRN at this time.

One of the diseases that can affect the brachial plexus, neuralgic amyotrophy (NA), also known as Parsonage–Turner syndrome, has been getting a new look thanks—in part—to MRN. Previously, the diagnosis of NA was largely made empirically in conjunction with an electrodiagnostic test, and the only treatment available was to provide symptomatic support. Clinical management of NA is now evolving as MRN has now revealed focal abnormalities in the nerves of patients with confirmed NA. MRN has shown abnormalities in the brachial plexus itself, toward the distal end of the brachial plexus (at the terminal branches) and/or in the more distal nerves beyond the brachial plexus [25, 26]. MRN abnormalities include increases in T2-hyperintensity, enlargement of the nerve, and/or hourglass-like constrictions of the nerve. Such abnormalities can be found on a single nerve or multiple nerves within the same patient. Of note, it appears that most abnormal findings are just beyond the plexus itself, so scanning nerves beyond the brachial plexus using MRN techniques should be considered especially if the brachial plexus is "normal." An important consideration is that ultrasound is also successfully being utilized to find abnormalities in cases of NA, which can detect pathologies such as focal or diffuse nerve/fascicle enlargement, incomplete nerve constriction, complete nerve constriction with torsion (hourglass-like appearance), and fascicular entwinement [27, 28]. Because of these diagnostic improvements, specialists in the treatment of NA are now offering surgical options, which are sometimes proving to be efficacious [29].

Dorsal Scapular Nerve

Patients with dorsal scapular (or dorsoscapular) nerve entrapment will present with pain between the scapula, just off midline that may be of a stabbing, sharp, burning quality. They can also present with arm/shoulder pain, arm/shoulder weakness, and/or winged scapula [30]. The dorsal scapular nerve emerges from the posterior aspect of the C5 nerve and runs inferiorly and laterally, piercing through the middle scalene and then coursing through the posterior triangle of the neck, which is bounded by the trapezius, sternocleidomastoid, and clavicle. In the neck, the nerve can be compressed or entrapped by various structures, including the cervical vertebrae and the surrounding muscles. After leaving the neck, the dorsal scapular nerve descends down the posterior aspect of the thorax. It provides innervation to the levator scapulae and rhomboid muscles, which are located between the scapula and the spine. In the upper back, the nerve can be compressed or entrapped by the rhomboid muscles, but the most common site of entrapment is thought to be a hypertrophied or fibrotic middle scalene [30, 31]. MRN may be able to show caliber and signal intensity change of the nerve in the area of entrapment. It will be important to image the contralateral asymptomatic nerve for comparison.

Suprascapular Nerve

As a mixed sensory and motor nerve, the suprascapular nerve can give rise to symptoms of posterolateral shoulder weakness and circumscapular/periscapular pain when injured or entrapped [21]. In general, individuals who perform repetitive overhead maneuvers are among those who sustain an injury to this nerve. Arising primarily from the fifth and sixth cervical nerve roots (with variable contribution from the 4th), the suprascapular nerve arises from the upper trunk of the brachial plexus to course through the posterior cervical triangle and eventually under the trapezius muscle and coracoclavicular ligament. The final segment of the nerve is exposed to two other points of impingement along its path, the suprascapular notch and the spinoglenoid notch, with the suprascapular notch being the more clinically significant as patients tend to complain of pain symptoms more consistently, especially since the sensory nerves generally exit proximal to the spinoglenoid notch [32]. With respect to the suprascapular notch, the variable morphologic appearance of the notch lends itself (with or without spasm or hypertrophy of the supraspinatus muscle) as a site of impingement of the nerve as the suprascapular nerve has been found to be mobile within the suprascapular notch, dynamically coming into contact with the suprascapular ligament and the bony inferior border of the notch during provocative maneuvers [33]. An additional site of suprascapular nerve entrapment is within the spinoglenoid notch, located downstream (posterior and inferior at the superior surface of the glenoid neck) to the suprascapular notch. Labral tears that give rise to paralabral cysts that extend from a superior labral tear to reside within the spinoglenoid notch can result in the compression of the suprascapular nerve [34–36]. More recently, scalene-piercing variants of the BP (as mentioned in the previous section) can also potentially give rise to dorsal scapular and long thoracic nerve problems as the altered relationships between the anterior scalene and the BP can place mechanical stress on these nerves [21].

Femoral Nerve

The femoral nerve (FN) originates in the lumbar plexus from the L2, L3, and L4 nerve roots, which combine to form the nerve at the L4–L5 disc level. In majority of cases, the nerve runs anterior to the iliacus and posterolateral to the psoas muscle and eventually passes deep to the inguinal ligament. It then divides into anterior and posterior divisions that provide the anterior thigh with the motor and sensory supply, in addition to the saphenous nerve.

There are several types of FN entrapment or impingement, which are rare. The more conventional or "classic" sites include the inguinal ligament or the femoral triangle in the proximal thigh [37]. Individuals who are obese or pregnant or have experienced a sudden increase in physical activity can experience the inguinal ligament form of entrapment. The femoral triangle is a triangular space in the upper thigh, bounded by the inguinal ligament superiorly, the sartorius muscle laterally, and the adductor longus muscle medially. In the femoral triangle, the FN can be entrapped by a tumor, an injury, or a narrowing of the femoral triangle due to scar tissue.

More recently, a number of psoas and iliacus muscle variants have been identified which have atypical relationships with the FN—many of which result in a spilt femoral or covered femoral nerve—and are prevalent in a fair proportion (5–30%) of cadaveric studies. While it is not known whether these aberrations contribute to or are solely responsible for femoral neuropathies, awareness of such anatomic variants is important for pain specialists as a possible explanation for one's lower extremity symptoms when all other possibilities have been exhausted. These FN/muscle variants are potentially amenable to image-guided injections to help further ascertain the role of these variants, if any at all. Furthermore, it is also important for surgeons who operate in this location to be aware of such variants since exposing and dissecting through the psoas muscle may lead to inadvertent transection of one of the branches of the split femoral nerve.

Vazquez et al., for example, found that approximately 8% of 242 specimens had a muscle slip from the iliacus or psoas major piercing the FN [37]. Among those specimens that had a muscle slip piercing the FN: a small subset had a psoas major muscular slip, another subset had an iliacus muscular slip piercing the FN, and there was the uncommon occurrence of a muscular slip covering the FN. Kirchmair et al. [38] and Anloague and Huijbregts [39] found that approximately 1/5–1/3 of the FNs were split into two or three parts by slips of the psoas muscles.

Psoas tertius muscle, which emerges from the first four transverse processes of the first four lumbar vertebrae as well as the inner part of the 12th rib before fusing with the iliopsoas tendon, has been involved in a rare case of "splitting" the femoral nerve [40]. In this specific case, the psoas tertius muscle punctured the FN before fusing with the iliopsoas tendon beyond this location. The FN was divided by this variant and then reunited with itself to continue its usual course prior to the inguinal ligament.

Iliac muscle variants have been found where a small iliacus muscle accessory slip "splits" the femoral nerve [41]. Accessory iliacus muscle, which originates from the iliac crest and inserts with the iliopsoas, has been found entrapping the L4 root of the FN. The accessory iliacus muscle may put pressure on the femoral nerve, causing pain to be transferred to the hip, knee, and the L4 dermatome.

A more rare iliacus muscle variant has been described, where a dominant segment of a branching FN penetrates deeply into the iliacus muscle before emerging distal to the iliopubic eminence and combining with the smaller branch that continued with the natural path anterior to the iliacus [42]. It is thought that this anatomic variant may predispose to FN compression against the iliopubic eminence as the nerve segment passes deep through the iliacus muscle with hip flexion and knee extension. Patients with this variant potentially experience anterior thigh weakness and anteromedial thigh sensory loss.

The clinical importance of these FN variations cannot be understated as the knowledge of these variations will certainly influence surgical techniques in this part of the body, lumbar plexus blocking, and other pelvic region procedures [38, 39]. Knowledge and visualization of such variant anatomy are likely to help improve the understanding of an individual's clinical presentation as it may explain FN compression and damage in certain split FN variants or help explain incomplete anesthetic blockade of the hip or thigh [43, 44]. It is hoped that MRN can identify these variants with relative consistency and thereby help improve the management of such individuals.

Lateral Femoral Cutaneous Nerve

The lateral femoral cutaneous nerve (LFCN) is a sensory nerve that originates from L2 and L3 at the lumbosacral plexus, courses through the retroperitoneum between the deep and superficial parts of the psoas muscle, and between the fascial layers of the iliacus muscle. The LFCN will then pass under the inguinal ligament, branch into anterior and posterior divisions, and supply the skin on the lateral aspect of the thigh, from the anterior superior iliac spine (ASIS) to the knee. The nerve can become compressed or inflamed as it passes through the inguinal ligament, resulting in a mononeuropathy known as *meralgia paresthetica* (MP), whereby patients have anterior and/or lateral thigh pain, burning, numbness, and diminished sensation that frequently interfere with everyday activities and sleep. MP can be caused by wearing tight clothing, belts, or injury. The incidence of MP increases in cases of diabetes, obesity, and advanced age [45, 46].

Following a confirmatory, positive anesthetic blockade test of the LFCN, treatment options for those individuals suffering from MP begin with nonoperative measures (including weight loss if needed), followed by anesthetic and steroid injection and then surgery (nerve decompression or transposition) [47–49]. While most patients respond to nonoperative measures or steroid treatment, the somewhat variable response to treatments could at least be partly explained by the rather variable relationship between the LFCN and the inguinal ligament, i.e., as the LFCN courses into the anterior portion of the thigh, the LFCN can pass anterior to, through, or posterior to the inguinal ligament. Additionally, the nerve will split into anterior and posterior divisions at a distance quite variable from the anterior superior iliac spine (ASIS) [49].

Five different anatomic relationships between the LFCN and inguinal ligament were demonstrated in a study of 79 cadavers [50]. Type A (4% of the cases) is superior and lateral to the ASIS, and Type B (27%) is medial to the ASIS and located within the inguinal ligament just *medial* to the origin of the sartorius muscle. Type C (23%) is similar to Type B, with the LFCN medial to the ASIS and within the inguinal ligament, but at the origin to the sartorius muscle. In Type D (26%), the LFCN is beneath the inguinal ligament and medial to the ASIS, and Type E (20%) places the LFCN beneath and medial to the ASIS but in a branching pattern. Knowledge of this anatomic variation is likely to help better understand an individual's presentation and help with outcomes as therapies can be potentially tailored to the individual variations. Indeed, those with Type A are at risk of trauma from car seat belts, work tool-belts, and sports injuries [51], while those with Type B and C are the types typically requiring surgical decompression in order to release the LFCN from entrapment within the inguinal ligament [52]. MRN using 3T magnets has been successfully used to identify neuropathic changes in the LFCN for a number of years now [53, 54]. Whether the different types of LFCN can be identified with MRN remains to be determined but should be possible with smaller FOV, high-resolution axial neurographic imaging dedicated to the area around the ASIS.

Summary

MRN is a valuable tool for the assessment of nerve impingement in the upper and lower limbs. By providing a noninvasive means of visualizing nerves, MRN can help identify areas of nerve impingement or other pathologies, guide the selection of appropriate treatment options, and monitor the effectiveness of treatment. MRN can also provide reassurance and reduce anxiety in patients with chronic pain, thus helping improve their overall quality of life.

References

1. Howe FA, Filler AG, Bell BA, Griffiths JR (1992) Magnetic resonance neurography. Magn Reson Med 28:328–338. https://doi.org/10.1002/mrm.1910280215
2. Filler AG, Howe FA, Hayes CE, Kliot M, Winn HR, Bell BA et al (1993) Magnetic resonance neurography. Lancet Lond Engl 341:659–661. https://doi.org/10.1016/0140-6736(93)90422-d
3. Chhabra A, Madhuranthakam AJ, Andreisek G (2018) Magnetic resonance neurography: current perspectives and literature review. Eur Radiol 28:698–707. https://doi.org/10.1007/s00330-017-4976-8
4. Johnson EM, Yoon D, Biswal S, Curtin C, Fox P, Wilson TJ et al (2021) Characteristics of patients with complex limb pain evaluated through an interdisciplinary approach utilizing magnetic resonance neurography. Front Pain Res Lausanne 2:689402. https://doi.org/10.3389/fpain.2021.689402
5. Dessouky R, Xi Y, Scott KM, Khaleel M, Gill K, Jones S et al (2018) Magnetic resonance neurography in chronic lumbosacral and pelvic pain: diagnostic and management impact-institutional audit. World Neurosurg 114:e77–e113. https://doi.org/10.1016/j.wneu.2018.02.072
6. Lutz AM, Gold G, Beaulieu C (2014) MR imaging of the brachial plexus. Neuroimaging Clin N Am 24:91–108. https://doi.org/10.1016/j.nic.2013.03.024
7. Chhabra A, Flammang A, Padua A Jr, Carrino JA, Andreisek G (2014) Magnetic resonance neurography: technical considerations. Neuroimaging Clin N Am 24:67–78. https://doi.org/10.1016/j.nic.2013.03.032
8. Fisher S, Wadhwa V, Manthuruthil C, Cheng J, Chhabra A (2016) Clinical impact of magnetic resonance neurography in patients with brachial plexus neuropathies. Br J Radiol 89:20160503. https://doi.org/10.1259/bjr.20160503
9. Wang X, Harrison C, Mariappan YK, Gopalakrishnan K, Chhabra A, Lenkinski RE et al (2017) MR Neurography of brachial plexus at 3.0 T with robust fat and blood suppression. Radiology 283:538–546. https://doi.org/10.1148/radiol.2016152842
10. Khalilzadeh O, Fayad LM, Ahlawat S (2021) 3D MR Neurography. Semin Musculoskelet Radiol 25:409–417. https://doi.org/10.1055/s-0041-1730909
11. Fereydooni A, Ho VT, Olson EM, Dyrek P, Harris T, Kussman A et al (2023) Impact of scalene muscle botulinum toxin injection with and without surgery in neurogenic thoracic outlet syndrome. Clin J Sport Med Off J Can Acad Sport Med 33:116–122. https://doi.org/10.1097/JSM.0000000000001094
12. Jones MR, Prabhakar A, Viswanath O, Urits I, Green JB, Kendrick JB et al (2019) Thoracic outlet syndrome: a comprehensive review of pathophysiology, diagnosis, and treatment. Pain Ther 8:5–18. https://doi.org/10.1007/s40122-019-0124-2
13. Freischlag J, Orion K (2014) Understanding thoracic outlet syndrome. Scientifica 2014:248163. https://doi.org/10.1155/2014/248163
14. Lum YW, Brooke BS, Likes K, Modi M, Grunebach H, Christo PJ et al (2012) Impact of anterior scalene lidocaine blocks on predicting surgical success in older patients with neurogenic thoracic outlet syndrome. J Vasc Surg 55:1370–1375. https://doi.org/10.1016/j.jvs.2011.11.132
15. Torriani M, Gupta R, Donahue DM (2010) Botulinum toxin injection in neurogenic thoracic outlet syndrome: results and experience using a ultrasound-guided approach. Skeletal Radiol 39:973–980. https://doi.org/10.1007/s00256-010-0897-1
16. Stewman C, Vitanzo PC, Harwood MI (2014) Neurologic thoracic outlet syndrome: summarizing a complex history and evolution. Curr Sports Med Rep 13:100–106. https://doi.org/10.1249/JSR.0000000000000038
17. Koh E (2021) Imaging of non-specific complaints of the arm, neck, and/or shoulder (CANS): role of the scalene muscles and piercing variants in neurogenic thoracic outlet syndrome. Clin Radiol 76:940.e17–940.e27. https://doi.org/10.1016/j.crad.2021.08.007
18. Leonhard V, Caldwell G, Goh M, Reeder S, Smith HF (2017) Ultrasonographic diagnosis of thoracic outlet syndrome secondary to brachial plexus piercing variation. Diagnostics 7:40. https://doi.org/10.3390/diagnostics7030040
19. Emamhadi M, Chabok SY, Samini F, Alijani B, Behzadnia H, Firozabadi FA et al (2016) Anatomical variations of brachial plexus in adult cadavers; a descriptive study. Arch Bone Jt Surg 4:253–258. PMID: 27517072; PMCID: PMC4969373
20. Orebaugh SL, Williams BA (2009) Brachial plexus anatomy: normal and variant. Sci World J 9:300–312. https://doi.org/10.1100/tsw.2009.39
21. Williams AA, Smith HF (2020) Anatomical entrapment of the dorsal scapular and long thoracic nerves, secondary to brachial plexus piercing variation. Anat Sci Int 95:67–75. https://doi.org/10.1007/s12565-019-00495-1
22. Guday E, Bekele A, Muche A (2017) Anatomical study of prefixed versus postfixed brachial plexuses in adult human cadaver: prefixed versus postfixed brachial plexuses in adult human cadaver. ANZ J Surg 87:399–403. https://doi.org/10.1111/ans.13534
23. Pellerin M, Kimball Z, Tubbs RS, Nguyen S, Matusz P, Cohen-Gadol AA et al (2010) The prefixed and postfixed brachial plexus: a review with surgical implications. Surg Radiol Anat 32:251–260. https://doi.org/10.1007/s00276-009-0619-3
24. Desai N, Merjavy P, Russon K (2017) Anatomical variation of the brachial plexus and its clinical implications. Anesth Tutor Week 369:1–9
25. Sneag DB, Saltzman EB, Meister DW, Feinberg JH, Lee SK, Wolfe SW (2017) MRI bullseye sign: an indicator of peripheral nerve con-

striction in parsonage-turner syndrome. Muscle Nerve 56:99–106. https://doi.org/10.1002/mus.25480
26. Sneag DB, Rancy SK, Wolfe SW, Lee SC, Kalia V, Lee SK et al (2018) Brachial plexitis or neuritis? MRI features of lesion distribution in Parsonage-Turner syndrome. Muscle Nerve 58:359–366. https://doi.org/10.1002/mus.26108
27. Arányi Z, Csillik A, Dévay K, Rosero M, Barsi P, Böhm J et al (2015) Ultrasonographic identification of nerve pathology in neuralgic amyotrophy: enlargement, constriction, fascicular entwinement, and torsion. Muscle Nerve 52:503–511. https://doi.org/10.1002/mus.24615
28. Glorioso D, Palestini R, Cuccagna C, Lauretti L, Padua L (2023) Nerve torsion as a pattern of Parsonage–Turner syndrome: literature review and two representative cases. J Clin Med 12:4542. https://doi.org/10.3390/jcm12134542
29. Gstoettner C, Mayer JA, Rassam S, Hruby LA, Salminger S, Sturma A et al (2020) Neuralgic amyotrophy: a paradigm shift in diagnosis and treatment. J Neurol Neurosurg Psychiatry 91:879–888. https://doi.org/10.1136/jnnp-2020-323164
30. Bishop KN, Varacallo M (2023) Anatomy, shoulder and upper limb, dorsal scapular nerve. In: StatPearls. StatPearls Publishing, Treasure Island (FL). [cited 2023 Apr 19]. Available from: http://www.ncbi.nlm.nih.gov/books/NBK459343/
31. Benedetti MG, Zati A, Stagni SB, Fusaro I, Monesi R, Rotini R (2016) Winged scapula caused by rhomboid paralysis: a case report. Joints 4:247–249. https://doi.org/10.11138/jts/2016.4.4.247
32. Shapiro BE, Preston DC (2009) Entrapment and compressive neuropathies. Med Clin North Am 93:285–315. https://doi.org/10.1016/j.mcna.2008.09.009
33. Yoo Y-S, Jang S-W, Kim YS, Choi J-A, Oh JH, Jeong JY (2022) Does the suprascapular nerve move within the suprascapular notch? Biomechanical perspective using the finite element method. Yonsei Med J 63:657–664. https://doi.org/10.3349/ymj.2022.63.7.657
34. Westrick RB, Fogarty BT, Johnson MP (2013) Posterior labral tear with a paralabral cyst causing suprascapular nerve compression. J Orthop Sports Phys Ther 43(7):511. https://doi.org/10.2519/jospt.2013.0412
35. Schroder CP, Skare O, Stiris M, Gjengedal E, Uppheim G, Brox JI (2008) Treatment of labral tears with associated spinoglenoid cysts without cyst decompression. J Bone Joint Surg Am 90:523–530. https://doi.org/10.2106/JBJS.F.01534
36. Clavert P, Thomazeau H (2014) Peri-articular suprascapular neuropathy. Orthop Traumatol Surg Res 100:S409–S411. https://doi.org/10.1016/j.otsr.2014.10.002
37. Vázquez MT, Murillo J, Maranillo E, Parkin IG, Sanudo J (2007) Femoral nerve entrapment: a new insight. Clin Anat N Y N 20:175–179. https://doi.org/10.1002/ca.20327
38. Kirchmair L, Lirk P, Colvin J, Mitterschiffthaler G, Moriggl B (2008) Lumbar plexus and psoas major muscle: not always as expected. Reg Anesth Pain Med 33:109–114. https://doi.org/10.1016/j.rapm.2007.07.016
39. Anloague PA, Huijbregts P (2009) Anatomical variations of the lumbar plexus: a descriptive anatomy study with proposed clinical implications. J Man Manip Ther 17:e107–e114. https://doi.org/10.1179/106698109791352201
40. Khalid S, Iwanaga J, Loukas M, Tubbs RS (2017) Split femoral nerve due to psoas tertius muscle: a review with other cases of variant muscles traversing the femoral nerve. Cureus 9:e1555. https://doi.org/10.7759/cureus.1555
41. D'Costa S, Ramanathan LA, Madhyastha S, Nayak SR, Prabhu LV, Rai R et al (2008) An accessory iliacus muscle: a case report. Romanian J Morphol Embryol Rev Roum Morphol Embryol 49:407–409
42. Vinson C, Pavlovsky E, Loomis M (2023) Variant femoral nerve: the path beneath the iliacus muscle and into neuropathic symptoms. Bull Natl Res Cent 47:35. https://doi.org/10.12669/pjms.38.1.4396
43. Tubbs RS, Oakes WJ, Salter EG (2006) The psoas quartus muscle. Clin Anat N Y N 19:678–680. https://doi.org/10.1002/ca.20288
44. Spratt JD, Logan BM, Abrahams PH (1996) Variant slips of psoas and iliacus muscles, with splitting of the femoral nerve. Clin Anat N Y N 9:401–404. https://doi.org/10.1002/(SICI)1098-2353(1996)9:6<401::AID-CA8>3.0.CO;2-D
45. Grothaus MC, Holt M, Mekhail AO, Ebraheim NA, Yeasting RA (2005) Lateral femoral cutaneous nerve: an anatomic study. Clin Orthop (437):164–168. https://doi.org/10.1097/01.blo.0000164526.08610.97
46. Kesserwani H (2021) Meralgia paresthetica: a case report with an update on anatomy, pathology, and therapy. Cureus 13:e13937. https://doi.org/10.7759/cureus.13937
47. Hanna AS (2017) Lateral femoral cutaneous nerve transposition: renaissance of an old concept in the light of new anatomy. Clin Anat N Y N 30:409–412. https://doi.org/10.1002/ca.22849
48. Greeneway GP, Page PS, Ammanuel SG, Hanna AS (2023) Lateral femoral cutaneous nerve transposition. Neurosurg Focus Video 8:V8. https://doi.org/10.3171/2022.10.FOCVID2289
49. Haim A, Pritsch T, Ben-Galim P, Dekel S (2006) Meralgia paresthetica: a retrospective analysis of 79 patients evaluated and treated according to a standard algorithm. Acta Orthop 77:482–486. https://doi.org/10.1080/17453670610046433
50. Aszmann OC, Dellon ES, Dellon LA (1997) Anatomical course of the lateral femoral cutaneous nerve and its susceptibility to compression and injury. Plast Reconstr Surg 100:600. https://doi.org/10.1097/00006534-199709000-00008
51. Dellon AL (2022) Discussion: anatomical analysis of the lateral femoral cutaneous nerve and its passage beneath the inguinal ligament. Plast Reconstr Surg 149:1152. https://doi.org/10.1097/PRS.0000000000009035
52. Lee CH, Dellon AL (2000) Surgical management of groin pain of neural origin1. No competing interest declared. J Am Coll Surg 191:137–142. https://doi.org/10.1016/s1072-7515(00)00319-7
53. Ally RM, Velleman MD, Suleman FE (2019) Meralgia paresthetica: now showing on 3T magnetic resonance neurography. SA J Radiol 23:1745. https://doi.org/10.4102/sajr.v23i1.1745
54. Chhabra A, Del Grande F, Soldatos T, Chalian M, Belzberg AJ, Williams EH et al (2013) Meralgia paresthetica: 3-Tesla magnetic resonance neurography. Skeletal Radiol 42:803–808. https://doi.org/10.1007/s00256-012-1557-4

Part III

Upper Body Nerves

Brachial Plexus, Supraclavicular Exposure

7

Amgad S. Hanna and Mark E. Ehlers

Surgical Anatomy

The supraclavicular brachial plexus includes the ventral rami of spinal nerves and the trunks. The brachial plexus is usually formed by the ventral rami of C5–T1. It forms between the scalenus anterior and scalenus medius muscles. It lies in the posterior triangle of the neck, bound by the sternocleidomastoid (SCM) anteriorly, trapezius posteriorly, and clavicle inferiorly (Fig. 7.1). C5 and C6 join to make the upper (superior) trunk, C7 continues as the middle trunk, and C8 and T1 join to make the lower (inferior) trunk. The suprascapular nerve (C5, 6) is the largest branch at the root/trunk level. It arises from the cranial aspect of the upper trunk, close to the divisions. The dorsal scapular nerve (to rhomboids and levator scapulae) comes off the C5 ventral ramus, the long thoracic nerve (to serratus anterior) comes off the C5, C6, and occasionally C7 ventral rami and usually runs through the scalenus medius muscle. The nerve to subclavius (C5 and C6) comes off the upper trunk.

Often, especially in thin people with tall neck, the divisions of the brachial plexus can be visualized during this exposure. The upper trunk typically ends in a trifurcation from cranial to caudal: suprascapular nerve (S), posterior division (P), and anterior division (A), respectively, hence the acronym SPA [1].

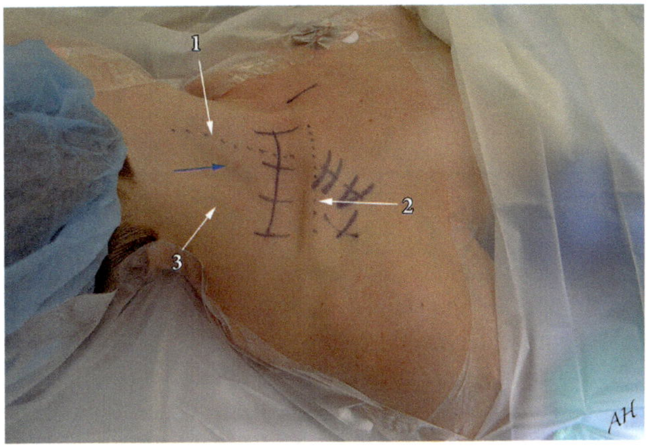

Fig. 7.1 Right supraclavicular brachial plexus exposure. (**a**) The patient is positioned supine with the head turned contralaterally, the back of the bed elevated, and the head slightly extended. *White arrows* show the boundaries of the posterior triangle of the neck: *1* posterior border of sternocleidomastoid (SCM), *2* clavicle, *3* anterior border of the trapezius. *Blue arrow* external jugular vein

Anatomical Variations

- Contribution to brachial plexus formation is very common from C4 (prefixed) and uncommon from T2 (postfixed) [2].
- There are different patterns of the termination of the upper trunk. Although it typically (70%) appears as a trifurcation (Fig. 7.2a), occasionally (25%), the suprascapular nerve comes off more distally from the posterior division (Fig. 7.2b) or less commonly (5%) from the upper trunk proper prior to the divisions (Fig. 7.2c) [1].

Supplementary Information The online version contains supplementary material available at https://doi.org/10.1007/978-3-031-73931-6_7.

A. S. Hanna (✉)
Department of Neurosurgery, University of Wisconsin School of Medicine and Public Health, Madison, WI, USA

M. E. Ehlers
Urology, Aurora Health Care Medical Group, Milwaukee, WI, USA
e-mail: mehlers@wisc.edu

A. S. Hanna (ed.), *Nerves: Anatomy, Exposures, and Techniques*, https://doi.org/10.1007/978-3-031-73931-6_7

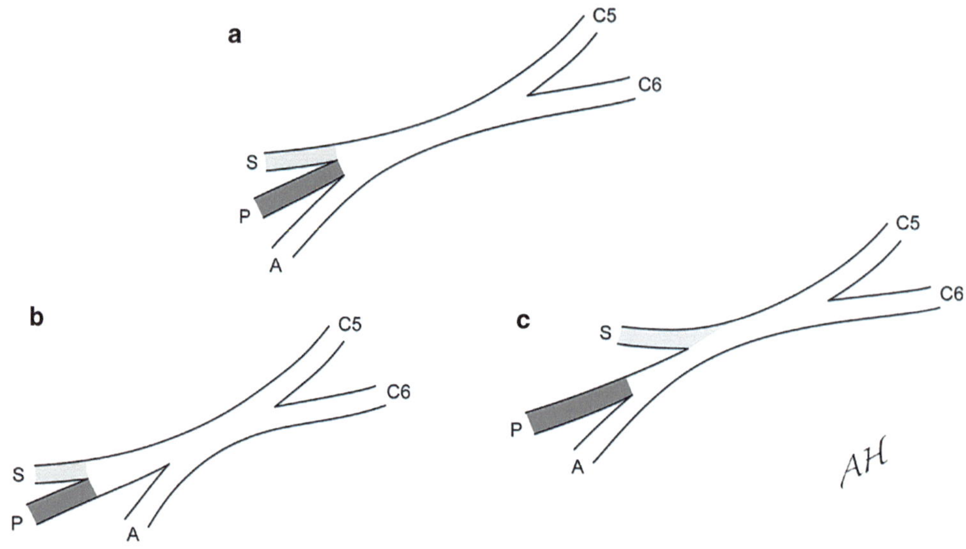

Fig. 7.2 Different patterns of upper trunk divisions. (**a**) Typical trifurcation (70%). (**b**) Suprascapular nerve comes off the posterior division (25%). (**c**) Suprascapular nerve comes off the upper trunk proper (5%). *S* suprascapular nerve, *P* posterior division, *A* anterior division. Copyright Amgad Hanna. Published with permission [1]

Exposure

1. Position: supine with the back of the table up, the head in a doughnut turned contralaterally, and the neck slightly extended (Fig. 7.3).
2. Incision: Horizontal curvilinear along or parallel to a skin crease (Fig. 7.1). This heals better esthetically (Fig. 7.4) than the more traditional oblique incision along the posterior border of SCM.
3. The skin flaps are elevated between the subcutaneous fat and platysma using DeBakey forceps and Metzenbaum or tenotomy scissors, while the assistant is lifting up the skin using two Senn retractors.
4. The platysma is opened along its fibers and undermined (Fig. 7.5).
5. The posterior border of the SCM is identified. Care should be taken not to injure the great auricular nerve (that winds around the posterior border of the SCM) or the spinal accessory nerve cranial to it. The external jugular vein can be ligated and cut if needed, this is usually well tolerated.
6. The fat pad is then dissected free from the posterior border of the SCM. The omohyoid muscle is found deep to the SCM and lies horizontally oblique (Fig. 7.6a). It is tagged with 2-0 Ethibond sutures, cut, and retracted (Fig. 7.6b). Cutaneous branches of the cervical plexus are usually encountered and may have to be sacrificed; but only the minimum needed to allow adequate exposure.
7. The transverse cervical and suprascapular vessels are also encountered and need to be ligated with 3-0 or 2-0 Silk ties then cut. They run horizontally in the caudal part of the exposure, sometimes behind the clavicle (Fig. 7.6c).

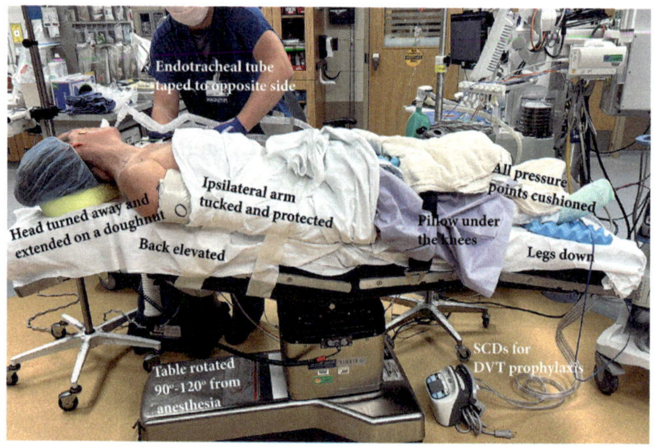

Fig. 7.3 The patient is positioned spine, back elevated, head extended in a doughnut, and turned contralaterally. It is also preferable to tape the endotracheal tube to the opposite side. *SCDs* sequential compression devices, *DVT* deep venous thrombosis. LMA (Laryngeal Mask Airway) should be discouraged since the cuff can compromise the surgical exposure

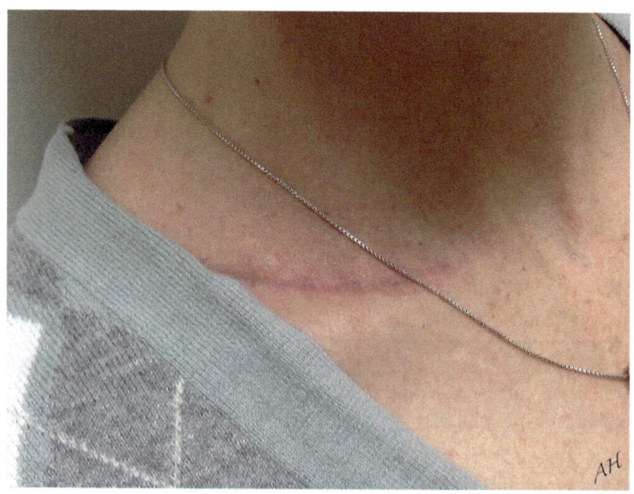

Fig. 7.4 Incision is horizontally curvilinear within or parallel to a skin crease. The healing of this is more esthetic than the traditional vertical one

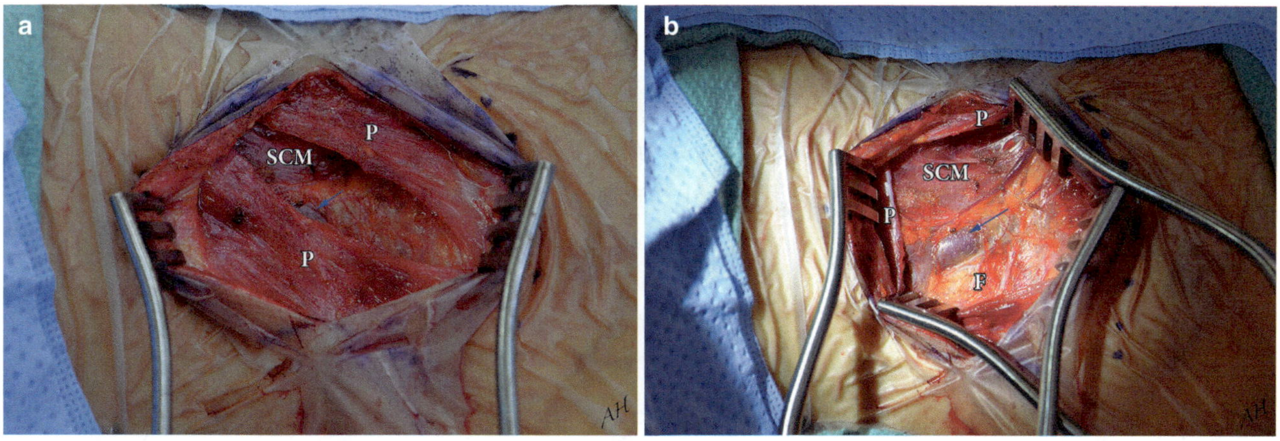

Fig. 7.5 Right brachial plexus exposure. The platysma (*P*) is divided along its fibers (**a**) and retracted (**b**). This reveals the posterior border of sternocleidomastoid (*SCM*), external jugular vein (*blue arrow*), and fat pad (*F*)

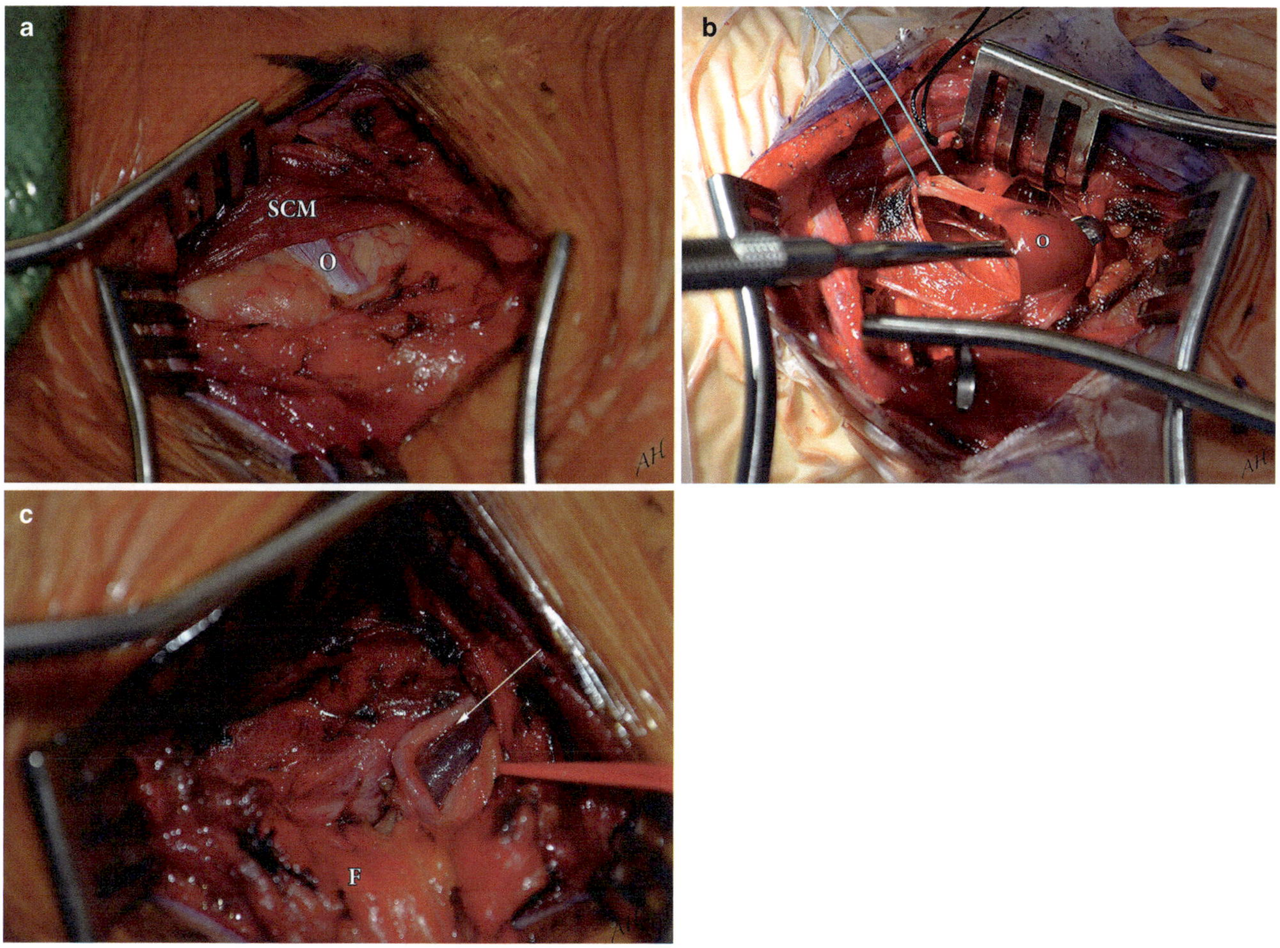

Fig. 7.6 (**a**) The omohyoid muscle (*O*) is identified deep to the *SCM*. (**b**) Omohyoid is tagged and cut. (**c**) The supraclavicular pad of fat (*F*) is dissected and retracted laterally. The transverse cervical vessels (*arrow*) are ligated and cut

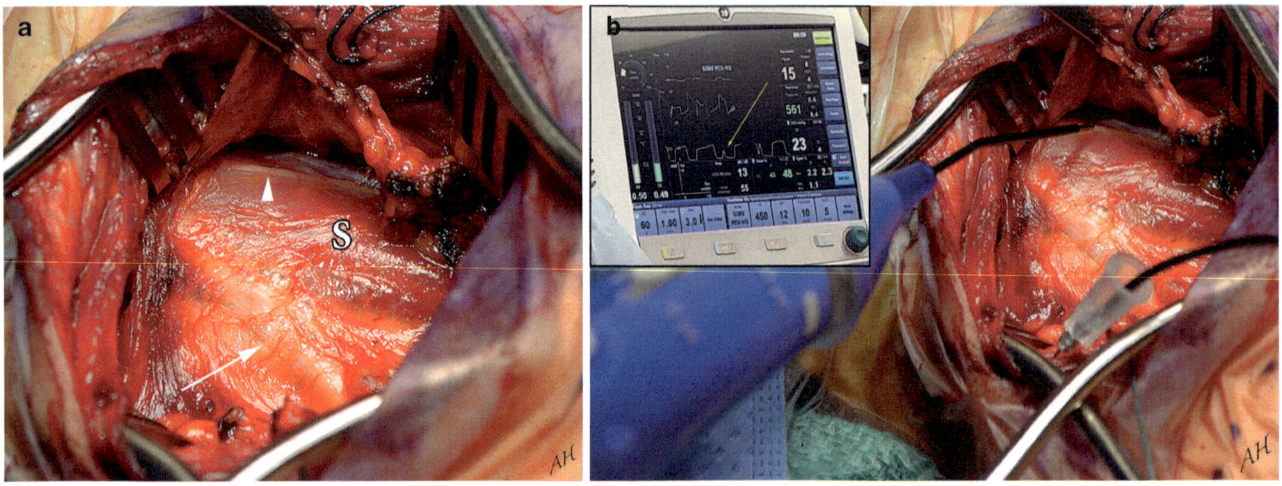

Fig. 7.7 (**a**) The phrenic nerve (*arrowhead*) is observed on the surface of the scalenus anterior muscle (*S*). The upper (superior) trunk (*arrow*) is seen through the fat; the upper trunk can usually be easily palpated through the fat even before seen. (**b**) Phrenic nerve stimulation leads to movement of the chest wall and change (*arrow*) in end tidal CO_2 curve (*inset*)

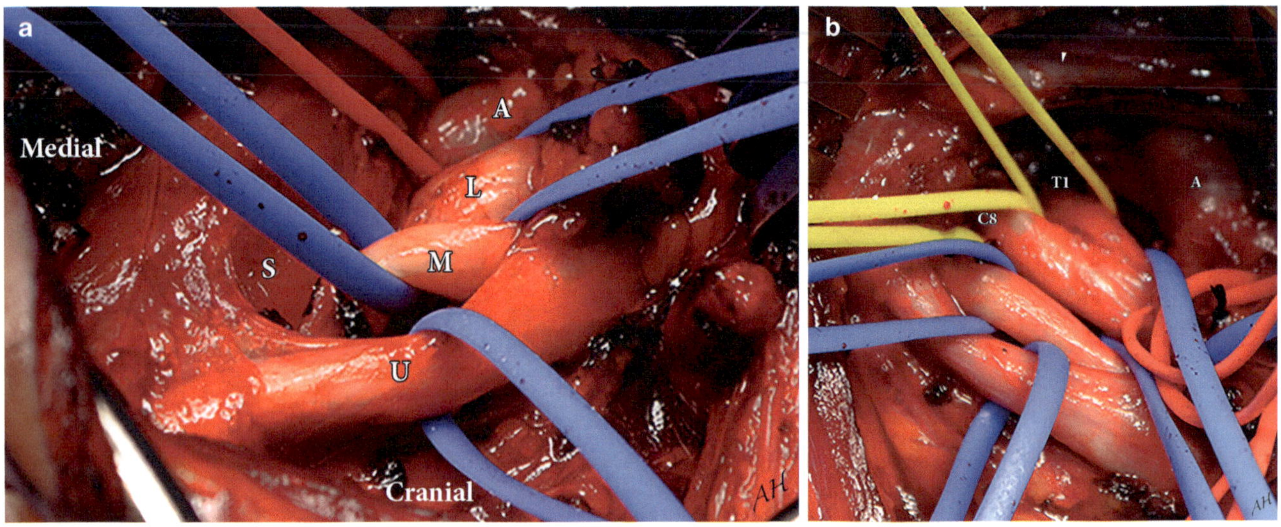

Fig. 7.8 (**a**) Identification of the trunks of the brachial plexus. *U* upper (superior) trunk (C5 and C6), *M* middle trunk (C7), *L* lower (inferior) trunk (C8 and T1), *A* subclavian artery, *S* scalenus anterior. (**b**) More medial exposure after anterior scalenectomy reveals C8 and T1 ventral rami. *Arrowhead* phrenic nerve

8. The scalenus anterior (anticus) muscle is then identified with the phrenic nerve anterior to it from cranio-lateral to caudo-medial (Fig. 7.7a). The nerve can also be tested by electrical stimulation (Fig. 7.7b).
9. In thoracic outlet cases, the upper trunk can usually be palpated through the fat, then visualized even before the phrenic nerve. In trauma cases, due to distorted anatomy, the phrenic nerve may be identified first, followed cranially to find C5. C5 followed distally will lead to the upper trunk, and the latter followed back proximally to separate C6 from C5, which is sometimes extremely challenging.
10. Caudal to the upper trunk and in a deeper plane is found the middle trunk formed by C7.
11. Caudal to the middle trunk is the subclavian artery, and posterior to it is the lower trunk (Fig. 7.8a). Following the lower trunk medially leads to the C8 nerve root. The latter is usually in line with the lower trunk. T1 ventral ramus ascends to meet C8 at an angle to form the lower trunk (Fig. 7.8b). T1 is sometimes easier to find by retracting the lower trunk anteriorly and looking for it in the back of the lower trunk.
12. The trunks usually divide behind the clavicle, however, especially with taller necks, at least the upper trunk trifurcation is easily identified above the clavicle.

13. The spinal accessory nerve, usually intact in brachial plexus injuries and used as a donor for nerve transfers, is found in the fat pad under the anterior border of the trapezius muscle. It can be identified by electrical stimulation.

Complications

1. Skin numbness is not uncommon in the infraclavicular area due to retraction or section of the supraclavicular nerves. Numbness of the ear lobule can occur from damage to the great auricular nerve Neuroma formation from transected cutaneous branches can be painful and may require reoperation (Chap. 63).
2. Diaphragmatic paralysis from phrenic nerve injury or use as a donor for nerve transfers. Usually well tolerated but can be complicated by exertional dyspnea, or rarely respiratory failure, that may require prolonged ventilation or even tracheostomy. Diaphragmatic plication can be done by a thoracic surgeon and has some success in improving ventilation. While transient phrenic nerve palsy was observed early on in our institution after thoracic outlet surgery, this complication has been completely eliminated by using minimal or *nonbipolar technique*. It is assumed that the heat generated by the bipolar coagulation during anterior scalenectomy may easily transmit to the phrenic nerve. Also, the phrenic nerve should not be skeletonized, the fascial plane between the anterior scalene and phrenic nerve should be preserved, and retraction should be kept to a minimum or preferably none.
3. Vascular injuries: to the subclavian artery, internal jugular vein, transverse cervical, or suprascapular vessels. Small vessels can be ligated or clipped. Large vessels require repair sometimes by a vascular surgeon. An expanding postoperative hematoma is a surgical emergency due to the risk of airway compromise.
4. Thoracic duct injury, mostly on the left side. Direct repair can be attempted, or patching with fat pad and supplementing with fibrin glue.
5. Pneumothorax, from injury to the pleura and possibly the lung apex. The pleura can be directly repaired. Chest tube may or may not be needed. If suspected, a chest X-ray should be obtained.
6. Brachial plexus injury. Most commonly neurapraxia from manipulation and retraction, which should be kept to a minimum. Very rarely accidental transection which should be avoided at all costs by meticulous dissection, knowledge of the anatomy, and not rushing through the surgery. Unfortunately, these are still seen when attention is focused on rib resection without adequate exposure of the plexus components.
7. Wound infection, very rare.

References

1. Hanna A (2016) The SPA arrangement of the branches of the upper trunk of the Brachial plexus: a correction of a longstanding misconception and a new diagram of the brachial plexus. J Neurosurg 125(2):350–354. https://doi.org/10.3171/2015.5.JNS15367
2. Pellerin M, Kimball Z, Tubbs RS, Nguyen S, Matusz P, Cohen-Gadol AA, Loukas M (2010) The prefixed and postfixed Brachial plexus: a review with surgical implications. Surg Radiol Anat 32(3):251–260. https://doi.org/10.1007/s00276-009-0619-3

Brachial Plexus, Infraclavicular Exposure

8

Amgad S. Hanna and Mark E. Ehlers

Surgical Anatomy

The infraclavicular brachial plexus includes the cords and the terminal branches. They correlate closely with the axillary artery. Posterior cord is formed by the junction of the posterior divisions of the three trunks, it first runs lateral and then posterior to the axillary artery. It gives off the thoracodorsal nerve (to latissimus dorsi), and the upper (to subscapularis) and lower subscapular nerves (to subscapularis and teres major). Terminal branches include the axillary and radial nerves. The lateral cord (fasciculus lateralis) forms by the junction of the anterior divisions of the upper and middle trunks, it first runs anterior and then lateral to the axillary artery. It gives off the lateral pectoral nerves. Terminal branches include the musculocutaneous nerve and the lateral contribution to the median nerve. The medial cord (fasciculus medialis) is the continuation of the anterior division of the lower trunk, which first runs posterior and then medial to the axillary artery. It gives off the medial pectoral nerve, medial brachial cutaneous, and medial antebrachial cutaneous nerves. Terminal branches include the ulnar nerve and medial contribution to the median nerve.

Anatomical Variations

Communications between lateral and medial cords may occur [1]. More than one contribution to the median nerve can be observed, especially from the lateral cord. The musculocutaneous nerve may arise more distally from the median nerve itself rather than the lateral cord.

Supplementary Information The online version contains supplementary material available at https://doi.org/10.1007/978-3-031-73931-6_8.

A. S. Hanna (✉)
Department of Neurosurgery, University of Wisconsin School of Medicine and Public Health, Madison, WI, USA

M. E. Ehlers
Urology, Aurora Health Care Medical Group, Milwaukee, WI, USA

Exposure

1. Position: supine, with the back of the table up, and the patient's head turned contralaterally. Exposure is easier if the arm is abducted to open the infraclavicular space, unless supraclavicular exposure required at the same time then the arm should be adducted.
2. Incision is made along the deltopectoral groove (Fig. 8.1).
3. The deltoid is separated from the pectoralis major muscle. In this interval, the cephalic vein is usually encountered (Fig. 8.2). It is important to preserve the vessels in this area if a free muscle flap is considered. If not, small vessels can be ligated and cut to facilitate the exposure.
4. The coracoid process is then palpated. Pectoralis minor inserts into the medial part of the coracoid process and the fibers originate from the ribs, while the short head of biceps brachii and coracobrachialis originate from the lateral part of the coracoid and head towards the arm, almost perpendicular to the pectoralis minor (Fig. 8.3). The pectoralis minor is tagged with 2-0 Ethibond sutures, transected, and then retracted. Underneath the pectoralis minor is a fatty layer that contains the brachial plexus.
5. Dissection through this fatty layer uncovers first the lateral cord as it gives off the musculocutaneous nerve (Fig. 8.4) and the lateral contribution to the median nerve.
6. Posterolateral to the lateral cord, the posterior cord can be found as it gives off the axillary and radial nerves.
7. The axillary artery is then found medial and posterior to the lateral cord and partially covers the medial cord.
8. The medial cord is located medial and posterior to the axillary artery as it gives off the ulnar nerve and medial contribution to the median nerve. Medial to the ulnar nerve are the medial antebrachial cutaneous (MABC) and medial brachial cutaneous (MBC) nerves (Figs. 8.5, 8.6 and 8.7). To find the medial cord, it's easier to follow the lateral contribution to median nerve distally until it meets the medial contribution, the latter is followed proximally to find the medial cord proper.

A. S. Hanna (ed.), *Nerves: Anatomy, Exposures, and Techniques*, https://doi.org/10.1007/978-3-031-73931-6_8

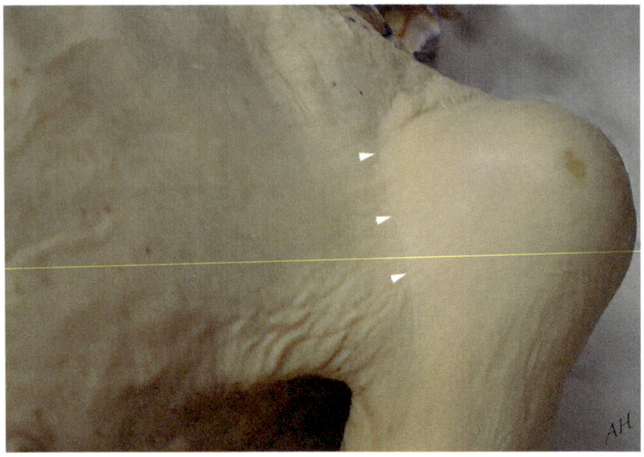

Fig. 8.1 Left infraclavicular brachial plexus exposure. Incision is made along the deltopectoral groove (*arrowheads*)

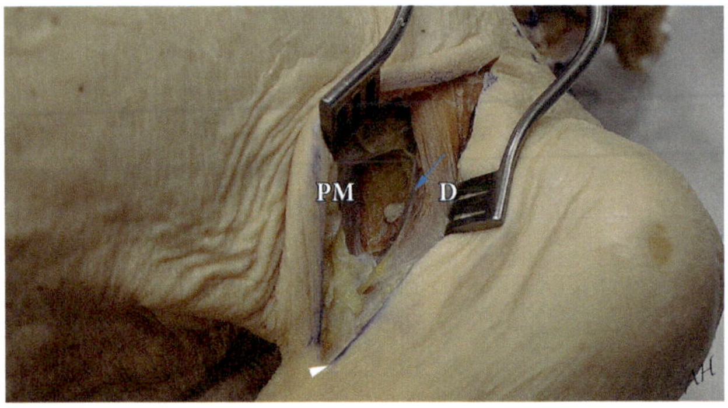

Fig. 8.2 The deltoid (*D*) and pectoralis major (*PM*) are retracted. The cephalic vein (*arrow*) is observed in-between

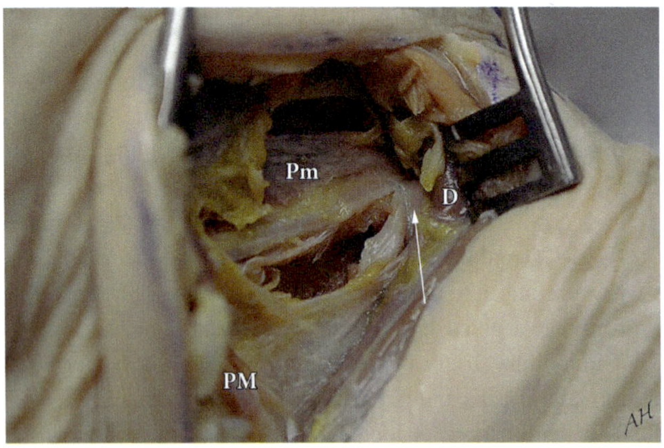

Fig. 8.3 Pectoralis minor (*Pm*) is defined, tagged, cut, and retracted. Note the common tendon of short head of biceps brachii and coracobrachialis (*arrow*) laterally, almost perpendicular to Pm. *PM* pectoralis major, *D* deltoid

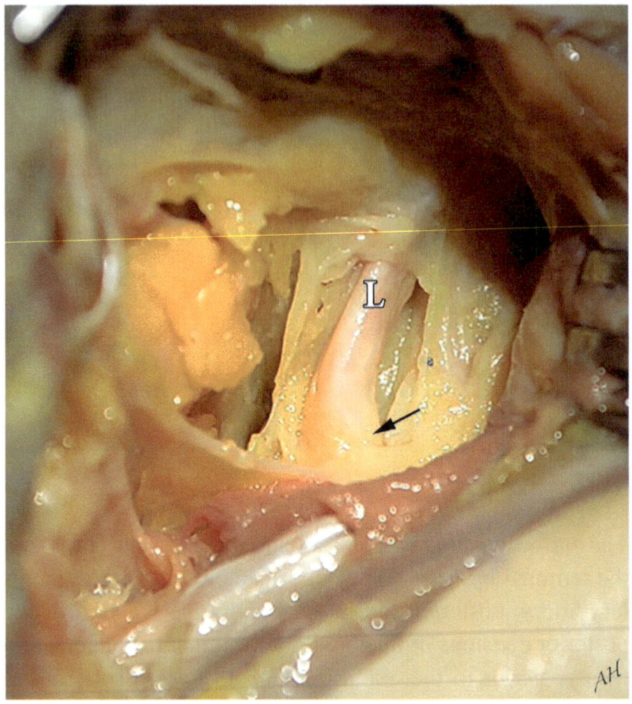

Fig. 8.4 The pad of fat deep to Pm contains the brachial plexus. The lateral cord (fasciculus lateralis, *L*) is first encountered as it gives off the musculocutaneous nerve (*arrow*)

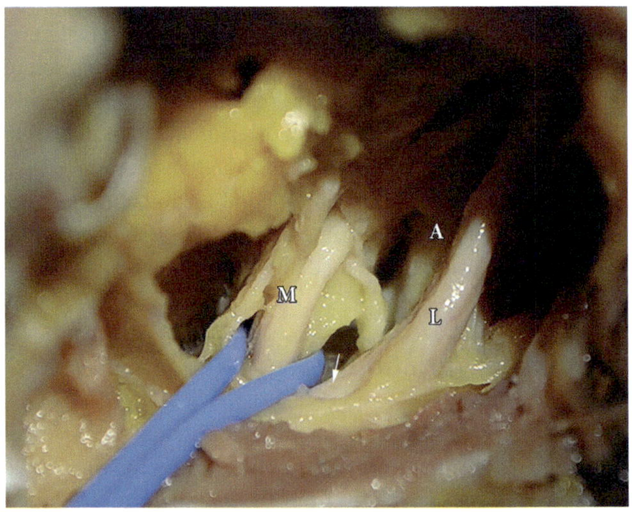

Fig. 8.5 Further dissection reveals the medial cord (fasciculus medialis, *M*). The lateral contribution to the median nerve (*arrow*) is also seen; usually more than one contribution is observed. *A* axillary artery, *L* lateral cord

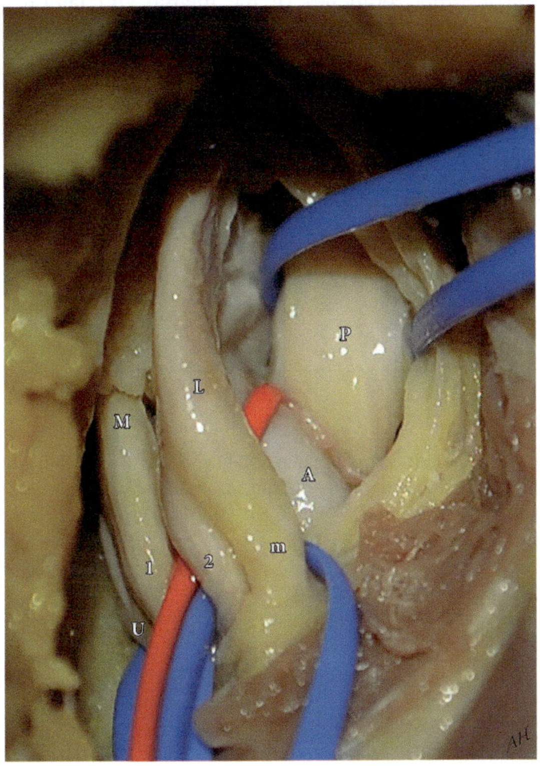

Fig. 8.6 The three cords are exposed. *M* medial cord, *L* lateral cord, *P* posterior cord, *A* axillary artery, *U* ulnar nerve, *m* musculocutaneous nerve, *1* medial contribution to median nerve, *2* lateral contribution to median nerve

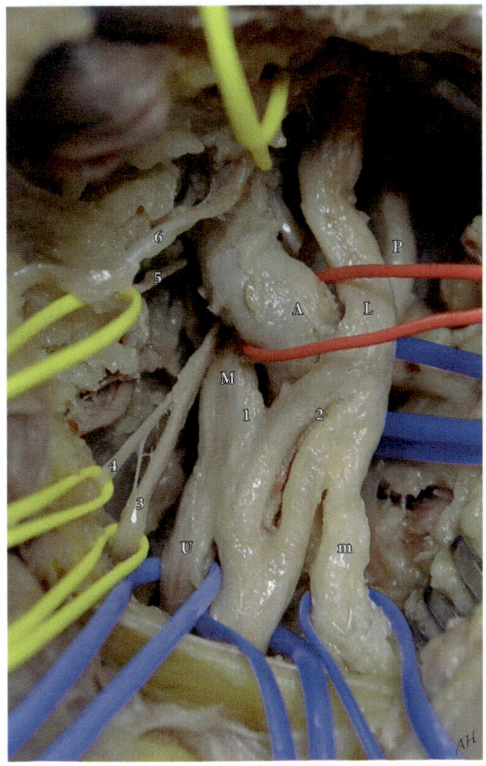

Fig. 8.7 The main branches of the medial (*M*) and lateral (*L*) cords are exposed. From the medial cord: medial contribution to the median nerve (*1*), ulnar nerve (*U*), medial antebrachial cutaneous nerve (*3*), medial brachial cutaneous nerve (*4*), and medial pectoral nerve (*5*). From the lateral cord: lateral contribution to the median nerve, here duplicated (*2*), musculocutaneous nerve (*m*), and lateral pectoral nerve (*6*). Note that the lateral and medial pectoral nerves join (ansa pectoralis). *P* posterior cord, *A* axillary artery

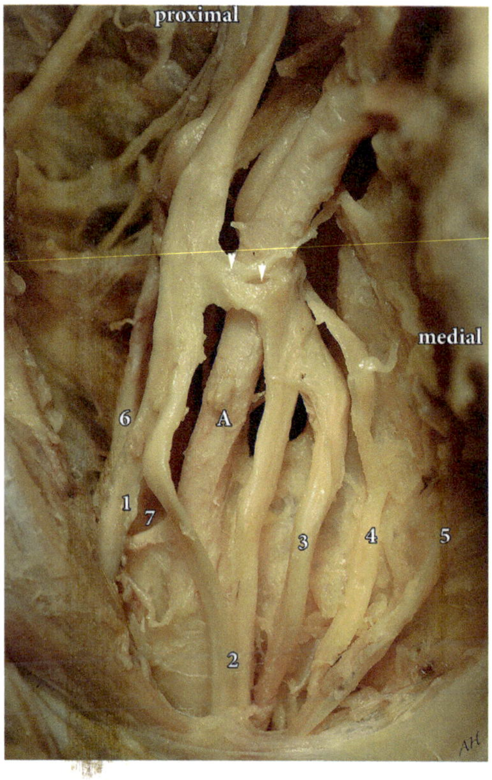

Fig. 8.8 Right infraclavicular exposure showing the components of "M": *1* musculocutaneous nerve, *2* median nerve, *3* ulnar nerve. *A* axillary artery, *4* medial antebrachial cutaneous (MABC) nerve, *5* medial brachial cutaneous (MBC) nerve, *6* axillary nerve, *7* radial nerve. Note the communication between the medial and lateral cords (*arrowheads*)

9. The terminal branches of the medial and lateral cords form an "M" and "hug" the axillary artery (Fig. 8.8).

Complications

1. Vascular injuries.
2. Pneumothorax.
3. Iatrogenic nerve injuries.
4. Wound infection.

Reference

1. Goel S, Rustagi SM, Kumar A, Mehta V, Suri RK (2014) Multiple unilateral variations in medial and lateral cords of brachial plexus and their branches. Anat Cell Biol 47(1):77–80. https://doi.org/10.5115/acb.2014.47.1.77

9 Brachial Plexus, Combined Supra- and Infraclavicular Exposures (Pan-Plexus Exposure)

Amgad S. Hanna and Mark E. Ehlers

Surgical Anatomy

The divisions of the three trunks are traditionally described posterior to the clavicle. However, almost universally, the upper trunk trifurcation can be seen cranial to the level of the clavicle.

Exposure

1. The incision can be planned in three different ways:
   (a) Two separate incisions, one curvilinear along a skin crease in the posterior triangle of the neck as described in Chap. 7 and another along the delto-pectoral groove as described in Chap. 8 (Fig. 9.1), leaving a skin bridge in between. The skin bridge is easy to retract and will not compromise visibility.
   (b) The lateral end of the supraclavicular incision can be connected to the cranial end of the infraclavicular one. Avoid narrow angles at the corners to maintain skin vitality.
   (c) A traditional Z-shaped incision, with the cranial part along the posterior border of sternocleidomastoid, middle segment along the clavicle, and caudal part along the deltopectoral groove, may still have a role in big tumors or trauma cases but is significantly less esthetic.

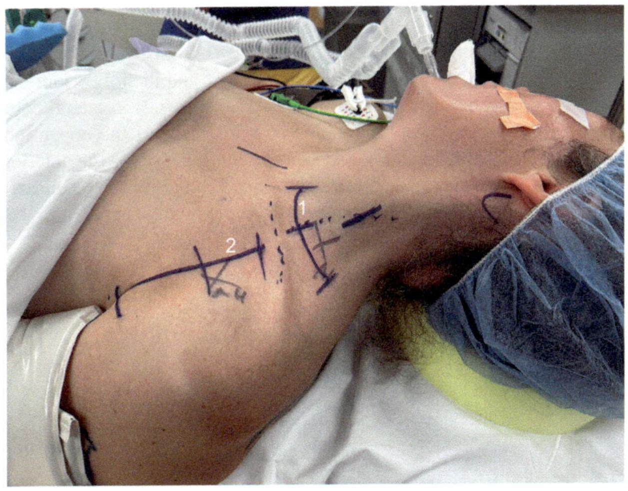

Fig. 9.1 Combined supra-and infraclavicular exposures. Two separate incisions are the most esthetic, in this case done for combined anterior scalenectomy (*1*) and pectoralis minor (*2*) release to treat the thoracic outlet syndrome

2. The clavicle can be dealt with in three different ways:
   (a) Left in place is feasible most of the time (Fig. 9.2). The clavicle is identified and surrounded by a lap sponge, umbilical tape [1], or a Penrose drain to allow retraction cranially and caudally.
   (b) A single osteotomy is made in the clavicle that is repaired at the end. The two parts of the clavicle are then retracted to expose the plexus.
   (c) A clavicular window is created by making two osteotomies and removing a segment of the clavicle that is put together at the end with a plate and screws. This avoids excessive retraction on the clavicle and soft tissues and may be beneficial in large tumors or extensive trauma cases. The screw holes for plating should be marked prior to osteotomies for better instrumentation at the end [2].
3. Supraclavicular dissection follows the steps described in Chap. 7.
4. Infraclavicular dissection is done as in Chap. 8 (Fig. 9.3).

Supplementary Information The online version contains supplementary material available at https://doi.org/10.1007/978-3-031-73931-6_9.

A. S. Hanna (✉)
Department of Neurosurgery, University of Wisconsin School of Medicine and Public Health, Madison, WI, USA

M. E. Ehlers
Urology, Aurora Health Care Medical Group, Milwaukee, WI, USA
e-mail: mehlers@wisc.edu

A. S. Hanna (ed.), *Nerves: Anatomy, Exposures, and Techniques*, https://doi.org/10.1007/978-3-031-73931-6_9

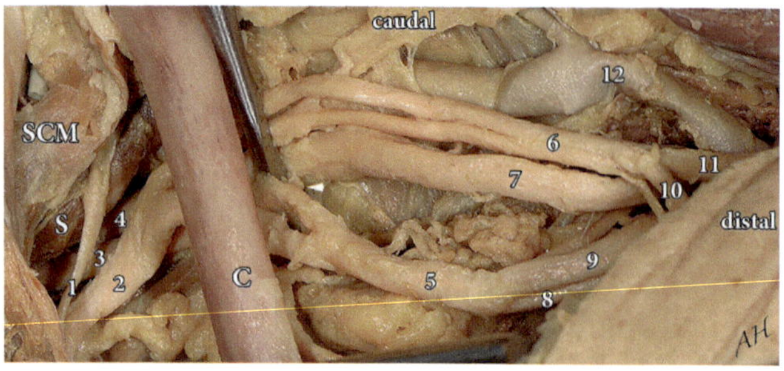

Fig. 9.2 For combined right supra- and infraclavicular exposures, the clavicle (*C*) can be exposed and retracted cranially or caudally as needed. In this particular case, the axillary artery (*12*) is more caudal than usual. *SCM* sternocleidomastoid, *S* scalenus anterior, *1* phrenic nerve, *2* upper (superior) trunk, *3* middle trunk, *4* lower (inferior) trunk, *5* posterior cord made by the junction of the posterior divisions of the three trunks. A small component (*arrowhead*) from the lower trunk joins the posterior division of the middle trunk, and then they join the posterior division of the upper trunk (see also Fig. 7.2). *6* lateral cord made by the junction between the anterior divisions of the upper and middle trunks, *7* medial cord made by the continuation of the anterior division of the lower trunk, *8* axillary nerve, *9* radial nerve, *10* musculocutaneous nerve, *11* lateral contribution to the median nerve

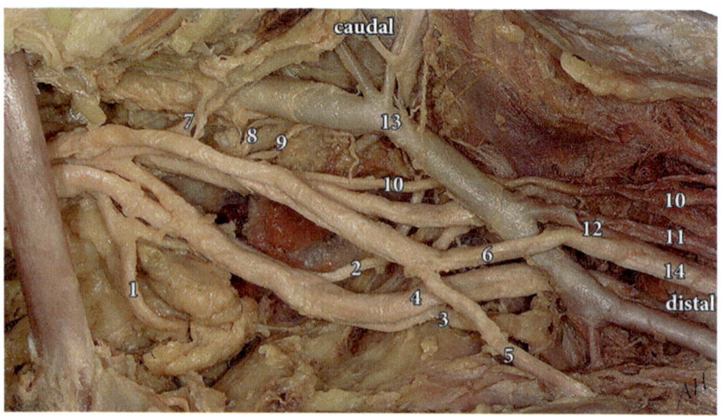

Fig. 9.3 Other branches of the same right brachial plexus. From the upper trunk, *1* suprascapular nerve. From the posterior cord, *2* thoracodorsal nerve, *3* axillary nerve, *4* radial nerve. From the lateral cord, *5* musculocutaneous nerve, *6* lateral contribution to the median nerve, *7* lateral pectoral nerve. From the medial cord, *8* medial pectoral nerve, *9* medial brachial cutaneous (MBC) nerve, *10* medial antebrachial cutaneous (MABC) nerve, *11* ulnar nerve, *12* medial contribution to the median nerve. *13* axillary artery, *14* median nerve

5. The upper trunk trifurcation is typically observed above the clavicle. The terminal branches are arranged from craniodorsal to caudoventral as follows: Suprascapular nerve, Posterior division, and then Anterior division, SPA [3] (Fig. 9.4).
6. The posterior divisions of the middle and lower trunks are also more cranial than the corresponding anterior divisions [4].
7. The posterior divisions of the three trunks form the posterior cord.
8. The anterior divisions of the upper and middle trunks join to make the lateral cord.

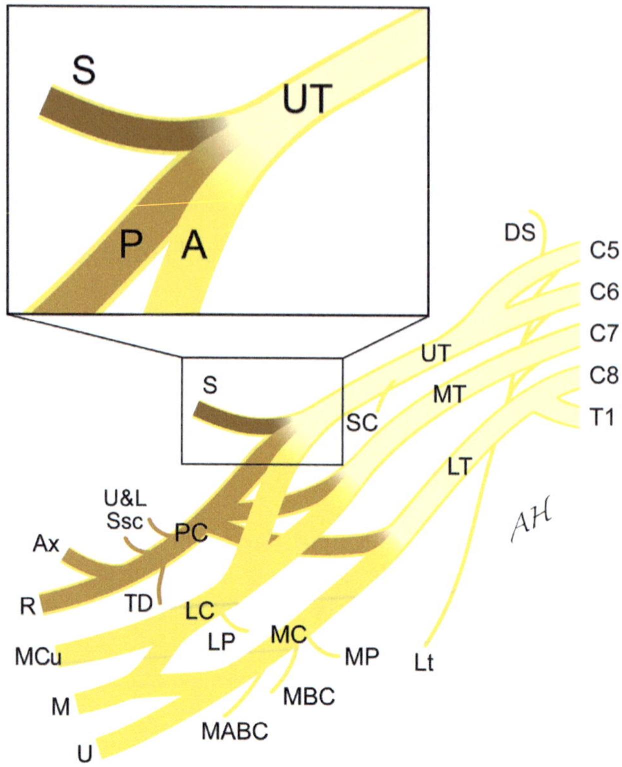

Fig. 9.4 Diagrammatic representation of the right brachial plexus. *DS* dorsal scapular nerve, *Lt* long thoracic nerve; *MT* middle trunk, *LT* lower (inferior) trunk, *SC* nerve to subclavius, *PC* posterior cord, *LC* lateral cord; *MC* medial cord, *LP* lateral pectoral nerve, *MP* medial pectoral nerve, *MBC* medial brachial cutaneous nerve, *MABC* medial antebrachial cutaneous nerve, *U & L Ssc* upper and lower subscapular nerves, *TD* thoracodorsal nerve, *Ax* axillary nerve, *R* radial nerve, *MCu* musculocutaneous nerve, *M* median nerve, *U* ulnar nerve. *Inset* the arrangement of the branches of the upper (superior) trunk (*UT*) from cranial to caudal: suprascapular nerve (*S*), posterior division (*P*), and then anterior division (*A*), hence the acronym SPA. Copyright Amgad Hanna. Published with permission [3]

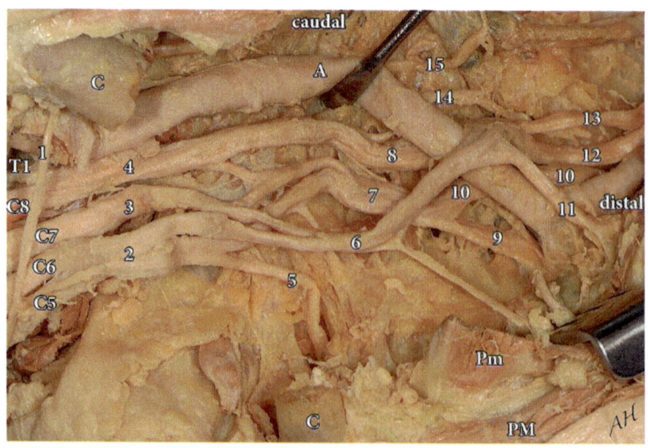

Fig. 9.5 Overview of the right brachial plexus from a different specimen after the division of the clavicle (*C*). *PM* pectoralis major, *Pm* pectoralis minor, *A* artery: subclavian → axillary, *1* phrenic nerve, *2* upper (superior) trunk, *3* middle trunk, *4* lower (inferior) trunk, *5* suprascapular nerve, *6* lateral cord, *7* posterior cord, *8* medial cord, *9* axillary nerve, *10* radial nerve, *11* musculocutaneous nerve, *12* median nerve, *13* ulnar nerve, *14* medial antebrachial cutaneous (MABC) nerve, *15* medial brachial cutaneous (MBC) nerve

9. The anterior division of the lower trunk continues as the medial cord.
10. The final view is depicted in Fig. 9.5.

References

1. Tse R, Pondaag W, Malessy M (2014) Exposure of the retroclavicular brachial plexus by clavicle suspension for birth brachial plexus palsy. Tech Hand Up Extrem Surg 18(2):85–88. https://doi.org/10.1097/BTH.0000000000000041
2. Hanna A (2024) Clavicular window for brachial plexus schwannoma removal. Surg Neurol Int 19(15):135. https://doi.org/10.25259/SNI_824_2023. eCollection 2024
3. Hanna A (2016) The SPA arrangement of the branches of the upper trunk of the brachial plexus: a correction of a longstanding misconception and a new diagram of the brachial plexus. J Neurosurg 125(2):350–354. https://doi.org/10.3171/2015.5.JNS15367
4. Neto JHS, Neto BC, Eiras ABD, Botelho RHS, Carmo JMM, Passos MARF (2022) The 2-dimensional and 3-dimensional anatomy of the adult brachial plexus divisions and cords. Hand (N Y) 17(1):50–54. https://doi.org/10.1177/1558944720906510

Brachial Plexus, Posterior Exposure

10

Amgad S. Hanna and Mark E. Ehlers

Surgical Anatomy

From a posterior approach, the brachial plexus is anterior to the following muscle planes from superficial to deep: trapezius, rhomboids and levator scapulae, serratus posterior superior, scalenus posterior, and scalenus medius. In this exposure, the subclavian artery is anterior to (deeper than) the lower trunk. This approach is very morbid and less commonly used than the anterior approaches. It still has a role in residual/recurrent thoracic outlet syndrome and tumors.

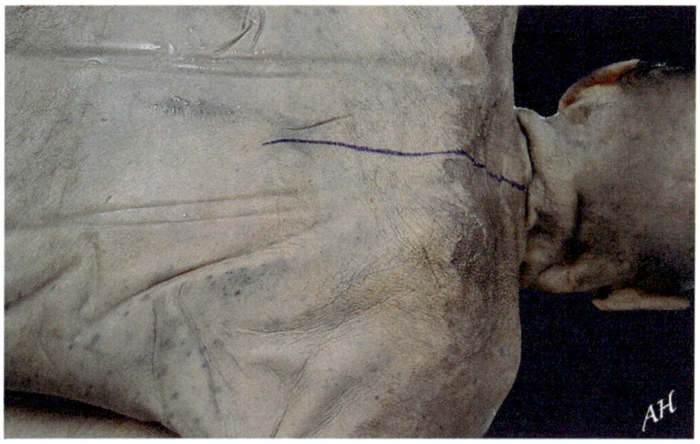

Fig. 10.1 Posterior exposure of the right brachial plexus. Position: prone. Incision: paramedian, between the midline and medial border of the scapula

Exposure [1]

1. Position prone on chest rolls.
2. Incision: paramedian, between midline and medial border of the scapula (Fig. 10.1).
3. The trapezius (Fig. 10.2) is incised vertically.
4. The rhomboids and levator scapulae (Fig. 10.3) are incised vertically.
5. This allows retraction of the scapula laterally.
6. The serratus posterior superior (Fig. 10.4) and posterior scalene muscles can be cut as they insert to the second rib. The middle scalene can be detached from the first rib. Care should be taken not to mistake the second rib for the first rib. Always palpate cranial and deeper to the most cranial rib to make sure it is indeed the first rib. X-ray confirmation can be obtained prior to rib resection.

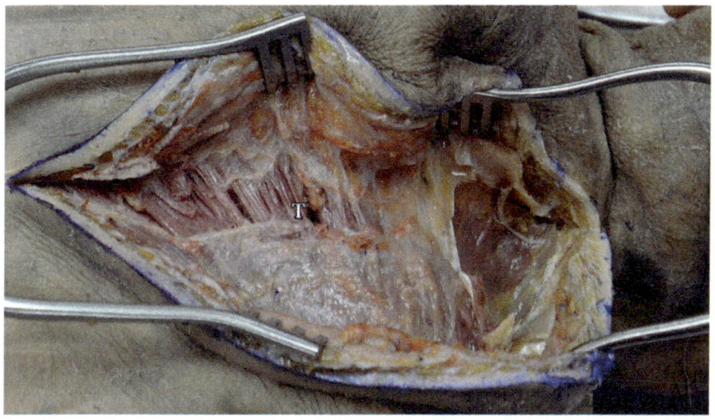

Fig. 10.2 The trapezius (*T*) is exposed and incised

7. Using a periosteal elevator (Doyen), the first rib is dissected, taking care not to injure the neurovascular bundle caudally, the subclavian vessels cranially, or the parietal pleura deep to it.
8. The first rib is then resected using a rib cutter or Leksell rongeur.
9. This should allow exposure of the trunks.
10. These can be followed proximally to the individual spinal nerves forming the trunks, where a bony foraminot-

Supplementary Information The online version contains supplementary material available at https://doi.org/10.1007/978-3-031-73931-6_10.

A. S. Hanna (✉)
Department of Neurosurgery, University of Wisconsin School of Medicine and Public Health, Madison, WI, USA

M. E. Ehlers
Urology, Aurora Health Care Medical Group, Milwaukee, WI, USA

A. S. Hanna (ed.), *Nerves: Anatomy, Exposures, and Techniques*, https://doi.org/10.1007/978-3-031-73931-6_10

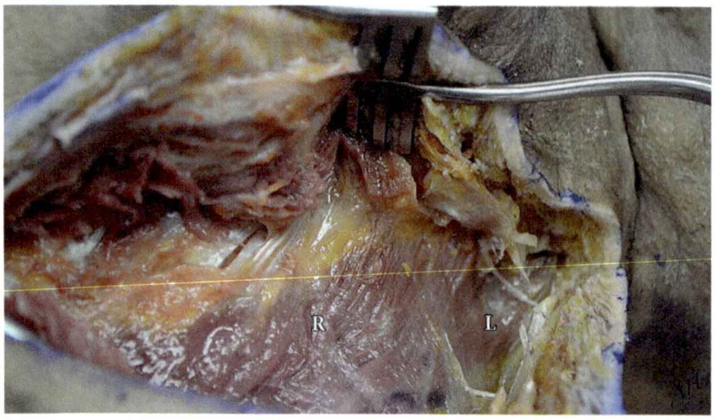

Fig. 10.3 The rhomboids (*R*) and levator scapulae (*L*) are exposed and incised

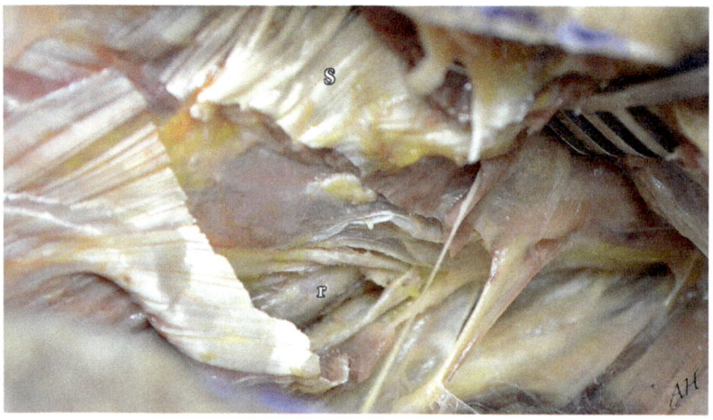

Fig. 10.4 The serratus posterior superior (*S*) is exposed and incised, thus exposing the ribs (*r*). The second rib is where scalenus posterior inserts, the first rib is more cranial and deeper than second rib

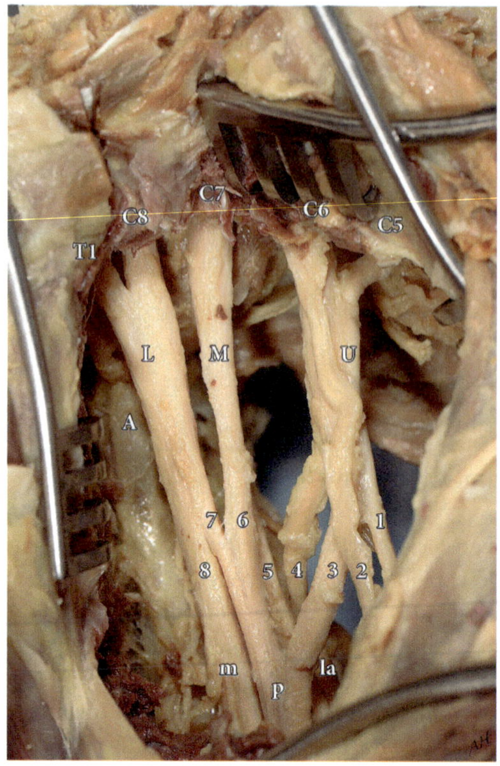

Fig. 10.5 Posterior view of the brachial plexus after resection of the first rib, posterior and middle scalenes. *U* upper (superior) trunk, *M* middle trunk, *L* lower (inferior) trunk, *A* subclavian artery, *la* lateral cord, *p* posterior cord, *m* medial cord, *1* suprascapular nerve, *2* long thoracic nerve, *3* upper trunk—posterior division, *4* upper trunk—anterior division, *5* middle trunk—anterior division, *6* middle trunk—posterior division, *7* lower trunk—posterior division, *8* lower trunk—anterior division

omy can be performed using Kerrison rongeurs. Venous bleeding is usually encountered in the foramen and can easily be tamponade with Gelfoam and thrombin.

11. The trunks can be followed distally to divisions (Fig. 10.5).
12. The suprascapular nerve can be identified coming off the upper trunk going toward the suprascapular notch.
13. The long thoracic nerve arises from the posterior aspect of the ventral rami of C5, 6, and occasionally 7, within scalenus medius, and travels toward the serratus anterior's outer surface.
14. The spinal accessory nerve can be found on the undersurface of the trapezius muscle at the superior angle of the scapula. It can be confirmed by electrical stimulation.
15. Variation: Alternatively, a horizontal incision is made above the spine of the scapula with a muscle splitting approach [2]. This is a less morbid procedure. However, care must be taken not to injure the spinal accessory nerve, which courses vertically at the superior angle of the scapula, deep to the trapezius (Fig. 10.6).

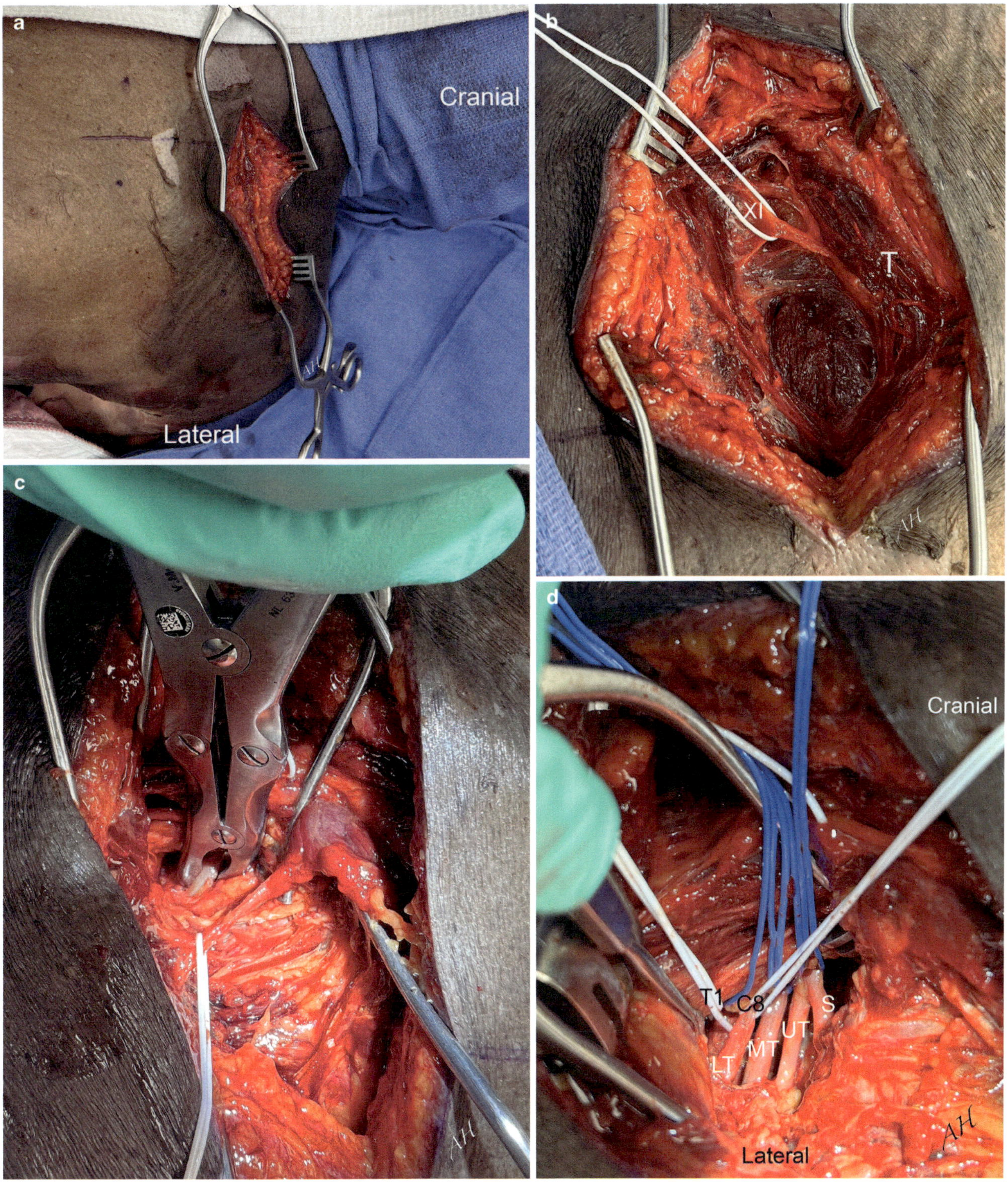

Fig. 10.6 Posterior exposure of the brachial plexus through a horizontal incision. (**a**) A horizontal incision is made cranial to the spine of the scapula. (**b**) The trapezius (*T*) is split along its fibers; care is taken not to injure the spinal accessory nerve (*white loop*, *XI*). (**c**) Once the first rib is exposed, a bone-biting forceps (Leksell rongeur) is used to resect the first rib. (**d**) Brachial plexus posterior view. *S* suprascapular nerve, *UT* upper (superior) trunk, *MT* middle trunk, *C8* and *T1* (*white loops*) form the lower (inferior) trunk (*LT*)

Complications

1. Pneumothorax.
2. Injury to the neurovascular bundle under the first rib.
3. Inadvertent resection of second rib (wrong level).
4. Vertebral artery injury.
5. Subclavian artery injury.
6. Wound infection.
7. Iatrogenic nerve injury.

References

1. Hager S, Backus TC, Futterman B, Solounias N, Mihlbachler MC (2014) Posterior subscapular dissection: an improved approach to the brachial plexus for human anatomy students. Ann Anat 196(2–3):88–91. https://doi.org/10.1016/j.aanat.2014.02.006
2. Aghayev K, Ciklatekerlio O (2018) Posterior upper rib excision for neurogenic thoracic outlet syndrome—feasibility and early outcomes. Oper Neurosurg (Hagerstown) 14(5):532–537. https://doi.org/10.1093/ons/opx143

Dorsal Scapular Nerve: Nervus Dorsalis Scapulae

11

Manuel Llusa-Pérez, Pablo Martínez-Collado, Marta Pérez-Montoya, Anton Fornieles-Espinel, and M. Rosa Morro-Martí

Indications

- Nerve sheath tumors, such as schwannomas and neurofibromas.
- Traumatic neuroma. Figure 11.1 shows a patient who had a neuroma resected from the distal portion of the nerve through a limited approach.
- Brachial plexitis (Parsonage–Turner syndrome). For nerve transfer.
- Scapula alata (winged scapula).
- Compression of the nerve in the minor interscalene triangle.
- Iatrogenic lesions such as the resection of the first rib or a cervical rib.
- Nerve transfer donor for upper brachial plexus injury.

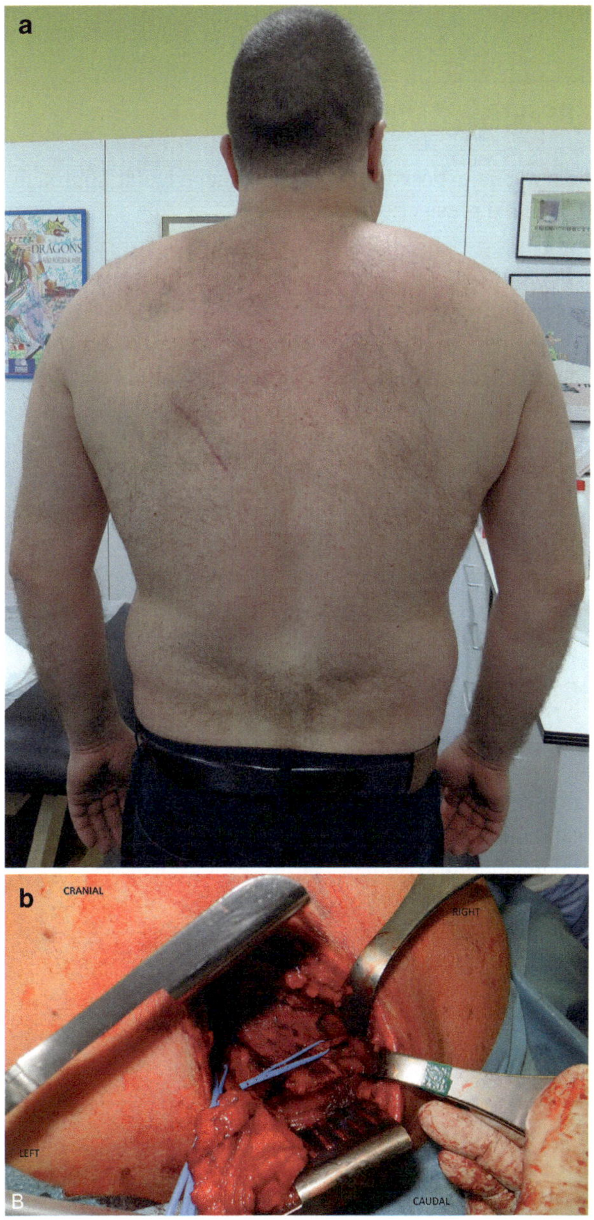

Fig. 11.1 Surgical exposure of the dorsal scapular nerve in its distal portion for neuroma resection. (**a**) Skin incision, left posterior thoracic region. (**b**) The nerve is exposed (blue loop, right)

Supplementary Information The online version contains supplementary material available at https://doi.org/10.1007/978-3-031-73931-6_11.

M. Llusa-Pérez · P. Martínez-Collado · A. Fornieles-Espinel
M. R. Morro-Martí (✉)
Department of Human Anatomy, University of Barcelona Medical School, Barcelona, Spain

Department of Orthopaedic Surgery and Traumatology, Vall d'Hebron Hospital, Barcelona, Spain
e-mail: mllusa@ub.edu; mrmorro@ub.edu

M. Pérez-Montoya
Department of Human Anatomy, University of Barcelona Medical School, Barcelona, Spain

Orthopaedic Surgery and Traumatology, Asepeyo Hospital, Sant Cugat del Vallès, Spain
e-mail: mperezmontoya@asepeyo.es

A. S. Hanna (ed.), *Nerves: Anatomy, Exposures, and Techniques*, https://doi.org/10.1007/978-3-031-73931-6_11

Surgical Anatomy

The dorsal scapular nerve is formed by small branches coming off the posterior aspect of C4 and C5; occasionally, C6 also participates. Its origin is within the substance of the scalenus medius. The anatomical pathway of the nerve is between the scalenus medius and posterior in the minor interscalene triangle. It descends obliquely in a posterolateral direction behind the first digitation of the serratus anterior muscle. From here, it goes posterolateral under and supplies the levator scapulae and the minor and major rhomboid muscles. In some preganglionic brachial plexus lesions, the nerve can still be functional because of C4 contribution [1].

Exposure

The nerve is exposed through a supraclavicular approach to the brachial plexus [2].

1. Position: supine, with the back of the table up and the head turned contralaterally.
2. Incision: L-shaped, following the posterior border of the sternocleidomastoideus and the inferior border of the clavicle. A limited transverse incision over the posterior triangle of the neck is also possible.
3. The skin flap is elevated including the subcutaneous fat and platysma, taking care not to lesion the vena jugularis externa, which can be ligated if necessary. Care must be taken to preserve the spinal accessory nerve at the anterior border of the trapezius (Fig. 11.2).
4. Identify the omohyoideus and pass a rubber band underneath to help retracting it. This approach takes place in the omotrapezius triangle (posterior to the omohyoid muscle).
5. Underneath the fat pad, the arteria transversa cervicis runs transversely over the brachial plexus in the supraclavicular area. It is ligated and sectioned.
6. Open the fascia covering the anterior interscalene triangle, taking special care not to lesion the phrenic nerve found underneath the fascia of the m. scalenus anterior in an oblique direction from lateral and cranial to medial and caudal.
7. Between the scalenus anterior and scalenus medius is located the superior trunk of the brachial plexus (Fig. 11.3).
8. Following the superior trunk proximally, C5 and C6 can be identified. In their posterior part, we can see the origin of the nervus dorsalis scapulae, which perforates the scalenus medius and travels distally between this muscle and the scalenus posterior (minor interscalene triangle) with the long thoracic nerve (Fig. 11.3). A nerve stimulator could be useful to localize the nerve [3].
9. Distally, the nervus dorsalis scapulae winds around the scalenus posterior and then travels deep to the levator scapulae which it innervates to join the deep branch of the transverse cervical artery along the medial border of the scapula to finally end in the rhomboideus minor and major [4] (Fig. 11.4).

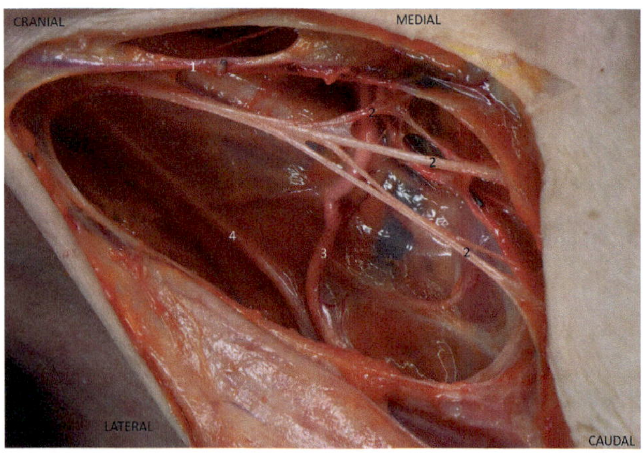

Fig. 11.2 Exposure of the right brachial plexus through a supraclavicular approach in an anatomical specimen. The jugular vein (*1*) is seen in the anterior aspect of the approach. The supraclavicular nerves (*2*) are found in a very superficial layer which should be preserved if possible. The transverse superficial cervical artery (*3*) (injected with red latex) is seen in a deeper layer and is used as a landmark. *4* spinal accessory nerve

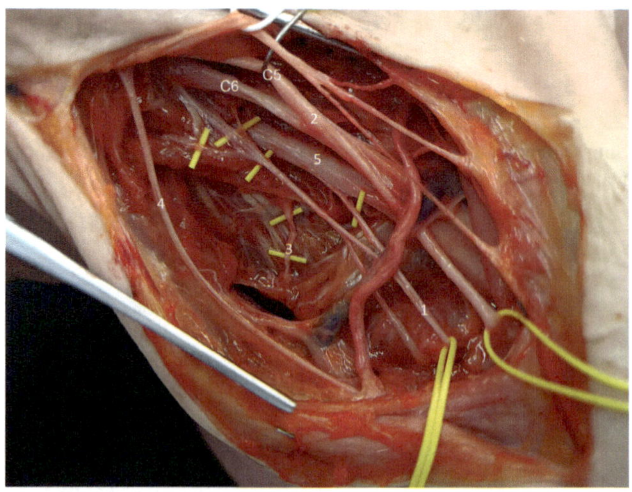

Fig. 11.3 Deep layer of the exposure of the brachial plexus through a supraclavicular approach in an anatomical specimen. The formation of the long thoracic nerve (*1*) can be seen in the posterior aspect of the superior trunk (*2*). The dorsal scapular nerve (*3*) is seen exiting through the posterior scalenus muscle. *4* spinal accessory nerve, *5* middle trunk

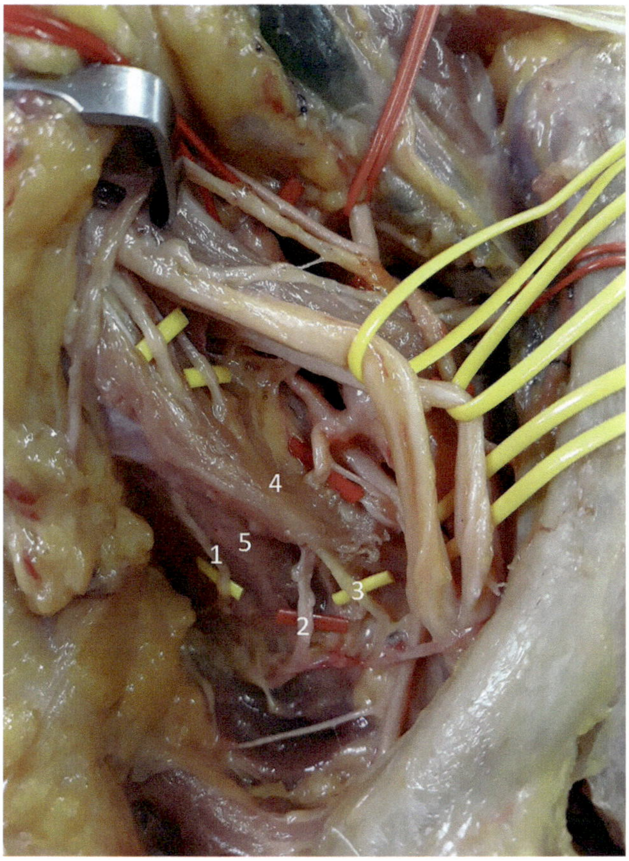

Fig. 11.4 The nervus dorsalis scapulae (*1*) and the deep branch of the transverse cervical artery (*2*) get to the medial border of the scapula. *3* long thoracic nerve, *4* middle scalene, *5* posterior scalene

Complications

1. Iatrogenic nerve injury: spinal accessory nerve or long thoracic nerve.
2. Vascular injury: transversa cervicis vessels (their superficial branch) superficially and transversa cervicis profunda or dorsalis scapulae vessels deeply.
3. Pneumothorax is also possible, although rare.

References

1. Llusa M, Palazzi S, Valer A (2013) Anatomía quirúrgica del plexo braquial y de los nervios periféricos de la extremidad superior. Médica Panamericana SA, Madrid
2. Hanna AS (2015) Anatomy and exposures of spinal nerves. Springer, Switzerland
3. Sunderland S (1972) Nerves and nerve injuries. Churchill Livingstone, Edinburgh
4. Frank DK, Wenk E, Stern JC, Gottlieb RD, Mostaello AL (1997) A cadaveric study of the motor nerves to the levator scapulae muscle. Otolaryngol Head Neck Surg 117:671–680. https://doi.org/10.1016/S0194-59989770051-2

12 Pectoral Nerves: Nervus Pectoralis Medialis and Lateralis

M. Rosa Morro-Martí, Joaquim Casañas-Sintes, Júlia Flores-Benítez, Pablo Martínez-Collado, and Manuel Llusa-Pérez

Indications

- Nerve transfer from either of these nerves, typically medial pectoral, to an anterior terminal branch of the brachial plexus such as the median or musculocutaneous nerve (Figs. 12.1, 12.2, and 12.3).
- Nerve sheath tumors such as schwannomas and neurofibromas.

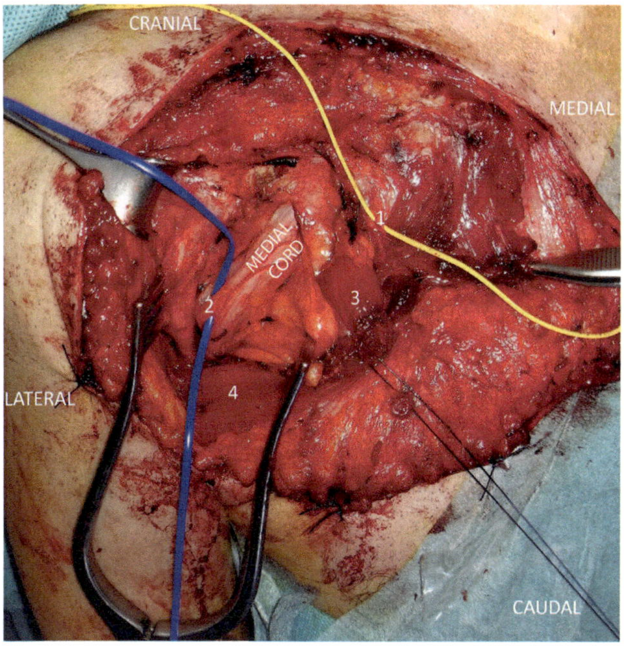

Fig. 12.1 Surgical exposure of the right lateral pectoral nerve (*1*) marked with a yellow rubber band through a deltopectoral approach. The anterior terminal branches of the brachial plexus are seen and marked with a blue rubber band. *2* median nerve, *3* pectoralis minor sectioned and retracted distally, *4* pectoralis major retracted distally

Supplementary Information The online version contains supplementary material available at https://doi.org/10.1007/978-3-031-73931-6_12.

M. R. Morro-Martí · P. Martínez-Collado · M. Llusa-Pérez (✉)
Department of Human Anatomy, University of Barcelona Medical School, Barcelona, Spain

Department of Orthopaedic Surgery and Traumatology, Vall d'Hebron Hospital, Barcelona, Spain
e-mail: mrmorro@ub.edu; mllusa@ub.edu

J. Casañas-Sintes
Teknon Hospital, Barcelona, Spain

Orthopaedic Surgery and Traumatology, Bellvitge Hospital, Barcelona, Spain

J. Flores-Benítez
Department of Human Anatomy, University of Barcelona Medical School, Barcelona, Spain

Orthopaedic Surgery and Traumatology, Bellvitge Hospital, Barcelona, Spain

A. S. Hanna (ed.), *Nerves: Anatomy, Exposures, and Techniques*, https://doi.org/10.1007/978-3-031-73931-6_12

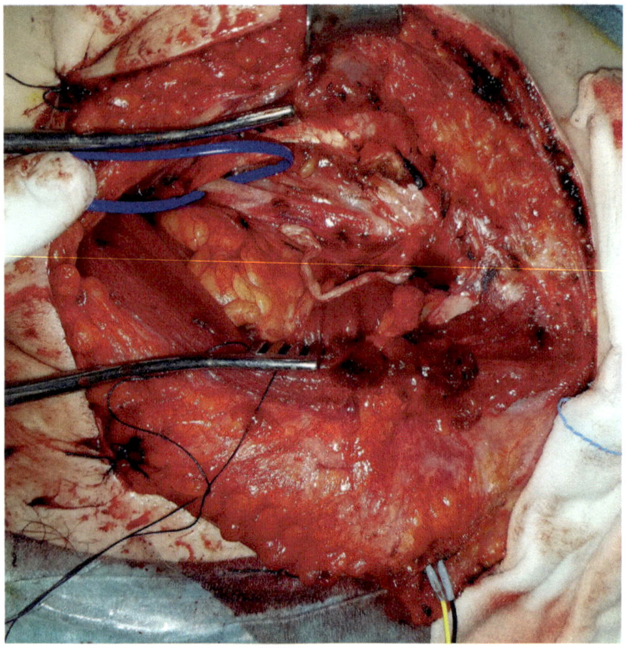

Fig. 12.2 Transfer of the lateral pectoral nerve to the median nerve. Note that there must be no tension on the transfer to ensure a full range of motion of the head and neck

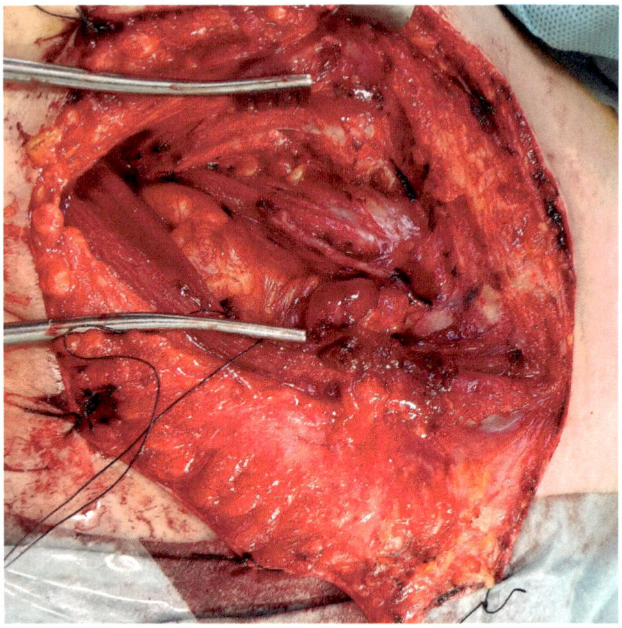

Fig. 12.3 An end-to-side suture of the lateral pectoral nerve to the median nerve

Surgical Anatomy

The nervus pectoralis lateralis originates from the anterior part of the lateral cord (fascicle), at the first portion of the axillary artery. It gives off a superior branch which perforates the clavipectoral fascia to get to the clavicular head of pectoralis major. The inferior branch joins the nervus pectoralis medialis forming the pectoral handle or ansa pectoralis [1, 2].

The n. pectoralis medialis originates from the anterior aspect of the medial cord (fascicle) at the level of the first portion of the axillary artery, located behind it. It curves around the artery passing between it and the axillary vein and joins the n. pectoralis lateralis forming the ansa pectoralis found in front of the second portion of the axillary artery, underneath the pectoralis minor muscle. The ansa pectoralis gives off several branches coming from the n. pectoralis medialis to innervate pectoralis minor, and some of them pass through it to reach the sternocostal head of pectoralis major [3] (Fig. 12.4).

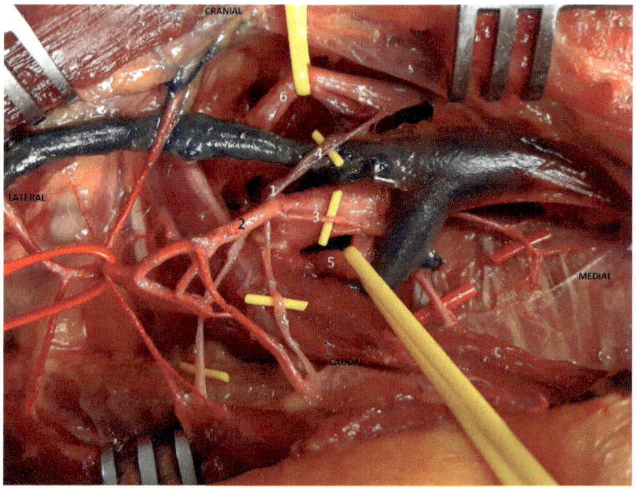

Fig. 12.4 Anatomical dissection of the right ansa pectoralis (*1*) formed around the thoracoacromial artery (*2*) by the medial (*3*) and lateral (*4*) pectoral nerves. Note the origin of the medial pectoral nerve from the medial cord (*5*) and the lateral pectoral nerve from the lateral cord (*6*)

Exposure

These nerves are exposed through an infraclavicular approach to the brachial plexus, in the clavicoracopectoral space through a deltopectoral approach.

1. Position: supine, occasionally with the back of the table up and the head turned contralaterally.
2. Incision: in the deltopectoral groove extended proximally over the clavicle (Fig. 12.5).
3. Two skin flaps are elevated including the subcutaneous fat and the deep fascia.
4. The cephalic vein is localized in the fat between the deltoid laterally and the pectoralis major medially. It can be retracted laterally with the deltoid or ligated if necessary.
5. Proceeding medially and deeper in this space, the branches of the thoracoacromial arterial trunk are found. Following them medially, they will bring us to the clavicoracopectoral space (Fig. 12.6).
6. For better access, partial deinsertion of the clavicular portion of the pectoralis major can be performed. If a wider exposure is necessary, a tenotomy of the pectoralis major can be performed, leaving 1–2 cm of tendon in the humerus to reattach at the end of the surgery. Now, the pectoralis major can be retracted medially, but care must be taken not to avulse the branches of the pectoral nerves to the pectoralis major.
7. The pectoralis minor tendon is sectioned near the coracoid process to allow the dissection of the clavipectoral fascia to localize the thoracoacromial vessels and the pectoralis lateralis nerve.
8. Dissection of the axillary vessels and their branches is very tedious as the axillary vein is easily injured since it is found anterior to the rest of the structures. The medial pectoral nerve is hidden by the axillary vein and passes between the axillary vein and artery to connect with the lateral pectoral nerve and forming the ansa pectoralis (Fig. 12.7). A nerve stimulator could be useful to localize the nerves and distinguish one nerve from the other and which portion of the muscle innervates.
9. The thoracoacromial artery is a key point at this level as it is easily recognized coming off the axillary artery in an anterior direction. Around this artery, the pectoral handle is found.
10. The lateral pectoral nerve gives off one or more branches which perforate the clavipectoral fascia to supply the clavicular portion of pectoralis major. The medial pectoral nerve gives off several branches to innervate pectoralis minor, and some of them pass through it to supply the sternocostal head of pectoralis major. Note that the lateral pectoral nerve is located medially in the axilla but carries the name of the cord it originates from, similarly, the medial pectoral nerve is located laterally but carries the name of its parent cord.

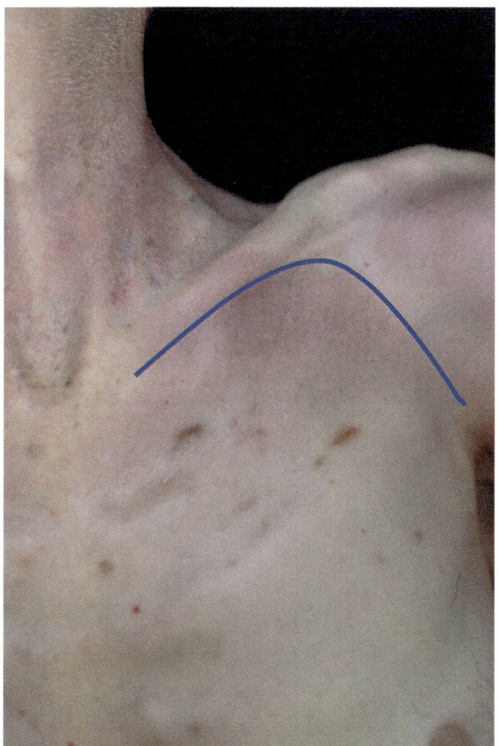

Fig. 12.5 Skin incision of the deltopectoral approach used to expose the pectoral nerves

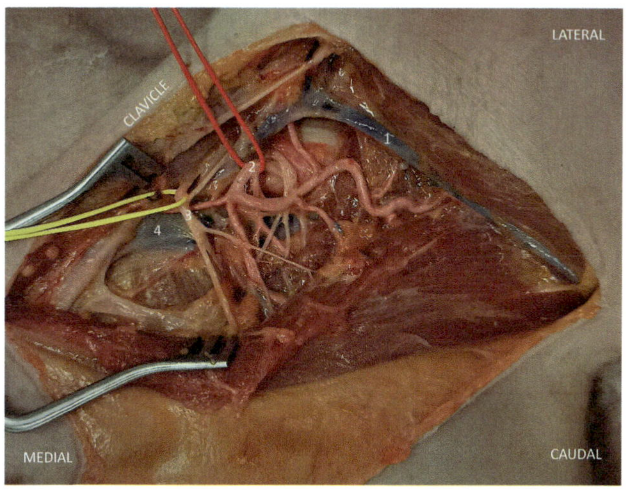

Fig. 12.6 Exposure of the pectoral nerves through a left deltopectoral approach in an anatomical specimen. The cephalic vein (*1*) has been retracted laterally with the deltoid so that the deeper layer can be exposed. The thoracoacromial artery (*2*), marked with a red rubber band, is used as a landmark as it has a very typical and unique pathway coming off the axillary artery in an anterior direction. The lateral pectoral nerve (*3*) is marked with a yellow rubber band. *4* axillary vein

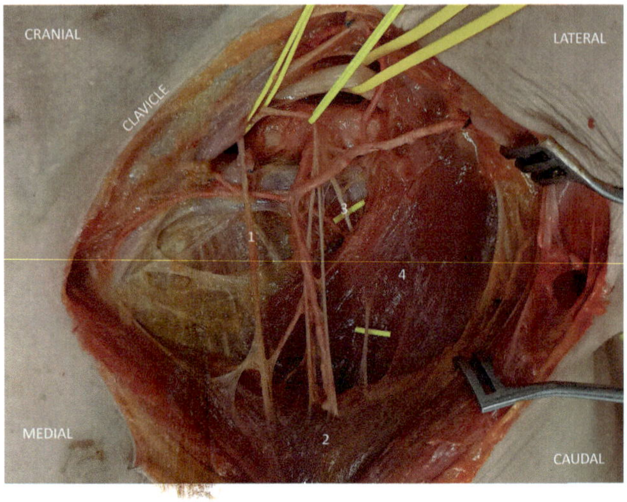

Fig. 12.7 A wider exposure of the pectoral nerves through a deltopectoral approach in an anatomical specimen. The different branches of the lateral pectoral nerve (*1*) can be seen innervating pectoralis major (*2*) and a branch of the medial pectoral nerve (*3*) perforating pectoralis minor (*4*) to reach pectoralis major

Complications

1. Partial denervation of the pectoralis major or minor muscles.
2. Injury to the lateral or medial cords.
3. Major bleeding from the axillary vessels or their branches/tributaries.
4. Minor bleeding from cephalic vein or thoracoacromial vessels.

References

1. Llusa M, Palazzi S, Valer A (2013) Anatomía quirúrgica del plexo braquial y de los nervios periféricos de la extremidad superior. Médica Panamericana SA, Madrid
2. Hanna AS (2015) Anatomy and exposures of spinal nerves. Springer, Switzerland
3. Aszmann OC, Rab M, Kamolz L, Frey M (2000) The anatomy of the pectoral nerves and their significance in brachial plexus reconstruction. J Hand Surg Am 25:942–947. https://doi.org/10.1053/jhsu.2000.17818

Subscapular Nerves: Nervi Subscapulares

13

Manuel Llusa-Pérez, Joaquim Casañas-Sintes, Pablo Martínez-Collado, and M. Rosa Morro-Martí

Indications

- Nerve sheath tumors such as schwannomas and neurofibromas.
- Brachial plexitis (Parsonage–Turner syndrome); for nerve transfer.
- Nerve transfer of one of these nerves to the axillary or long thoracic nerve (Fig. 13.1) in lesions of the latter or in brachial plexus injuries.

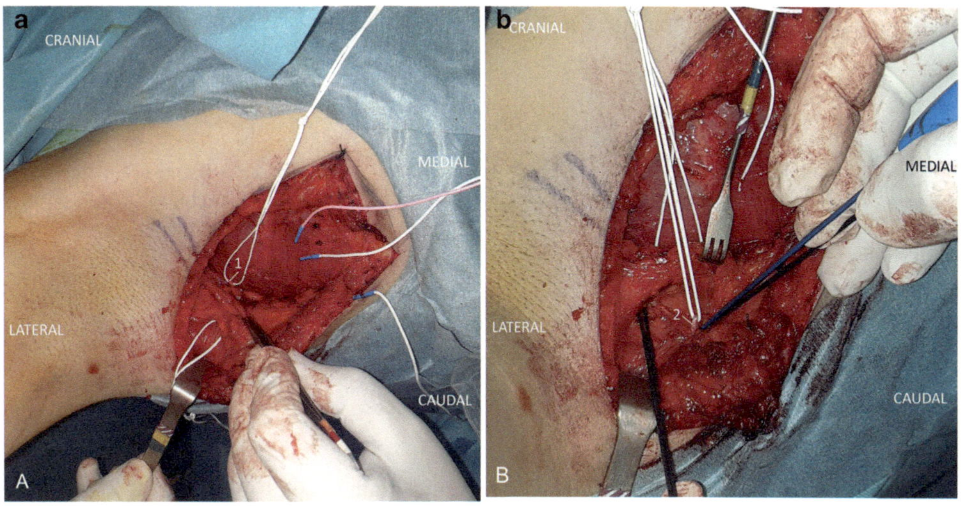

Fig. 13.1 Lower subscapular to long thoracic nerve transfer on a right upper extremity in a lateral decubitus position. Intraoperative recordings used to localize the nerves, the pink and white needles are in teres major. (**a**) Surgical approach to the distal portion of the subscapular nerves (*1*). (**b**) Localization and dissection of the long thoracic nerve (*2*)

Supplementary Information The online version contains supplementary material available at https://doi.org/10.1007/978-3-031-73931-6_13.

M. Llusa-Pérez · P. Martínez-Collado · M. R. Morro-Martí (✉)
Department of Human Anatomy, University of Barcelona Medical School, Barcelona, Spain

Department of Orthopaedic Surgery and Traumatology, Vall d'Hebron Hospital, Barcelona, Spain
e-mail: mllusa@ub.edu; mrmorro@ub.edu

J. Casañas-Sintes
Teknon Hospital, Barcelona, Spain

Orthopaedic Surgery and Traumatology, Bellvitge Hospital, Barcelona, Spain

A. S. Hanna (ed.), *Nerves: Anatomy, Exposures, and Techniques*, https://doi.org/10.1007/978-3-031-73931-6_13

Surgical Anatomy

The posterior branches of the infraclavicular plexus include the upper and lower subscapular nerves and the thoracodorsal nerve, they arise from the posterior cord (fasciculus posterior), occasionally from the axillary nerve. The subscapular nerves are two, one proximal and one distal; the thoracodorsal nerve is located in between the two [1, 2]. The upper subscapular nerve lies on and supplies the subscapularis, whereas the lower subscapular nerve is directed vertically to innervate the inferior aspect of the subscapularis and teres major.

The thoracodorsal nerve arises between the two subscapular nerves and proceeds distally over the subscapularis, along with the thoracodorsal artery. It finally reaches and supplies the latissimus dorsi. It is the biggest of the posterior branches at this level [3, 4].

Exposure

The subscapular nerves are exposed through an infraclavicular approach to the brachial plexus, extended to the deltopectoral space.

1. Position: supine, with the upper extremity free for movement.
2. Incision: infraclavicular approach to the brachial plexus extended to the deltopectoral groove.
3. Two skin flaps are elevated, including the subcutaneous fat and the deep fascia.
4. The cephalic vein is localized in the fat found between the deltoid laterally and the pectoralis major medially. It can be ligated or retracted laterally with the deltoid muscle.
5. Proceeding deeper in this space, the main elements of the infraclavicular plexus and axillary vessels are found (Fig. 13.2).
6. Deinsertion of the clavicular portion of the pectoralis major gives access to the infraclavicular plexus and axillary vessels. To have a wider exposure, a tenotomy of the pectoralis major can be performed, leaving 1–2 cm of tendon on the humerus to reattach at the end of surgery. Now, the pectoralis major can be retracted medially, but care must be taken not to lesion the branches of the pectoral nerves to the pectoralis major.

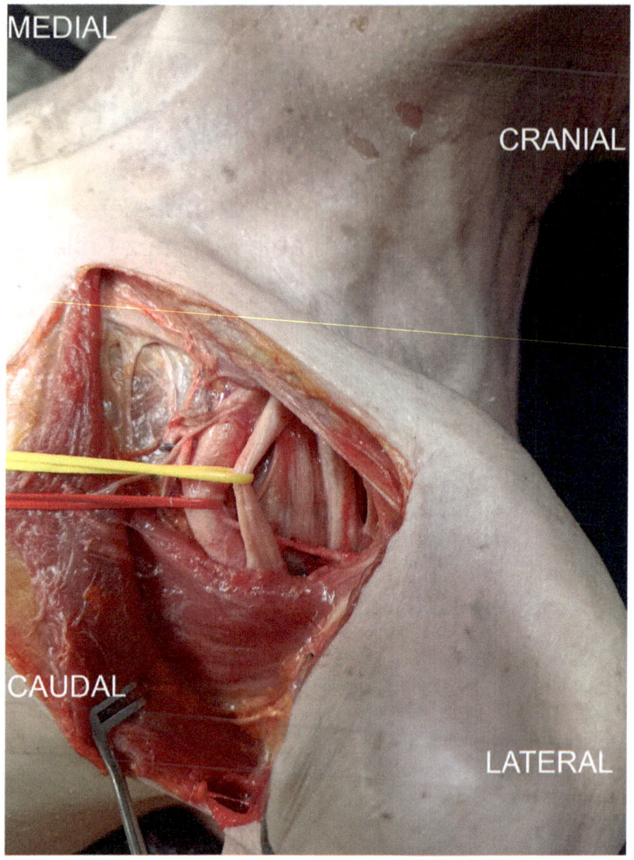

Fig. 13.2 Exposure of the infraclavicular brachial plexus in an anatomical specimen. Identification of the axillary artery marked with a red rubber band and its branches retracted medially and distally. Identification of the lateral cord of the brachial plexus marked with a yellow rubber band also retracted medially and distally

7. It could be necessary to section the pectoralis minor tendon near the coracoid process to allow the dissection of the clavipectoral fascia.
8. Retracting the axillary vessels and the lateral cord anteriorly and inferiorly, the posterior cord (posterior fascicle) can be reached avoiding the tedious dissection of the axillary artery and vein (Figs. 13.3 and 13.4). This maneuver gives a cranial access to the posterior cord, avoiding all the vascular and neural anterior structures.
9. In the posterior aspect of the posterior cord (occasionally, they can come from the axillary nerve) can be found the nervus subscapularis superior, nervus thoracodorsalis, and nervus subscapularis inferior [5] (Figs. 13.5 and 13.6). A nerve stimulator could be useful to localize the nerves.

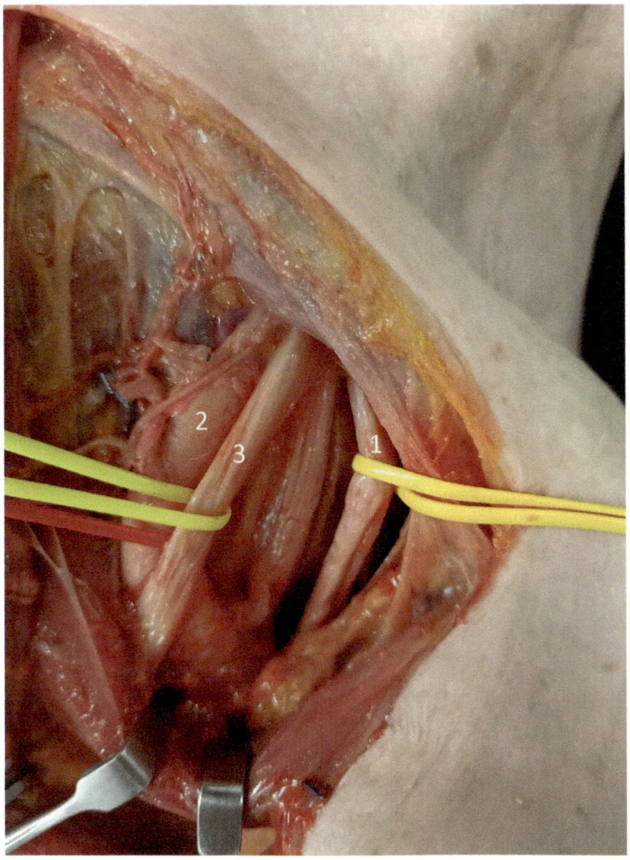

Fig. 13.3 Exposure of the infraclavicular brachial plexus in an anatomical specimen. Identification of the posterior cord (fasciculus posterior, *1*) of the brachial plexus by retracting inferomedially the axillary artery (*2*) and the lateral cord (*3*)

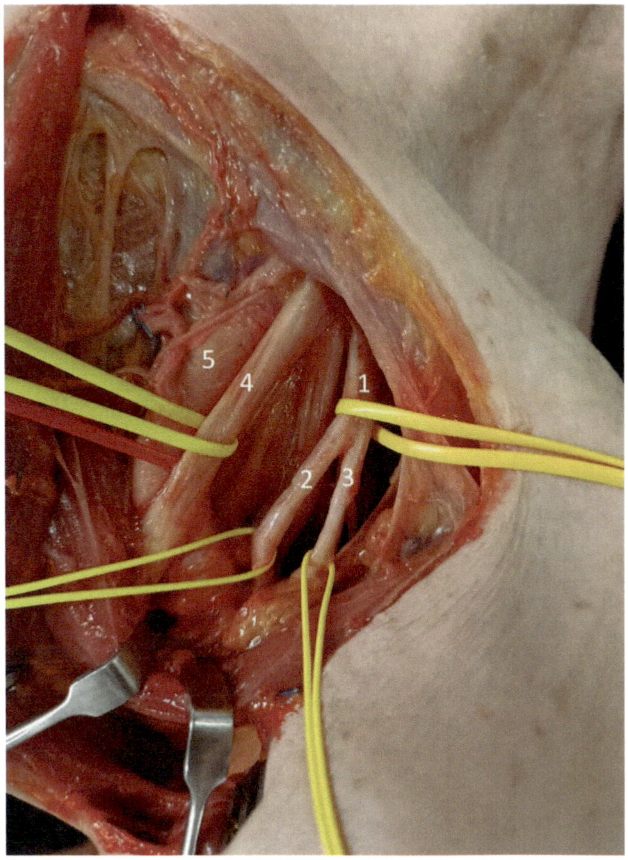

Fig. 13.4 Exposure of the infraclavicular brachial plexus in an anatomical specimen. Identification of the terminal branches of the posterior cord (*1*) of the brachial plexus: the radial (*2*) and axillary (*3*) nerves. The radial nerve is thicker and more medial, and the axillary nerve is thinner and more lateral. *4* lateral cord (fascicle), *5* axillary artery

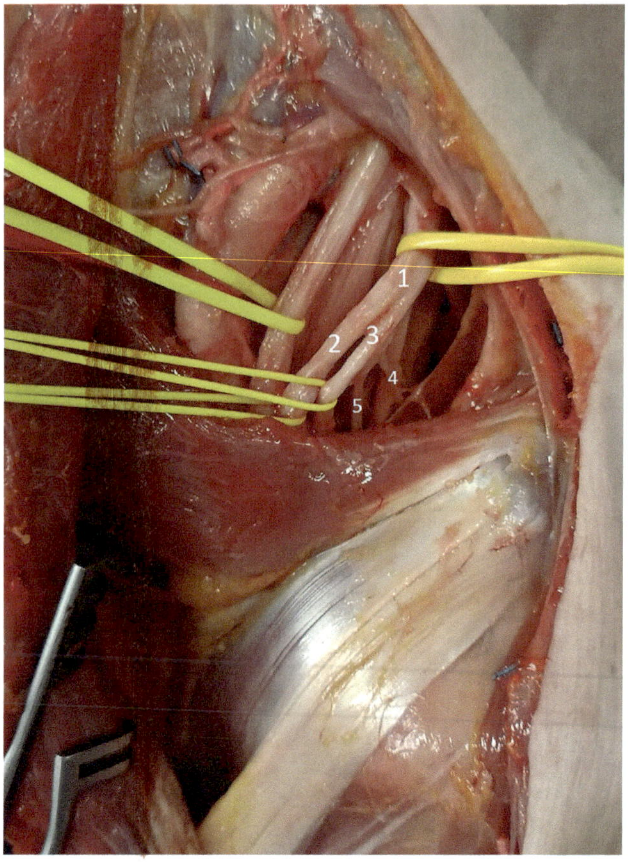

Fig. 13.5 Exposure of the infraclavicular brachial plexus in an anatomical specimen. The posterior cord (*1*) of the brachial plexus divides into the radial (*2*) and axillary (*3*) nerves. Coming off the posterior aspect of the posterior cord or the axillary nerve (as in this case), the thoracodorsal (*4*) and lower subscapular (*5*) nerves are found

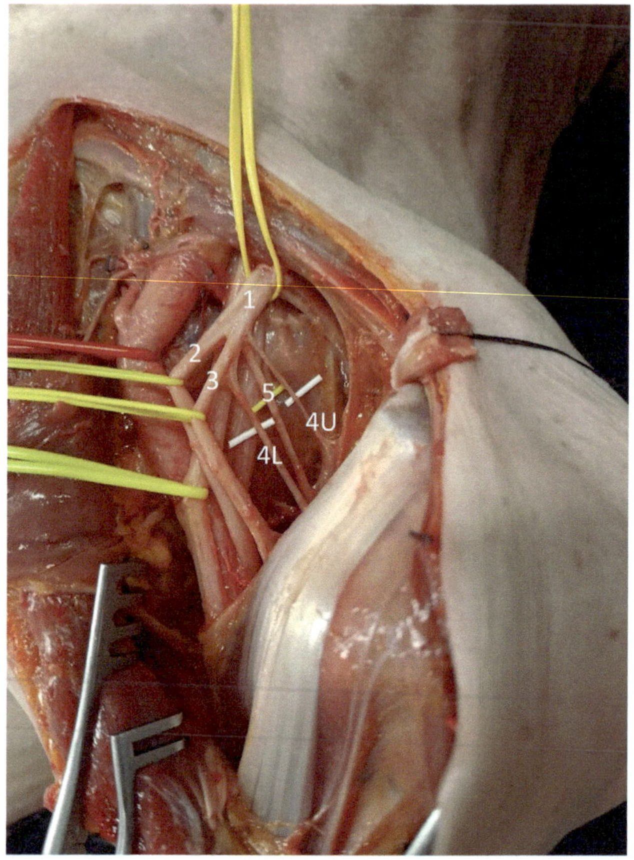

Fig. 13.6 Anatomical dissection of the posterior cord (*1*) and its divisions, radial (*2*) and axillary (*3*) nerves. Identification of the upper subscapular nerve (*4U*), lower subscapular nerve (*4L*) (white rubber bands), and the thoracodorsal nerve (*5*) (yellow rubber band) in between

Alternatively, a limited approach to the lower part of the lower subscapular nerve can be achieved through an axillary incision used, for instance, for a nerve transfer of the teres major branch to the axillary nerve or the long thoracic nerve (Fig. 13.1).

Complications

1. Major bleeding from the axillary vessels.
2. Minor bleeding from cephalic vein or thoracoacromial vessels.
3. Lesion of the lateral or medial cords and their branches.
4. Lesion of the posterior cord and its branches, especially the axillary nerve.
5. Lesion of the long thoracic nerve.
6. Special attention to the branch of the thoracodorsal nerve for the latissimus dorsi.

References

1. Llusa M, Palazzi S, Valer A (2013) Anatomía quirúrgica del plexo braquial y de los nervios periféricos de la extremidad superior. Médica Panamericana SA, Madrid
2. Hanna AS (2015) Anatomy and exposures of spinal nerves. Springer, Switzerland
3. Kim DI, Lee KS, Kim HJ, Chae HK, Yu KH (2008) The spinal root origins and clinical implications of the lower subscapular nerve. Clin Anat 21:416–419. https://doi.org/10.1002/ca.20630
4. Chen LZ, Chen L, Zhu Y, Gu YD (2013) Semiquantifying of fascicles of the C7 spinal nerve in the upper and lower subscapular nerves innervating de subscapularis and its clinical inference in Erb's palsy. Clin Anat 26:470–475. https://doi.org/10.1002/ca.22064
5. Tubbs RS, Loukas M, Shahid K, Judge T, Pinyard J, Shoja MM et al (2007) Anatomy and quantitation of the subscapular nerves. Clin Anat 20:656–659. https://doi.org/10.1002/ca.20478

14 Axillary Nerve

Amgad S. Hanna

Surgical Anatomy

The axillary nerve (C5 and C6) comes off the posterior cord at the level of the coracoid process [1]. Fibers originate mainly from the posterior division of the upper trunk. It lies posterior to the axillary artery and then the musculocutaneous nerve. It leaves the axilla to enter the posterior aspect of the upper arm through the quadrangular space, accompanied by the posterior circumflex humeral vessels. The quadrangular space is bound by subscapularis and teres minor superiorly, teres major inferiorly, long head of triceps medially, and humerus laterally. Teres major separates the axillary nerve from the radial nerve. The axillary nerve supplies teres minor and deltoid. It has anterior and posterior divisions, the anterior division is deeper and in closer relationship to the humerus. The posterior division gives off the upper lateral cutaneous nerve of the arm.

Clinical Significance

The axillary nerve is frequently injured with shoulder dislocations or humeral neck fractures. This causes inability to abduct the arm. The axillary nerve may be surgically exposed as a recipient in radial to axillary nerve transfers (Chap. 32) or a donor for spinal cord injury to neurotize the triceps (Chap. 60).

Supplementary Information The online version contains supplementary material available at https://doi.org/10.1007/978-3-031-73931-6_14.

A. S. Hanna (✉)
Department of Neurosurgery, University of Wisconsin School of Medicine and Public Health, Madison, WI, USA

Exposure

Anterior Approach

1. Infraclavicular exposure, as in Chap. 8.
2. The axillary nerve comes off the posterior cord at the level of the coracoid process (Fig. 14.1). It is lateral in relation to the radial nerve.
3. Followed laterally, it enters the quadrangular space with the posterior circumflex humeral vessels.
4. The axillary nerve then enters the posterior aspect of the arm.

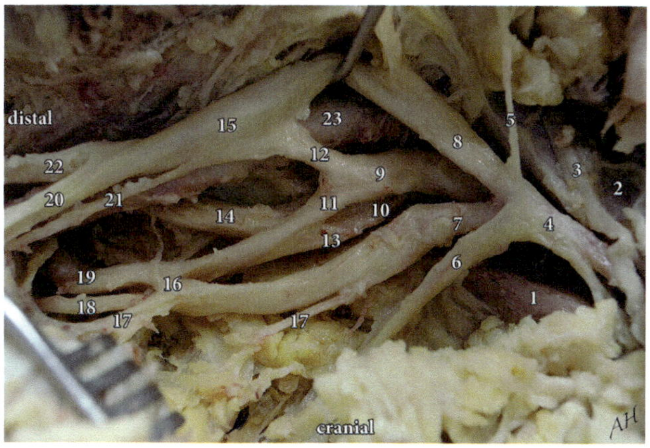

Fig. 14.1 Origins of the axillary and radial nerves from the posterior cord (fasciculus posterior) of the left brachial plexus. *1* scalenus medius, *2* scalenus anterior, *3* phrenic nerve, *4* upper (superior) trunk, *5* nerve to subclavius, *6* suprascapular nerve, *7* upper trunk—posterior division, *8* upper trunk—anterior division, *9* middle trunk, *10* lower (inferior) trunk, *11* middle trunk—posterior division, *12* middle trunk—anterior division, *13* lower trunk—posterior division, *14* lower trunk—anterior division → medial cord, *15* lateral cord, *16* posterior cord, *17* upper and lower subscapular nerves, *18* axillary nerve, *19* radial nerve, *20* musculocutaneous nerve, *21* early coracobrachialis branch, *22* median nerve—lateral contribution

A. S. Hanna (ed.), *Nerves: Anatomy, Exposures, and Techniques*, https://doi.org/10.1007/978-3-031-73931-6_14

Posterior Approach

1. The patient can be positioned supine with a bump under the shoulder, lateral, or prone.
2. Incision along the posterior border of the deltoid muscle extends halfway through the posterior aspect of the arm in the direction of the olecranon (Fig. 14.2a).
3. The incision is deepened through the superficial and deep fasciae.
4. The posterior border of the deltoid is identified with the cutaneous branch winding around it from deep to superficial.
5. This branch is important to identify. It is then followed deeply under the deltoid to find its origin from the posterior division of the axillary nerve.
6. The posterior division can be followed proximally to find the main stem of the axillary nerve coming out of the quadrangular space and giving off also the anterior division after a very short course and a branch to teres minor (typically from posterior division) (Fig. 14.2b).

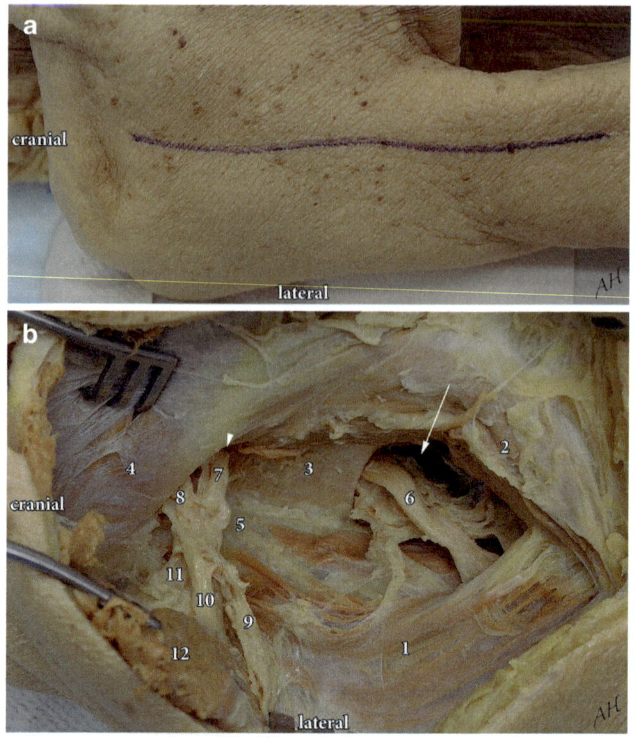

Fig. 14.2 Left axillary and radial nerve exposure in the posterior arm. (**a**) Position: prone, lateral, or supine with a shoulder bump. Incision, along the posterior border of the deltoid, extends distally between the long and lateral heads of the triceps. (**b**) The radial nerve (*6*) is exposed between the lateral (*1*) and long (*2*) heads of the triceps and then followed proximally till the lower triangular space (triangular interval) (arrow). To expose the axillary nerve, one may first encounter the upper lateral cutaneous nerve of the arm (*9*) around the posterior border of the deltoid (*12*). Followed proximally, it will lead to the posterior division (*10*) of the axillary nerve, and this will lead to the main trunk of the axillary nerve (*7*) toward the quadrangular space (arrowhead). The anterior division (*11*) of the axillary nerve is deep toward the humerus (*5*). The teres minor (*4*) nerve (*8*) can also be dissected. Teres major (*3*) separates the radial nerve from the axillary nerve

Reference

1. Kang MS, Woo JS, Hur MS, Lee KS (2014) Spinal nerve compositions and innervations of the axillary nerve. Muscle Nerve 50(5):856–858. https://doi.org/10.1002/mus.24297. Epub 2014 Sep 24.

Radial Nerve

15

Amgad S. Hanna and Thomas M. Staniszewski

Surgical Anatomy

The radial nerve (C5, C6, C7, C8, and T1) arises from the posterior cord (fasciculus posterior) at the level of the coracoid process, posterior to the axillary artery and lateral cord. It exits the axilla toward the posterior arm through the lower triangular space (triangular interval) bound by the teres major cranially, the long head of triceps medially, and the humerus laterally. The triceps branches come off the radial nerve high in the axilla. The nerve then courses in the posterior arm, in the spiral groove along with the profunda brachii vessels. It then enters the anterior compartment of the arm between the biceps brachii and triceps and then between the biceps tendon and brachioradialis. It gives off the brachioradialis, extensor carpi radialis longus and brevis (ECRL and ECRB) branches. It then splits into deep and superficial radial nerves. The superficial radial nerve emerges from under the brachioradialis tendon and supplies the skin of the dorsum of the hand laterally as well as the lateral three-and-a-half fingers up to the middle phalanx. The deep radial nerve supplies the supinator muscle and then continues as the posterior interosseous nerve (PIN), passes deep to the supinator (arcade of Fröhse), and supplies the remaining muscles of the posterior forearm.

Clinical Significance

- Radial nerve injury in the spiral groove spares the triceps branches and results in wrist drop (Fig. 15.1). Sensory loss is limited to the skin overlying the anatomical snuffbox. Injury could occur with humeral shaft fractures or during their surgical repair (Fig. 15.1).
- PIN injury spares ECRL and ECRB branches resulting in wrist extension with radial deviation, finger drop, and no loss of cutaneous sensation. Compression can occur at the arcade of Fröhse [1] or the leash of Henry (vascular) [2]. Hanna et al. described the Window Test as a simple bedside test to detect the radial deviation of the wrist (Fig. 15.2) [3]. PIN palsy could also be inflammatory, like Parsonage–Turner syndrome.
- Wartenberg's disease (Cheiralgia paresthetica) is caused by compression of the superficial radial nerve in the lower forearm [4]. It can complicate the use of handcuffs (handcuff neuropathy).
- Radial tunnel syndrome causes pain along the lateral aspect of the elbow and can be hard to differentiate from lateral epicondylitis (tennis elbow) [5–7].
- The radial nerve can be used as a donor to neurotize the deltoid in the upper arm (Chap. 32) or AIN in the forearm (Chap. 35), or as a recipient in cervical spinal cord injury (teres minor to triceps, supinator to PIN) (Chap. 60).

Supplementary Information The online version contains supplementary material available at https://doi.org/10.1007/978-3-031-73931-6_15.

A. S. Hanna (✉)
Department of Neurosurgery, University of Wisconsin School of Medicine and Public Health, Madison, WI, USA

T. M. Staniszewski
Department of Neurological Surgery, University of Wisconsin School of Medicine and Public Health, Madison, WI, USA
e-mail: staniszewski@neurosurgery.wisc.edu

A. S. Hanna (ed.), *Nerves: Anatomy, Exposures, and Techniques*, https://doi.org/10.1007/978-3-031-73931-6_15

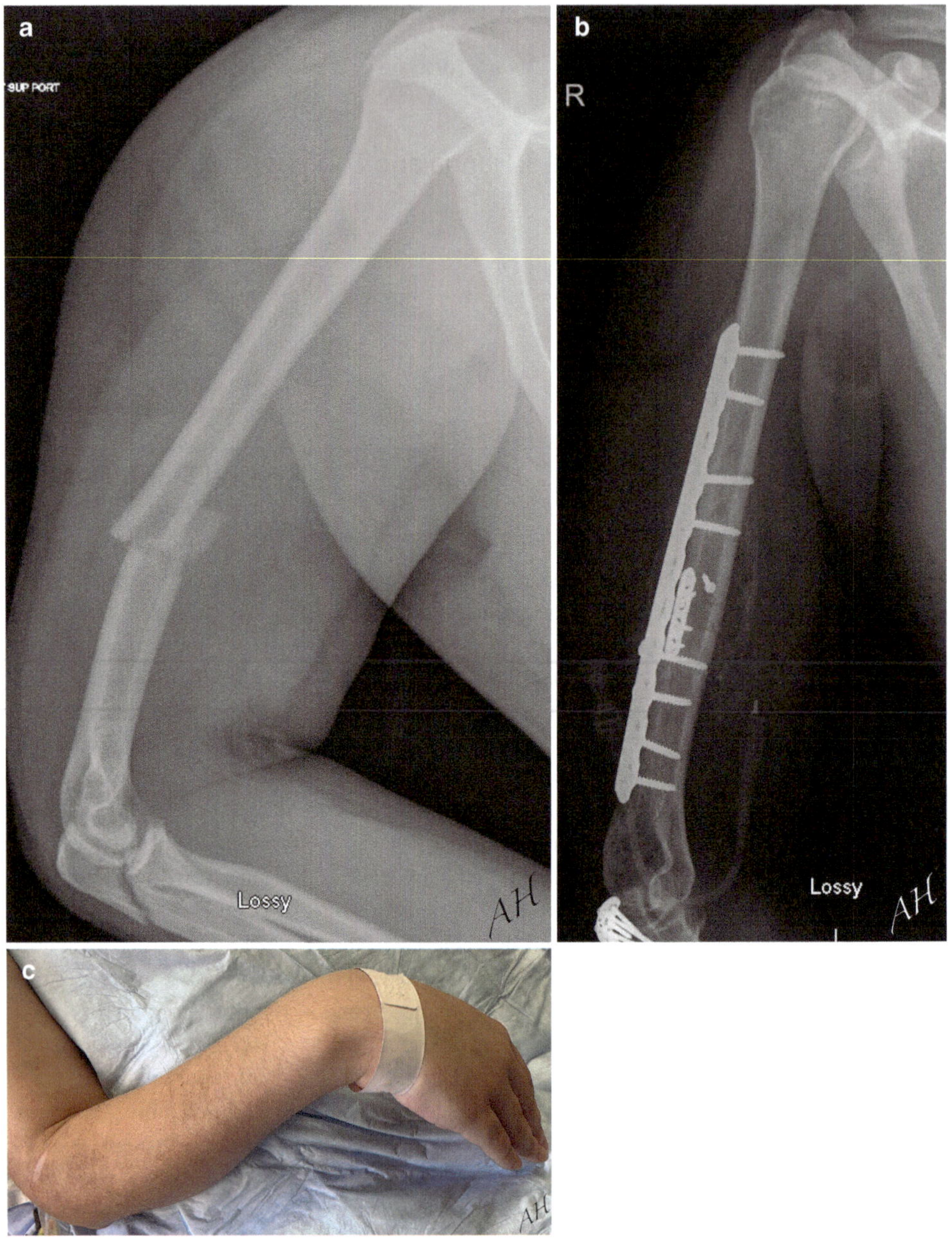

Fig. 15.1 A 19-year-old male was involved in a severe motor vehicle crash. He sustained a mid-shaft humerus fracture (**a**) that required open reduction and internal fixation (ORIF) (**b**). This resulted in a complete right wrist drop from radial nerve palsy with preservation of the triceps (**c**)

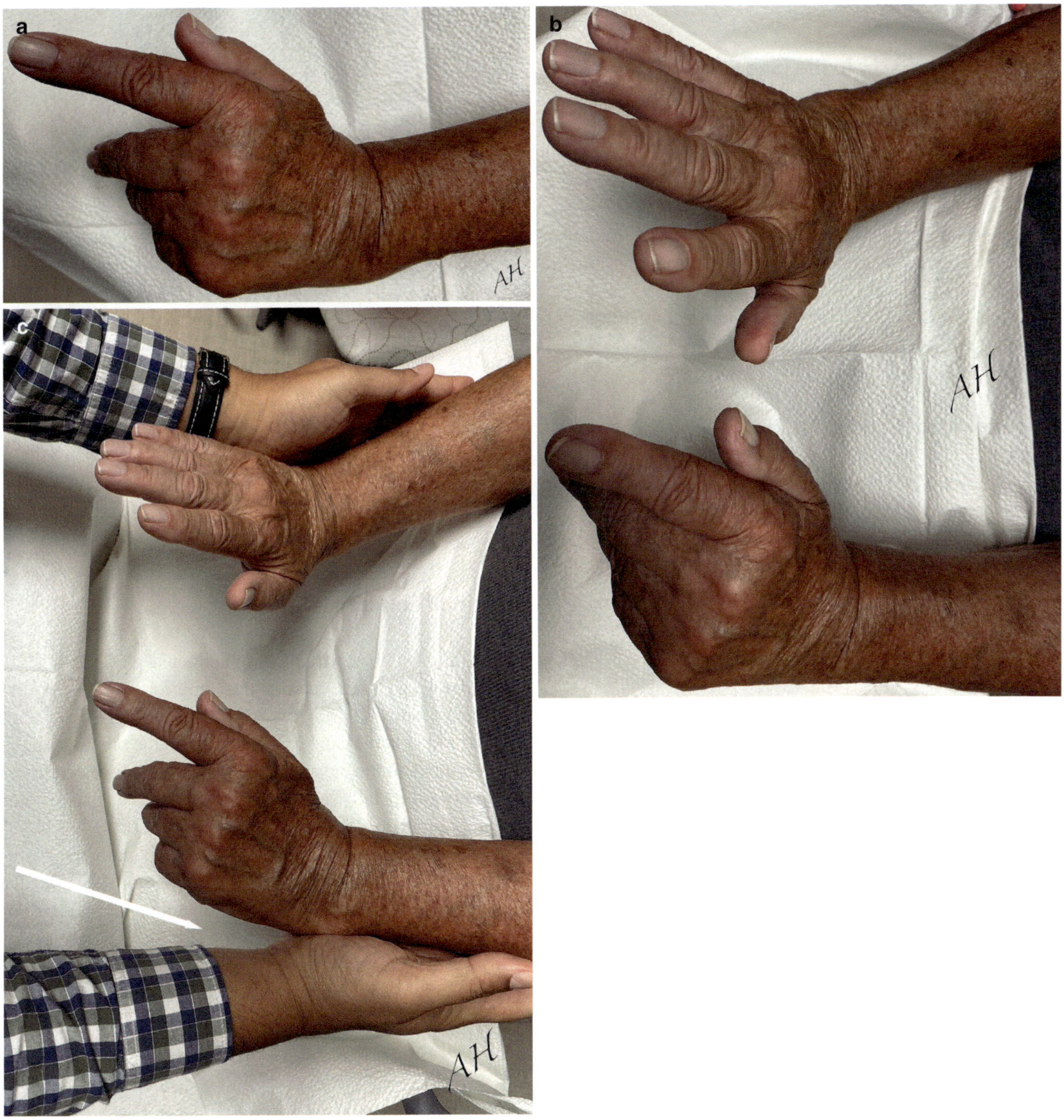

Fig. 15.2 Left PIN palsy. Note the radial deviation when the patient attempts to extend the wrist as well as finger drop (**a**). This becomes more obvious when compared to the normal right hand (**b**). The Window Test (**c**) is a simple bedside test to detect radial deviation: the examiner's wrists are applied against the patient's wrists, and the patient is asked to extend the wrists and fingers. A positive Window Test is reported when a gap (arrow) is observed between the examiner's forearm and the patient's hand [3]

Exposure

Anterior Approach, Axilla (See Fig. 14.1)

1. Infraclavicular exposure as in Chap. 8.
2. The radial nerve is identified at the level of the coracoid process as it comes off the posterior cord as the more medial of its two terminal branches.
3. It is followed distally as it enters the lower triangular space (triangular interval) with the profunda brachii vessels.
4. The radial nerve then enters the posterior compartment of the arm.

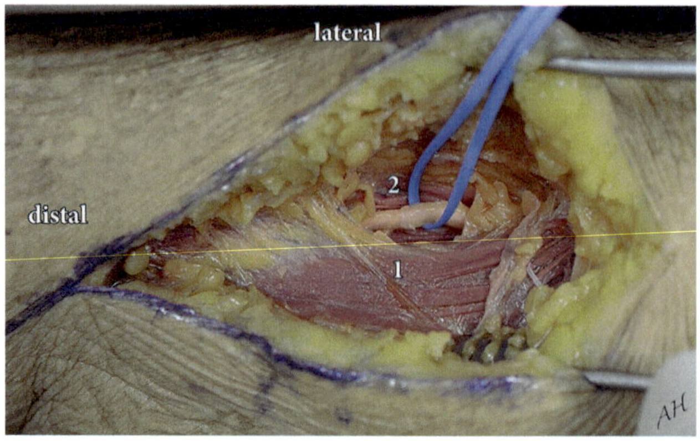

Fig. 15.4 In the distal arm, the radial nerve (blue loop) is found between the biceps brachii (*1*) medially and the triceps (*2*) laterally

Posterior Arm (See Fig. 14.2)

1. The patient can be positioned supine with a bump under the shoulder, lateral, or prone.
2. Incision is made in the posterior aspect of the arm along the posterior border of the deltoid and then extended distally in the mid-posterior arm.
3. The incision is deepened through the superficial and deep fasciae.
4. We then identify the raphe between the long and lateral heads of the triceps.
5. The raphe is opened, and the two heads of triceps are separated.
6. This reveals the radial nerve and its different triceps branches.
7. It can be followed more distally between the lateral and medial heads of the triceps in the spiral groove.

Distal Arm and Anterior Elbow (Figs. 15.3 and 15.4)

1. Position: supine, with the arm abducted.
2. Incision is made in the anterior aspect of the lower arm between the biceps brachii medially and the triceps laterally; then, more distally between the biceps tendon medially and brachioradialis laterally.
3. The superficial and deep fasciae are opened.
4. The radial nerve can be found in the interval between the biceps brachii medially and the triceps laterally.
5. Followed distally, the nerve is between the biceps tendon medially and the brachioradialis laterally.

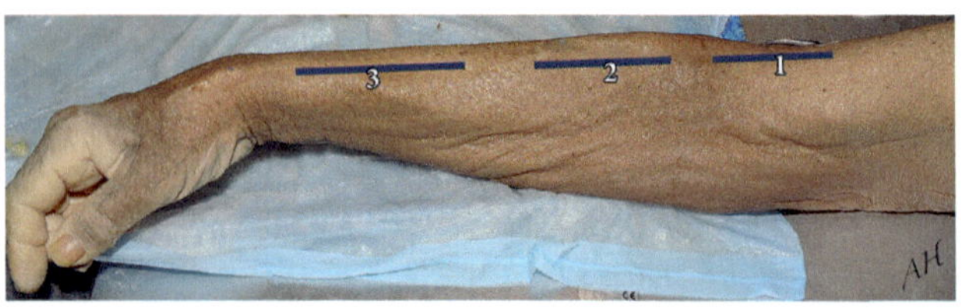

Fig. 15.3 Incisions for radial nerve exposures in the distal arm (*1*), proximal (*2*), and distal forearm (*3*)

Proximal Forearm (Fig. 15.5)

1. Position: supine, with the arm abducted.
2. Incision is made along the anterior border of the brachioradialis.
3. The radial nerve can be found between the brachioradialis laterally and the biceps brachii and brachialis medially.
4. Followed distally, one can identify the branches to brachioradialis, ECRL, and ECRB.
5. The PIN comes off the radial nerve and enters the posterior forearm under the aponeurotic edge of the supinator (arcade of Fröhse). Vessels could come in close relationship with the PIN in this location (Leash of Henry).
6. Variation: posterior approach can be used between brachioradialis and ECRL; it provides direct access to the PIN but does not allow proximal extension to radial tunnel (Chap. 54).

Distal Forearm, Superficial Radial Nerve (Fig. 15.6)

1. Position: supine, with the arm abducted.
2. Incision along the lateral border of the radius.
3. The superficial radial nerve is found in the superficial fascia accompanied by the cephalic vein.
4. Followed proximally, it can be seen entering the deep fascia and then disappears under the tendon of brachioradialis.
5. Distally, the superficial radial nerve enters the lateral aspect of the dorsum of the hand and branches into its terminal digital branches.

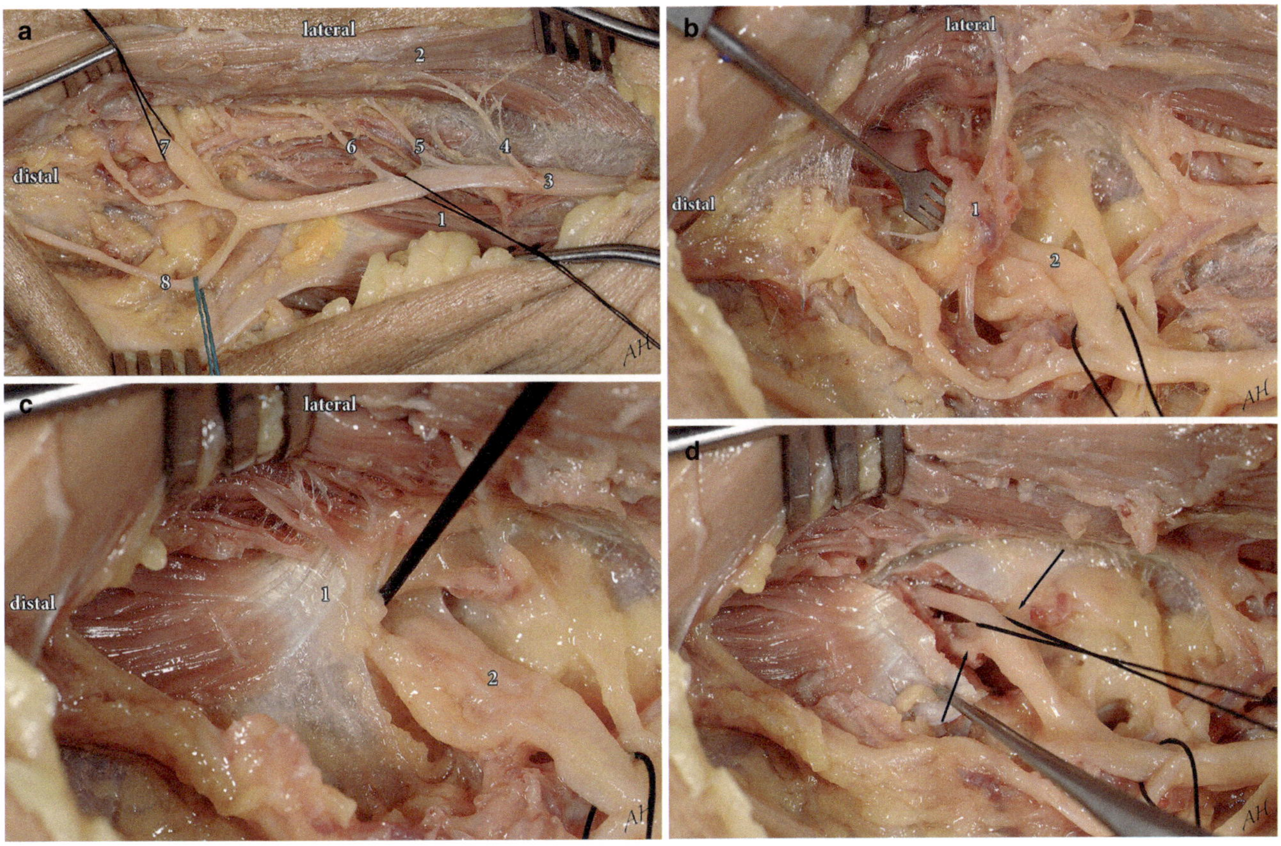

Fig. 15.5 Right radial nerve exposure in the proximal forearm. (**a**) The radial nerve (*3*) is found between the biceps brachii (*1*) medially and the brachioradialis (*2*) laterally. The two main terminal branches are the deep radial which becomes the PIN (*7*) and the superficial radial nerve (*8*). Note the branches to the brachioradialis (*4*), ECRL (*5*), and ECRB (*6*) take off before the origin of the PIN. (**b**) A vascular leash (leash of Henry) (*1*) can be compressive to the PIN (*2*) and should be ligated and cut. (**c**) The arcade of Fröhse (*1*) is the sharp aponeurotic edge of the supinator; it can also be compressive to the PIN (*2*) and should be released. (**d**) PIN seen after full decompression. Note supinator branches (arrows)

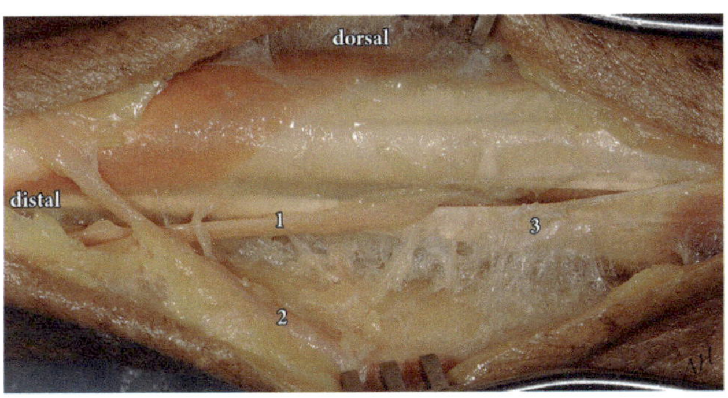

Fig. 15.6 Right superficial radial nerve (*1*) exposure in the distal forearm. *2* cephalic vein, *3* tendon of brachioradialis

References

1. Kinni V, Craig J, van Holsbeeck M, Ditmars D (2009) Entrapment of the posterior interosseous nerve at the arcade of Frohse with sonographic, magnetic resonance imaging, and intraoperative confirmation. J Ultrasound Med 28(6):807–812. https://doi.org/10.7863/jum.2009.28.6.807
2. Loizides A, Peer S, Ostermann S, Henninger B, Stampfer-Kountchev M, Gruber H (2011) Unusual functional compression of the deep branch of the radial nerve by a vascular branch (leash of Henry): ultrasonographic appearance. Rofo 183(2):163–166. https://doi.org/10.1055/s-0029-1245738. Epub 2010 Oct 11.
3. Hanna AS, Omuro PM, Hutchinson JR, Fofana ML, Hellenbrand DJ (2022) The Window Test: a simple bedside method to detect radial deviation of the wrist commonly seen in posterior interosseous nerve palsy. World Neurosurg 158:e369–e376. https://doi.org/10.1016/j.wneu.2021.10.186. Epub 2021 Nov 7.
4. Sprofkin BE (1954) Cheiralgia paresthetica; Wartenberg's disease. Neurology 4(11):857–862. https://doi.org/10.1212/wnl.4.11.857
5. Tang JBO (2020) Radial tunnel syndrome: definition, distinction and treatments. J Hand Surg Eur 45(8):882–889. https://doi.org/10.1177/1753193420953990
6. Naam NH, Nemani S (2012) Radial tunnel syndrome. Orthop Clin North Am 43(4):529–536. https://doi.org/10.1016/j.ocl.2012.07.022
7. Johns N, Shridhar V (2020) Lateral epicondylitis: current concepts. Aust J Gen Pract 49(11):707–709. https://doi.org/10.31128/AJGP-07-20-5519

16 Musculocutaneous Nerve

Amgad S. Hanna

Surgical Anatomy

The musculocutaneous nerve (C5, C6, and C7) arises as one of the main terminal branches of the lateral cord at the level of the coracoid process. It is lateral to the axillary artery. It supplies several branches to the coracobrachialis muscle before piercing it. More distally, it runs between the biceps brachii and the brachialis, supplies them, and then continues as the lateral antebrachial cutaneous nerve (LABC) to supply the skin of the lateral aspect of the forearm.

Anatomical Variations

Various communications could occur between the median and musculocutaneous nerves in the arm [1]. The musculocutaneous nerve may originate more distally from the median nerve rather than from the lateral cord (Fig. 16.1) [2].

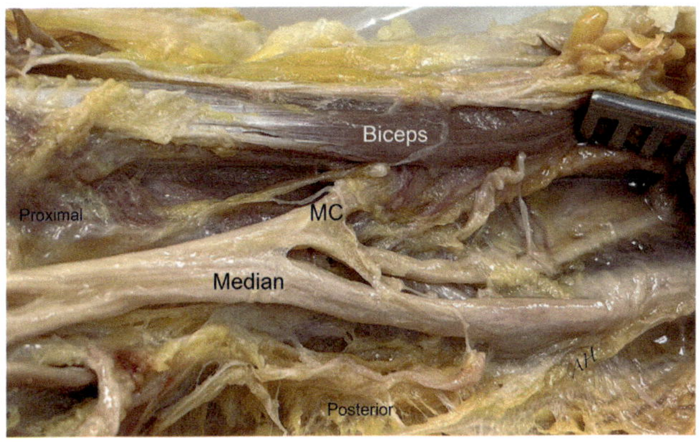

Fig. 16.1 Musculocutaneous nerve (MC) arising distally from the median nerve

Clinical Significance

Musculocutaneous nerve injury causes loss of elbow flexion. This typically occurs at the level of the lateral cord or the upper trunk. It could also be caused by avulsion of the C5 and C6 nerve roots. The musculocutaneous nerve can be compressed in the distal arm by an accessory muscle or bicipital aponeurosis [3].

Exposure

In the Axilla (Fig. 16.2)

1. Infraclavicular exposure as in Chap. 8.
2. The nerve is then followed laterally, which will require retracting or transecting the pectoralis major tendon.
3. It courses laterally to pierce the coracobrachialis muscle after giving off several branches to supply that muscle (Fig. 16.3).

Supplementary Information The online version contains supplementary material available at https://doi.org/10.1007/978-3-031-73931-6_16.

A. S. Hanna (✉)
Department of Neurosurgery, University of Wisconsin School of Medicine and Public Health, Madison, WI, USA

A. S. Hanna (ed.), *Nerves: Anatomy, Exposures, and Techniques*, https://doi.org/10.1007/978-3-031-73931-6_16

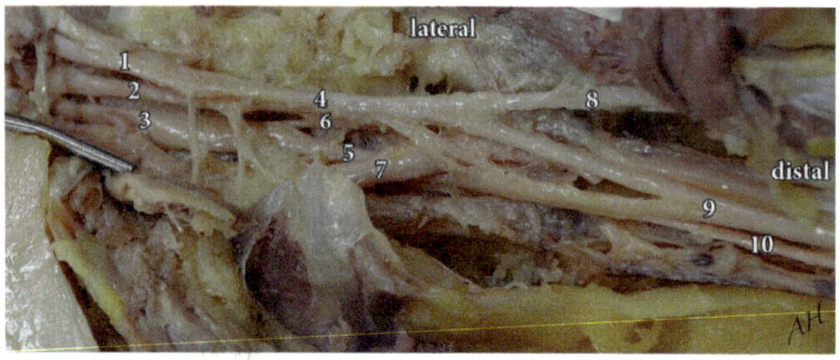

Fig. 16.2 The left musculocutaneous nerve (*8*) is one of the two terminal branches of the lateral cord (*4*). It pierces the coracobrachialis after supplying it. The ulnar nerve (*10*) is one of the terminal branches of the medial cord (*5*). The median nerve (*9*) arises from one or more contributions of the lateral and medial cords. *1* upper (superior) trunk, *2* middle trunk, *3* lower (inferior) trunk, *6* posterior cord, *7* axillary artery

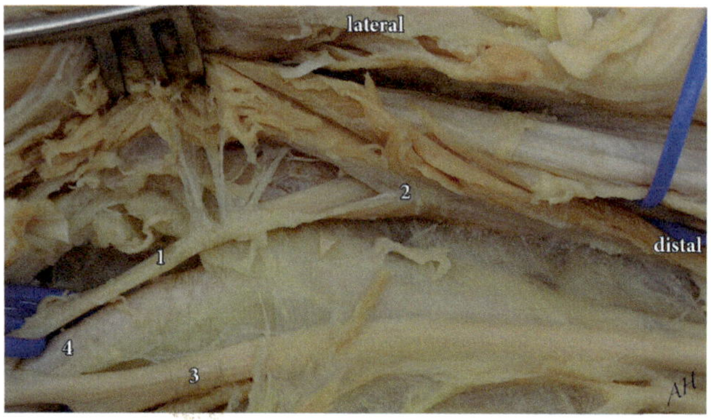

Fig. 16.3 The musculocutaneous nerve (*1*) as it enters the coracobrachialis (*2*). Note the comb-like appearance of the branches to the coracobrachialis. Early branching can occur from a higher location on the musculocutaneous nerve or the lateral cord. *3* median nerve, *4* axillary artery

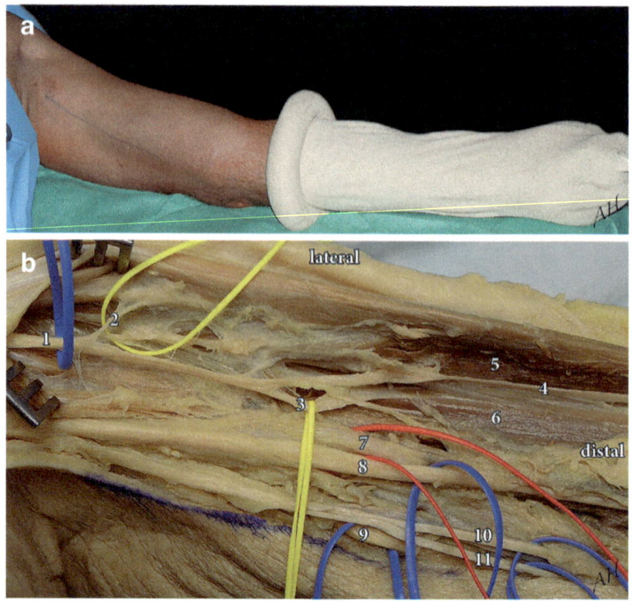

Fig. 16.4 (**a**) Musculocutaneous, median, and ulnar nerve exposure in the inner aspect of the left arm. The patient is positioned supine, with the arm abducted on a hand table. Incision is made along the medial aspect of the arm with the neurovascular bundle. The brachial pulse can be palpated to mark the incision. (**b**) The musculocutaneous (*1*), median (*8*), and ulnar (*9*) nerves are exposed in the arm. The median and ulnar nerves have no major branches in the arm. The musculocutaneous nerve gives off a biceps brachii branch (*2*), a brachialis branch (*3*), and the lateral antebrachial cutaneous (LABC) nerve (*4*). It courses between the biceps brachii (*5*) and brachialis (*6*) muscles. *7* brachial artery, *10* medial antebrachial cutaneous (MABC) nerve, *11* medial brachial cutaneous (MBC) nerve

In the Arm (Fig. 16.4)

1. Skin incision along the medial border of the biceps brachii muscle. One may try to palpate the brachial artery pulse to mark the incision.
2. The incision is deepened through the superficial and deep fasciae.
3. The medial aspect of the biceps brachii is identified and retracted laterally; this uncovers the interval between the biceps brachii and brachialis muscles. The musculocutaneous nerve is found in that interval.
4. Followed proximally, we can identify the biceps brachii branch along the medial and deep surface of the muscle and the main musculocutaneous nerve trunk as it passes between the two heads of the coracobrachialis.
5. Distally, the brachialis branch comes off and courses over the anterior surface of the muscle.
6. The main nerve continues laterally and distally as the lateral antebrachial cutaneous nerve. It pierces the deep fascia lateral and distal to the tendon of the biceps brachii.

References

1. Kumar N, Guru A, D'Souza MR, Patil J, Nayak BS (2013) Incidences and clinical implications of communications between musculocutaneous nerve and median nerve in the arm—a cadaveric study. West Indian Med J 62(8):744–747. https://doi.org/10.7727/wimj.2013.175
2. Kubwimana O, Ndata A, Ivang A, Ndahimana P, Nzayisenga A, Byiringiro JC et al (2022) Musculocutaneous and median nerve branching: anatomical variations. Case series from UR clinical anatomy and literature review. Afr Health Sci 22(1):263–268. https://doi.org/10.4314/ahs.v22i1.33
3. Kraemer MR, Corriveau MD, Tuite MJ, Hanna AS (2021) Surgical decompression of an accessory bicipital aponeurosis associated with median neuropathy in the antecubital fossa: a case report. Surg Neurol Int 12:615. https://doi.org/10.25259/SNI_520_2021

Median Nerve

17

Amgad S. Hanna and Amruth K. V. Addanki

Surgical Anatomy

The median nerve (C5, C6, C7, C8, and T1) is formed by contributions from the medial and lateral cords in the axilla. It courses anterior to the axillary and then brachial arteries. It enters the cubital fossa anterior to the brachialis and deep to the bicipital aponeurosis (lacertus fibrosus). It gives off its first branches in the upper forearm. It supplies most of the flexor muscles of the forearm: pronator teres, flexor carpi radialis, palmaris longus, and flexor digitorum superficialis (sublimis). The anterior interosseous nerve (AIN) comes off the deep lateral aspect of the median nerve and supplies the flexor pollicis longus, lateral half of flexor digitorum profundus, and pronator quadratus; it has no cutaneous distribution. The median nerve courses between the two heads of pronator teres and then the two heads of flexor digitorum superficialis. It then enters the carpal tunnel with the flexor tendons under the flexor retinaculum (transverse carpal ligament). The palmar cutaneous branch typically arises proximal to the wrist and courses superficial to the flexor retinaculum. In the hand, the median nerve gives off the palmar recurrent branch that supplies the muscles of the thenar eminence: flexor pollicis brevis, abductor pollicis brevis, and opponens pollicis. It also supplies the lateral two lumbrical muscles and then divides into digital cutaneous branches that supply the palmar surface of the lateral three and a half fingers and the dorsal surface of their distal phalanges.

Anatomical Variations

Martin–Gruber anastomosis is a connection from median to ulnar nerves in the forearm. Marinacci communication is an ulnar-to-median connection in the forearm. Riche–Cannieu anastomosis is a deep ulnar-to-thenar recurrent in the hand. Berretini anastomosis is a connection between ulnar and median digital nerves in the palm [1]. Anatomical variations in the course of the median nerve could cause it to travel deep to the flexor tendons in the carpal tunnel instead of the typical superficial course (see Fig. 67.7) [2].

Hanna classified the palmar recurrent branch (motor) of the median nerve based on the zone of origin (I–IV) and angle with the median nerve (A–D), with the most dangerous being type IVD (most medial and most perpendicular to the median nerve, Fig. 17.1) [3].

Supplementary Information The online version contains supplementary material available at https://doi.org/10.1007/978-3-031-73931-6_17.

A. S. Hanna (✉)
Deparment of Neurosurgery, University of Wisconsin School of Medicine and Public Health, Madison, WI, USA

A. K. V. Addanki
Doris Duke Clinical Research Continuum, Duke University, Durham, NC, USA

University of Wisconsin–Madison, Madison, WI, USA
e-mail: amruth.addanki@duke.edu

A. S. Hanna (ed.), *Nerves: Anatomy, Exposures, and Techniques*, https://doi.org/10.1007/978-3-031-73931-6_17

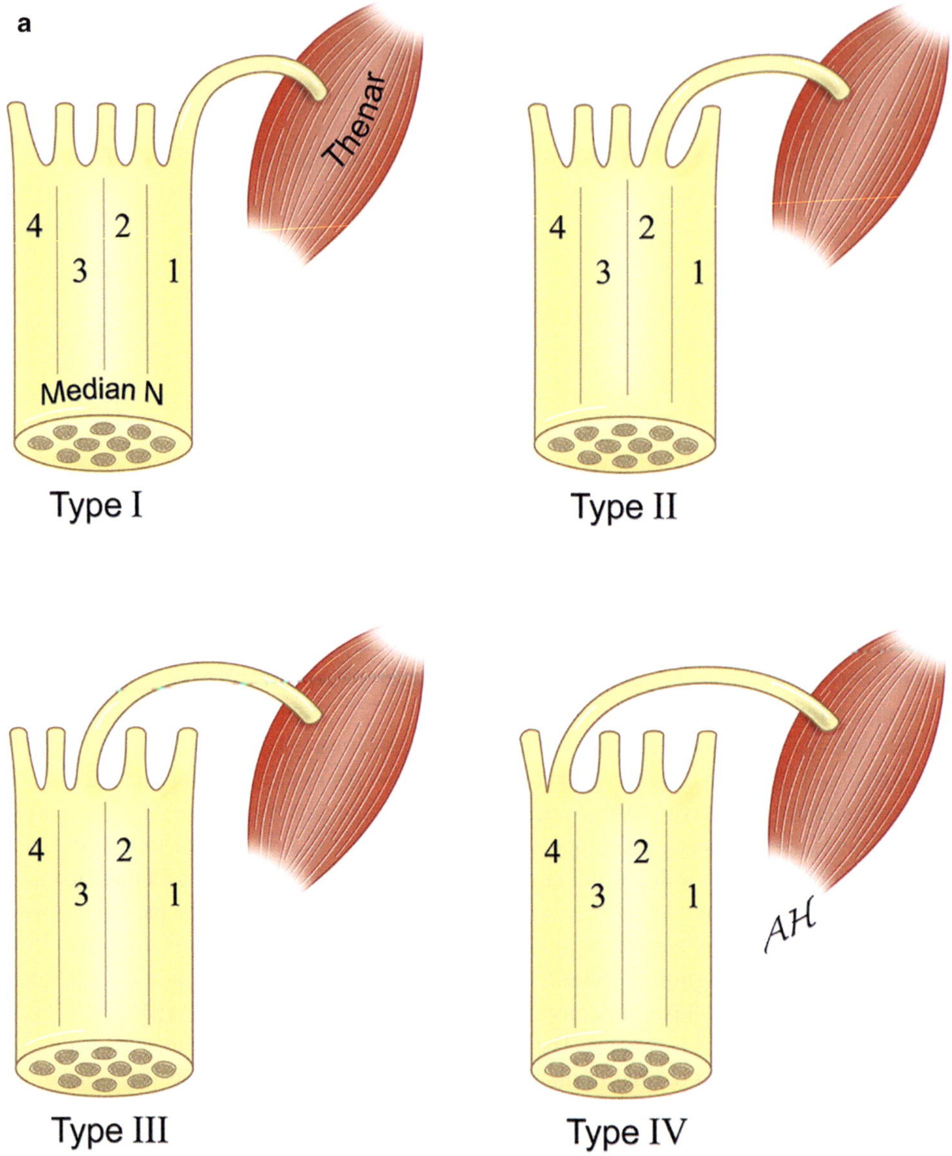

Fig. 17.1 Palmar recurrent branch of the median nerve. (**a**) From lateral to medial; types I–IV correspond to zones 1–4, respectively. The more medial the origin, the more risky it is for iatrogenic injury. (**b**) Axial and (**c**) oblique axial views showing the angle this motor branch makes with the axial plane of the median nerve. Type A = 0°, type B = 45°, type C = 60°, and type D = 90°. The most dangerous type is type D. (Copyright Amgad Hanna. Published with permission)

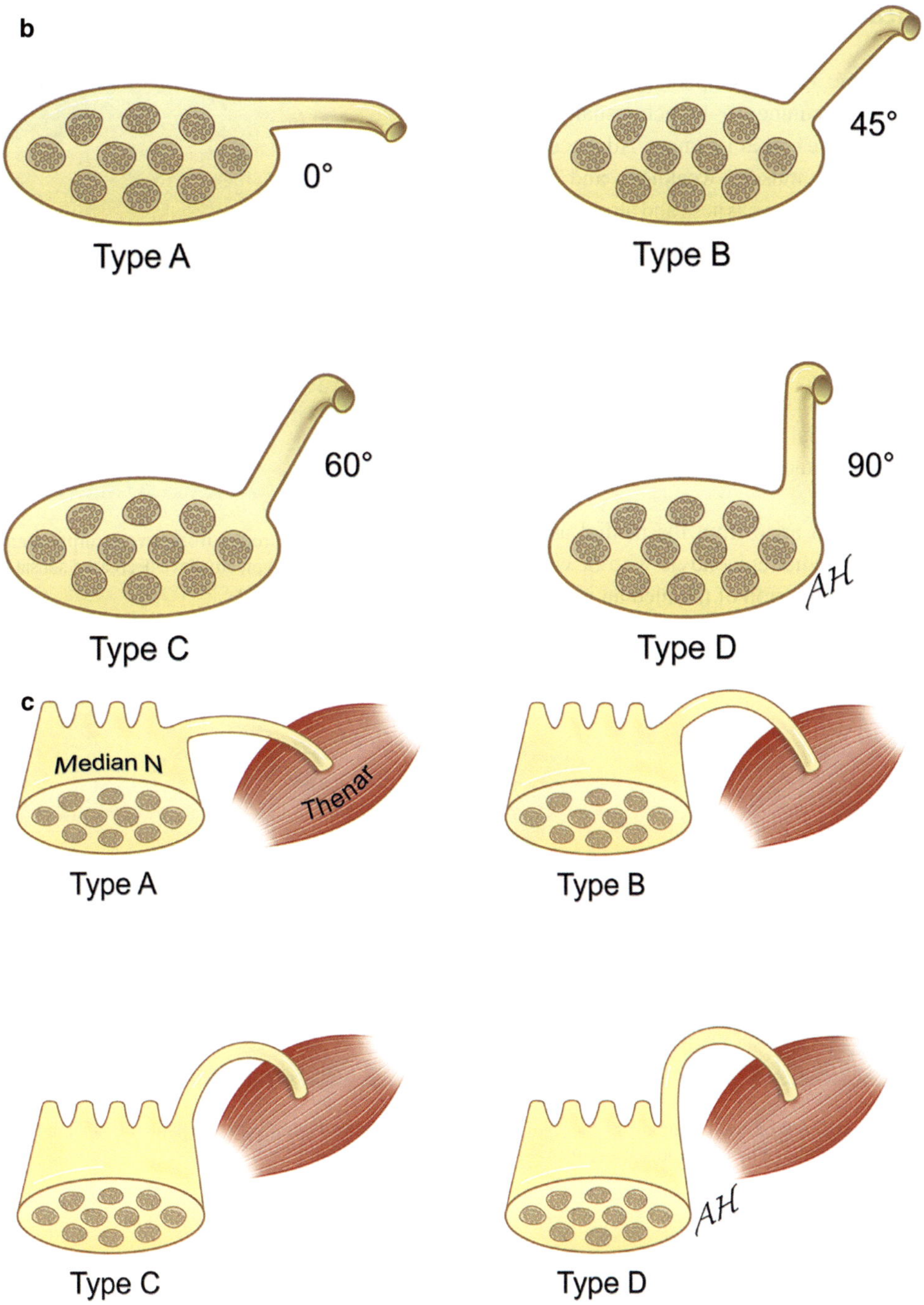

Fig. 17.1 (continued)

Clinical Significance

Carpal tunnel syndrome typically spares sensation in the palm since the palmar cutaneous branch usually passes superficial to the transverse carpal ligament. Advanced cases can present with thenar muscle weakness and atrophy (Fig. 17.2). However, if thenar weakness and atrophy develop postoperatively, this should raise suspicion for palmar recurrent branch injury. AIN lesions cause inability to flex the interphalangeal joint (IPJ) of the thumb and the distal interphalangeal joint (DIP) of the index finger, resulting in the inability to make the "OK" sign (Fig. 17.3). There is no sensory loss. More proximal median nerve lesions cause inability to make a fist. The medial two fingers are still able to flex since the ulnar nerve is intact, resulting in the Benediction hand (Fig. 17.4).

Struthers' ligament can arise from the medial aspect of the humerus above the medial epicondyle with or without a bony spur and cause compression of the median nerve [4].

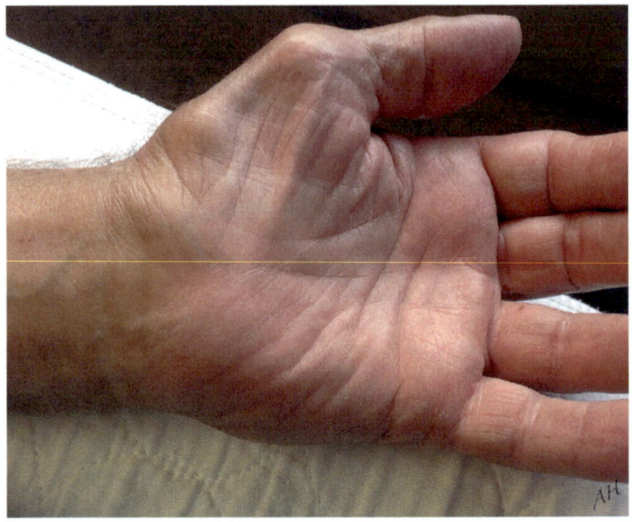

Fig. 17.2 Thenar atrophy from severe carpal tunnel syndrome. Such patients would also typically have decreased sensation in the lateral 3.5 fingers, sparing the palm

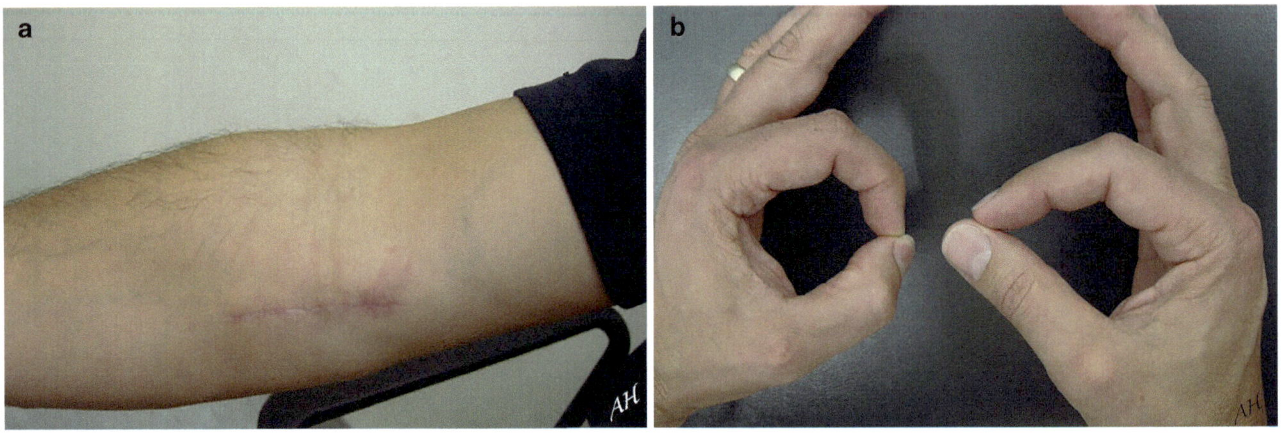

Fig. 17.3 (**a**) Incision for removal of a schwannoma of the right median nerve. (**b**) Postoperatively, the patient is unable to make the "OK" sign with the right hand from AIN palsy. There was no sensory loss

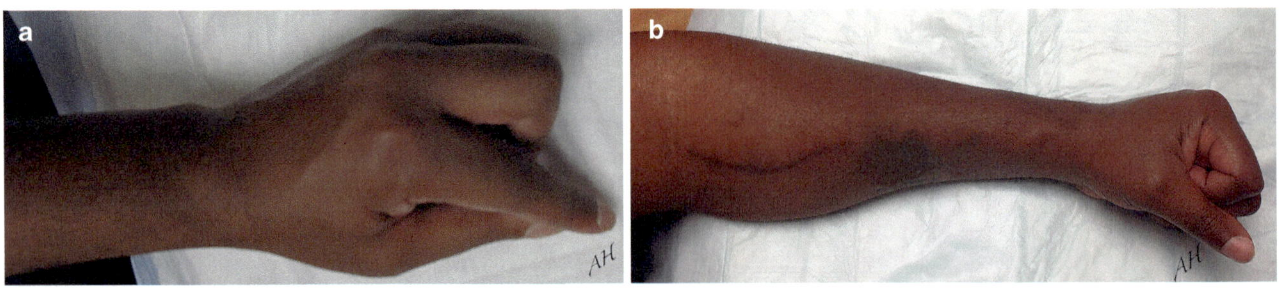

Fig. 17.4 (**a**) Following a stab wound to the axilla involving the median nerve, the patient is unable to make a fist with the left hand: Benediction sign. (**b**) Significantly improved grip 6 months after surgical repair: sural nerve grafting to the median nerve in the upper arm as well as distal nerve transfers; extensor carpi radialis brevis to AIN

Exposures

In the Arm (See Fig. 16.3)

1. Skin incision along the medial border of the biceps brachii muscle. One may try to palpate the brachial artery pulse to mark the incision.
2. The incision is deepened through the superficial and deep fasciae.
3. The median nerve is usually found superficial to the brachial artery.
4. Followed proximally toward the axilla under the pectoralis major tendon, it can be traced back to the contributions from the medial and lateral cords.
5. Distally, it can be followed between the biceps brachii and brachialis muscles.

In the Cubital Fossa (Fig. 17.5)

1. Midline anterior incision, z-shaped, to avoid crossing the elbow crease. Alternatively, one may use 2 incisions leaving a skin bridge at the elbow crease.
2. The antecubital vein may be encountered in the superficial fascia.
3. The deep fascia is opened and then the bicipital aponeurosis.
4. This exposes the contents of the cubital fossa, with the brachial artery dividing into radial and ulnar arteries and the median nerve medial to the artery. From lateral to medial, TAN: biceps Tendon, brachial Artery, median Nerve.
5. The median nerve gives off branches to the superficial flexor muscles except flexor carpi ulnaris.
6. The AIN comes off the deep radial aspect of the median nerve.
7. The median nerve and AIN leave the cubital fossa between the two heads of pronator teres and then course under the tendinous origin of flexor digitorum superficialis (i.e., sublime bridge) [5].

Carpal Tunnel Release (Open Technique) (Fig. 17.6)

1. Tourniquet is optional.
2. Anterior midline incision from the distal wrist crease to the thenar crease along the radial aspect of the ring finger.
3. The palmar cutaneous branch, if encountered, should be protected. It may course superficial to or pass through the transverse carpal ligament.
4. The palmar aponeurosis is the extension of the palmaris longus tendon. It can be opened along the skin incision and retracted.

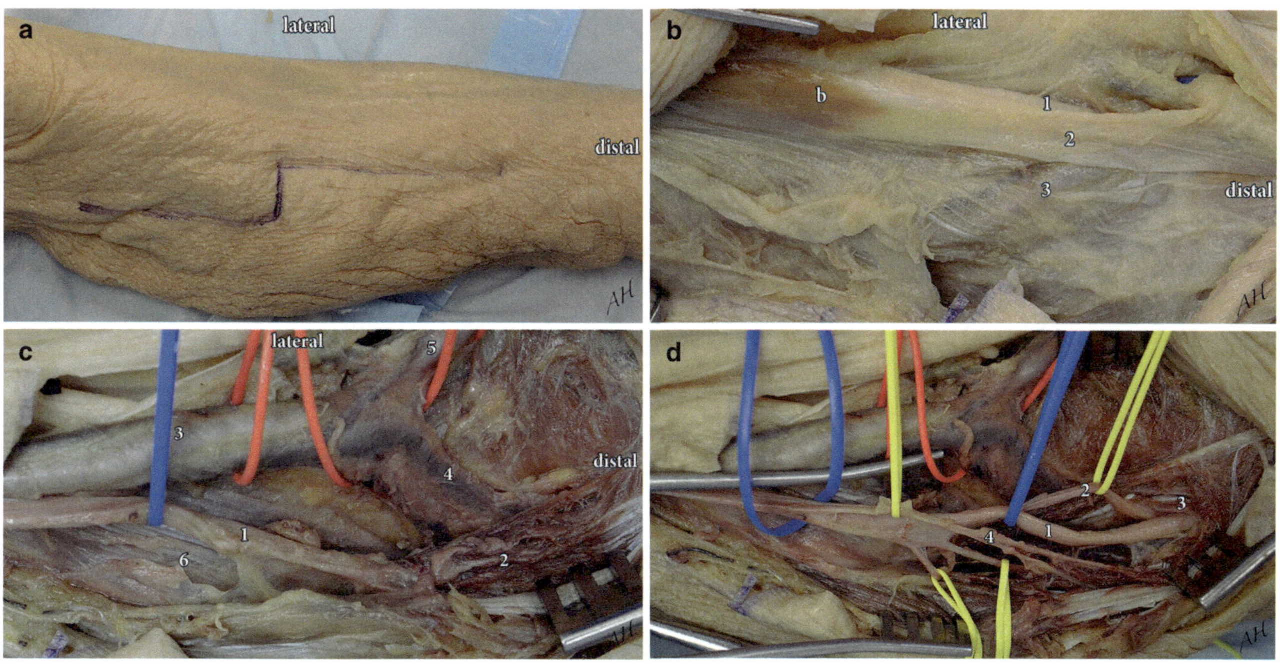

Fig. 17.5 Median nerve exposure in the left cubital fossa. (**a**) Skin incision. (**b**) *b* biceps brachii, *1* biceps tendon, *2* bicipital aponeurosis (lacertus fibrosus), *3* brachial artery. (**c**) The bicipital aponeurosis has been opened, exposing the median nerve (*1*) as it enters the pronator teres (*2*), the brachial artery (*3*) and its venae comitantes, as well as its bifurcation into ulnar (*4*) and radial (*5*) vessels. The brachialis (*6*) is seen in the floor of the cubital fossa. (**d**) Median nerve (*1*) branches are identified: *2* anterior interosseous nerve (AIN), typically arises from the radial and deep aspect of the median nerve. Both median nerve and AIN travel between the two heads of flexor digitorum superficialis (*3*) (sublime bridge). Pronator teres branches (*4*) are the first ones to arise from the median nerve

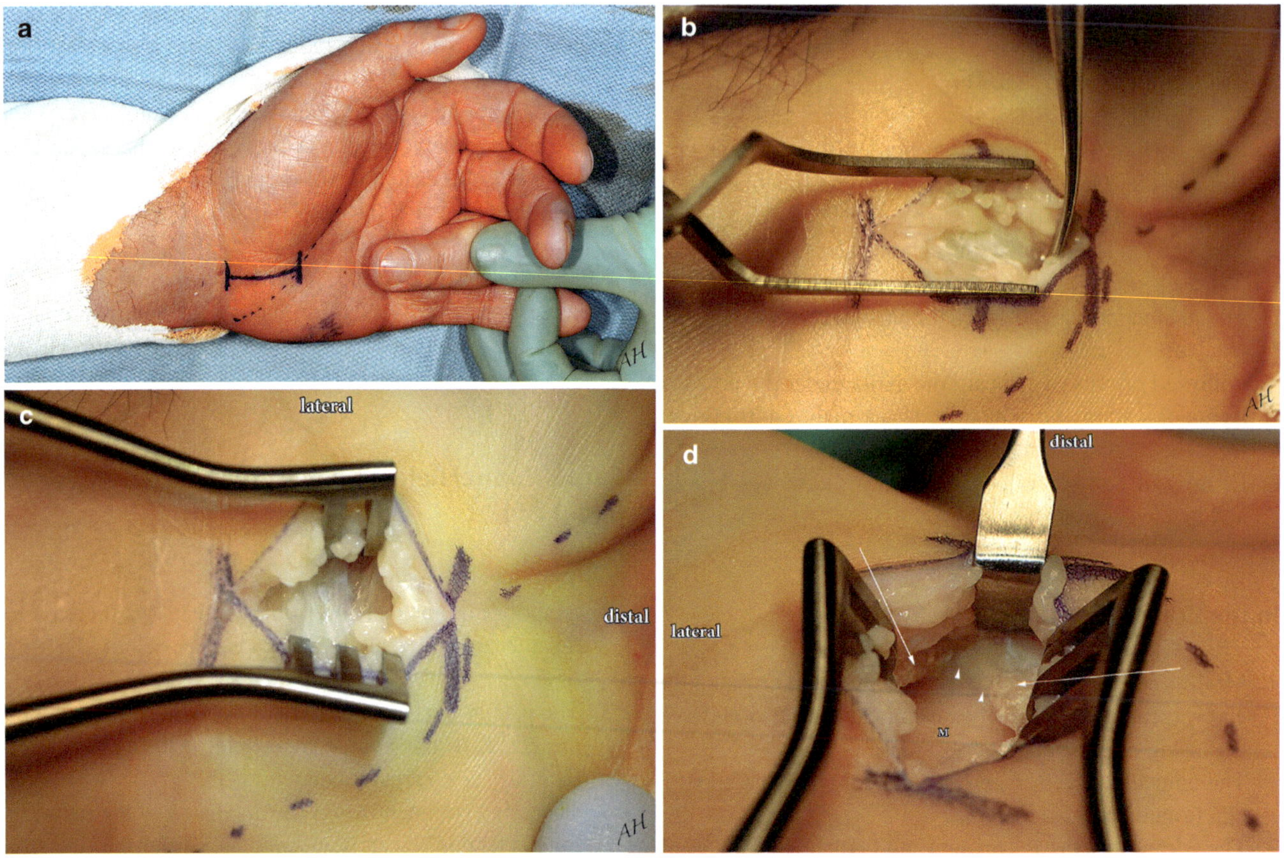

Fig. 17.6 Left carpal tunnel release. (**a**) Incision is made from the distal wrist crease till Kaplan's cardinal line (from the thenar crease to the pisiform bone), in line with the radial aspect of the ring finger. (**b**) The palmar aponeurosis is exposed, cut, and retracted. (**c**) The transverse carpal ligament is now exposed. Thenar muscle fibers are seen attaching laterally. (**d**) The transverse carpal ligament (arrows) has been opened, thus decompressing the median nerve (M). Note that the fat (arrowheads) around the nerve distally marks the distal extent of the decompression. If a tourniquet is used, it is our preference to release it before closure, for adequate hemostasis

5. The transverse carpal ligament is then sharply opened using a 15-blade scalpel.
6. This exposes the median nerve. A Woodson tool or Penfield #4 is then introduced under the ligament to protect the nerve, while the remaining part of the ligament is being cut with the scalpel. Dissection should remain on the ulnar side of the nerve to protect the palmar recurrent branch.
7. The decompression is then extended proximally and distally using Metzenbaum scissors.
8. Once the perineural fat is identified, this delineates the distal extent of decompression to protect the superficial palmar arch.
9. The epineurium can be opened if thick or scarred.
10. Closure in one layer of nonabsorbable sutures.
11. The procedure could be performed endoscopically [6] or using ultrasound-guided looped thread [7] or mini-open.

In the Hand

1. Incisions in the hand and fingers are made in a zigzag fashion (Bruner's) to avoid contractures.
2. The digital nerves course along the medial and lateral aspects of the fingers along with the digital vessels.

Complications of Carpal Tunnel Release

1. Failure to improve the symptoms from incomplete release of the transverse carpal ligament.
2. Recurrent symptoms from scar tissue.
3. Pain from injury to the palmar cutaneous branch.
4. Thumb paralysis from injury to the palmar recurrent branch.
5. More rarely injury to the median or ulnar nerves.
6. Vascular injury to the superficial palmar arch.
7. Wound infection or wound dehiscence, especially in diabetic patients.

References

1. Unver Dogan N, Uysal II, Karabulut AK, Seker M, Ziylan T (2010) Communications between the palmar digital branches of the median and ulnar nerves: a study in human fetuses and a review of the literature. Clin Anat 23(2):234–241. https://doi.org/10.1002/ca.20906
2. Hanna AS, Wei Z, Hanna BA (2020) Median nerve variation: a complete spin before terminal branching. J Brachial Plex Peripher Nerve Inj 15(1):e1–e4. https://doi.org/10.1055/s-0039-3402734. eCollection 2020 Jan.
3. Hanna A (2020) Classification of the variations of the palmar recurrent branch of the median nerve with special emphasis on angulation. J Neurosurg 133(2):556–563. https://doi.org/10.3171/2019.4.JNS19516. Epub July 2019.
4. Bilecenoglu B, Uz A, Karalezli N (2005) Possible anatomic structures causing entrapment neuropathies of the median nerve: an anatomic study. Acta Orthop Belg 71(2):169–176
5. Tubbs RS, Marshall T, Loukas M, Shoja MM, Cohen-Gadol AA (2010) The sublime bridge: anatomy and implications in median nerve entrapment. J Neurosurg 113(1):110–112. https://doi.org/10.3171/2009.10.JNS091251
6. Li Y, Luo W, Wu G, Cui S, Zhang Z, Gu X (2020) Open versus endoscopic carpal tunnel release: a systematic review and meta-analysis of randomized controlled trials. BMC Musculoskelet Disord 21(1):272. https://doi.org/10.1186/s12891-020-03306-1
7. Guo D, Guo D, Guo J, Schmidt SC, Lytie RM (2017) A clinical study of the modified thread carpal tunnel release. Hand (N Y) 12(5):453–460. https://doi.org/10.1177/1558944716668831. Epub 2016 Sep 12.

18 Ulnar Nerve

Amgad S. Hanna and Amruth K. V. Addanki

Surgical Anatomy

The ulnar nerve (C8, T1, and often C7) is one of the terminal branches of the medial cord of the brachial plexus in the axilla. It courses medial to the axillary artery and then posterior to the brachial artery. It enters the posterior compartment of the arm dorsal to the medial intermuscular septum and the medial epicondyle. It enters the forearm between the two heads of flexor carpi ulnaris (when the ulnar head is present), to course between it and the flexor digitorum profundus, medial to the ulnar artery. The first motor branches arise in the forearm supplying flexor carpi ulnaris and the medial half of flexor digitorum profundus. It enters Guyon's canal at the wrist, lateral to the pisiform bone. It gives off a superficial branch that supplies the palmaris brevis and the skin of the palmar aspect of the medial one and a half fingers as well as the medial aspect of the palm and a deep motor branch that supplies the hypothenar muscles: abductor digiti minimi, flexor digiti minimi, and opponens digiti minimi. It also supplies the medial two lumbricals, interossei, adductor pollicis, as well as part of the flexor pollicis brevis. The dorsal cutaneous branch arises in the lower forearm to supply the dorsum of the medial one-and-half fingers as well as the medial aspect of the hand; this branch is spared in cases of ulnar neuropathy at the wrist. Another palmar cutaneous branch may arise just proximal to Guyon's canal and supply the ulnar aspect of the palm proximally.

Supplementary Information The online version contains supplementary material available at https://doi.org/10.1007/978-3-031-73931-6_18.

A. S. Hanna (✉)
Deparment of Neurosurgery, University of Wisconsin School of Medicine and Public Health, Madison, WI, USA

A. K. V. Addanki
Doris Duke Clinical Research Continuum, Duke University, Durham, NC, USA

University of Wisconsin–Madison, Madison, WI, USA
e-mail: amruth.addanki@duke.edu

Clinical Significance

Ulnar nerve injuries at the wrist spare the dorsal sensation on the medial hand and the medial one-and-half fingers, flexor carpi ulnaris, and the medial half of flexor digitorum profundus. It results in *ulnar claw hand* (Fig. 18.1) with the inability to extend the interphalangeal joints of the medial two fingers (lumbrical paralysis), hypothenar atrophy, and atrophy of the first dorsal interosseous space. Paradoxically, with

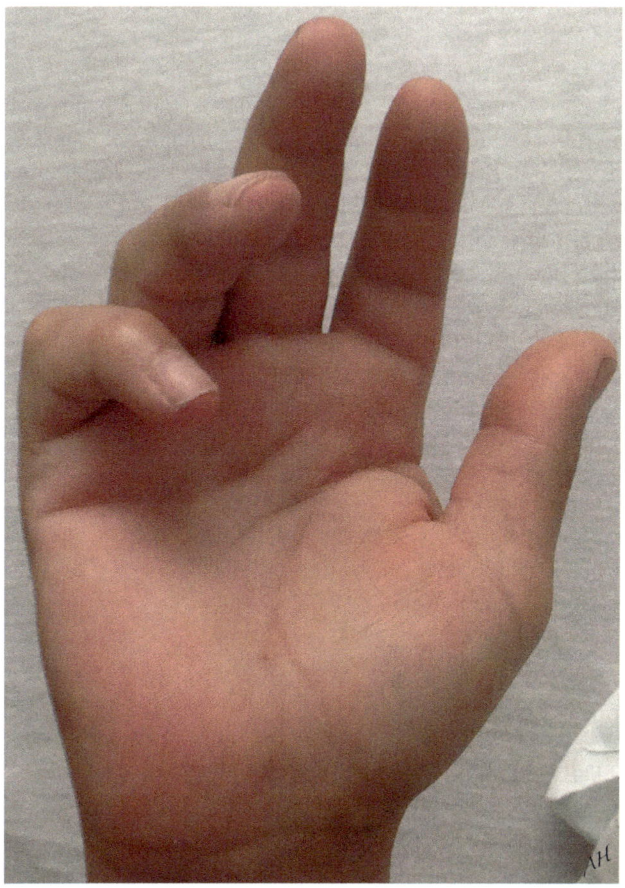

Fig. 18.1 Ulnar claw hand. The patient is unable to extend the medial two fingers due to lumbrical paralysis

A. S. Hanna (ed.), *Nerves: Anatomy, Exposures, and Techniques*, https://doi.org/10.1007/978-3-031-73931-6_18

a more proximal lesion at the elbow, the clawing is less pronounced due to the loss of flexor digitorum profundus function (ulnar nerve paradox). *Wartenberg's sign* (Fig. 18.2a): persistent abduction of the little finger by the extensor digiti minimi (quinti) (radial nerve) in the absence of the palmar interossei function. *Froment's sign* (Fig. 18.2b): flexion of the interphalangeal joint of the thumb by flexor pollicis longus, supplied by anterior interosseous nerve (AIN) from the median nerve to compensate for the weakness of the adductor pollicis, when the patient tries to hold a flat object between the thumb and index fingers. **Anconeus epitrochlearis** (Fig. 18.3) is an anomalous accessory muscle that attaches to the medial epicondyle and olecranon process. It can cause ulnar nerve compression at the elbow [1]. The **arcade of Struthers** is between the medial head of triceps and medial intermuscular septum. It can cause persistent or recurrent symptoms after ulnar nerve surgery. Its presence is controversial. **Osborne's band** is the fascia between the two heads of flexor carpi ulnaris. Recent research suggests that Osborne's band may represent rudimentary anconeus epitrochlearis (Tubbs). **Ulnar nerve subluxation** occurs when the ulnar nerve dislocates anteriorly around the medial epicondyle with elbow flexion. In **triceps snapping**, the medial head of triceps dislocates (snaps) around the medial epicondyle with elbow flexion, thus pushing and compressing the ulnar nerve. Predominantly neurogenic thoracic outlet syndrome is an important differential diagnosis for ulnar neuropathy. It can manifest with Gilliatt–Sumner hand with atrophy of thenar, hypothenar, and interossei muscles (Fig. 18.4). Amyotrophic lateral sclerosis (ALS) can present with hand atrophy, fasciculations, and no sensory loss. For ulnar nerve entrapment at the elbow, most randomized trials did not show benefit for transposition over simple decompression [2].

Most cases of de novo ulnar nerve entrapment at the elbow would benefit from simple decompression. Transposition should be reserved for cases of

- Revision surgery
- Subluxation
- Severe motor involvement with atrophy
- Elbow deformity (tardy ulnar nerve palsy)
- Triceps snapping (Fig. 18.5)

In cases of severe ulnar neuropathy or a high nerve injury in the upper arm, distal nerve transfer can be considered (Chap. 37). In this case, distal AIN (proximal to pronator quadratus) is transferred to the ulnar motor branch end-to-end or end-to-side (supercharge; babysitting).

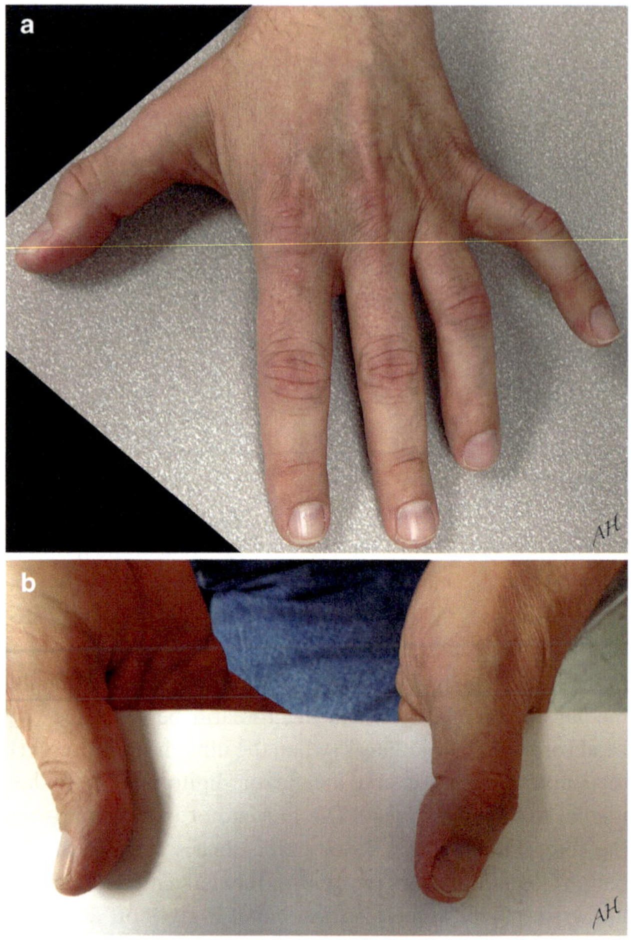

Fig. 18.2 (**a**) Wartenberg's sign. The patient is unable to adduct the little finger from paralysis of the interossei. Note also atrophy of the first dorsal interosseous and the hypothenar muscles. All are signs of ulnar neuropathy. (**b**) Positive Froment's sign in the left hand. The patient is unable to adduct the thumb from ulnar neuropathy; he is flexing the interphalangeal joint of the thumb instead (intact flexor pollicis longus supplied by AIN)

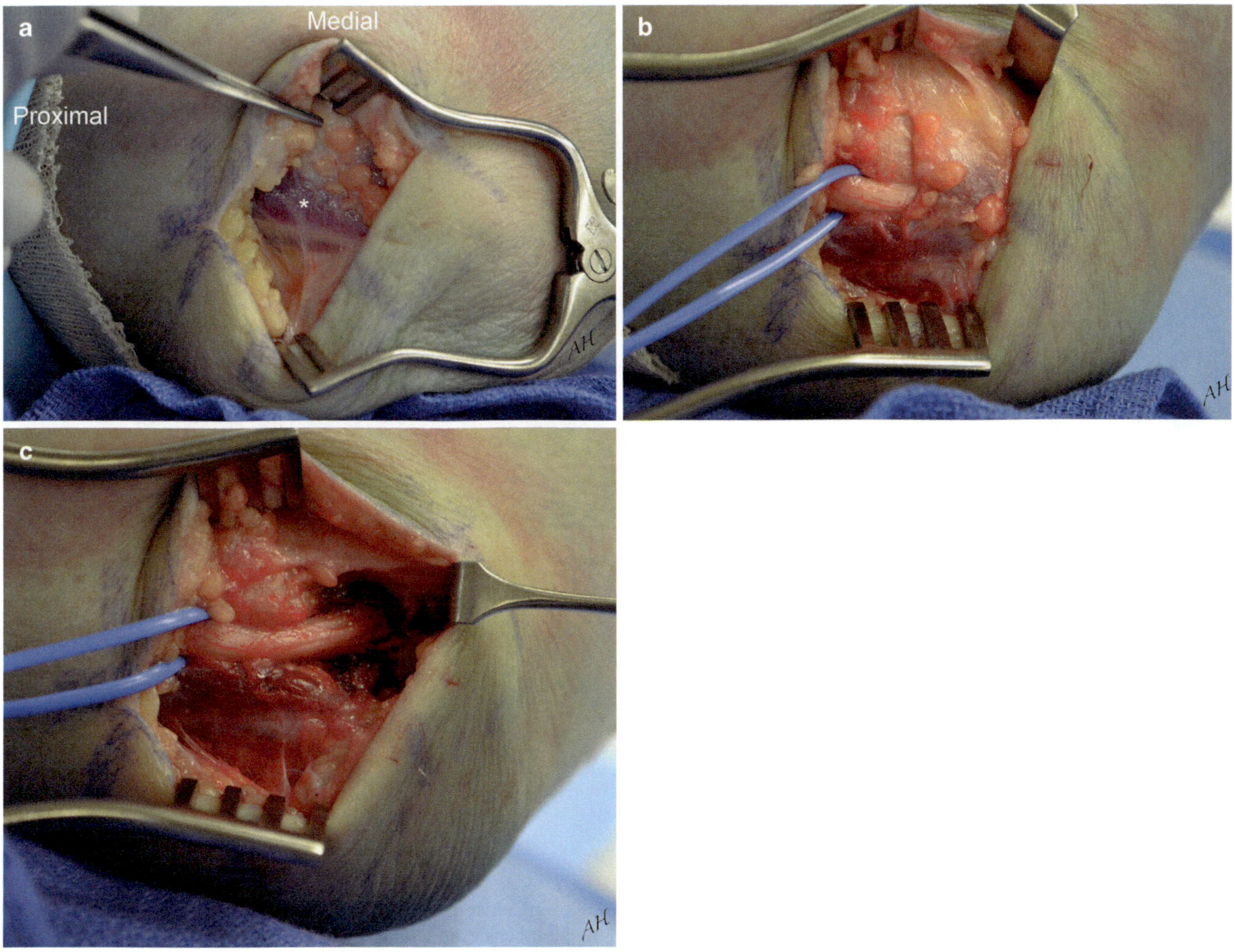

Fig. 18.3 Left Anconeus epitrochlearis (*) before (**a**), during (**b**), and after (**c**) resection. Blue loop ulnar nerve

Fig. 18.4 Gilliatt–Sumner hand with atrophy of the thenar eminence (**a**) and interossei (**b**). These are supplied by the median and ulnar nerves, respectively. This localizes the lesion to the lower trunk, as seen in predominantly neurogenic thoracic outlet syndrome

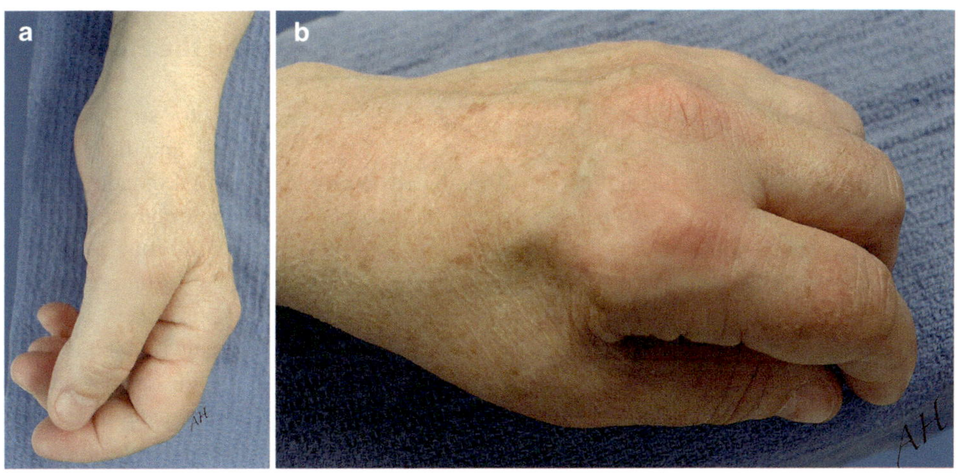

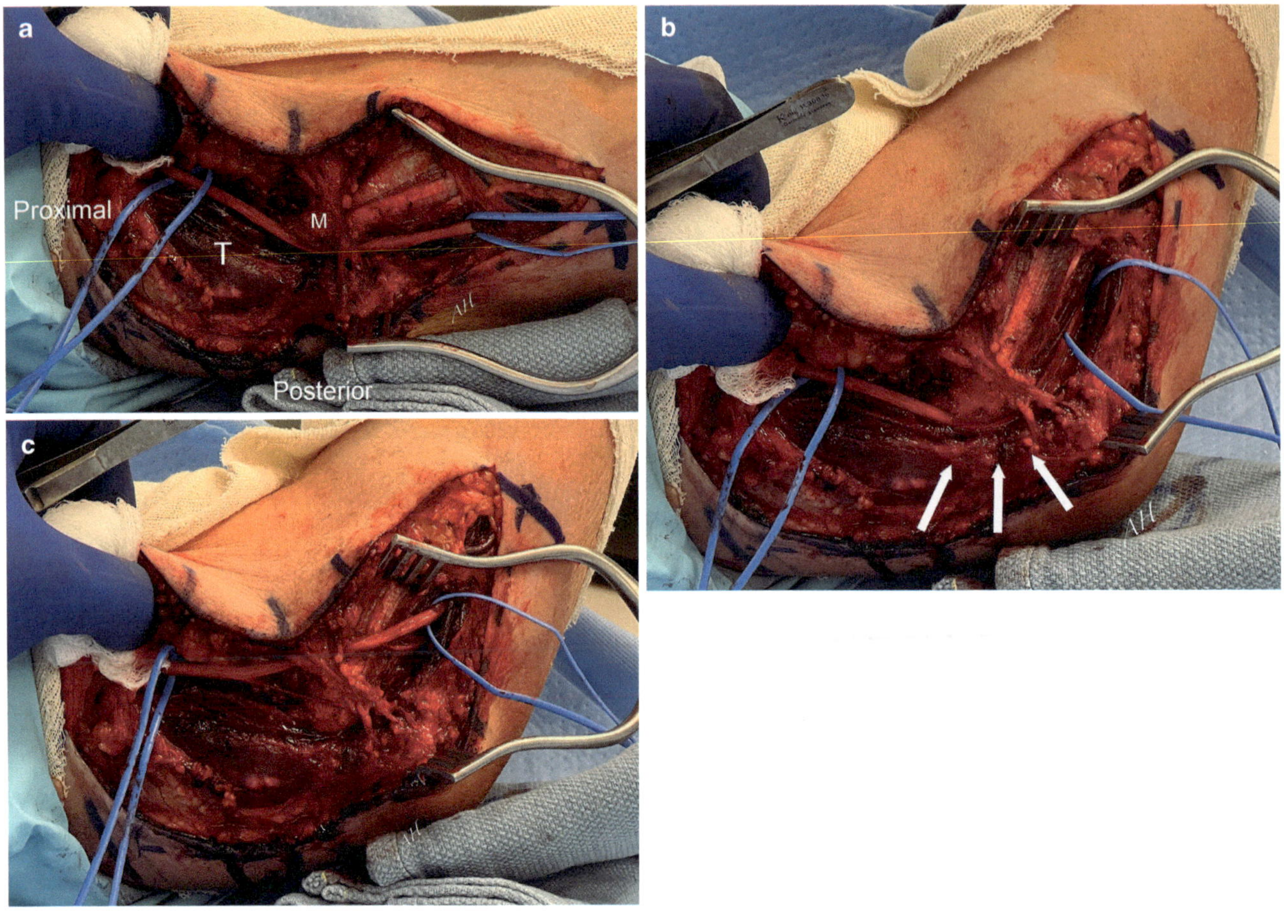

Fig. 18.5 Triceps snapping. (**a**) The left ulnar nerve (blue loops) is exposed behind the medial epicondyle (*M*) and in front of the triceps (*T*). (**b**) With elbow flexion, the triceps is observed riding over the ulnar nerve and compressing it against the medial epicondyle (arrows). (**c**) Following ulnar nerve transposition, the nerve is free from compression by the triceps even with elbow flexion. Partial triceps resection could also be performed

Exposures

In the Arm (See Fig. 16.3)

1. Skin incision along the medial border of the biceps brachii muscle. One may try to palpate the brachial artery pulse to plan the incision.
2. The incision is deepened through the superficial and deep fasciae.
3. The ulnar nerve is usually found posterior to the brachial artery.
4. Followed proximally toward the axilla under the pectoralis major tendon, one can trace it to its origin from the medial cord.
5. Distally, it enters the posterior arm behind the medial intermuscular septum and then travels posterior to the medial epicondyle, in the retrocondylar groove.

Around the Elbow

1. Position: supine with the arm abducted, externally rotated, and the elbow flexed.
2. Incision is made between the medial epicondyle and the olecranon process. It is extended cranially and caudally along the course of the nerve. Short incision is used for a simple decompression, but longer incision is used for a transposition.
3. The superficial fascia is opened. Care is taken not to injure the medial antebrachial cutaneous nerve (located ~2.5 cm distal to the medial epicondyle).
4. Before opening the deep fascia, one should palpate the ulnar nerve against the retrocondylar groove. It is important to open the deep fascia right on top of the nerve to avoid missing the nerve. Using forceps to lift up the fascia and tenotomy scissors, the incision in the deep fascia is

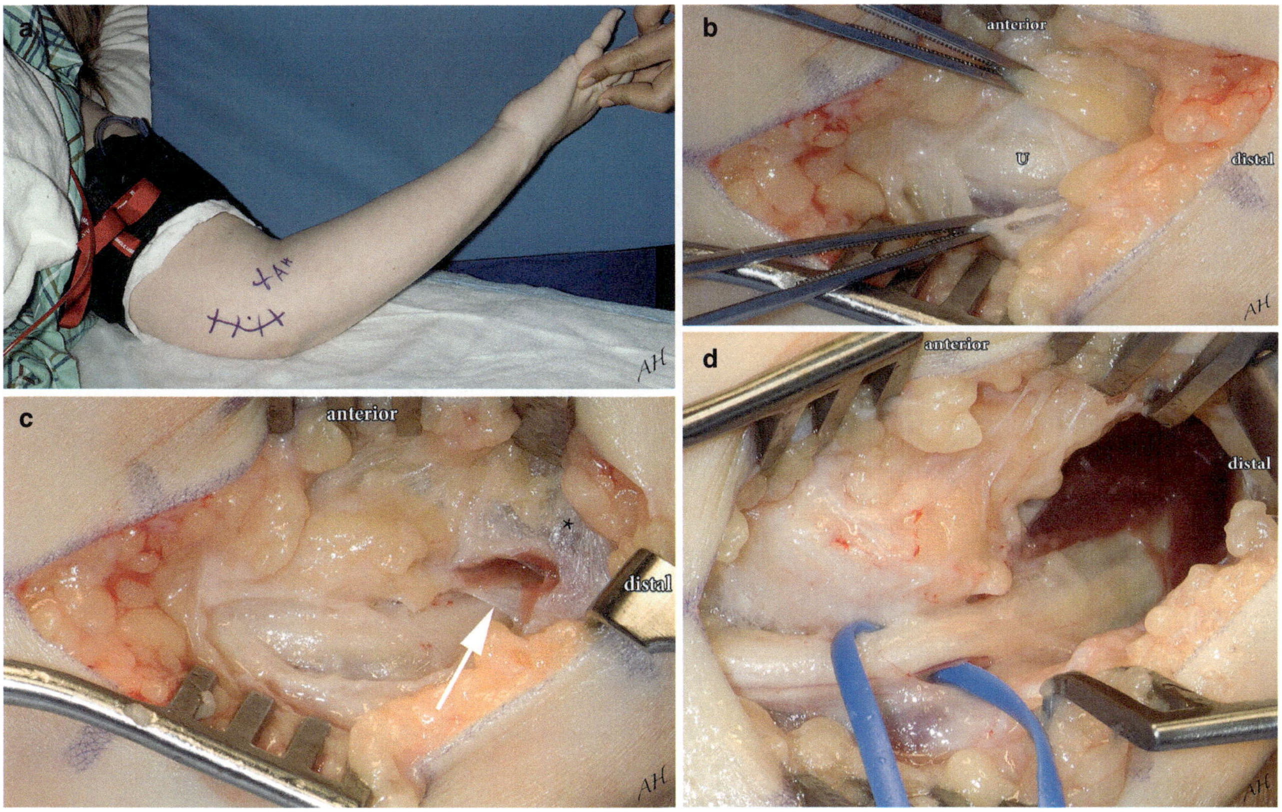

Fig. 18.6 Ulnar decompression at the elbow. (**a**) The patient is positioned supine with the arm abducted, externally rotated, and the elbow flexed. Incision is made between the medial epicondyle and the olecranon. Tourniquet use is optional. (**b**) The nerve sheath is opened, and the ulnar nerve (*U*) is exposed. (**c**) The fascia (*) superficial to flexor carpi ulnaris is opened, the two heads separated from each other, and the fascia (arrow) deep to the muscle is also opened. (**d**) The ulnar nerve (blue loop) is completely unroofed proximally and distally. There is no need for a 360° decompression; this may cause iatrogenic subluxation

deepened until the nerve sheath is opened and the nerve is exposed. It is not uncommon to encounter an anconeus epitrochlearis in this location, it should be carefully dissected off the nerve (Fig. 18.3).

5. Once in the right plane, the nerve can be unroofed proximally and distally. Ulnar nerve branches start below the medial epicondyle. To protect these, dissection should mainly be on the surface of the nerve and not on its sides.
6. Distally, the fascia overlying the flexor carpi ulnaris is opened, the two heads of the muscle separated, and the fascia underneath it opened (Fig. 18.6).
7. For a transposition (Fig. 18.7), the medial intermuscular septum should be resected, and the ulnar branches dissected off the nerve in an interfascicular fashion, to avoid tension, and then the nerve is transposed anteriorly. Sometimes, an FCU branch would straddle the ulnar nerve to supply the two heads preventing a free excursion of the nerve anteriorly. In this case, the branch to one of the heads can be cut, the nerve moved and then the branch sutured together or left unrepaired. For subcutaneous transposition, a pocket is created between subcutaneous fat and the deep fascia covering the flexor muscle origin, and the nerve is transposed into that pocket and secured in place. For submuscular (intramuscular) transposition, the fascia overlying the flexor origin is opened, and a soft muscular bed is created by cutting through the superficial layers of the flexor muscle origin. The nerve is transposed to the new muscular bed, and the deep fascia is closed, usually with a z-plasty for lengthening. Care should be taken not to dissect too lateral to avoid injury of the median nerve while creating the new bed for the transposed ulnar nerve.

At Guyon's Canal (Fig. 18.8)

1. Position: supine, with the arm abducted and supinated.
2. Incision is made lateral to the flexor carpi ulnaris tendon and pisiform, crossing the wrist obliquely and then along the hypothenar eminence.
3. The flexor carpi ulnaris tendon is identified at the proximal part of the incision and retracted medially. The ulnar nerve with the artery lateral to it enters Guyon's canal lateral to the pisiform bone.
4. Guyon's canal is then unroofed, and the nerve is followed until it branches.
5. The deep motor branch is followed under the hypothenar muscle arch, which is released for full decompression.

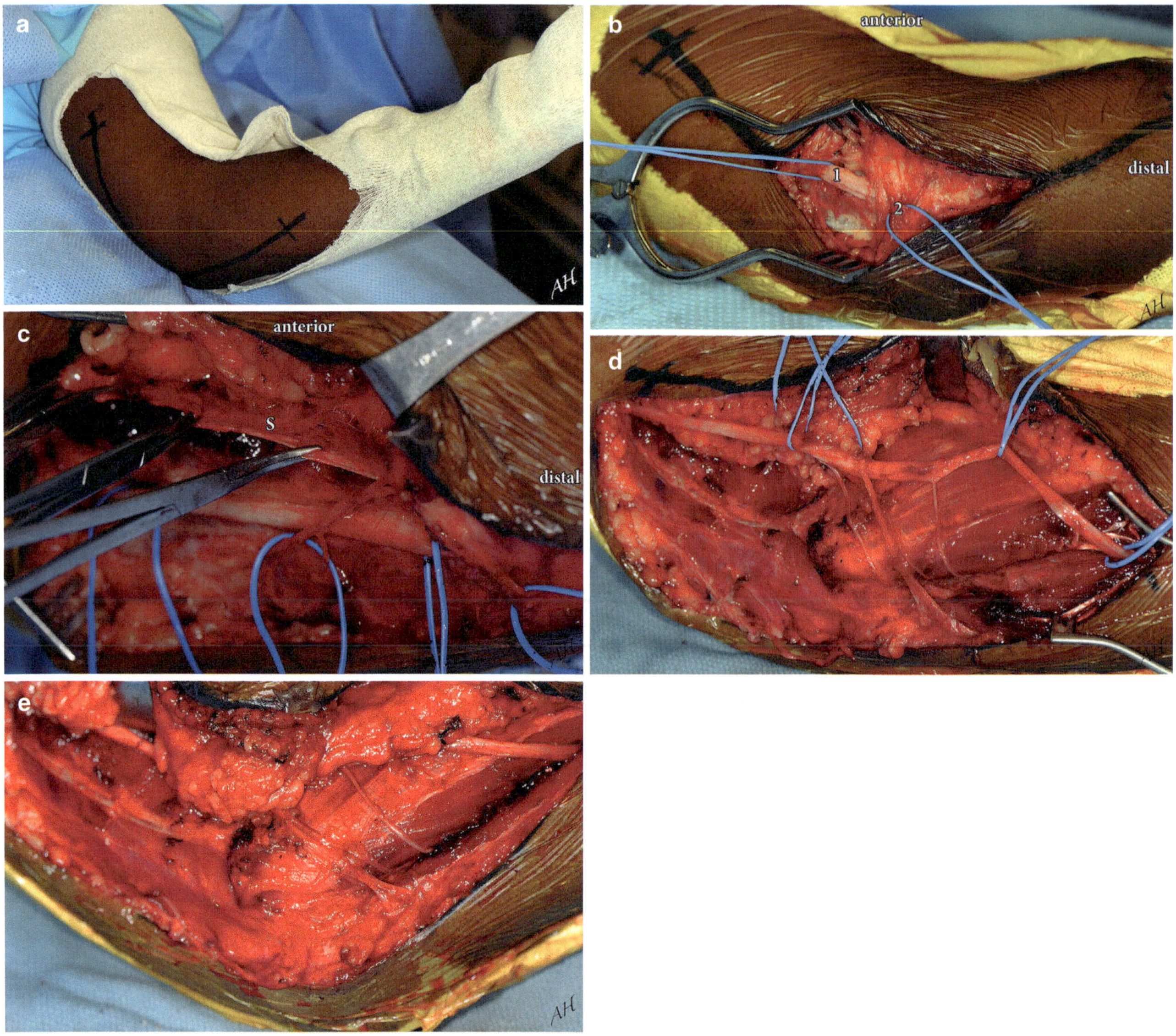

Fig. 18.7 Subcutaneous transposition of the ulnar nerve. (**a**) Position is the same as for a decompression, and the incision is longer. (**b**) The ulnar nerve (*1*) is exposed as above; the medial antebrachial cutaneous nerve (*2*) is identified and protected. (**c**) The medial intermuscular septum (*S*) is dissected free and resected. (**d**) Interfascicular dissection of the ulnar nerve branches increases their length, thus allowing transposition without tension. Note the subcutaneous pocket created between the subcutaneous fat and the fascia overlying the flexor muscles. (**e**) Once the nerve is transposed, it is kept in place by suturing the fat to the fascia

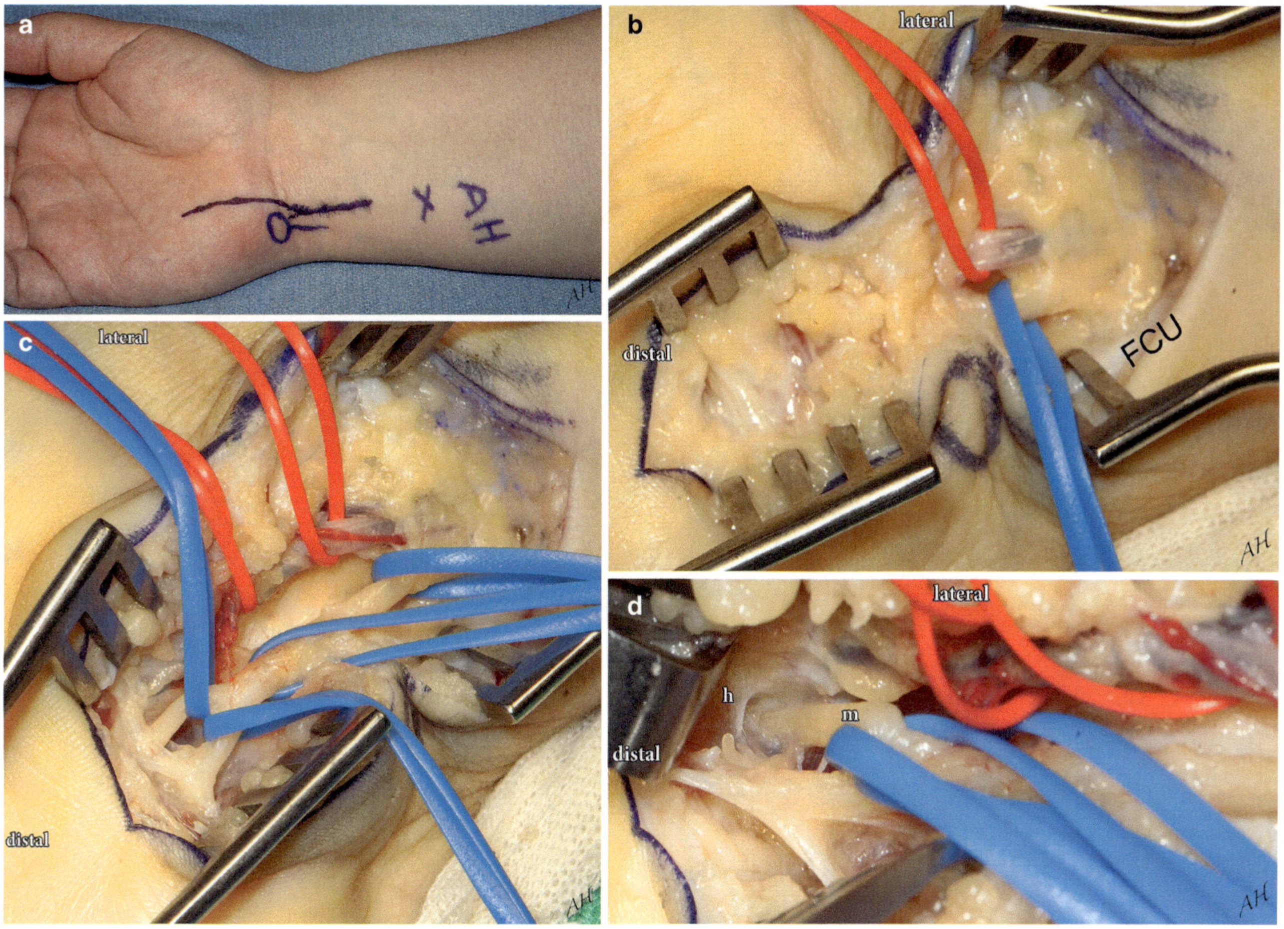

Fig. 18.8 Right Guyon's canal decompression. (**a**) The patient is positioned supine with the arm abducted and supinated on a hand table. The incision is lateral to the flexor carpi ulnaris (FCU) tendon and pisiform bone and extended into the palm lateral to the hypothenar eminence. (**b**) The *FCU* tendon is retracted medially, and the ulnar nerve (blue loop) and vessels (red loop) are exposed. These are seen entering the Guyon's canal distally. (**c**) After opening the Guyon's canal, the ulnar nerve and vessels are decompressed. (**d**) The deep motor branch (*m*) is followed until it enters under the hypothenar arch (*h*), which needs to be decompressed as well

In the Hand

1. Incisions in the hand and fingers are made in a zigzag fashion (Bruner's type) to avoid contractures.
2. The digital nerves course along the medial and lateral aspects of the fingers with the digital vessels.

References

1. Nellans K, Galdi B, Kim HM, Levine WN (2014) Ulnar neuropathy as a result of anconeus epitrochlearis. Orthopedics 37(8):e743–e745. https://doi.org/10.3928/01477447-20140728-92
2. Bartels RH, Verhagen WI, van der Wilt GJ, Meulstee J, van Rossum LG, Grotenhuis JA (2005) Prospective randomized controlled study comparing simple decompression versus anterior subcutaneous transposition for idiopathic neuropathy of the ulnar nerve at the elbow: Part 1. Neurosurgery 56(3):522–530; discussion 522–30. https://doi.org/10.1227/01.neu.0000154131.01167.03

Suprascapular Nerve

19

Amgad S. Hanna

Surgical Anatomy

The suprascapular nerve arises from the upper trunk (superior trunk) of the brachial plexus, predominantly from C5, with occasional small contribution from C6 [1, 2]. The upper trunk division typically forms a trifurcation with the suprascapular nerve, posterior division, and then anterior division arranged from cranial to caudal, respectively (SPA). It travels posteriorly toward the suprascapular notch, which it enters underneath the suprascapular ligament, which typically separates the nerve from the suprascapular artery. Occasionally, the suprascapular ligament is completely ossified, transforming the notch into a foramen [3, 4]. The nerve then travels deep to the supraspinatus, which it supplies, then through the spinoglenoid notch to the undersurface of the infraspinatus, which it also supplies. It is responsible for shoulder stability, initiation of abduction, and external rotation.

Clinical Significance

The suprascapular nerve can be damaged by entrapment at the suprascapular notch, which affects the supraspinatus and infraspinatus muscles. More distal compression at the spinoglenoid notch would involve the infraspinatus only. It can also be damaged in the upper trunk stretch or avulsion injuries, which would also affect the deltoid, biceps brachii, and brachialis muscles. Nerve entrapment is treated by sectioning the suprascapular ligament (below). Nerve trauma can be treated by nerve transfer from the spinal accessory nerve via anterior or posterior approach (see Chap. 33).

Supplementary Information The online version contains supplementary material available at https://doi.org/10.1007/978-3-031-73931-6_19.

A. S. Hanna (✉)
Deparment of Neurosurgery, University of Wisconsin School of Medicine and Public Health, Madison, WI, USA

Exposure

Anterior

See Chap. 7.

Posterior

1. The patient is positioned laterally on a beanbag (Fig. 19.1) or prone.
2. The suprascapular notch is located at the level of the medial aspect of the coracoid process. It is also almost halfway between the superior angle of the scapula and acromion.
3. Skin incision along the upper border of the spine of the scapula. Take the incision over the acromion (you are never lateral enough).
4. The incision is deepened through the superficial and deep fasciae.
5. The trapezius is opened horizontally along its fibers, above the spine of the scapula (Fig. 19.2), some trape-

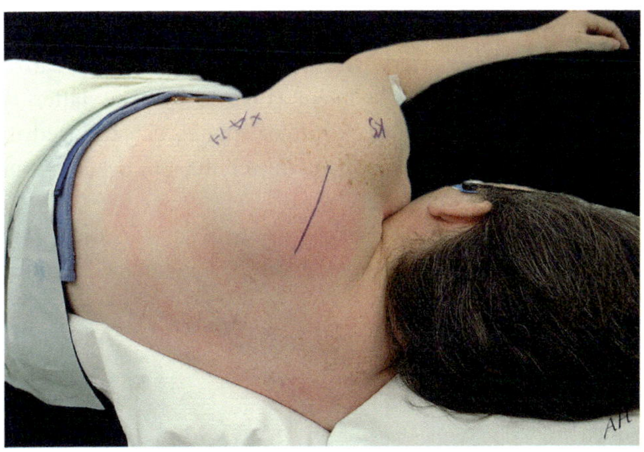

Fig. 19.1 The patient is positioned lateral on a beanbag for left suprascapular decompression. Prone position could also be used

A. S. Hanna (ed.), *Nerves: Anatomy, Exposures, and Techniques*, https://doi.org/10.1007/978-3-031-73931-6_19

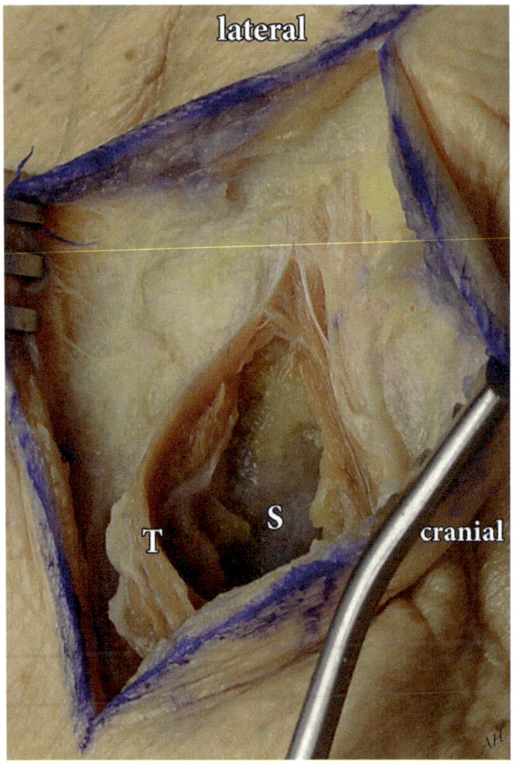

Fig. 19.2 Cadaveric dissection of left suprascapular nerve. The trapezius (*T*) is opened along its fibers. This exposes the fascia covering the supraspinatus (*S*)

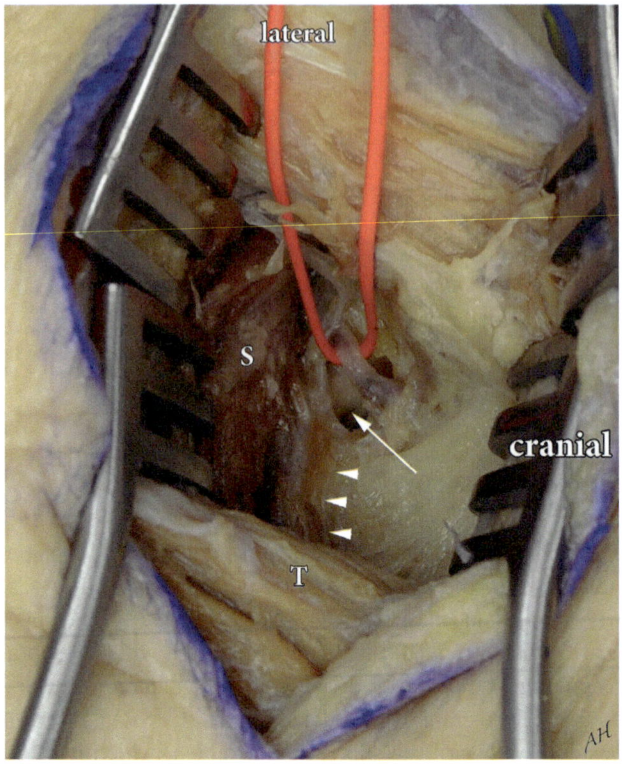

Fig. 19.3 The supraspinatus (*S*) is retracted caudally, exposing the upper border of the scapula (arrowheads). The suprascapular artery (red loop) is observed superficial to the transverse scapular (suprascapular) ligament (arrow) and suprascapular notch. *S* supraspinatus, *T* trapezius

zius fibers, especially laterally, will have to be cut for the approach and repaired during closure. A self-retaining retractor is placed.

6. Another layer of deep fascia is encountered; once opened, this exposes the supraspinatus muscle.
7. The supraspinatus muscle is retracted caudally; this exposes the upper border of the scapula. Followed laterally, one can feel the suprascapular notch. As the finger moves laterally over the upper border of the scapula, you may feel a dip as you feel the notch, and the hard bony feeling gives way to the firm ligament feeling.
8. A Doppler ultrasound probe can be used to identify the suprascapular artery. The artery is retracted to visualize the suprascapular ligament (Fig. 19.3). The latter is white and glistening. A kittner sponge can be used to better identify the ligament, detach the soft tissues from it, and retract the artery.
9. The ligament is opened sharply with scissors or, if it is ossified, with Kerrison rongeurs. The notch itself can be enlarged with Kerrison rongeurs for full decompression. The author finds it easier to place a grooved Woodson tool (dental) inside the notch, under the ligament, protecting the nerve, and the assistant uses a #15 scalpel blade to cut the ligament on top of the Woodson.
10. The suprascapular nerve can then be identified and followed proximally and distally (Fig. 19.4).
11. At the spinoglenoid notch: the supraspinatus muscle is retracted cranially to expose the nerve as it enters the spinoglenoid notch (Fig. 19.5). More inferior exposure would require separation of the infraspinatus muscle from the undersurface of the spine of the scapula. The nerve can be identified as it passes from the spinoglenoid notch to the undersurface of the infraspinatus muscle (Fig. 19.6). Using Kerrison rongeurs, the spinoglenoid notch can be enlarged for further decompression.

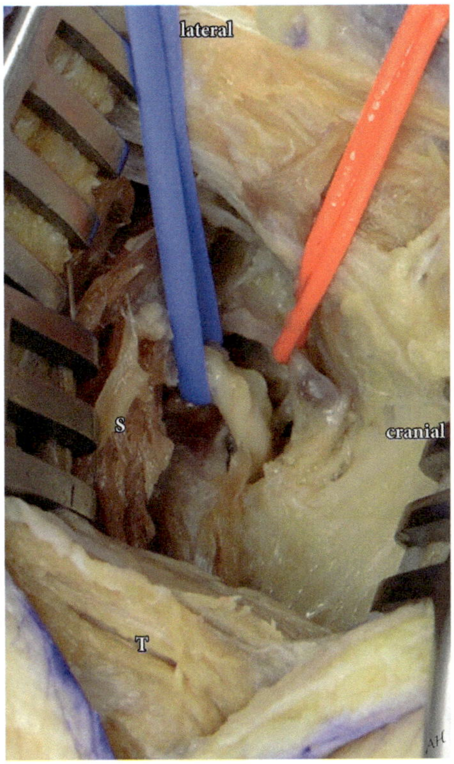

Fig. 19.4 The suprascapular ligament has been opened. The suprascapular nerve (blue loop) is now decompressed. *S* supraspinatus, *T* trapezius

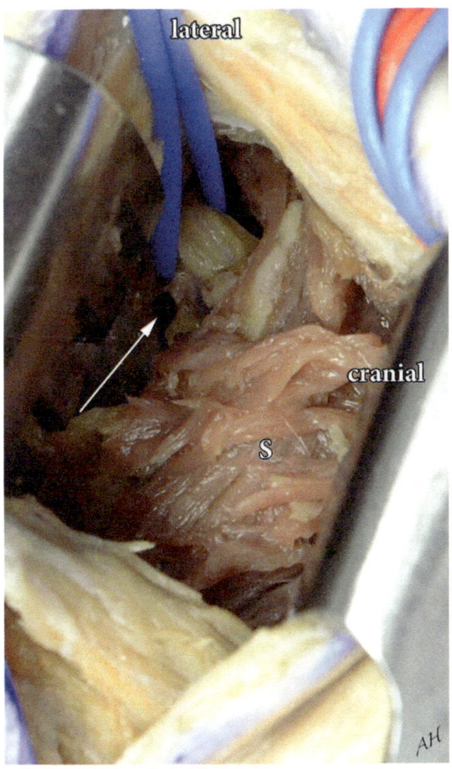

Fig. 19.5 If further decompression is needed, the supraspinatus (*S*) is retracted cranially, thus exposing the suprascapular nerve (blue loop) in the spinoglenoid notch (arrow)

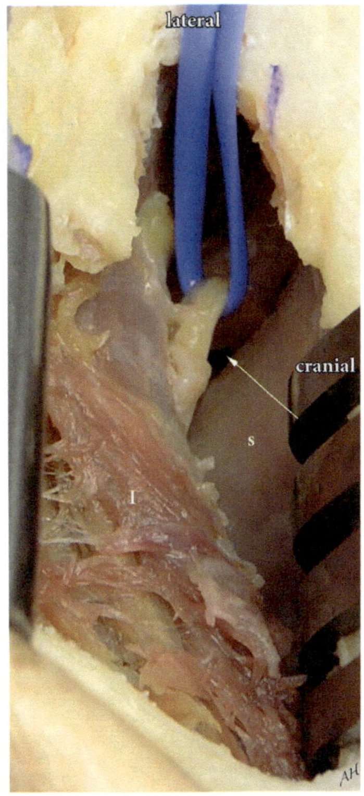

Fig. 19.6 More caudally, the infraspinatus (*I*) can be separated from the spine of the scapula (*s*), thus exposing the suprascapular nerve (blue loop) coming out of the spinoglenoid notch (arrow)

References

1. Siqueira MG, Foroni LHL, Martins RS, Chadi G, Malessy MJA (2010) Fascicular topography of the suprascapular nerve in the C5 root and upper trunk of the brachial plexus: a microanatomic study from a nerve surgeon's perspective. Neurosurgery 67(2 Suppl Operative):402–406. https://doi.org/10.1227/NEU.0b013e3181f74297
2. Hanna A (2021) Letter: Fascicular topography of the suprascapular nerve in the C5 root and upper trunk of the brachial plexus: a microanatomic study from a nerve surgeon's perspective. Neurosurgery 89(1):E88. https://doi.org/10.1093/neuros/nyab132
3. Polguj M, Sibinski M, Grzegorzewski A, Waszczykowski M, Majos A, Topol M (2014) Morphological and radiological study of ossified superior transverse scapular ligament as potential risk factor of suprascapular nerve entrapment. Biomed Res Int 2014:613601. https://doi.org/10.1155/2014/613601. Epub 2014 Apr 3.
4. Kumar A, Sharma A, Singh P (2014) Anatomical study of the suprascapular notch: quantitative analysis and clinical considerations for suprascapular nerve entrapment. Singapore Med J 55(1):41–44. https://doi.org/10.11622/smedj.2014009

Spinal Accessory Nerve

20

Amgad S. Hanna

Surgical Anatomy

The spinal accessory nerve arises from the upper cervical spinal cord (C1–C5), ascends between the dentate ligament and the posterior cervical rootlets, then through the foramen magnum joins the cranial part and then exits through the jugular foramen. It runs through or deep to the sternocleidomastoid (SCM). It courses subcutaneously in the posterior triangle of the neck from the posterior border of the SCM cranially to the anterior border of the trapezius muscle caudally [1]. It supplies both the SCM and the trapezius. There are frequent contributions from C2 and C3 medial to SCM [2]. The cranial portion arises from the medulla oblongata and eventually joins the vagus nerve [3].

Clinical Significance

The spinal accessory nerve usually remains intact after brachial plexus injuries. It can be used as a donor (distal to some trapezius branches) for nerve transfers to the suprascapular nerve (anterior vs posterior approach) (Chap. 33) or a free muscle flap (Chap. 41). More distal targets like musculocutaneous nerve can be neurotized using a nerve graft. The nerve can be injured in the posterior triangle of the neck during lymph node biopsies or removal of masses like lipomas, causing shoulder pain and paralysis of the trapezius muscle. This can result in scapular winging, especially with the elbows flexed (Fig. 20.1) and the inability to abduct the shoulder beyond 90°. Selective denervation of the SCM is used to treat cervical dystonia (Chap. 61): contralateral SCM in torticollis, and ipsilateral SCM in laterocollis.

Supplementary Information The online version contains supplementary material available at https://doi.org/10.1007/978-3-031-73931-6_20.

A. S. Hanna (✉)
Department of Neurosurgery, University of Wisconsin School of Medicine and Public Health, Madison, WI, USA

A. S. Hanna (ed.), *Nerves: Anatomy, Exposures, and Techniques*, https://doi.org/10.1007/978-3-031-73931-6_20

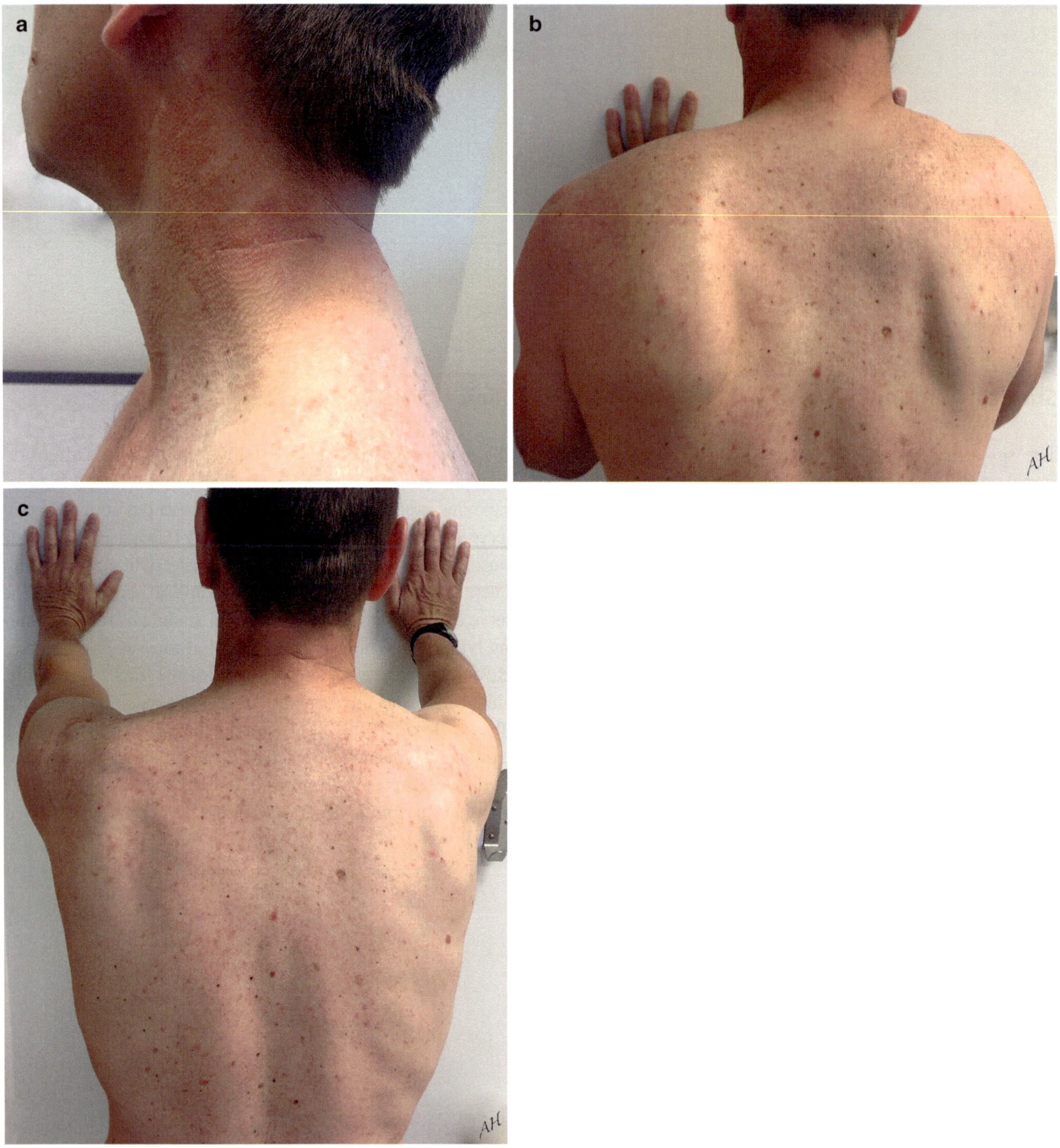

Fig. 20.1 (**a**) Incision for resection of a subcutaneous lipoma of the neck. (**b**) This resulted in partial injury of the spinal accessory nerve and left scapular winging. Note the winging is more pronounced with elbow flexion, rather than with elbow extension (**c**)

Exposure

During Brachial Plexus Exposure (Fig. 20.2)

1. Supraclavicular brachial plexus exposure as in Chap. 7.
2. The nerve is searched for within the fat pad along the anterior border of the trapezius muscle.
3. Dissection is carried along the undersurface of the trapezius using Metzenbaum scissors. Electrical stimulation can be used to identify the nerve.
4. If used as a donor, the nerve should be harvested distal to some trapezius branches to avoid postoperative weakness.

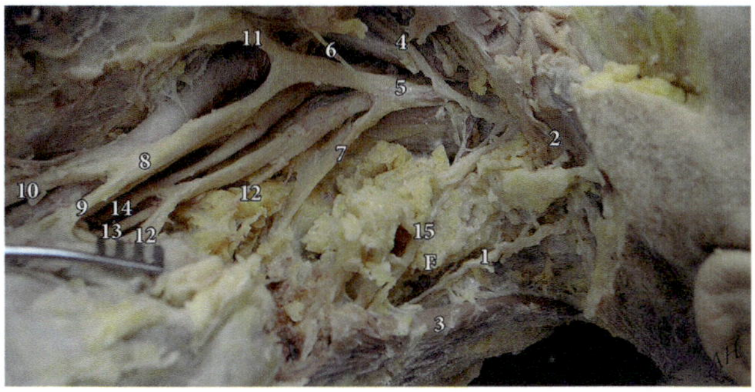

Fig. 20.2 Left spinal accessory nerve (*1*) exposure during a brachial plexus exposure. The nerve is found within the fat (*F*) anterior and deep to the trapezius muscle (*3*). Note the wavy course of the nerve. *2* sternocleidomastoid, *4* phrenic nerve, *5* brachial plexus—upper trunk, *6* nerve to subclavius, *7* suprascapular nerve, *8* lateral cord, *9* musculocutaneous nerve, *10* median nerve, *11* lateral pectoral nerve, in this specimen arising from the anterior division of the upper trunk rather than the lateral cord, *12* upper and lower subscapular nerves, *13* axillary nerve, *14* radial nerve. Branches of the cervical plexus (*15*), not to be mistaken for the spinal accessory nerve

Anterior Approach to the Spinal Accessory Nerve

1. Position: supine, with the head turned to the contralateral side.
2. The nerve trajectory in the posterior triangle of the neck should be drawn first. This is represented by a line joining the posterior border of the SCM about 5 cm below the mastoid process and the anterior border of the trapezius about 5 cm above the midpoint of the clavicle (Fig. 20.3) [1].
3. Incision is made along this line, or curvilinear along a skin crease, through the skin and superficial fascia.
4. The nerve is found in the superficial fascia as it courses from ventral and cranial to dorsal and caudal. At the posterior border of the SCM, the nerve is about 1.5 cm cranial to the great auricular nerve. The great auricular nerve winds around the posterior border of SCM from deep to superficial and ascends vertically toward the angle of the mandible and ear.
5. The spinal accessory nerve can be followed anteriorly until the undersurface of the SCM and posteriorly until the undersurface of the trapezius muscle.

Posterior Approach

See Chap. 33.

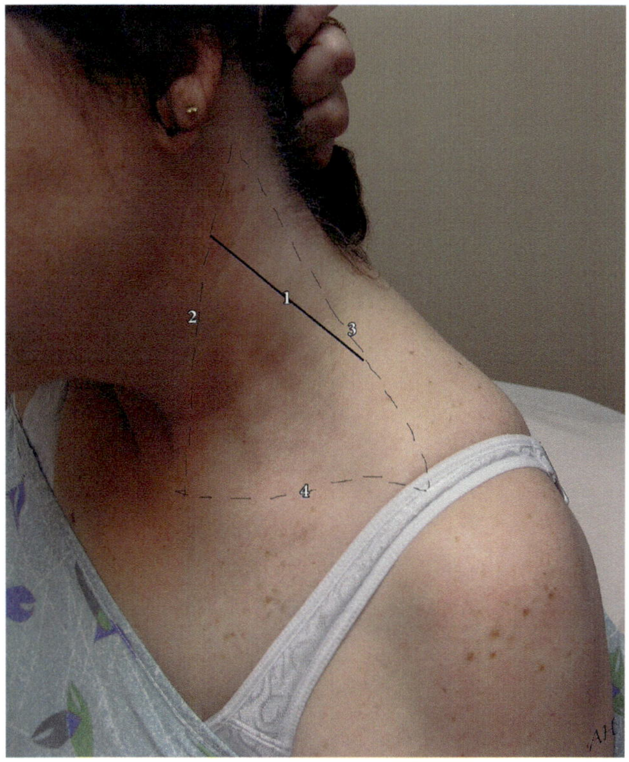

Fig. 20.3 Trajectory of the spinal accessory nerve (*1*) in the posterior triangle of the neck. It travels from 5 cm below the mastoid process along the posterior border of sternocleidomastoid (*2*) to the anterior border of trapezius (*3*), 5 cm above the mid-clavicular point. *4* clavicle

References

1. Tubbs RS, Salter EG, Wellons JC III, Blount JP, Oakes WJ (2005) Superficial landmarks for the spinal accessory nerve within the posterior cervical triangle. J Neurosurg Spine 3(5):375–378. https://doi.org/10.3171/spi.2005.3.5.0375
2. Tubbs RS, Maldonado AA, Stoves Y, Fries FN, Li R, Loukas M et al (2018) A novel method of lengthening the accessory nerve for direct coaptation during nerve repair and nerve transfer procedures. J Neurosurg 128(1):272–276. https://doi.org/10.3171/2016.10.JNS161106. Epub 2017 Mar 3
3. Johal J, Iwanaga J, Tubbs K, Loukas M, Oskouian RJ, Tubbs RS (2019) The accessory nerve: a comprehensive review of its anatomy, development, variations, landmarks and clinical considerations. Anat Rec (Hoboken) 302(4):620–629. https://doi.org/10.1002/ar.23823. Epub 2018 Apr 23

Long Thoracic and Thoracodorsal Nerves

21

Amgad S. Hanna

Surgical Anatomy

The long thoracic nerve arises from the posterior aspect of C5, C6, and often C7 ventral rami. It travels within the scalenus medius. It then runs over the lateral surface of the serratus anterior (SA), supplying it with multiple branches.

The thoracodorsal nerve (C6, C7, and C8) arises from the posterior cord. It courses anterior to the latissimus dorsi (LD) along with the corresponding vessels and supplies the muscle.

Clinical Significance

Injury to the long thoracic nerve can occur during mastectomies. The nerve is also usually involved in brachial plexitis (Parsonage–Turner syndrome). This causes scapular winging, especially with the arms in full extension (Fig. 21.1). The long thoracic and thoracodorsal nerves course close enough to each other that one of them can be used to neurotize the other, usually the posterior division of the thoracodorsal nerve to the long thoracic nerve [1]. LD and its neurovascular pedicle can be used for the reconstruction of elbow flexion after brachial plexus injury [2]. The thoracodorsal nerve has also been used to reinnervate the triceps branch of the radial nerve [3].

This chapter focuses on more distal exposures in the axilla and chest wall. For more proximal exposure, refer to Chaps. 7, 8, 9, 11, and 13.

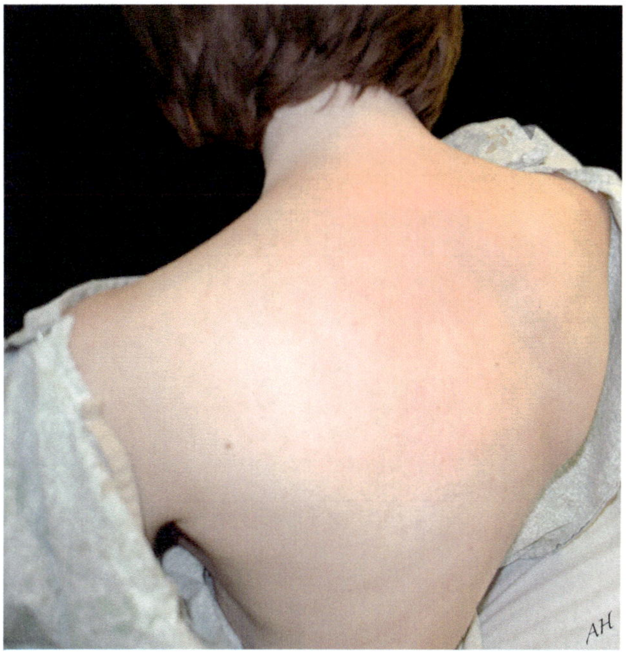

Fig. 21.1 Right scapular winging from long thoracic neuropathy

Supplementary Information The online version contains supplementary material available at https://doi.org/10.1007/978-3-031-73931-6_21.

A. S. Hanna (✉)
Department of Neurosurgery, University of Wisconsin School of Medicine and Public Health, Madison, WI, USA

A. S. Hanna (ed.), *Nerves: Anatomy, Exposures, and Techniques*, https://doi.org/10.1007/978-3-031-73931-6_21

Exposure

1. Position: supine, with the arm abducted 90°.
2. Incision in the midaxillary line (Fig. 21.2).
3. The superficial fascia is opened.
4. The deep fascia overlying the SA is opened.
5. The long thoracic nerve can be seen on the surface of the SA, sequentially giving off branches to supply different digitations of the muscle (Fig. 21.3).
6. To expose the thoracodorsal nerve, the deep fascia overlying the LD is opened (Fig. 21.3). The micro-Doppler effect can be used to locate the corresponding vessels that typically travel along the nerve.
7. Once identified, the nerve can be followed proximally and distally until its anterior and posterior divisions. The posterior division can be used as a donor, end-to-end versus end-to-side (Fig. 21.4).

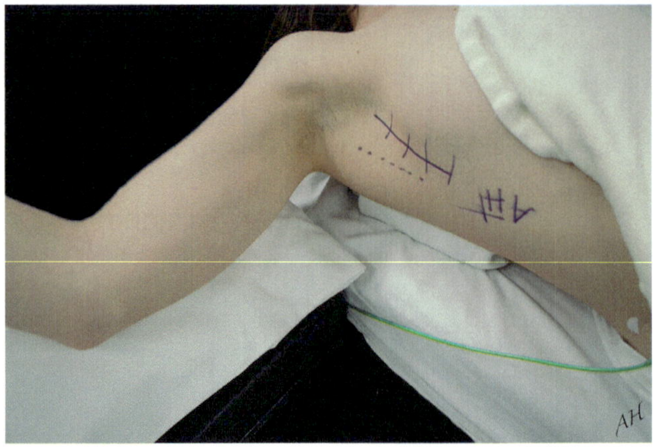

Fig. 21.2 Position and incision for exposure of the long thoracic and thoracodorsal nerves

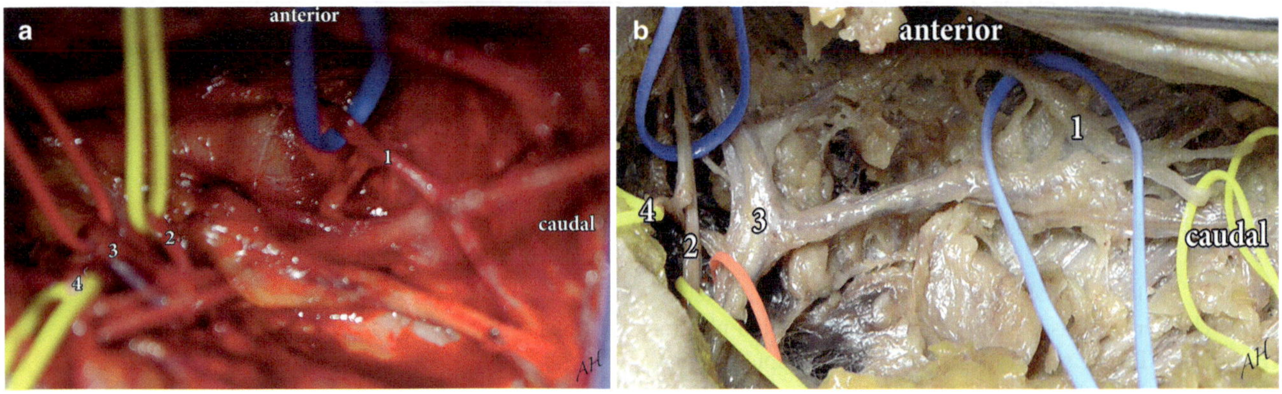

Fig. 21.3 The long thoracic nerve (*1*) is found anteriorly deep to the fascia covering the serratus anterior. The thoracodorsal nerve, with its anterior (*2*) and posterior (*4*) branches, is found along the thoracodorsal vessels (*3*) toward the posterior axillary fold. (**a**) Surgical view. (**b**) Cadaveric dissection

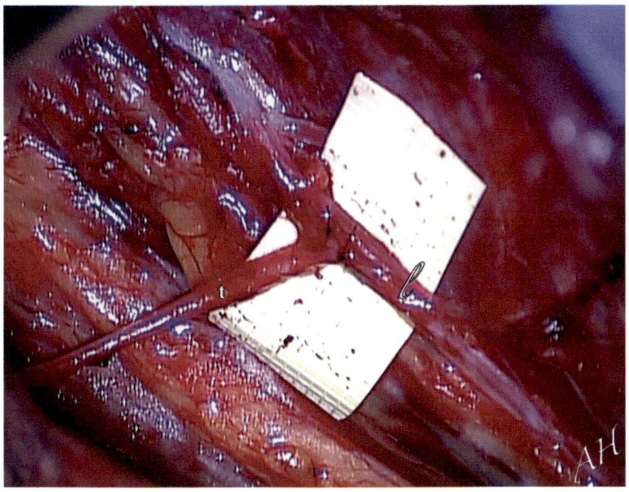

Fig. 21.4 End-to-side neurorrhaphy from the posterior division of the thoracodorsal nerve (*t*) to the long thoracic nerve (*l*). End-to-side was chosen in this case because long thoracic nerve stimulation evoked muscle contraction

References

1. Ray WZ, Pet MA, Nicoson MC, Yee A, Kahn LC, Mackinnon SE (2011) Two-level motor nerve transfer for the treatment of long thoracic nerve palsy. J Neurosurg 115(4):858–864. https://doi.org/10.3171/2011.5.JNS101615. Epub 2011 Jun 24
2. Azab AAH, Alsabbahi MS (2017) Bipolar transfer of latissimus dorsi myocutaneous flap for restoration of elbow flexion in late traumatic brachial plexus injury: evaluation of 13 cases. Ann Plast Surg 78(2):198–201. https://doi.org/10.1097/SAP.0000000000000907
3. Pet MA, Ray WZ, Yee A, Mackinnon SE (2011) Nerve transfer to the triceps after brachial plexus injury: report of four cases. J Hand Surg Am 36(3):398–405. https://doi.org/10.1016/j.jhsa.2010.11.024

22 Intercostal Nerves

Amgad S. Hanna and Thomas M. Staniszewski

Surgical Anatomy

The intercostal nerves arise from the ventral rami of the corresponding thoracic nerves. They run on the undersurface of the lower border of the rib in a neurovascular bundle with the following arrangement from cranial to caudal: vein, artery, and nerve (VAN).

They typically follow the course of the rib from dorsal to ventral. They supply the intercostal muscles and give off two cutaneous branches, one laterally and one anteriorly. They also send a collateral branch that follows the upper border of the next rib. Exceptions to this are the first and second thoracic ventral rami: T1 main contribution joins the brachial plexus lower trunk, and a smaller branch continues as the first intercostal nerve. T2 lateral cutaneous branch forms the intercostobrachial nerve that supplies the skin of the floor of the axilla and medial upper arm.

Clinical Significance

The intercostal nerves are usually used to reinnervate the brachial plexus. They are good donors for nerve transfers. They can be used for the musculocutaneous nerve [1], radial nerve [2, 3], axillary nerve [3], or to a free gracilis muscle flap (obturator nerve branch mobilized with the muscle). The cutaneous component can be used to neurotize the median nerve (lateral cord contribution) in an attempt to regain protective sensation in the hand.

Supplementary Information The online version contains supplementary material available at https://doi.org/10.1007/978-3-031-73931-6_22.

A. S. Hanna (✉)
Department of Neurosurgery, University of Wisconsin School of Medicine and Public Health, Madison, WI, USA

T. M. Staniszewski
Department of Neurological Surgery, University of Wisconsin School of Medicine and Public Health, Madison, WI, USA
e-mail: staniszewski@neurosurgery.wisc.edu

This chapter focuses on the subperiosteal technique. See also Chap. 38 for the transmuscular approach.

Exposure

1. Incision along the midaxillary line curving anteriorly along the ribs at about the sixth intercostal space (Fig. 22.1).
2. The incision is deepened through the superficial and deep fasciae.
3. A flap is raised separating the pectoralis major then minor from the chest wall.
4. The ribs are identified. Typically, intercostal nerves 3–6 are the usual donors (Fig. 22.2).
5. The periosteum is opened sharply with a scalpel blade. A periosteal elevator is used to achieve a subperiosteal dis-

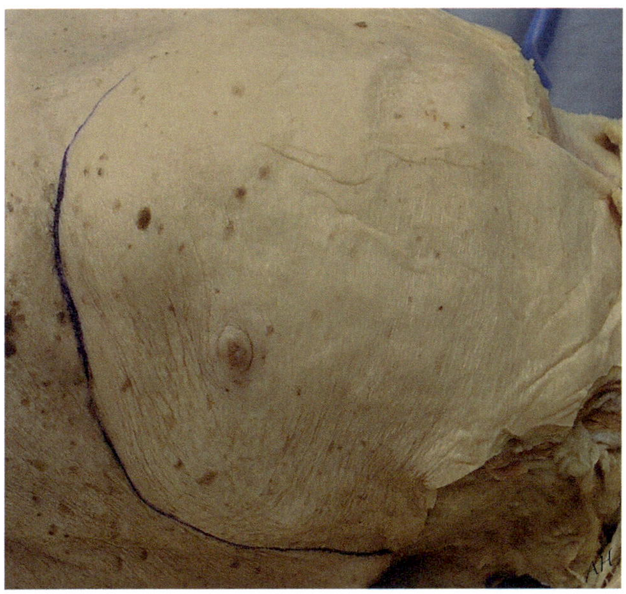

Fig. 22.1 Incision for intercostal nerve harvesting

A. S. Hanna (ed.), *Nerves: Anatomy, Exposures, and Techniques*, https://doi.org/10.1007/978-3-031-73931-6_22

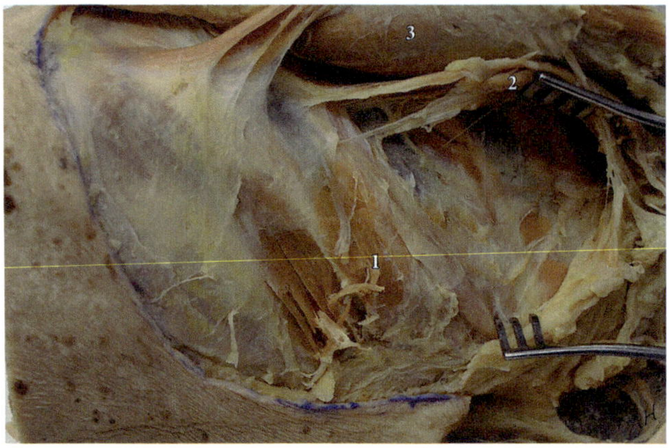

Fig. 22.2 Once pectoralis major (*3*) and minor (*2*) are separated from the chest wall, the ribs with overlying serratus anterior (*1*) can be exposed

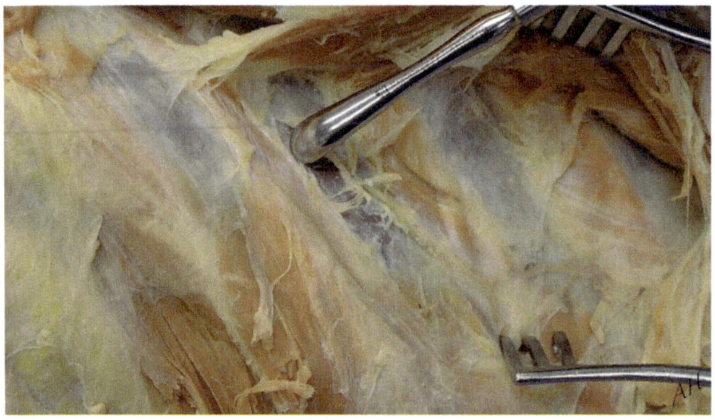

Fig. 22.3 A periosteal elevator is used to dissect the periosteum off the rib

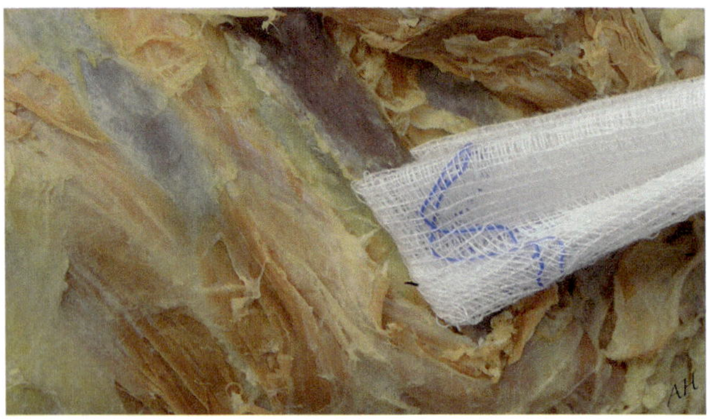

Fig. 22.4 A Ray-Tec sponge can be used to retract the rib cranially to expose the neurovascular bundle. Of note, it is not necessary to completely skeletonize the rib; caudal exposure with retraction cranially can be sufficient

section of the anterior surface and the upper and lower borders of the rib (Fig. 22.3).

6. A Doyen rib dissector is used to strip the periosteum from the undersurface of the rib. The pleura is very thin, and care should be taken not to violate the pleura. A Ray-Tec

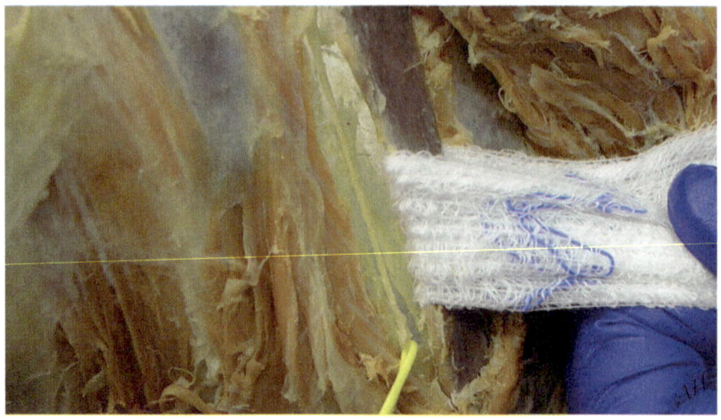

Fig. 22.5 The intercostal nerve (*yellow loop*) has been dissected free. A nerve stimulator can be used to find the motor component

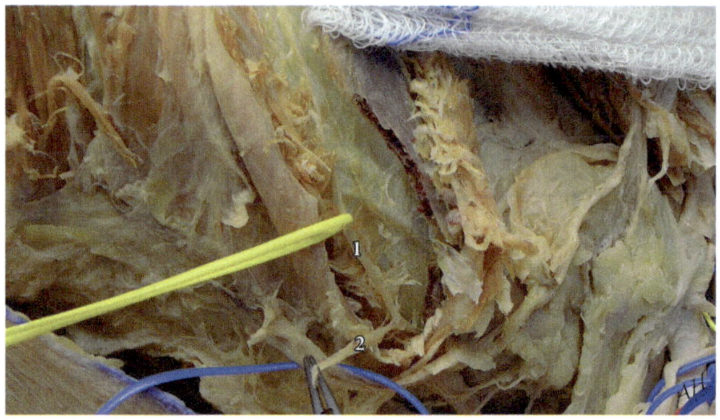

Fig. 22.6 Both the motor (*1*) and sensory (*2*) branches have been dissected

sponge can then be used to retract the rib cranially (Fig. 22.4). Alternatively, the rib needs not be skeletonized completely; caudal exposure with retraction cranially using a Regnell or Heiss retractor can be sufficient.

7. The neurovascular bundle can then be identified at the lower border of the rib. The deep periosteum overlying the neurovascular bundle is opened sharply. Electrical stimulation can be used to find the nerve.
8. The nerve is then followed medially (anteriorly) and laterally (posteriorly) to gain as much length as possible (Fig. 22.5).
9. The lateral cutaneous branch takes off laterally almost perpendicular to the main nerve and can just be pulled through the superficial tissues (Fig. 22.6).

Complications

Pneumothorax: If the pleura is violated, it can be closed with a 3-0 Vicryl stitch over a small feeding tube. The tube can be pulled out during a Valsalva maneuver at the end. Postoperative chest X-ray should be obtained. Larger pneumothorax will warrant a chest tube placement.

References

1. Xiao C, Lao J, Wang T, Zhao X, Liu J, Gu Y (2014) Intercostal nerve transfer to neurotize the musculocutaneous nerve after traumatic brachial plexus avulsion: a comparison of two, three, and four nerve transfers. J Reconstr Microsurg 30(5):297–304. https://doi.org/10.1055/s-0033-1361840. Epub 2014 Mar 28
2. Kittithamvongs P, Leechavengvongs S, Malungpaishrope K, Pongpinyopap W, Anantavorasakul N, Uerpairojkit C (2023) The intercostal nerves transfer to the radial nerve branch to the long head triceps muscle: influencing factor and outcome of 55 cases. J Hand Surg Am 48(7):733.e1–733.e7. https://doi.org/10.1016/j.jhsa.2022.01.014. Epub 2022 Mar 7
3. Malungpaishrope K, Leechavengvongs S, Witoonchart K, Uerpairojkit C, Boonyalapa A, Janesaksrisakul D (2012) Simultaneous intercostal nerve transfers to deltoid and triceps muscle through the posterior approach. J Hand Surg Am 37(4):677–682. https://doi.org/10.1016/j.jhsa.2011.12.034. Epub 2012 Feb 28

Part IV

Lower Body Nerves

Lumbosacral Plexus

23

Amgad S. Hanna and Mark E. Ehlers

Surgical Anatomy

The lumbar plexus arises from the ventral rami of L1–L5 nerve roots. It forms within the psoas major muscle. The nerves are divided into three groups based on their relationship to the psoas muscle as they enter the retroperitoneal space.

Anterior to the Psoas Major Muscle

- Genitofemoral nerve (L1 and L2)

Lateral to the Psoas Major Muscle, from Cranial to Caudal

- Iliohypogastric (T12 and L1)
- Ilioinguinal (L1)
- Lateral femoral cutaneous nerve (L2 and L3, posterior division)
- Femoral nerve (L2–L4, posterior division)

Medial to the Psoas Major Muscle, from Cranial to Caudal

- Obturator nerve (L2–L4, anterior division)
- Accessory obturator nerve (seen in ~10% of cases) (L2–L4, anterior division)
- Lumbosacral trunk (L4 and L5)

Supplementary Information The online version contains supplementary material available at https://doi.org/10.1007/978-3-031-73931-6_23.

A. S. Hanna (✉)
Department of Neurosurgery, University of Wisconsin School of Medicine and Public Health, Madison, WI, USA

M. E. Ehlers
Urology, Aurora Health Care Medical Group, Milwaukee, WI, USA

The sacral plexus arises from the ventral rami of L4–S4. It forms in the pelvis anterior to the piriformis muscle. The nerves are divided into four groups depending on their destination:

Buttock

They exit the pelvis through the greater sciatic foramen:

- Superior gluteal nerve (L4, L5, and S1 above the piriformis, to gluteus medius, gluteus minimus, and tensor fasciae latae)
- Inferior gluteal nerve (L5, S1, and S2 below piriformis, to gluteus maximus)

Lower Extremity

They exit the pelvis through the greater sciatic foramen below the piriformis muscle:

- Sciatic nerve: tibial nerve, anterior division L4–S3 and common peroneal (fibular) nerve , posterior division L4–S2
- Posterior cutaneous nerve of the thigh (S1–S3)

Perineum

- Pudendal nerve (S2–S4): exits the pelvis through the greater sciatic foramen and enters the perineum through the lesser sciatic foramen

A. S. Hanna (ed.), *Nerves: Anatomy, Exposures, and Techniques*, https://doi.org/10.1007/978-3-031-73931-6_23

Local

Three groups:

- Muscular:
  - Piriformis
  - Obturator internus and superior gemellus
  - Quadratus femoris and inferior gemellus
- Cutaneous:
  - Perforating cutaneous branches
  - Perineal branch of fourth sacral
- Parasympathetic:
  - Pelvic splanchnic nerves, nervi erigentes (S2–S4)

Clinical Significance

The need to expose the lumbosacral plexus is much less common than the brachial plexus. Pathologies include tumors and less commonly trauma. The approach usually involves an access surgeon (general, trauma, vascular, gynecology, or colorectal surgeon). Occasionally, proximal lesions close to spinal foramina could be approached posteriorly via a paraspinal (Wiltse) approach, with various degrees of facetectomies depending on the intraspinal extent of the lesion, which may warrant spinal instrumentation.

Iatrogenic injuries to the lumbosacral plexus can occur during hip surgery (sciatic, femoral, and lateral femoral cutaneous nerves) or lateral transpsoas approaches for interbody fusion of the lumbar spine (femoral nerve).

Perineurial spread of pelvic cancer could cause involvement of the lumbosacral nerves that can mimic sciatic pain [1].

Piriformis syndrome can cause deep gluteal and sciatic pain from the compression of the sciatic nerve at the piriformis (see also Chap. 26) [2, 3].

Surgical Approaches

Retroperitoneal [4]

1. An access surgeon is usually required. The procedure can be done open or laparoscopic. The open approach is described here.
2. Position: supine (Fig. 23.1) or lateral on a beanbag.
3. Incision through the skin and superficial fascia: superficial fatty (Camper's) and deep membranous (Scarpa's).
4. Incision through the abdominal wall muscles: external oblique, internal oblique, and transversus abdominis; can be muscle splitting (Fig. 23.2) or cutting depending on the size of the incision.
5. Once the transversalis fascia is opened, the glistening yellow extraperitoneal fat is recognized. Further dissection in this plane will expose the quadratus lumborum and iliacus laterally and the psoas major medially.
6. Nerves lateral to the psoas muscle from cranial to caudal include: iliohypogastric, ilioinguinal, lateral femoral cutaneous, and femoral nerves. The fascia overlying the posterior abdominal wall muscles needs to be opened to expose the nerves. In addition, for the femoral nerve, the psoas muscle needs to be separated from the iliacus muscle.
7. Anterior to the psoas major muscle is the genitofemoral nerve, which bifurcates to its femoral and genital components; occasionally, it arises as two separate nerves.
8. Medial to the psoas muscle are the obturator nerve and the lumbosacral trunk. Their exposure will likely require mobilization of the iliac vessels (Fig. 23.3).

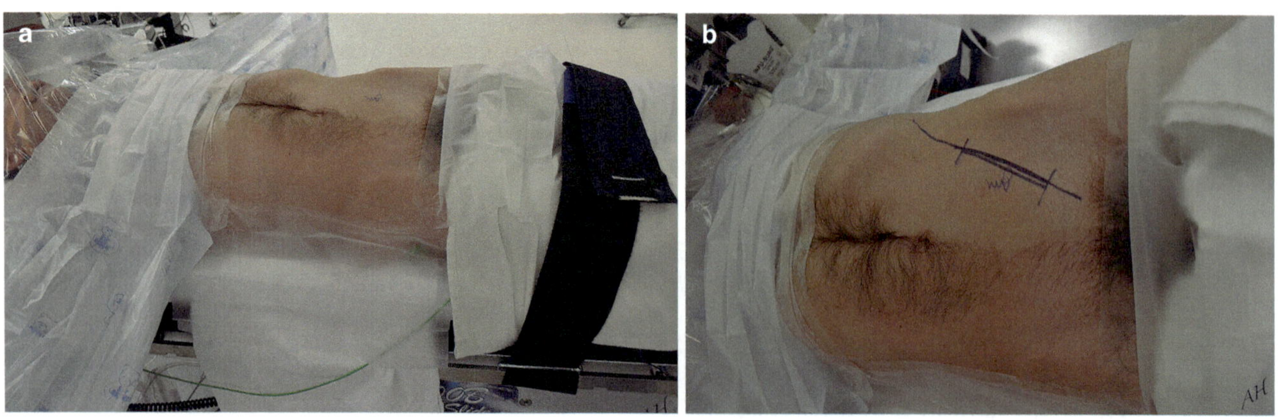

Fig. 23.1 Left lumbosacral plexus exposure. (**a**) The patient is positioned supine. (**b**) Oblique incision parallel to the inguinal ligament. The size and level of the incision depend on the pathology and location to be addressed. Large incisions can be muscle cutting. Small incisions should be muscle splitting

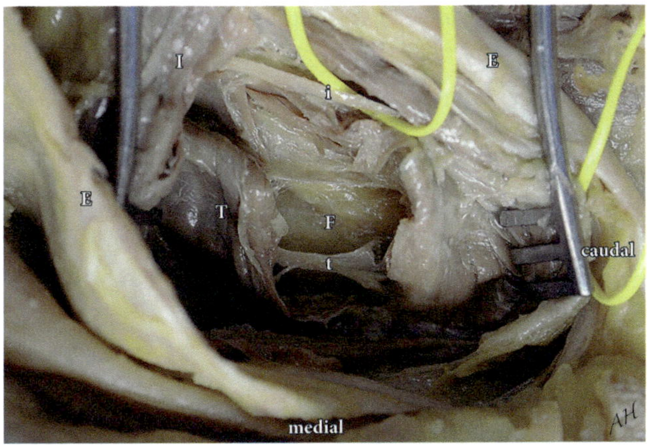

Fig. 23.2 Left muscle splitting approach in a cadaver. *E* external oblique, *I* internal oblique, *T* transversus abdominis, *t* transversalis fascia, *F* extraperitoneal fat, *i* ilioinguinal nerve

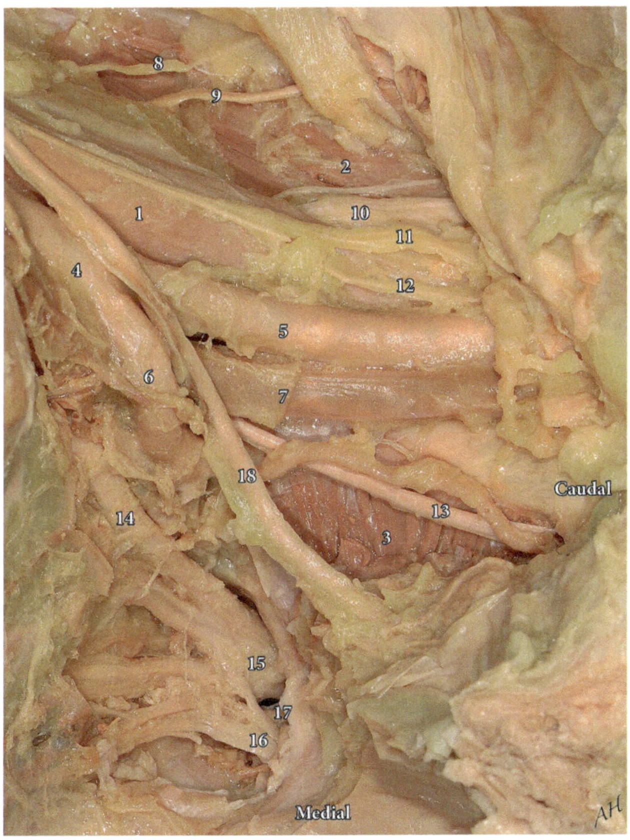

Fig. 23.3 Retroperitoneal view of the left lumbosacral plexus in a cadaver. *1* psoas major, *2* iliacus, *3* obturator internus, *4* common iliac artery, *5* external iliac artery, *6* internal iliac artery, *7* external iliac vein, *8* ilioinguinal nerve, *9* lateral femoral cutaneous nerve, *10* femoral nerve. 8–10 exit at the lateral border of the psoas muscle. *11* femoral branch of the genitofemoral nerve, *12* genital branch of the genitofemoral nerve. 11 and 12 are anterior to the psoas muscle. *13* obturator nerve, *14* lumbosacral trunk. 13 and 14 are medial to the psoas muscle. *15* sciatic nerve, *16* pudendal nerve, *17* posterior cutaneous nerve of the thigh, *18* ureter

9. The sacral plexus is deep in the pelvis anterior to the piriformis muscle. Exposure would require mobilization of the colon and rectum in addition to the vessels.

Posterior Paraspinal Approach (Wiltse) [5]

1. Position prone.
2. X-ray localization is usually required prior to skin incision.
3. Incision is about 4 cm lateral to the midline.
4. Incision is deepened through the superficial and deep fasciae.
5. The paraspinal muscles are opened to expose the transverse processes of the corresponding vertebrae. A self-retaining retractor is placed.
6. The intertransverse membrane is opened.
7. Electrical stimulation can be used to identify different nerves. Muscle response can be visual, tactile, or through needle recordings.
8. A partial or complete facetectomy can be performed as needed.

Complications

Retroperitoneal Approach

- Vascular, ureter, or bowel injury
- Nerve injuries
- Ileus
- Incisional hernia, especially with muscle cutting approaches

Wiltse Approach

- Neuropathic pain from manipulating the dorsal root ganglion (DRG)

General

- Wound infection
- Bleeding
- Anesthesia complications

References

1. Hébert-Blouin MN, Amrami KK, Myers RP, Hanna AS, Spinner RJ (2010) Adenocarcinoma of the prostate involving the lumbosacral plexus: MRI evidence to support direct perineural spread. Acta Neurochir (Wien) 152(9):1567–1576. https://doi.org/10.1007/s00701-010-0682-x. Epub 2010 May 15
2. Filler AG (2008) Piriformis and related entrapment syndromes: diagnosis and management. Neurosurg Clin N Am 19(4):609–622, vii. https://doi.org/10.1016/j.nec.2008.07.029
3. Tiel RL (2008) Piriformis and related entrapment syndromes: myth & fallacy. Neurosurg Clin N Am 19(4):623–627, vii. https://doi.org/10.1016/j.nec.2008.07.028
4. McAfee PC, Bohlman HH, Yuan HA (1985) Anterior decompression of traumatic thoracolumbar fractures with incomplete neurological deficit using a retroperitoneal approach. J Bone Joint Surg Am 67-A(1):89–104
5. Wiltse LL, Spencer CW (1988) New uses and refinements of the paraspinal approach to the lumbar spine. Spine 13(6):696–706

Femoral Nerve

24

Amgad S. Hanna and Mark E. Ehlers

Surgical Anatomy

The femoral nerve arises from the posterior division of the ventral rami of L2–L4. It forms within the psoas muscle and exits lateral to the muscle supplying it and the iliacus muscle. It courses in the retroperitoneum and then enters the thigh below the inguinal ligament with the corresponding vessels. The vein (V) is the most medial, then the artery (A), and then the nerve (N) (VAN). The femoral nerve proper is short. It divides into multiple muscular branches to the quadriceps femoris and sartorius, medial, and intermediate cutaneous nerves of the thigh, as well as the saphenous nerve. The saphenous nerve courses along the femoral artery in the adductor canal (subsartorial canal) and then along the long saphenous vein on the medial aspect of the leg. The nerve also typically supplies the pectineus muscle, which could also be supplied by obturator or accessory obturator nerves.

Clinical Significance

The saphenous nerve, similar to the sural and the superficial radial nerves, can be used for nerve biopsies (~6 cm) or as a donor for nerve grafts, but has a relatively smaller diameter. Neuromas of the infrapatellar branch of the saphenous nerve are a common cause of pain following knee replacement [1].

Exposure

In the Femoral Triangle

1. A vertical incision is made just lateral to the pulse of the femoral artery and below the inguinal ligament (Fig. 24.1).
2. The incision is deepened through the superficial and deep fasciae.
3. Cutaneous branches of the femoral nerve are usually encountered first; followed deeply, they lead to the main stem of the nerve. Alternatively, the femoral artery can be exposed first; the nerve is just lateral to the artery outside of the femoral sheath (Fig. 24.2).
4. The fascia overlying the psoas and iliacus muscles needs to be opened to expose the nerve.
5. The nerve is followed proximally under the inguinal ligament as indicated.

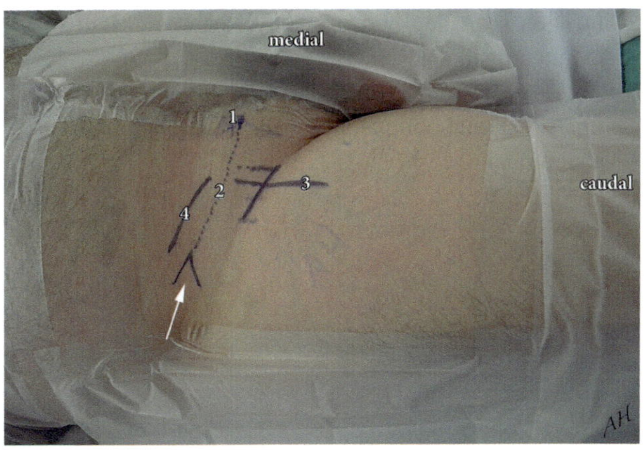

Fig. 24.1 Exposure of the right femoral nerve. The patient is positioned supine. *Arrow* anterior superior iliac spine (ASIS), *1* pubic tubercle, *2* inguinal ligament (*dotted line*), *3* incision for the exposure of the femoral nerve in the femoral triangle (thigh). It starts at the midpoint of the inguinal ligament, just lateral to the femoral pulse. *4* incision for retroperitoneal exposure of the femoral nerve. A hip bump can be used to facilitate retroperitoneal exposure

Supplementary Information The online version contains supplementary material available at https://doi.org/10.1007/978-3-031-73931-6_24.

A. S. Hanna (✉)
Department of Neurosurgery, University of Wisconsin School of Medicine and Public Health, Madison, WI, USA

M. E. Ehlers
Urology, Aurora Health Care Medical Group, Milwaukee, WI, USA

A. S. Hanna (ed.), *Nerves: Anatomy, Exposures, and Techniques*, https://doi.org/10.1007/978-3-031-73931-6_24

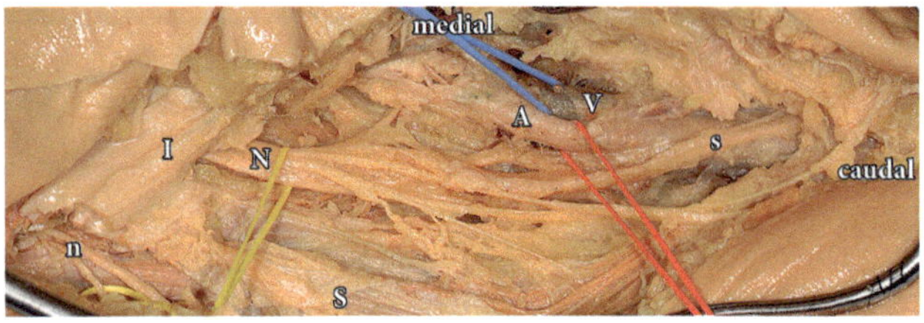

Fig. 24.2 Cadaveric dissection of the right femoral nerve in the thigh. *V* femoral vein, *A* femoral artery, *N* femoral nerve, *I* inguinal ligament, *n* lateral femoral cutaneous nerve, *S* sartorius, *s* saphenous nerve

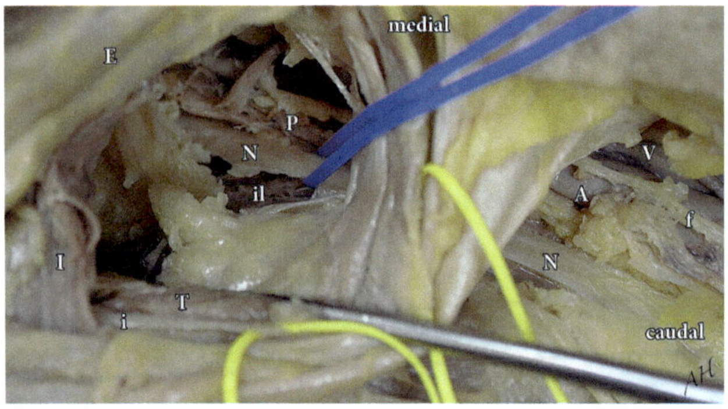

Fig. 24.3 Another cadaver specimen showing combined exposure of the right femoral nerve in the retroperitoneum and thigh. *E* external oblique, *I* internal oblique, *i* ilioinguinal nerve, *T* transversus abdominis, *P* psoas major, *il* iliacus, *N* femoral nerve, *A* femoral artery, *V* femoral vein, *f* femoral branch of the genitofemoral nerve

In the Retroperitoneum (Fig. 24.3; See Also Figs. 23.1–23.3)

1. Open (described here) or laparoscopic.
2. Incision is made obliquely above the lateral half of the inguinal ligament.
3. The abdominal wall muscles can be split along their fibers: external oblique, internal oblique, and transversus abdominis.

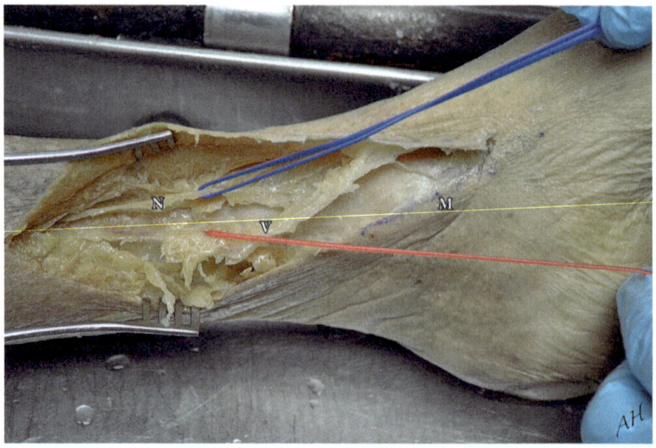

Fig. 24.4 Saphenous nerve (*N*) exposure along the medial aspect of the left lower leg. *M* medial malleolus, *V* long saphenous vein

4. The transversalis fascia is opened, the extraperitoneal fat is then encountered. Blunt dissection allows swiping the peritoneum with its contents medially exposing the retroperitoneal space.
5. The fascia overlying the iliacus and psoas muscles is opened.
6. We first encounter the lateral femoral cutaneous nerve that crosses in front of the iliacus muscle from the lateral border of the psoas toward the anterior superior iliac spine (ASIS).
7. The femoral nerve is found by opening the groove between the psoas major and iliacus muscles.

Saphenous Nerve

It is a small cutaneous branch that can be exposed in the superficial fascia, along the long saphenous vein anterior to the medial malleolus (Fig. 24.4), on the medial aspect of the leg and knee joint. Followed proximally, it travels deep to the sartorius, and then accompanies the femoral artery in the adductor (Hunter's) canal (Fig. 24.5).

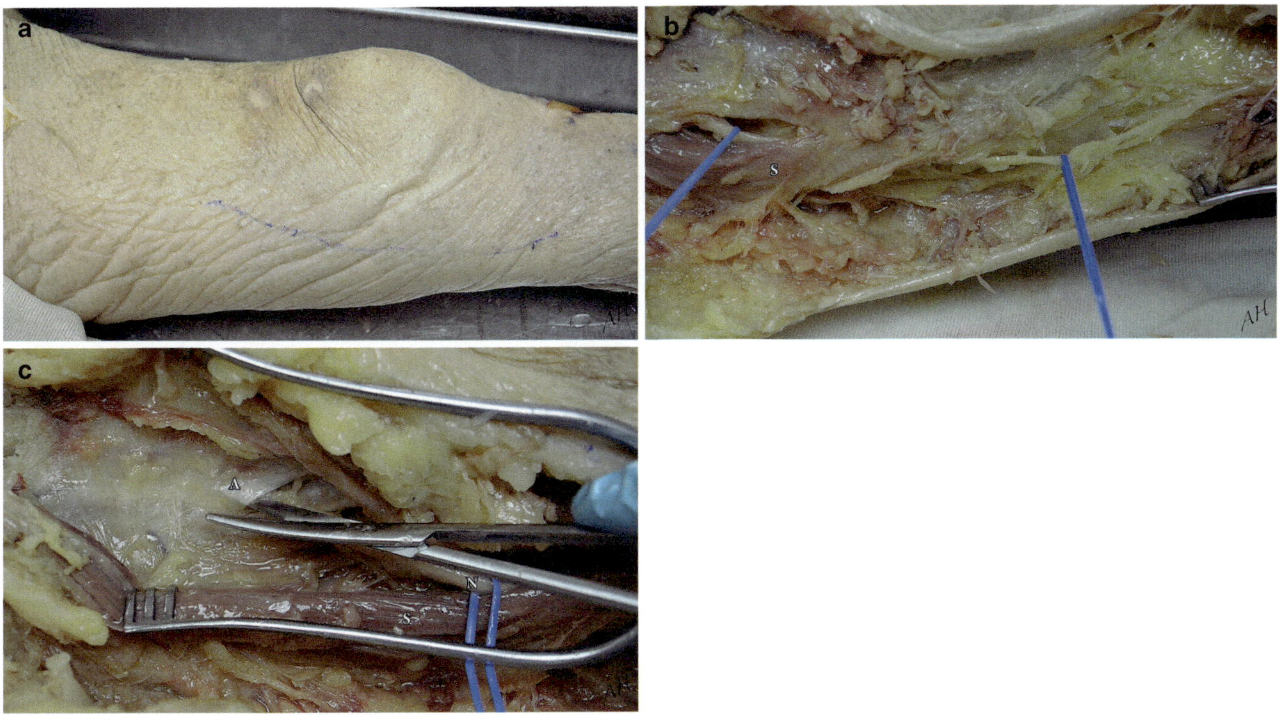

Fig. 24.5 (**a**) Saphenous nerve exposure along the medial aspect of the left knee. (**b**) The saphenous nerve (*blue loops*) is observed crossing deep to the sartorius (*S*). (**c**) The aponeurotic roof (*A*) of the adductor (Hunter's) canal can be opened for further exposure. *S* sartorius, *N* saphenous nerve (*blue loop*)

Reference

1. Nahabedian MY, Johnson CA (2001) Operative management of neuromatous knee pain: patient selection and outcome. Ann Plast Surg 46(1):15–22. https://doi.org/10.1097/00000637-200101000-00004

25 Lateral Femoral Cutaneous Nerve

Amgad S. Hanna and Thomas M. Staniszewski

Surgical Anatomy

The lateral femoral cutaneous nerve (LFCN) arises from the posterior divisions of the ventral rami of L2–L3. It emerges lateral to the psoas muscle between the femoral nerve medially and the ilioinguinal nerve laterally (see Fig. 23.3). It travels ventral to the iliacus muscle within the duplication of fascia iliaca. It enters the thigh typically under the lateral aspect of the inguinal ligament. The nerve is surrounded 360° by its own fascial canal, the LFCN canal (Fig. 25.1) [1, 2]. Within the canal, the nerve is cushioned by fat, loosely in the retroperitoneum and tightly under the inguinal ligament and in the thigh. It supplies an area of skin in the anterolateral aspect of the thigh, which typically tapers toward the iliac crest (Fig. 25.2), sometimes a small branch supplies a strip of skin in the buttock.

Supplementary Information The online version contains supplementary material available at https://doi.org/10.1007/978-3-031-73931-6_25.

A. S. Hanna (✉)
Department of Neurosurgery, University of Wisconsin School of Medicine and Public Health, Madison, WI, USA

T. M. Staniszewski
Department of Neurological Surgery, University of Wisconsin School of Medicine and Public Health, Madison, WI, USA
e-mail: staniszewski@neurosurgery.wisc.edu

A. S. Hanna (ed.), *Nerves: Anatomy, Exposures, and Techniques*, https://doi.org/10.1007/978-3-031-73931-6_25

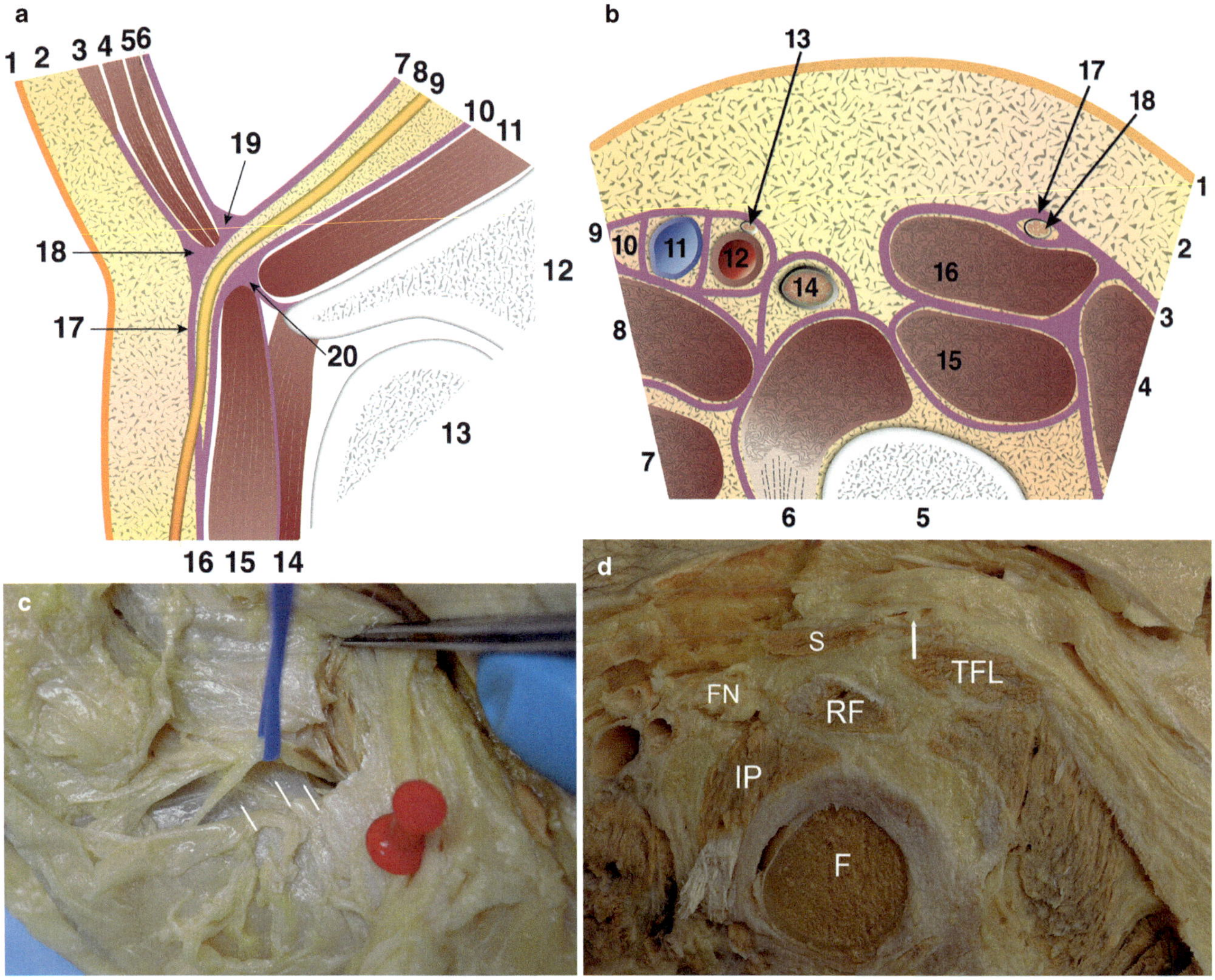

Fig. 25.1 The LFCN canal. (**a**) Diagrammatic oblique sagittal view at the level of the anterior inferior iliac spine. *1* skin, *2* subcutaneous tissue, *3* external oblique muscle and aponeurosis, *4* internal oblique, *5* transversus abdominis, *6* transversalis fascia, *7* fascia iliaca superficial lamina, *8* retroperitoneal fat, *9* LFCN, *10* fascia iliaca deep lamina, *11* iliacus, *12* iliac bone, *13* femur, *14* rectus femoris, *15* sartorius, *16* fascia lata, *17* LFCN canal, *18* inguinal ligament, *19* iliopubic tract, *20* thickening of the fascia deep to the LFCN (here, by the tendinous origin of the sartorius; can also be a slip from the inguinal ligament, or periosteum if the nerve is riding over the ASIS or iliac crest) (Copyright Amgad Hanna. Published with permission [1]). (**b**) Diagrammatic axial view. *1* skin, *2* subcutaneous fat, *3* fascia lata, *4* tensor fasciae latae, *5* femur, *6* iliopsoas, *7* adductor magnus, *8* pectineus, *9* femoral sheath, *10* femoral canal, *11* femoral vein, *12* femoral artery (10-12, from medial to lateral respectively), *13* femoral branch of genitofemoral nerve, *14* femoral nerve, *15* rectus femoris, *16* sartorius, *17* LFCN canal, *18* LFCN (Copyright Amgad Hanna. Published with permission [1]). (**c**) Cadaveric dissection of the left LFCN (*blue loop*) showing white glistening fascia deep to the nerve (*arrows*) separating it from the underlying muscle. *Red pin* anterior superior iliac spine (ASIS). (**d**) Cadaveric axial cut showing left LFCN (*arrow*) in its canal. *S* sartorius, *RF* rectus femoris, *TFL* tensor fasciae latae, *IP* iliopsoas, *F* femur, *FN* femoral nerve

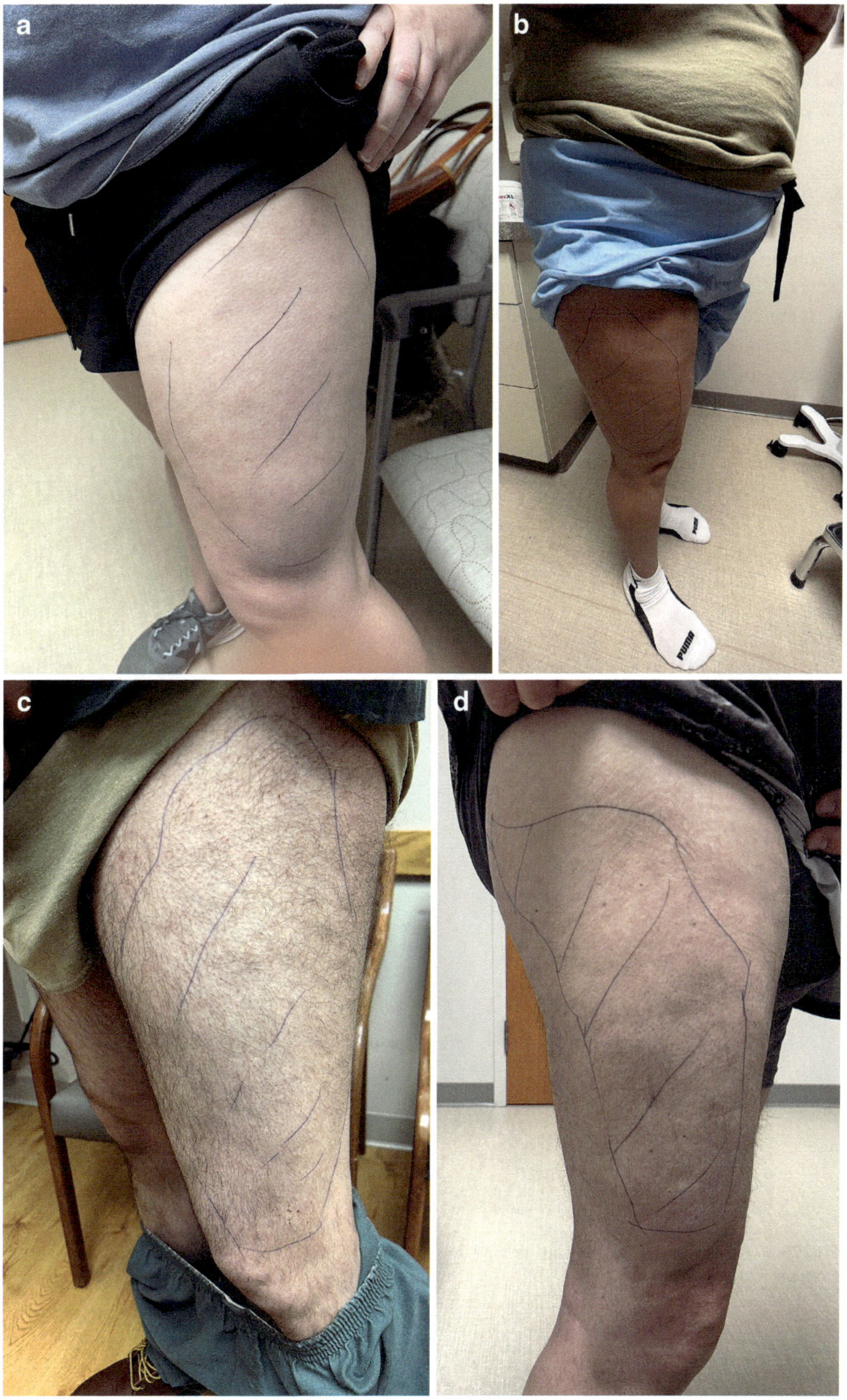

Fig. 25.2 (**a**–**c**) Typical area of burning, tingling, numbness, and hypesthesia in meralgia paresthetica patients. Note tapering toward the iliac crest (as if a pear is hanging from the iliac crest) and stopping above the knee which help differentiate from lumbar radiculopathy. The disease is common in overweight males. (**d**) Occasionally, a posterior branch of the nerve extends the area of the involved skin further toward the buttock

Anatomical Variations

Anatomical variabilities of the LFCN are the rule rather than the exception. The nerve has the most fascinating and intriguing anatomy.

- Bilateral symmetry is rare.
- Typically, the LFCN originates from the lumbosacral plexus, but occasionally it branches off the femoral nerve (Fig. 25.3) and rarely ilioinguinal nerve.
- It enters the thigh typically medial to the anterior superior iliac spine (ASIS), but occasionally over the ASIS (especially in cases of meralgia paresthetica), or lateral to it (Fig. 25.4), sometimes forming a groove in the bone (supra-iliac groove) [1].
- The nerve can be duplicate (Fig. 25.5).

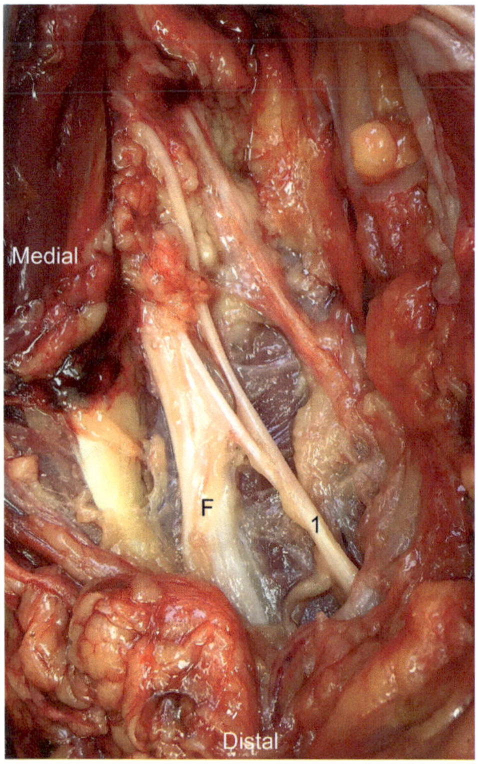

Fig. 25.3 Postmortem specimen showing left LFCN (*1*) originating from the femoral nerve (*F*)

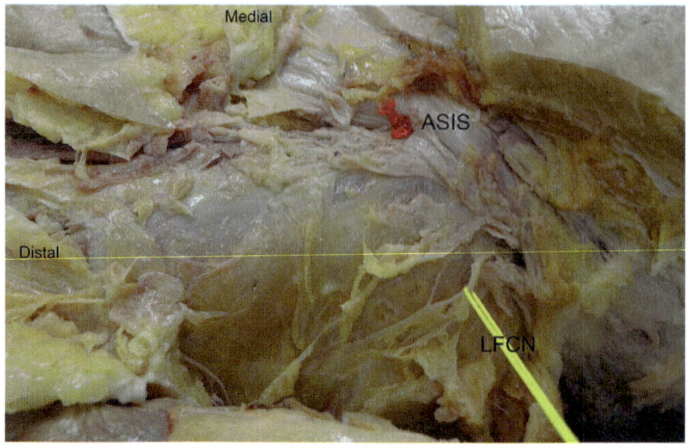

Fig. 25.4 Left LFCN (*yellow loop*) passing lateral to ASIS (*red pin*)

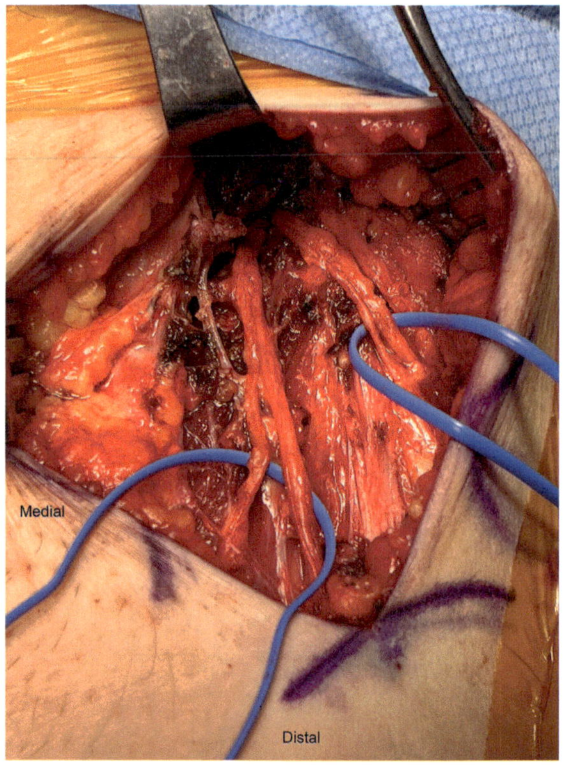

Fig. 25.5 Duplicate left LFCN (*blue loops*) in a meralgia paresthetica patient

Clinical Significance

Meralgia paresthetica (MP) is a nerve entrapment affecting the LFCN at the groin. It manifests by pain, typically burning, allodynia, and hypesthesia in the anterolateral thigh (Fig. 25.2). Although commonly idiopathic, it can follow trauma, including iatrogenic injuries from open surgery like anterior hip surgery or positioning from prolonged surgery in the prone position [3] or even prone ventilation in the ICU

(Intensive Care Unit) [4]. Despite traditionally being described in obese males, MP can occur in any age, any sex, and any body habitus. The typical clinical scenario is key to the diagnosis, together with ultrasound (US)-guided injections. Electrodiagnostic studies are rarely helpful.

Nonoperative treatment includes avoiding tight belts, tight clothes, and weight loss. The latter is usually challenging if most activities aggravate the pain. Injections usually help but are short-lived. Surgical treatment includes nerve decompression (neurolysis), neurectomy, and transposition. Simple decompression has a high failure rate even after an initial good response due to scar tissue formation (see Fig. 47.1) [5, 6]. Neurectomy can be complicated by deafferentation pain, neuroma formation, and is always associated with sensory loss in the LFCN distribution. In our institution, we have adopted LFCN transposition since 2013 [7–10]. The procedure is detailed in Chap. 47. It consists of releasing all fascial planes around the nerve, namely the fascia superficial to the nerve, the fascia deep to the nerve, and the septum medial to the sartorius. The nerve is mobilized medially away from the ASIS for about 2 cm (Fig. 25.6). At the end of the procedure, the nerve has a straighter course, is not tethered, has a softer muscular bed, and is away from any bony compression. Transposition is the only procedure that addresses the nerve proximity to bone which is a common problem in MP patients. Success rate is >90%. There were previous attempts at LFCN transposition (Table 25.1), with neither large series nor long-term follow-up.

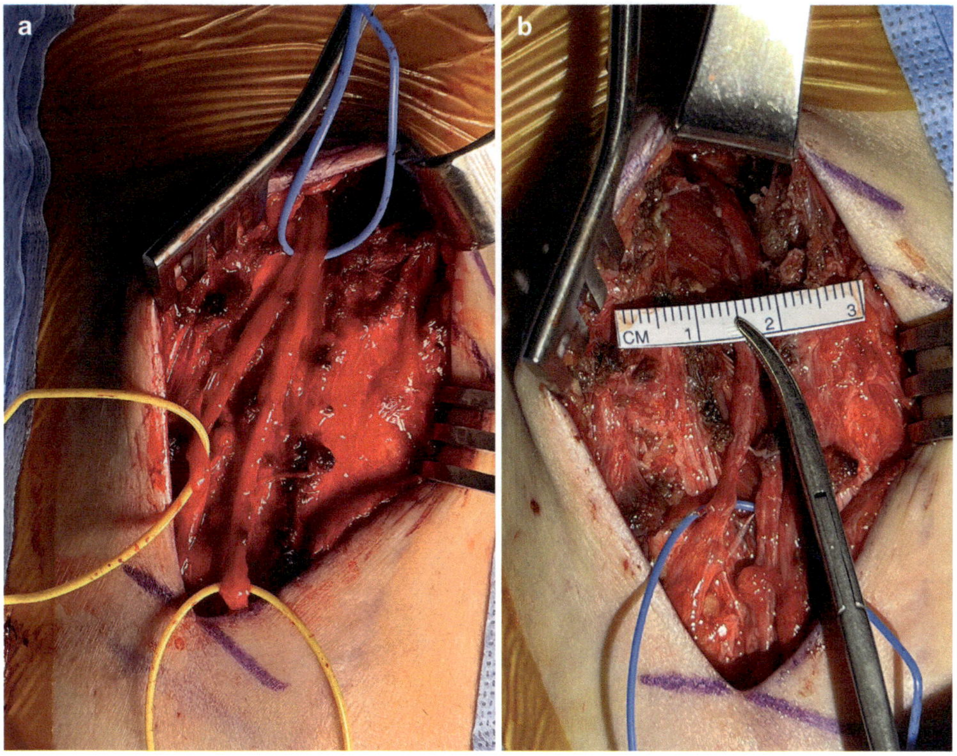

Fig. 25.6 Right LFCN (*blue loop*) and branches (*yellow loops*) before (**a**) and after (**b**) transposition. Note that both fasciae superficial and deep to the nerve are opened resulting in a soft muscular bed. The nerve is typically mobilized medially by about 2 cm

Table 25.1 Different techniques of LFCN transposition in the literature

Author	Lee [11]	Keegan [12]	Aldrich [13]	Hanna [7–10]
Year	1936 (published 1941)	1962	1989	2013 (published 2017)
Direction	Lateral in a bony notch	Medial	Medial	Medial
Excursion	1 inch posterior to ASIS	Half-an-inch	Unknown	2 cm
Approach	Thigh	Thigh	Suprainguinal	Thigh with retroperitoneal extension
Incision	Horizontal	Horizontal	Horizontal	Vertical (oblique)
Deep decompression	Yes, at the level of the inguinal ligament	Yes, at the level of the inguinal ligament	Unknown (all fascial bands)	Yes, throughout the thigh and into retroperitoneum
Release of the septum medial to sartorius	No	Not described	Unknown (all fascial bands)	Yes
Number of cases	1 (+1 more case by Mack [14])	2	None reported	50 (2013–2023)
Follow-up	2 years (2 months for Mack 1946)	6 and 2 months	None	1 year

Preoperative Ultrasound (US)-Guided Localization [15–17]

Due to anatomical variabilities of the LFCN, we have adopted the preoperative US-guided localization of the LFCN since 2011. Carai reports as high as 8.8% rate of not finding the nerve and aborting the procedure [18]. The nerve is readily visible in its canal on US (Fig. 25.7). Our initial approach was to deploy a wire under the nerve (Fig. 25.8). More recently (since 2022), we have used the Envisio navigation system (Elucent Medical) (Fig. 25.7, Table 25.2, Video 25.1). In most cases, it takes less than 10 min to find the nerve.

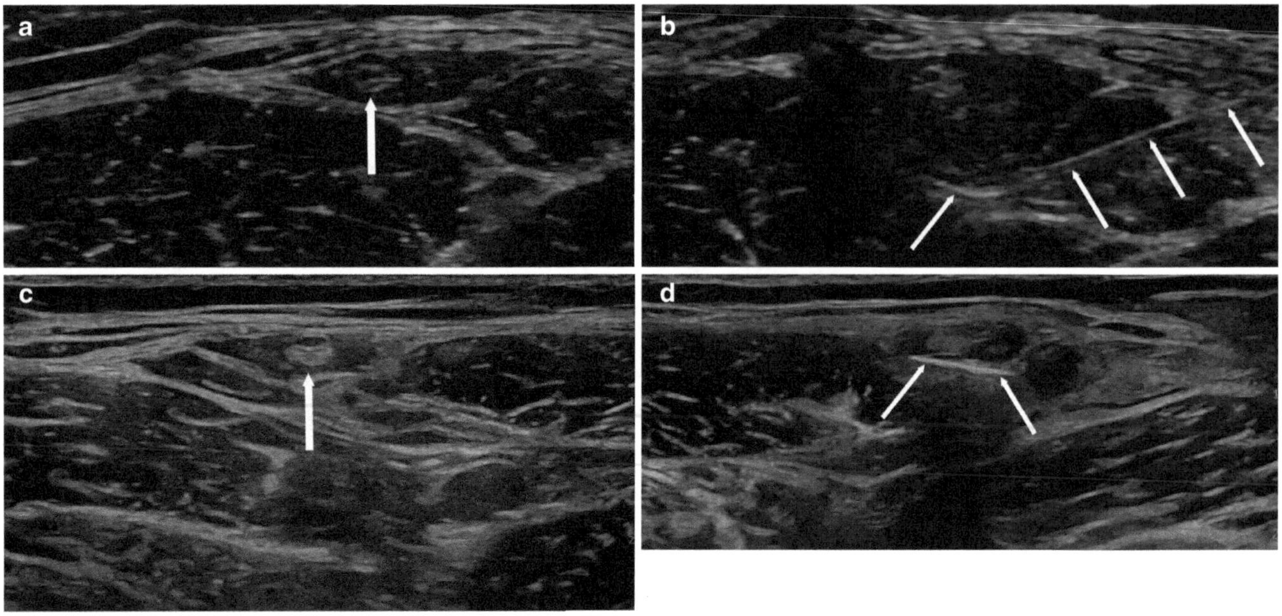

Fig. 25.7 Preoperative US-guided localization of the LFCN. (**a**, **c**) Diagnostic US in two different cases showing LFCN (*arrow*) in its canal. (**b**) Wire (*arrows*) localization. (**d**) Smart clip (*arrows*) localization (Envisio system)

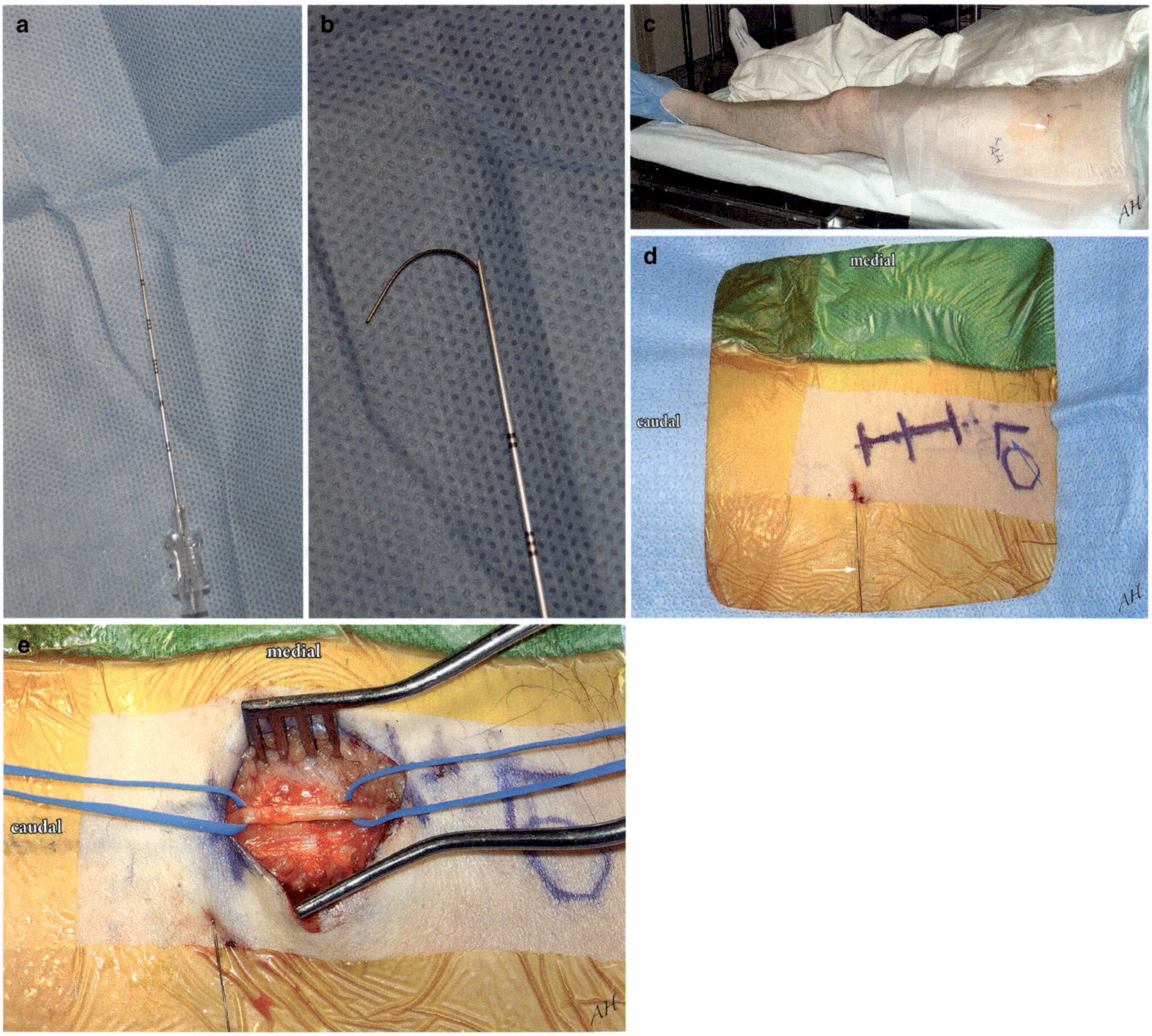

Fig. 25.8 Wire used for localization showing pre- (**a**) and post- (**b**) deployment of the Homer needle. (**c**) Patient positioned for surgery. Note the wire (*white arrow*) exit from the skin. The incision is planned based on US measurements from the wire tip projection on the skin. (**d**) The incision is marked medial to the ASIS (*blue arrow*), along the nerve trajectory mapped by preoperative US. Measurements taken in the US suite will show how deep the nerve is from the skin surface (light pressure applied on the skin by the US probe to avoid falsely smaller measured depth) and the distance from the wire (*white arrow*) entry point to the tip projection on the skin. The latter distance is used to mark the incision. (**e**) The LFCN is exposed by opening the nerve sheath (LFCN canal)

Table 25.2 Data analysis of cases of MP performed by senior author between 2011 and 2023 using preoperative US-guided localization of LFCN comparing wire vs. clip

	Wire localization	Clip localization
Number of cases	51	9
Skin-to-nerve time (min)	8.1	7.7
<10 min to find the nerve	69%	77.7%
Misplaced marker (*n*)	5 /51 (~10%)	0/9 (0%)
Marker dislodgement (*n*)	1/51 (1.96%)	0/9 (0%)
Timing of placement	The day of nerve surgery	A few days prior until the day of nerve surgery
Soft tissue migration	None	None, if placed within a few days of surgery*
Cost	– Ultrasound machine – Wire: ~$187	– Ultrasound machine – Smart clip, applicator needle: ~$350 – Navigation probe (sensor): ~$495 – Envisio® Navigation System (reusable): ~$85,000

*In more recent cases, we have observed some clip migration if the clip is placed between the deep fascia and the muscle, ideal placement should be between the nerve and the fascia deep to it, this keeps it snug in place until the date of surgery

Retroperitoneal Approach (See Chaps. 23, 24, 53, and 54)

This can be used for occasional cases where the nerve has to be transected in the retroperitoneum, like traumatic injury, neuroma, or recurrent cases of MP (Fig. 25.9). The approach can be used for nerve sheath tumors of the LFCN as well.

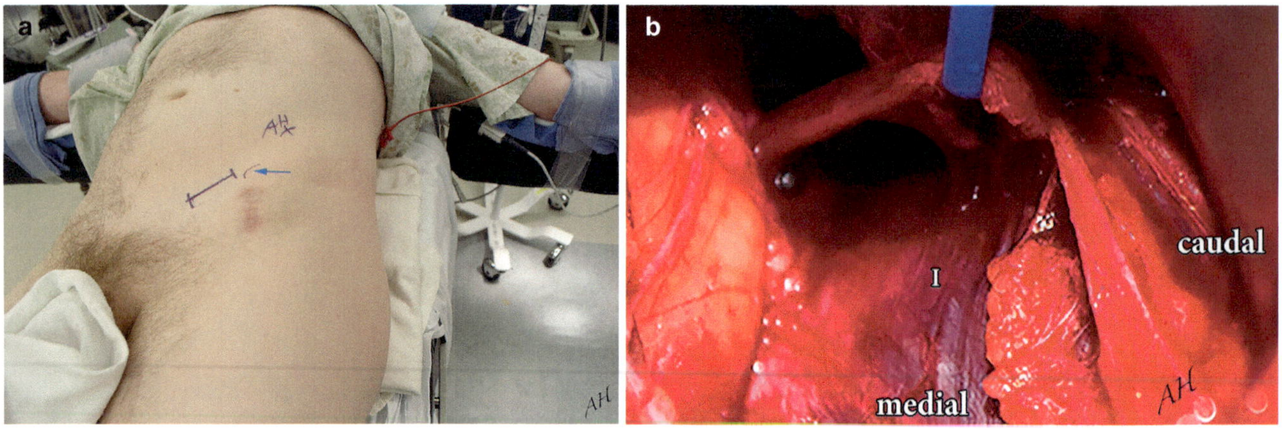

Fig. 25.9 (**a**) Positioning and incision for retroperitoneal exposure of the left LFCN. The incision is cranial and parallel to the inguinal ligament, medial to the ASIS (*blue arrow*). (**b**) The left LFCN (*blue loop*) is exposed in the retroperitoneum. *I* iliacus

References

1. Hanna A (2017) The lateral femoral cutaneous nerve canal. J Neurosurg 126(3):972–978. https://doi.org/10.3171/2016.1.JNS152262. Epub 2016 Apr 22
2. Xu Z, Tu L, Zheng Y, Ma X, Zhang H, Zhang M (2018) Fine architecture of the fascial planes around the lateral femoral cutaneous nerve at its pelvic exit: an epoxy sheet plastination and confocal microscopy study. J Neurosurg 131(6):1860–1868. https://doi.org/10.3171/2018.7.JNS181596
3. Yoshida S, Oya S, Matsui T (2021) Risk factors of meralgia paresthetica after prone position surgery: possible influence of operating position, laminectomy level, and preoperative thoracic kyphosis. J Clin Neurosci 89:292–296. https://doi.org/10.1016/j.jocn.2021.05.022. Epub 2021 May 21
4. Marinelli L, Mori L, Avanti C, Cotellessa F, Fabbri S, Schenone C et al (2020) Meralgia paraesthetica after prone position ventilation in a patient with COVID-19. Eur J Case Rep Intern Med 7(12):002039. https://doi.org/10.12890/2020_002039. eCollection 2020
5. de Ruiter GC, Wurzer JA, Kloet A (2012) Decision making in the surgical treatment of meralgia paresthetica: neurolysis versus neurectomy. Acta Neurochir (Wien) 154:1765–1772. https://doi.org/10.1007/s00701-012-1431-0. Epub 2012 Jul 6
6. van Eerten PV, Polder TW, Broere CA (1995) Operative treatment of meralgia paresthetica: transection versus neurolysis. Neurosurgery 37:63–65. https://doi.org/10.1227/00006123-199507000-00009
7. Hanna AS (2017) Lateral femoral cutaneous nerve transposition: renaissance of an old concept in the light of new anatomy. Clin Anat 30(3):409–412. https://doi.org/10.1002/ca.22849
8. Hanna A (2020) Letter to the Editor. Meralgia paresthetica: what to do? J Neurosurg 132(6):2020–2021. https://doi.org/10.3171/2019.10.JNS192708
9. Hanna A, Hanna B (2018) Response to: Anatomical considerations on transposition of the lateral femoral cutaneous nerve. Clin Anat 31(8):1222–1224. https://doi.org/10.1002/ca.23070. Epub 2018 Apr 30
10. Hanna A (2019) Transposition of the lateral femoral cutaneous nerve. J Neurosurg 130(2):496–501. https://doi.org/10.3171/2017.8.JNS171120. Epub 2018 Apr 13
11. Lee FC (1941) An osteoplastic neurolysis operation for the cure of meralgia paresthetica. Ann Surg 113(1):85–94. https://doi.org/10.1097/00000658-194101000-00012
12. Keegan JJ, Holyoke EA (1962) Meralgia paresthetica. An anatomical and surgical study. J Neurosurg 19:341–345. https://doi.org/10.3171/jns.1962.19.4.0341
13. Aldrich EF, van den Heever CM (1989) Suprainguinal ligament approach for surgical treatment of meralgia paresthetica. Technical note. J Neurosurg 70(3):492–494. https://doi.org/10.3171/jns.1989.70.3.0492

14. Mack EW (1946) Meralgia paresthetica; new causal observations. West J Surg Obstet Gynecol 54:390
15. Hanna AS, Ehlers ME, Lee KS (2017) Preoperative ultrasound-guided wire localization of the lateral femoral cutaneous nerve. Oper Neurosurg (Hagerstown) 13(3):402–408. https://doi.org/10.1093/ons/opw009
16. Frinkelstein ER, Buitrago J, Jose J, Levi AD, Xu KY, Burks SS (2023) Lower extremity peripheral nerve pathology: utility of preoperative ultrasound-guided needle localization before operative intervention. Skeletal Radiol 52(10):1997–2002. https://doi.org/10.1007/s00256-023-04347-y. Epub 2023 Apr 15
17. Haldeman CL, Baggott CD, Hanna AS (2015) Intraoperative ultrasound-assisted peripheral nerve surgery. Neurosurg Focus 39(3):E4. https://doi.org/10.3171/2015.6.FOCUS15232
18. Carai A, Fenu G, Sechi E, Crotti FM, Montella A (2009) Anatomical variability of the lateral femoral cutaneous nerve: findings from a surgical series. Clin Anat 22(3):365–370. https://doi.org/10.1002/ca.20766

Sciatic Nerve

26

Amgad S. Hanna, Thomas M. Staniszewski,
Ahmed H. Omar, Natalia Guevara-Moriones,
and Luis Rafael Moscote-Salazar

Surgical Anatomy

The sciatic nerve has two major components: tibial nerve from the anterior division of L4–S3 and the common peroneal (common fibular) nerve from the posterior division of L4–S2. It forms in front of the piriformis in the pelvis and exits the greater sciatic notch usually below the piriformis and then enters the thigh between the ischial tuberosity and the greater trochanter. Occasionally, an accessory piriformis head would split the sciatic nerve into two. Structures superficial to the sciatic nerve in the buttock: piriformis and gluteus maximus; in the thigh: the long head of biceps femoris crosses the nerve from medial to lateral. The nerve supplies the hamstrings: biceps femoris, semimembranosus, and semitendinosus, as well as the ischial part of adductor magnus. The nerve ends by splitting into tibial and common peroneal components, typically in the lower thigh.

Supplementary Information The online version contains supplementary material available at https://doi.org/10.1007/978-3-031-73931-6_26.

A. S. Hanna (✉) · L. R. Moscote-Salazar
Department of Neurosurgery, University of Wisconsin School of Medicine and Public Health, Madison, WI, USA

T. M. Staniszewski
Department of Neurological Surgery, University of Wisconsin School of Medicine and Public Health, Madison, WI, USA
e-mail: staniszewski@neurosurgery.wisc.edu

A. H. Omar
Department of Neurosurgery, University of Wisconsin School of Medicine and Public Health, Madison, WI, USA

Department of Neurosurgery, Cairo University, Giza, Egypt
e-mail: Ahmed-hussein@kasralainy.edu.eg

N. Guevara-Moriones
Faculty of Medicine, Universidad Juan N. Corpas, Bogotá, Colombia
e-mail: nataliam-guevara@juanncorpas.edu.co

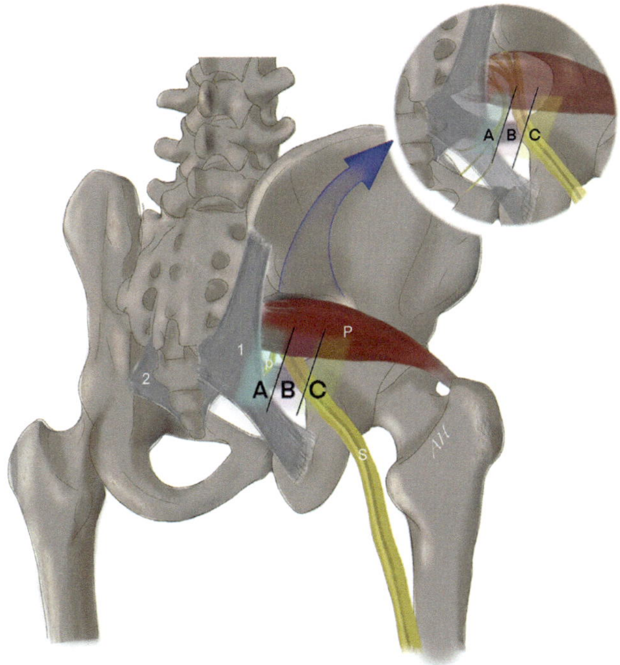

Fig. 26.1 Hanna classification of the zones of exit of sciatic and pudendal nerves from the greater sciatic foramen. Zone A medial to ischial spine (entirely on the sacrospinous ligament), zone B on the ischial spine, zone C lateral to the ischial spine (entirely on the ischial bone). *P* piriformis, *S* sciatic nerve, *p* pudendal nerve, *1* sacrotuberous ligament, *2* sacrospinous ligament [1]. (Copyright Amgad Hanna, published with permission)

Hanna classified the zones of exit of the sciatic and pudendal nerves through the greater sciatic foramen into zone A medial to ischial spine, zone B on the ischial spine, and zone C lateral to the ischial spine (Fig. 26.1) [1].

Clinical Significance

The sciatic nerve is most vulnerable around the hip, where it can be injured with hip dislocations, hip or pelvic fractures, or stretched during hip arthroplasty [2]. The peroneal com-

A. S. Hanna (ed.), *Nerves: Anatomy, Exposures, and Techniques*, https://doi.org/10.1007/978-3-031-73931-6_26

ponent is more frequently and more severely involved. It is also the less likely to recover [3]. The last branch of the peroneal component in the thigh is the short head of biceps femoris. This is important for lesion localization.

Exposures

In the Buttock

Transgluteal

1. Position: prone or lateral on a beanbag.
2. Incision: oblique, along the fibers of the gluteus maximus muscle (Fig. 26.2).
3. The incision is deepened through the superficial and deep fasciae.
4. The gluteus maximus muscle is split along its fibers. This can be done using Bovie cautery or Metzenbaum scissors and bipolar coagulation. A self-retaining retractor (Gelpi or cerebellar) is placed.
5. The fat layer deep to the gluteus maximus is then identified (Fig. 26.3). Palpation through the fat pad will reveal the big cord-like sciatic nerve. A nerve stimulator can also help find the nerve.
6. Vertical dissection along the course of the sciatic nerve allows identification of the nerve (Fig. 26.4), with the posterior cutaneous nerve of the thigh superficial to it.
7. The nerve can be followed proximally until the piriformis.
8. In cases of piriformis syndrome, a segment of the muscle should be transected and if possible its nerve supply, which is deep to the muscle. Before cutting the muscle, it's lifted up away from the sciatic nerve using sutures or a right-angled hemostat.
9. The pudendal nerve can be accessed through the same approach. It is deeper and more medial to the sciatic nerve.
10. For a fascicular biopsy, the nerve sheath is opened. An interfascicular dissection is performed. A grossly abnormal fascicle should be the target for the biopsy; otherwise, a randomly selected fascicle is taken, preferably after nerve stimulation reveals no motor response. The fascicle is dissected cranially and caudally until a good size (4–6 cm) is exposed and harvested.

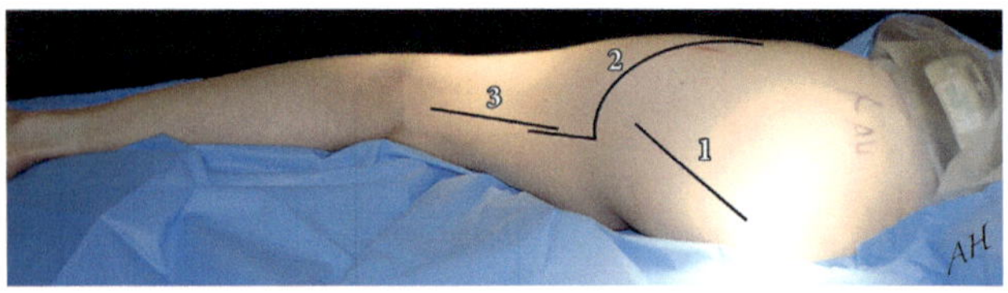

Fig. 26.2 Different incisions for left sciatic nerve exposure. *1* transgluteal, *2* gluteal flap, *3* posterior thigh. This patient is positioned lateral. Alternatively, this can be done in the prone position

Gluteal Flap (More Morbid, Less Favorable)

1. Position: prone.
2. Question mark incision, starting along the lateral aspect of the hip, around the buttock, then vertically along the middle of upper thigh (Figs. 26.2 and 26.5).
3. The incision is deepened through the superficial and deep fasciae.
4. The gluteus maximus is cut along its insertion, leaving a cuff to stitch to during closure (Fig. 26.6).
5. The gluteus maximus is then lifted up as a flap and reflected medially.
6. This exposes the next muscle layer: gluteus medius, gluteus minimus, and piriformis.
7. The fat pad below the piriformis is identified. Palpation through the fat pad will reveal the big cord-like sciatic nerve.

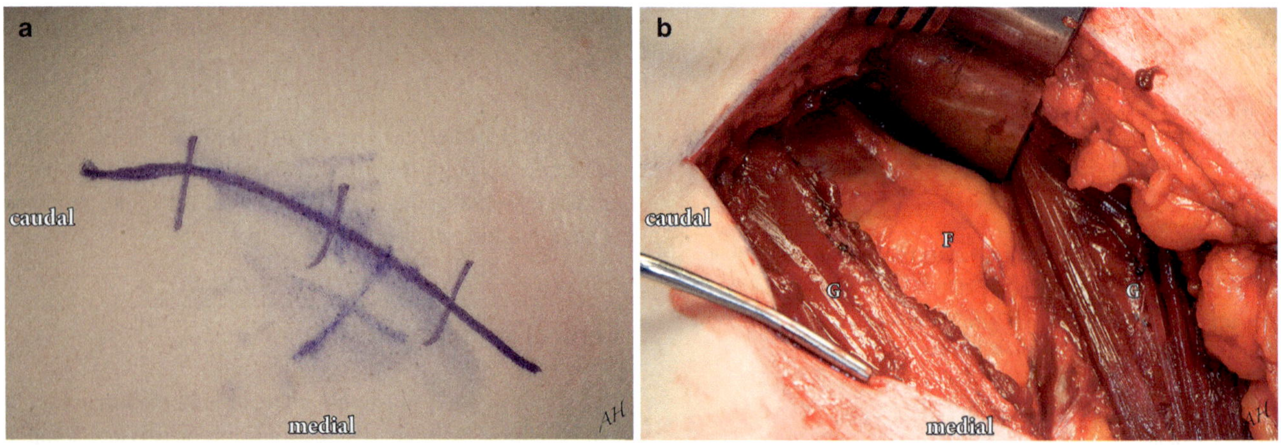

Fig. 26.3 (**a**) The incision is marked for a left transgluteal approach. (**b**) Separation of the gluteus maximus fibers (*G*) allows identification of the fat pad (*F*) underneath

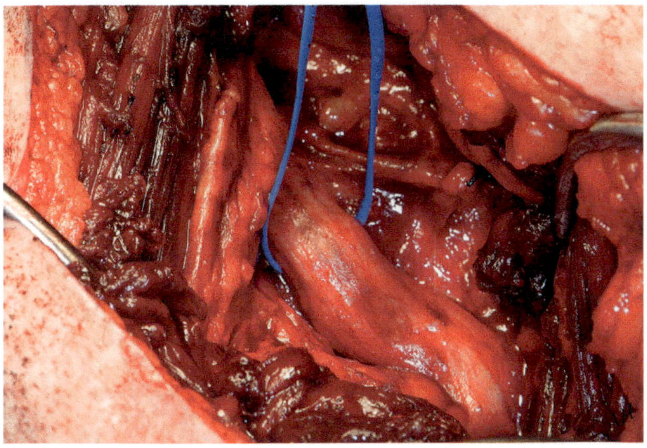

Fig. 26.4 The sciatic nerve (*blue loop*) is found within the fat pad. A nerve stimulator can be used to help find it

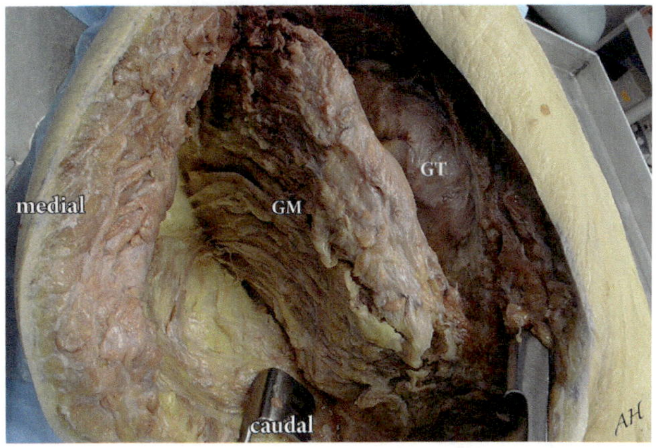

Fig. 26.6 The gluteus maximus (*GM*) flap is elevated. *GT* greater trochanter

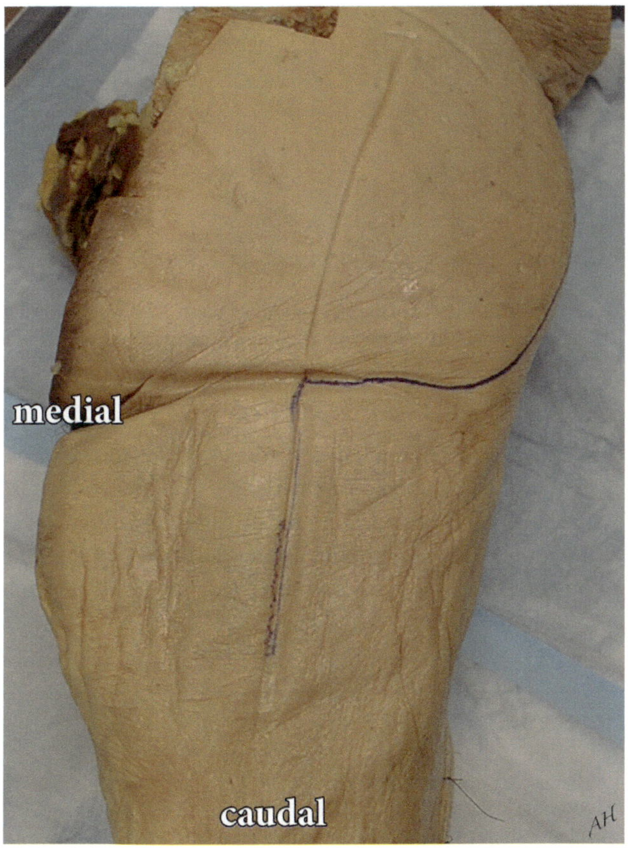

Fig. 26.5 Incision for a right gluteal flap in a cadaver

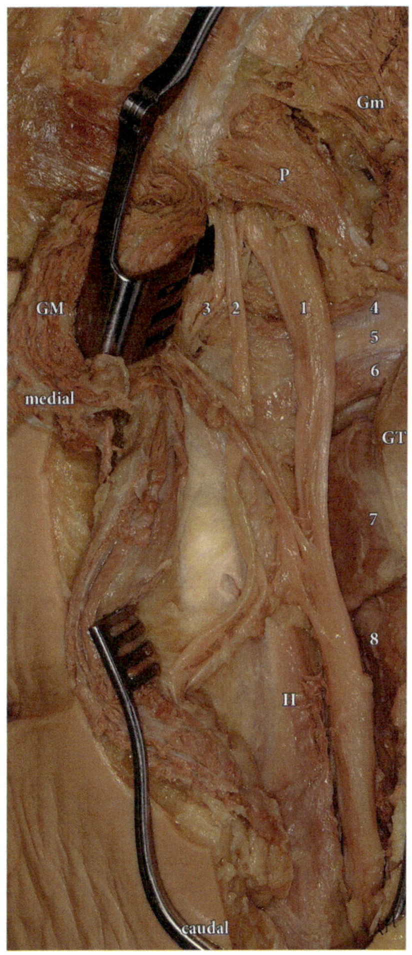

Fig. 26.7 The sciatic nerve (*1*) is found in the fat pad deep to the gluteus maximus (*GM*). *Gm* gluteus minimus, *P* piriformis, *GT* greater trochanter, *H* hamstrings, *2* posterior cutaneous nerve of the thigh, *3* pudendal nerve, *4–8* sciatic nerve bed: *4* gemellus superior, *5* obturator internus, *6* gemellus inferior, *7* quadratus femoris, *8* adductor magnus

8. Vertical dissection along the course of the sciatic nerve allows identification of the nerve, with the posterior cutaneous nerve of the thigh superficial to it and the pudendal nerve deep and medial to it.
9. The bed of the sciatic nerve (deep structures), from cranial to caudal, is made of: gemellus superior, obturator internus, gemellus inferior, quadratus femoris, and adductor magnus (Fig. 26.7).

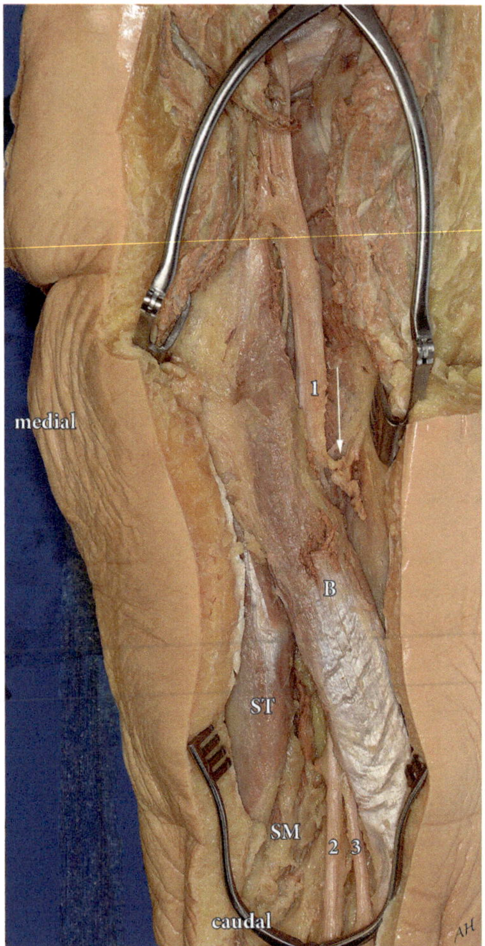

Fig. 26.8 In the posterior thigh, the sciatic nerve (*1*) is crossed by the long head of biceps femoris (*B*) and then divides in the popliteal fossa into tibial (*2*) and common peroneal (common fibular) (*3*) nerves. *ST* semitendinosus, *SM* semimembranosus, *arrow* peroneal branch to the short head of biceps, last branch in the thigh

10. The nerve can be followed proximally until the piriformis muscle.
11. The nerve can also be followed distally until it is crossed by the long head of the biceps femoris (Fig. 26.8).

In the Lower Thigh

1. Position: prone.
2. Posterior midline thigh incision (Fig. 26.2).
3. Incision is deepened through superficial and deep fasciae.
4. The hamstrings are separated with the biceps femoris laterally and the semitendinosus and semimembranosus medially (Fig. 26.9). A self-retaining retractor is placed.
5. The fat layer deep to the muscles is then identified. Palpation through the fat pad will reveal the big cord-like sciatic nerve.

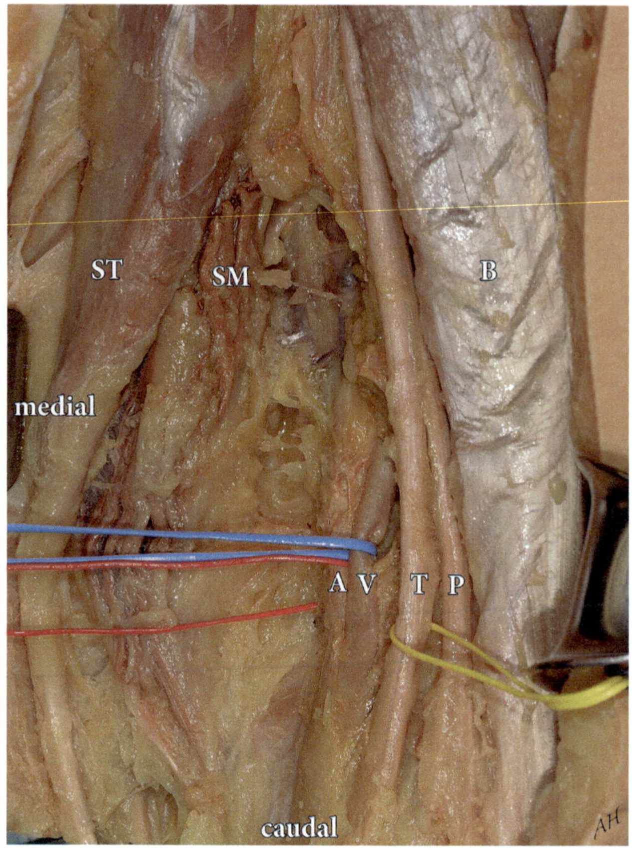

Fig. 26.9 Sciatic nerve in the right popliteal fossa. *ST* semitendinosus, *SM* semimembranosus, *B* biceps, *P* common peroneal nerve, *T* tibial nerve, *V* popliteal vein, *A* popliteal artery

6. Vertical dissection along the course of the sciatic nerve allows identification of the nerve.
7. The nerve can be followed distally until its bifurcation.
8. It can be followed proximally until crossed by the long head of biceps femoris and then under the gluteus maximus in the buttock.

References

1. Hanna AS, Staniszewski T, Omar AH, Guevara-Moriones N, Moscote-Salazar LR, Hilger KH, Hellenbrand D (2024) Anatomical relationships of the sciatic nerve and pudendal nerve to the ischial spine as they exit the greater sciatic foramen. World Neurosurg. 2024;183:e564-e570. https://doi.org/10.1016/j.wneu.2023.12.147. Epub 2024 Jan 3. PMID: 38181879. https://doi.org/10.1016/j.wneu.2023.12.147. pii: S1878-8750(23)01880-6
2. Lee PT, Lakstein DL, Lozano B, Safir O, Backstein J, Gross AE (2014) Mid-to long-term results of revision total hip replacement in patients aged 50 years or younger. Bone Joint J 96-B(8):1047–1051. https://doi.org/10.1302/0301-620X.96B8.31587
3. Burks SS, Levi DJ, Hayes S, Levi AD (2014) Challenges in sciatic nerve repair: anatomical considerations. J Neurosurg 121(1):210–218. https://doi.org/10.3171/2014.2.JNS131667. Epub 2014 Apr 11

Tibial Nerve

27

Amgad S. Hanna

Surgical Anatomy

The tibial nerve separates from the sciatic nerve, typically at the lower third of the thigh, the proximal part of the popliteal fossa. It continues in the midline, posterior to the popliteal vessels. In the upper leg, it passes between the two heads of the gastrocnemius and then under the soleal arch. It supplies all the muscles of the calf and a cutaneous contribution to the sural (medial sural cutaneous) nerve. It then travels in the medial aspect of the ankle, where it gives off a calcaneal branch, enters the tarsal tunnel, and divides into medial and lateral plantar nerves. These enter their individual tunnels under the abductor hallucis, and supply the intrinsic muscles of the foot, and the skin of the sole of the foot. In the tarsal tunnel, the tendons are deeper than the neurovascular plane and are typically not seen in a standard tarsal tunnel surgery since they are encased in their own fascia. From anterior to posterior, the structures in the tarsal tunnel include: Tibialis posterior, flexor Digitorum longus, posterior tibial Vessels, tibial Nerve, flexor Hallucis longus. Hence the acronym: *Tom Does Very Nice Hats*.

Clinical Significance

The tibial nerve can be entrapped at the soleal arch or the tarsal tunnel. Tarsal tunnel is much less common than carpal tunnel and is more difficult to diagnose. Decompression can improve foot sensation and enhance healing of diabetic ulcers [1, 2]. Morton's neuroma is a misnomer since it is not a true neuroma but a reaction to nerve entrapment; it affects the digital branches of the medial plantar nerve in the second or third web spaces [3]. The tibial nerve can be injured with knee dislocation and/or fractures. It tends to recover better and faster than the peroneal nerve.

Popliteal artery entrapment syndrome (PAES) could occur separately or concomitantly with the tibial nerve entrapment at the soleal arch. Functional PAES occurs in young athletics and causes exertional pain [4–6].

Exposures

In the Popliteal Fossa and Upper Leg (Fig. 27.1)

1. Position: prone.
2. Incision in the posterior midline of the lower thigh and upper leg. If the knee crease is to be crossed, this should be done obliquely or in a Z-shaped fashion. Two incisions can be used leaving a skin bridge at the knee crease.
3. The superficial and deep fasciae are opened.
4. The tibial nerve is found in the midline, while the common peroneal nerve can be found in the lateral aspect along the biceps femoris and its tendon. More than often, the sural nerve contribution is encountered first, followed proximally it leads to the main tibial nerve.
5. The tibial nerve can be followed distally, where it gives off multiple branches to the calf muscles, as well as a contribution to the sural nerve. It passes between the two heads of gastrocnemius and then under the soleal arch. The latter should be split open for decompression of the tibial nerve.
6. In addition, for full vascular decompression, especially in cases of functional PAES, the plantaris is resected as well as the aponeurotic fascia deep to the soleus muscle fibers.

Supplementary Information The online version contains supplementary material available at https://doi.org/10.1007/978-3-031-73931-6_27.

A. S. Hanna (✉)
Department of Neurosurgery, University of Wisconsin School of Medicine and Public Health, Madison, WI, USA

A. S. Hanna (ed.), *Nerves: Anatomy, Exposures, and Techniques*, https://doi.org/10.1007/978-3-031-73931-6_27

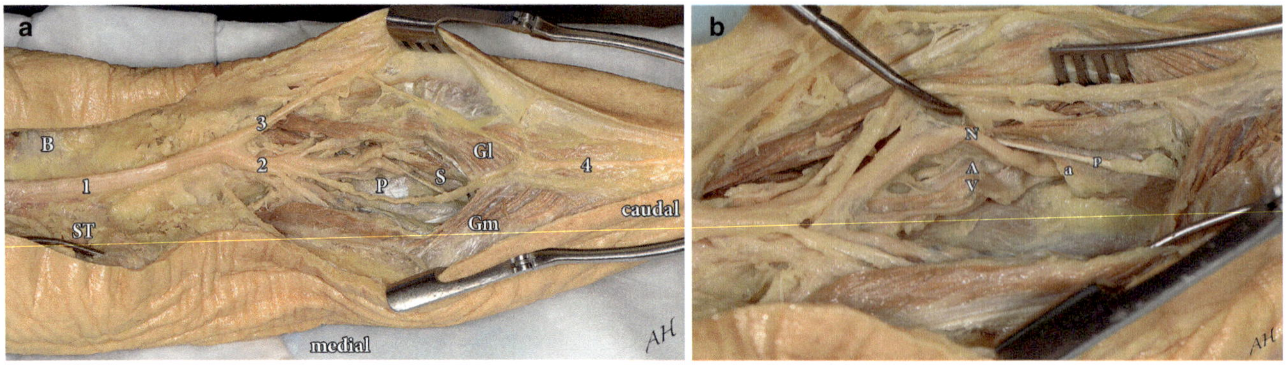

Fig. 27.1 (**a**) Sciatic (*1*), tibial (*2*), and common peroneal (common fibular) (*3*) nerve exposure in the right popliteal fossa. Position: prone. *B* biceps, *ST* semitendinosus, *Gm* gastrocnemius, medial head, *Gl* gastrocnemius, lateral head, *S* soleus, *P* popliteus, *4* sural nerve with contributions from both the tibial and common peroneal nerves. (**b**) Close-up showing the popliteal artery (*A*), popliteal vein (*V*), and tibial nerve (*N*) exiting the popliteal fossa under the soleal arch (*a*). *p* plantaris tendon

In the Tarsal Tunnel (Fig. 27.2) [7]

1. Position: supine, with the hip externally rotated and the knee slightly flexed.
2. A tourniquet can be used.
3. A curvilinear incision is made midway between the medial malleolus and the calcaneus.
4. The incision is deepened through the superficial and deep fasciae.
5. The flexor retinaculum is opened sharply. This allows exposing the tibial nerve and posterior tibial vessels.
6. The calcaneal branch arises from the posterior aspect of the tibial nerve and runs posteriorly and caudally.
7. In the distal part of the tarsal tunnel, the tibial nerve splits into medial and lateral plantar nerves.
8. These are followed distally under the abductor hallucis.
9. They enter their individual tunnels. These should be individually decompressed, and then the septum between the two tunnels should be resected.
10. Closure with nonabsorbable sutures, and the patient is kept non-weight-bearing (on crutches) for 3 weeks for better wound healing.

In the Foot (for Morton's Neuroma) (Fig. 27.3)

1. This is a pseudoneuroma, a reaction to nerve compression. Treatment should be decompression rather than neurectomy.
2. Position: supine, with the hip and knee flexed. The foot can be stabilized using sandbags and tape; tourniquet is preferred to improve visibility.
3. Incision on the dorsum of the foot between the second and third toes or the third and fourth.
4. The dorsal digital nerves (branches of superficial peroneal nerve) are first encountered and should be protected. A small self-retaining retractor (Heiss, small Gelpi, or laminar spreader) is placed between the metatarsal bones of the affected space; this is a key step in opening the space. It allows exposure and stretching of the intermetatarsal ligament.
5. Dissection is carried deeply until the common plantar digital nerve (branch of medial plantar nerve) is identified.
6. The intermetatarsal ligament is then transected, and the digital nerve is thus fully decompressed.

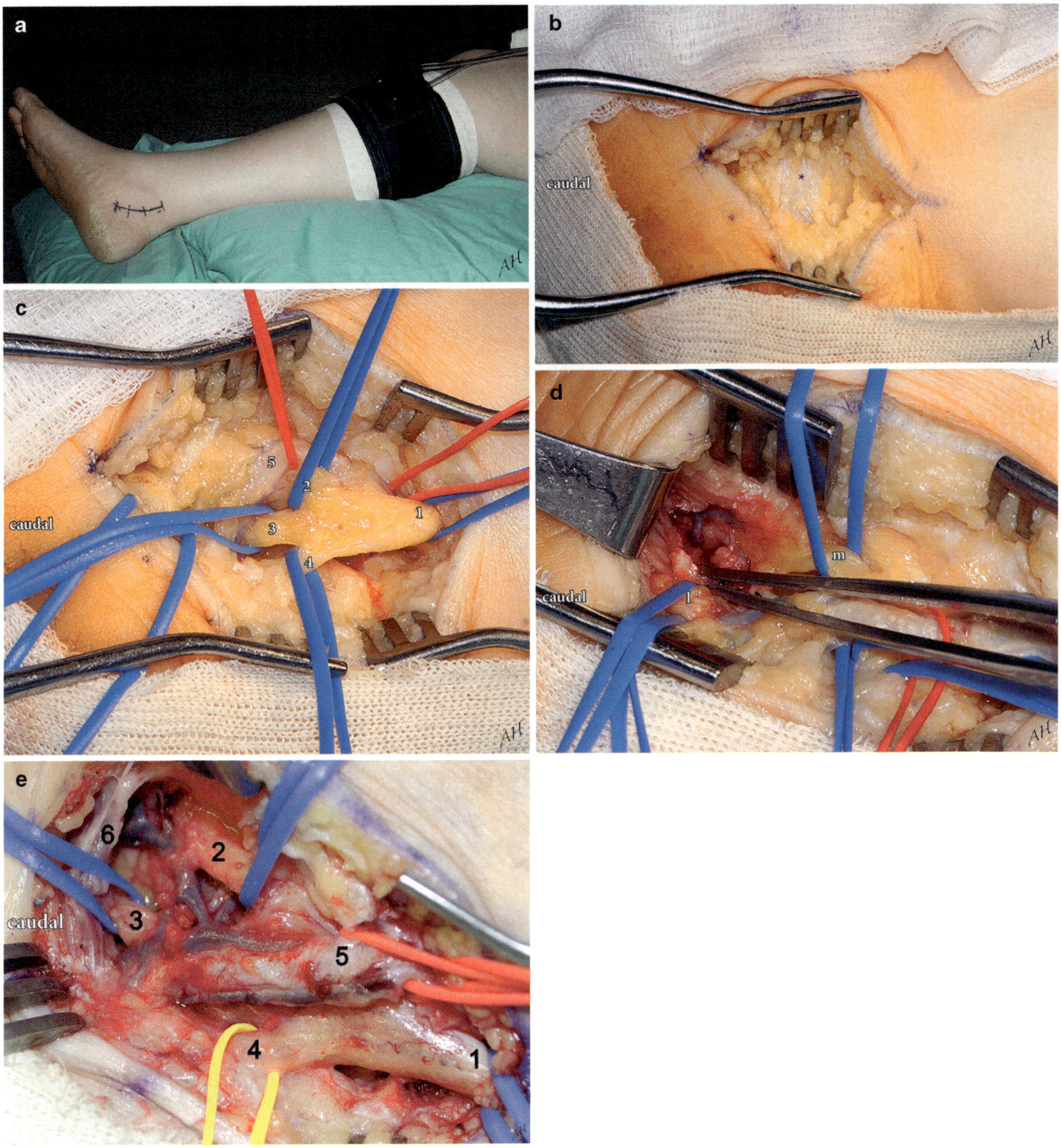

Fig. 27.2 Right tarsal tunnel release. (**a**) The patient is positioned supine, with the hip externally rotated and the knee slightly flexed. A tourniquet can be used. Incision is made between the medial malleolus and the calcaneus. (**b**) The flexor retinaculum (*) is exposed and then opened. (**c**) The tibial (*1*), medial plantar (*2*), and lateral plantar (*3*) nerves are exposed, as well as the calcaneal branch (*4*). The posterior tibial vessels (*5*) are also dissected free. (**d**) The medial (*m*) and lateral (*l*) plantar nerves are followed distally into their individual tunnels under the abductor hallucis. The septum in between (held with a forceps) needs to be resected for full decompression. (**e**) Final view after tarsal tunnel decompression and tourniquet release. *1* tibial nerve, *2* medial plantar nerve, *3* lateral plantar nerve, *4* calcaneal branch, *5* posterior tibial vessels, *6* abductor hallucis

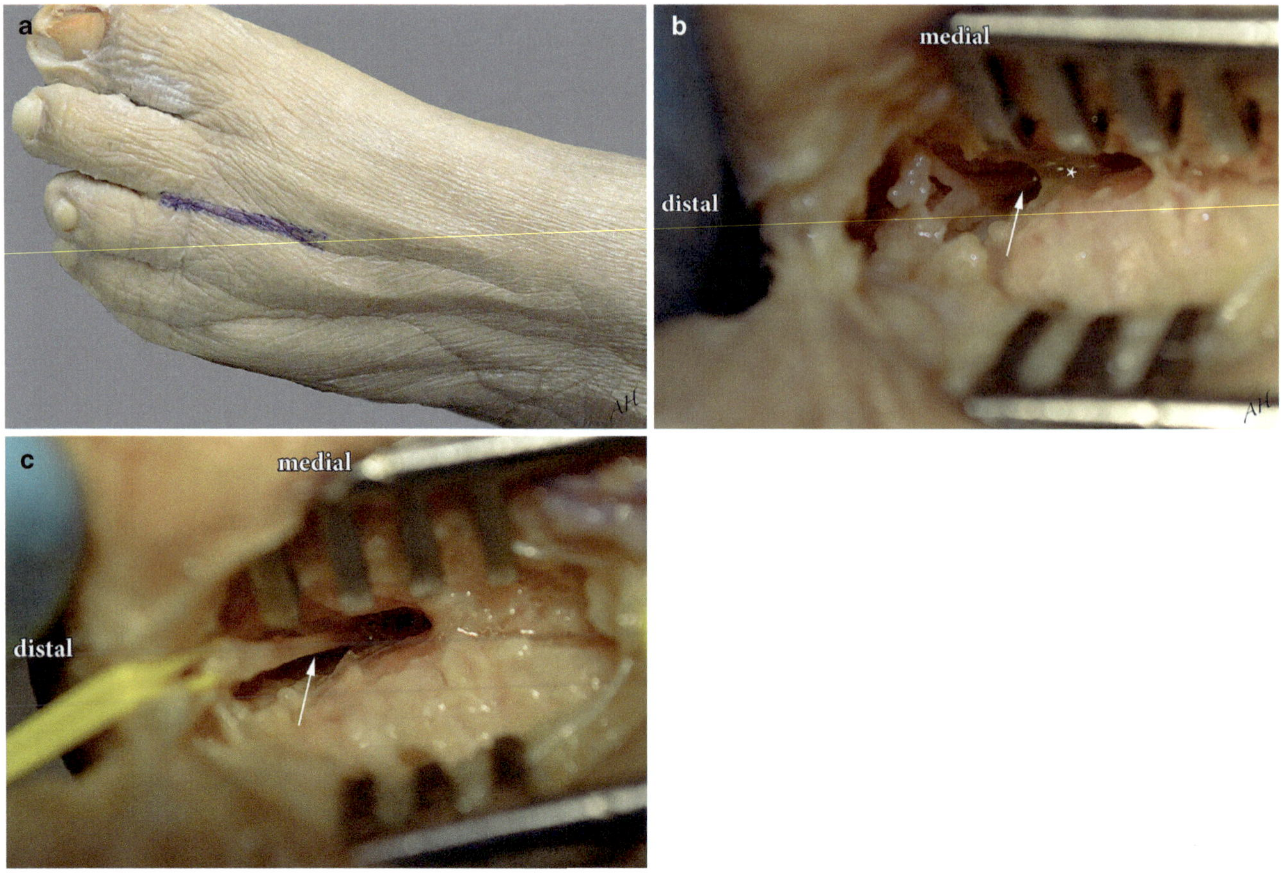

Fig. 27.3 Cadaveric illustration of surgery for left Morton's neuroma. (**a**) Incision is made between the second and third toes, or third and fourth, depending on the location of the pseudoneuroma. (**b**) The common plantar digital (branch of medial plantar) nerve (*arrow*) is observed deep to the intermetatarsal ligament (*white star*). (**c**) The nerve (*arrow*) after full decompression

Complications of Tarsal Tunnel Release

1. Pain from injury to the saphenous nerve anteriorly or the calcaneal branch posteriorly.
2. Residual symptoms from inadequate distal decompression.
3. Vascular injury to the posterior tibial vessels.
4. Wound infection or dehiscence, especially in diabetic patients. Keeping the patient non-weight bearing on crutches for 2–3 weeks should help protect the wound.

References

1. Nickerson DS (2017) Nerve decompression and neuropathy complications in diabetes: are attitudes discordant with evidence? Diabet Foot Ankle 8(1):1367209. https://doi.org/10.1080/2000625X.2017.1367209. eCollection 2017
2. Sessions J, Nickerson DS (2014) Biologic basis of nerve decompression surgery for focal entrapments in diabetic peripheral neuropathy. J Diabetes Sci Technol 8(2):412–418. https://doi.org/10.1177/1932296814525030. Epub 2014 Feb 27
3. Levitsky KA, Alman BA, Jevsevar DS, Morehead J (1993) Digital nerves of the foot: anatomic variations and implications regarding the pathogenesis of interdigital neuroma. Foot Ankle 14(4):208–214. https://doi.org/10.1177/107110079301400406
4. Hislop M, Kennedy D, Cramp B, Dhupelia S (2014) Functional popliteal artery entrapment syndrome: poorly understood and frequently missed? A review of clinical features, appropriate investigations, and treatment options. J Sports Med (Hindawi Publ Corp) 2014:105953. https://doi.org/10.1155/2014/105953. Epub 2014 Sep 7
5. Lovelock T, Claydon M, Dean A (2021) Functional popliteal artery entrapment syndrome: an approach to diagnosis and management. Int J Sports Med 42(13):1159–1166. https://doi.org/10.1055/a--1524-1703. Epub 2021 Aug 2
6. Turnipseed WD (2009) Functional popliteal artery entrapment syndrome: a poorly understood and often missed diagnosis that is frequently mistreated. J Vasc Surg 49(5):1189–1195. https://doi.org/10.1016/j.jvs.2008.12.005
7. Dellon AL (2008) The Dellon approach to neurolysis in the neuropathy patient with chronic nerve compression. Handchir Mikrochir Plast Chir 40(6):351–360. https://doi.org/10.1055/s-2008-1039216. Epub 2008 Dec 2

Common Peroneal Nerve

28

Amgad S. Hanna, Thomas M. Staniszewski, and Asma Eslami

Surgical Anatomy

The common peroneal (fibular) nerve is one of the two terminal branches of the sciatic nerve in the lower third of the thigh. It runs laterally, medial to the biceps femoris tendon, then posterior to the fibular head, and lateral to the fibular neck. It gives off the sural communicating branch (lateral sural cutaneous nerve). This typically joins the contribution from the tibial nerve to form the sural nerve. The latter descends along the lateral aspect of the leg anterior to the Achilles tendon. The lateral dorsal cutaneous nerve is one of its terminal branches. The common peroneal nerve then divides into superficial peroneal, deep peroneal, and articular (recurrent genicular) branches. The articular trunk gives off a tibialis anterior motor branch before becoming a pure sensory articular branch.

The superficial peroneal nerve supplies the peroneus longus and peroneus brevis muscles. It gives off two terminal cutaneous branches: medial dorsal cutaneous and intermediate dorsal cutaneous nerves. These pierce the deep fascia at the lower third of the leg and supply the dorsal surface of the foot and toes except the first web space and the lateral aspect of the little toe.

The deep peroneal nerve supplies the tibialis anterior, extensor hallucis longus, extensor digitorum longus, and peroneus tertius. It continues under the extensor retinaculum in the anterior tarsal tunnel and then divides in the dorsum of the foot into a lateral muscular branch supplying the extensor digitorum brevis and a medial cutaneous branch supplying the adjacent sides of the first and second toes.

Clinical Significance

The common peroneal nerve is easily injured with knee dislocations and/or fractures. It is slow to recover, and the prognosis is generally poor, especially with longer lesions. Injury can result in a foot drop with intact inversion, unless there is concomitant involvement of the tibial nerve (Fig. 28.1). The recurrent genicular branch supplies the superior tibio-fibular joint. Inflammation of this joint can result in retrograde synovial filling of the articular branch and the peroneal nerve, especially deep component, thus creating an intraneural ganglion cyst that usually causes foot drop (see Chap. 55). Tibial to peroneal nerve transfers have been used to treat foot drop with limited success (see Chap. 42). Hanna used the cross-

Supplementary Information The online version contains supplementary material available at https://doi.org/10.1007/978-3-031-73931-6_28.

A. S. Hanna (✉) · A. Eslami
Department of Neurosurgery, University of Wisconsin School of Medicine and Public Health, Madison, WI, USA
e-mail: Aeslami@wisc.edu

T. M. Staniszewski
Department of Neurological Surgery, University of Wisconsin School of Medicine and Public Health, Madison, WI, USA
e-mail: staniszewski@neurosurgery.wisc.edu

A. S. Hanna (ed.), *Nerves: Anatomy, Exposures, and Techniques*, https://doi.org/10.1007/978-3-031-73931-6_28

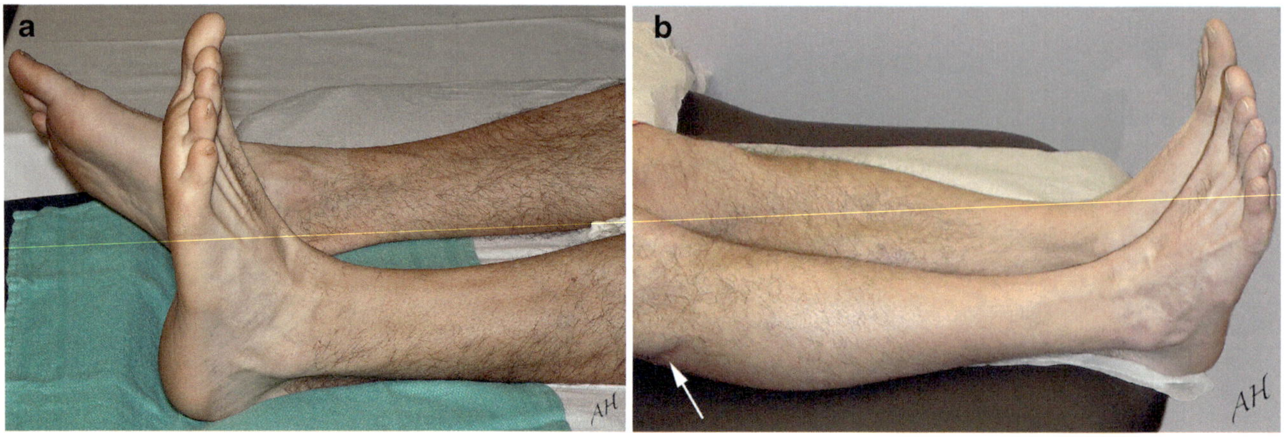

Fig. 28.1 Pre- (**a**) and postoperative (**b**) photos from a patient with right foot drop from common peroneal nerve entrapment at the fibular neck. *Arrow* scar from peroneal decompression surgery

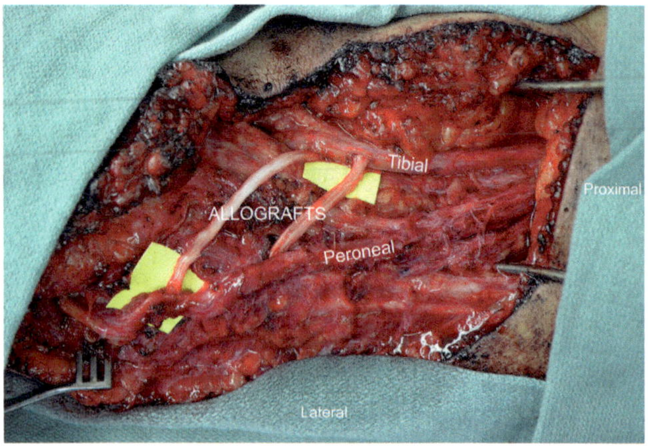

Fig. 28.2 In cases of peroneal nerve injury or high sciatic with only recovery of tibial component, cross-bridge grafts can be placed end-to-side from tibial to peroneal nerves. At the end, the construct looks like a ladder [1]. Alternatively, end-to-end can be used from lateral gastrocnemius branch to deep peroneal nerve using locally harvested sural nerve as a graft

bridge ladder technique from tibial to peroneal end-to-side with good results (Fig. 28.2) [1].

The cutaneous branches of the superficial peroneal nerve can be injured during fasciotomies for compartment syndrome. Different cutaneous branches in the area are also vulnerable during ankle surgery [2].

Exposures

In the Popliteal Fossa

1. Position: prone.
2. Incision oblique along the posterior border of biceps femoris.
3. The superficial and deep fasciae are opened.
4. The common peroneal nerve is found within the popliteal fossa fat medial to the biceps femoris tendon (see Fig. 27.1).

Around the Fibular Neck (Fig. 28.3)

1. Position: lateral on a beanbag.
2. Incision: curvilinear, posterior to the fibular head and lateral to the fibular neck. A common mistake is to palpate the knee joint and think it is fibular head. Operator should palpate the tibial tuberosity anteriorly (insertion of patellar tendon) and draw a line posteriorly and laterally; this will lead to the fibular neck.
3. The superficial and deep fasciae are opened. The common peroneal nerve can be felt against the head of fibula.
4. The nerve sheath is opened sharply using Metzenbaum scissors.
5. The nerve is followed proximally toward the popliteal fossa and decompressed.
6. The nerve is followed distally under the peroneal fascia, which is opened for full decompression: first the fascia on top of the muscle is opened, and then the muscle is

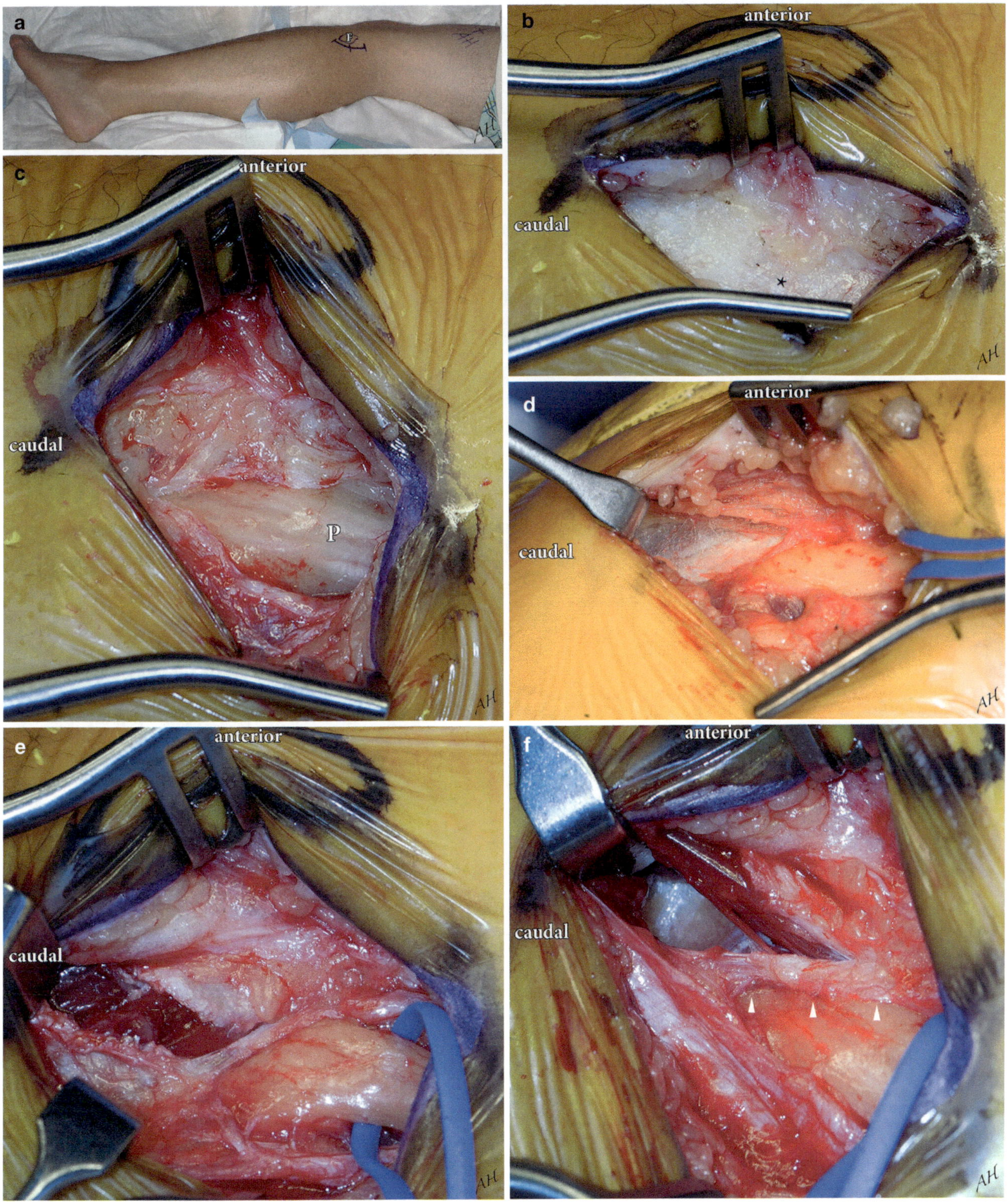

Fig. 28.3 Another patient undergoing left common peroneal nerve decompression at the fibular neck. (**a**) Position is lateral on a beanbag, and incision is posterior to the fibular head (*F*) and lateral to the fibular neck. (**b**) The nerve sheath is exposed (*), and opened (**c**), thus exposing the common peroneal (common fibular) nerve (*P*). (**d**) The fascia overlying the peronei muscles is exposed and opened (**e**). (**f**) The muscle is retracted, thus exposing the fascia deep to it, with its sharp edge (*arrowheads*) compressing the nerve. (**g**) This fascia is opened, achieving full distal decompression. The three terminal branches of the common peroneal nerve are exposed: *S* superficial peroneal, *D* deep peroneal, and *A* articular trunk. (**h**) Full proximal decompression medial to the tendon of biceps femoris (*B*)

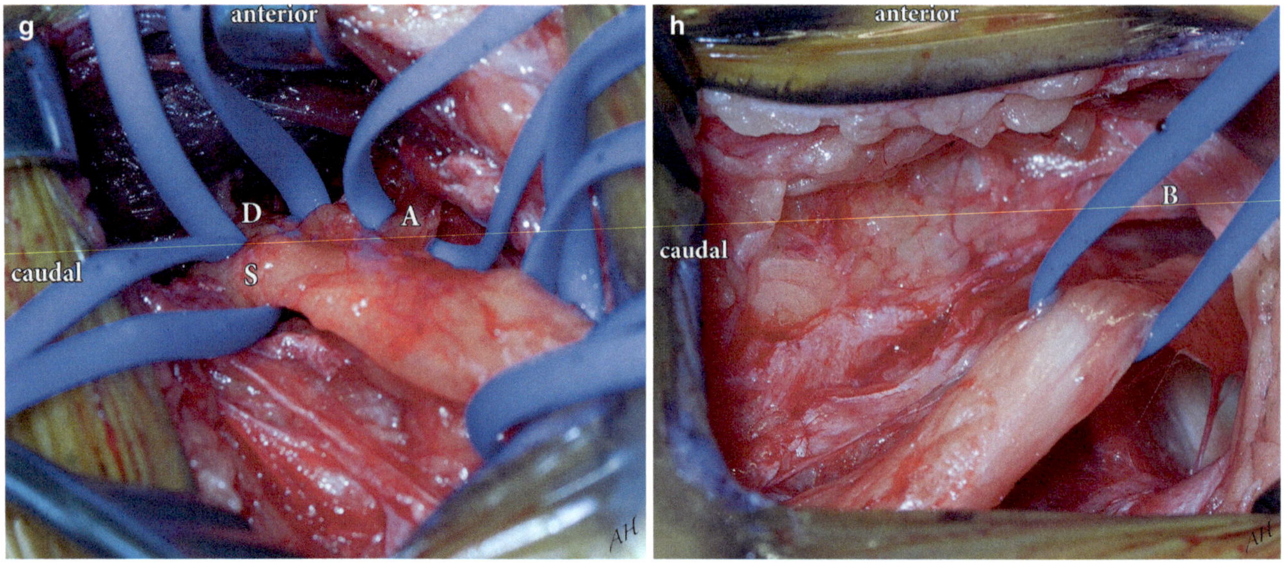

Fig. 28.3 (continued)

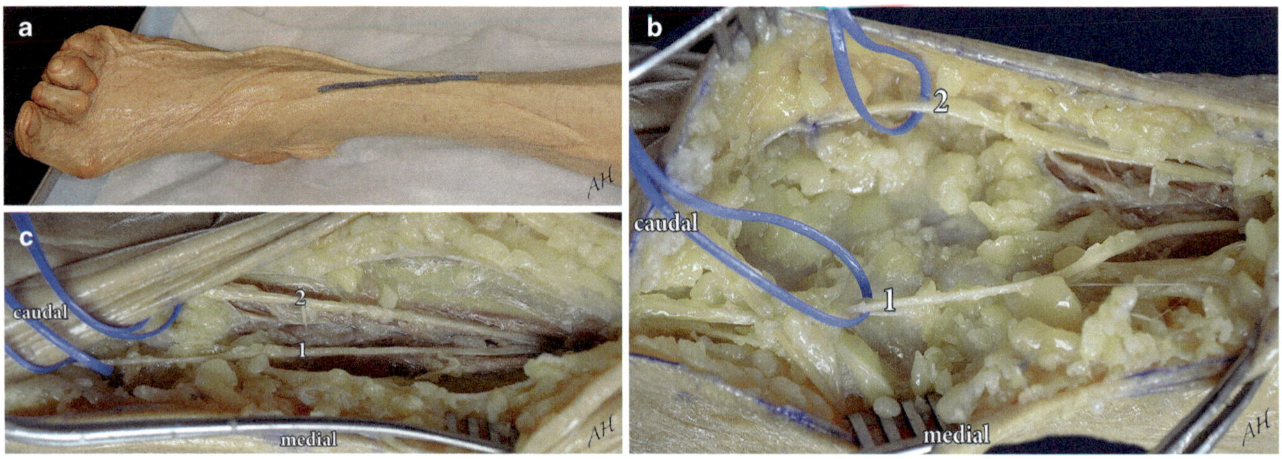

Fig. 28.4 (**a**) Incision for exposure of the cutaneous branches of the right superficial peroneal (superficial fibular) nerve. The medial (*1*) and intermediate (*2*) dorsal cutaneous nerves are observed in the subcutaneous fat distally (**b**) and deep to the peroneal fascia proximally (**c**)

retracted exposing the deeper fascial layer. This is opened as well.

7. This exposes the three branches of the peroneal nerve: superficial peroneal, deep peroneal, and articular branches.

In the Lower Leg and Anterior Ankle

Superficial Peroneal (Fig. 28.4)

1. Position: supine.
2. Oblique incision along the lateral aspect of the leg and dorsum of ankle.
3. The terminal dorsal cutaneous branches can be found piercing the deep fascia in the lower third of the leg. Then, they course in the subcutaneous fat, with the medial branch medially and the intermediate branch laterally.
4. Ultrasound assistance could be used to localize these small cutaneous nerves.

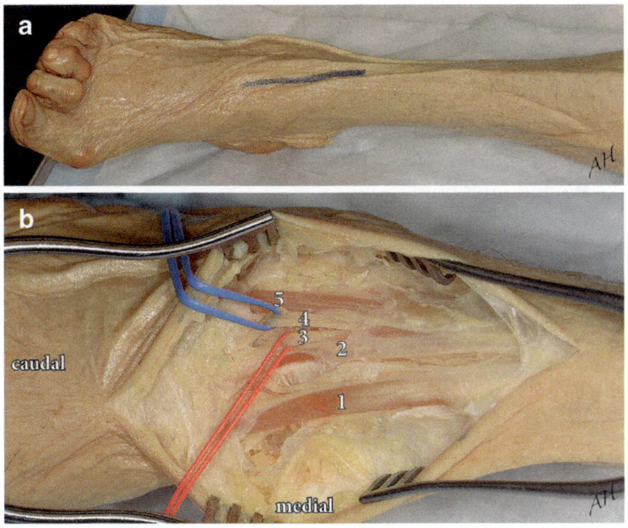

Fig. 28.5 (a) Incision for anterior tarsal tunnel release. (b) Once the extensor retinaculum is opened, the following structures can be identified from medial to lateral: *1* Tibialis anterior, *2* extensor Hallucis longus, *3* anterior tibial artery (Vessels), *4* deep peroneal (deep fibular) Nerve, *5* extensor Digitorum longus

Deep Peroneal (Anterior Tarsal Tunnel) (Fig. 28.5)

1. Position: supine.
2. Incision: midline dorsum of the ankle.
3. The extensor retinaculum is opened.
4. The deep peroneal Nerve is found with the anterior tibial Vessels. Tibialis anterior and extensor Hallucis longus tendons are medial to it, and extensor Digitorum longus and Peroneus tertius are lateral to it. Hence, the acronym *Tom Has Very Nice Dogs and Pigs*, from medial to lateral.
5. The extensor retinaculum separates the superficial peroneal nerve branches in the subcutaneous fat from the deep peroneal nerve in the anterior tarsal tunnel.

Sural Nerve (Fig. 28.6)

1. Position: depends on the indication—for a nerve biopsy, the patient is positioned lateral under local anesthesia and sedation. For nerve grafting, the position is dictated by

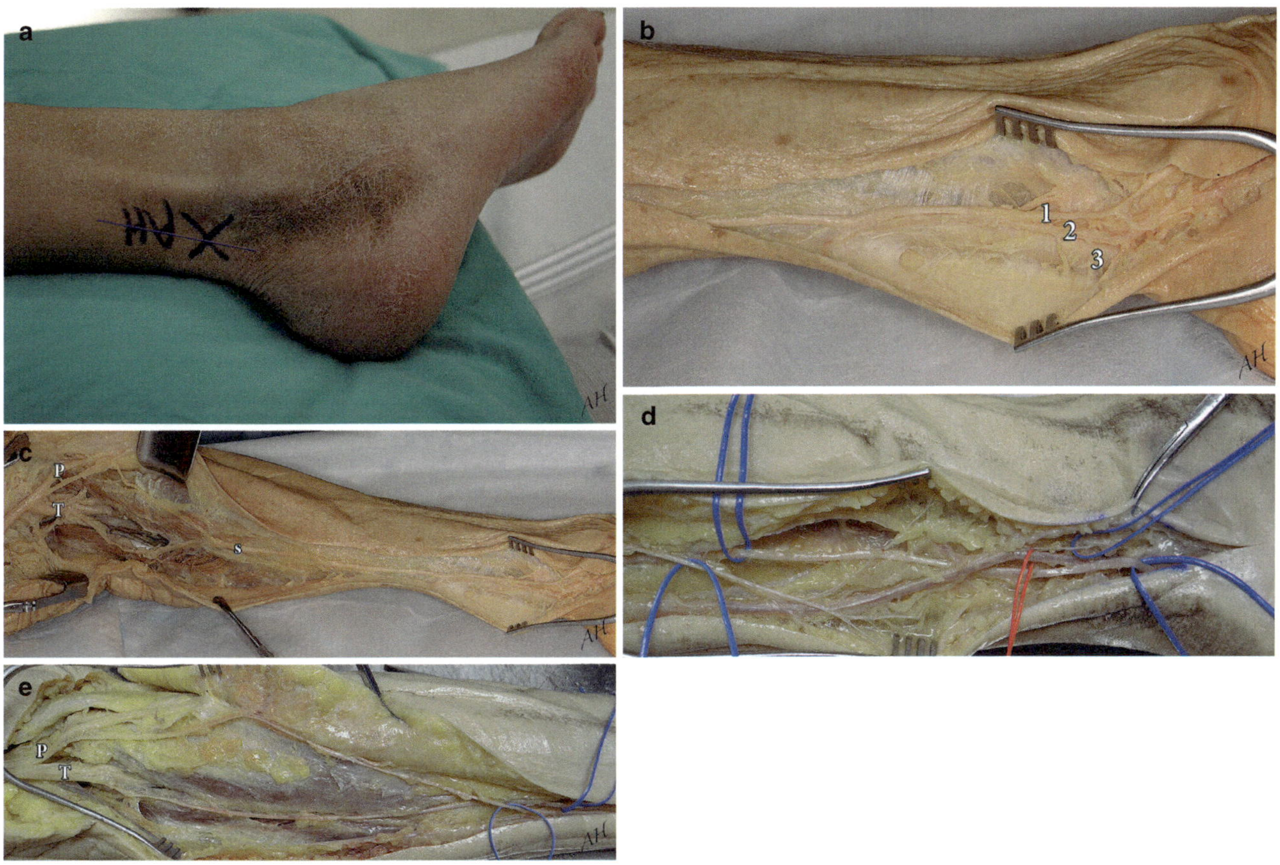

Fig. 28.6 Sural nerve exposure. (a) Position is lateral, and the incision is made laterally, anterior to the Achilles tendon. (b) The skin is opened; within the fat is the sural nerve (*1*), along the short saphenous vein (*2*), anterior to the Achilles tendon (*3*). (c) As needed, the sural nerve (*s*) can be followed proximally until its origins from the tibial (*T*) and common peroneal (*P*) nerves. (d, e) Occasionally, the two components of the sural nerve never meet and remain as two distinct nerves (*blue loops*) until their origins from the tibial (*T*) and common peroneal (*P*) nerves. *Red loop* short saphenous vein

the primary nerve to be repaired. Sural nerve can even be harvested in a supine position, with the leg elevated by an assistant, or bent at the knee. There are four different ways to harvest sural nerve:
   (a) One long incision
   (b) Skip incisions with tunneling in between
   (c) Use a nerve stripper [3]
   (d) Endoscopic [4]
2. Incision is made lateral and anterior to the Achilles tendon.
3. Once a self-retaining retractor is placed, the short saphenous vein can be seen within the subcutaneous fat. The sural nerve could have multiple branches and runs along the short saphenous vein.
4. Dissection is carried longitudinally along the nerve, to free it 360°.
5. The nerve can be followed proximally until its origin in the upper leg from both the tibial and peroneal nerves. Occasionally, these two contributions to the sural nerve remain separate and continue as two distinct nerves.
6. Some surgeons prefer to repair the sural nerve with an allograft after a nerve biopsy to avoid neuroma formation.

Complications of Sural Nerve Harvest

1. Loss of sensation on the lateral aspect of the dorsum of the foot and little toe
2. Pain from neuroma formation
3. Wound infection

References

1. Ammanuel S, Burkett D, Kim JJ, Bond ES, Hanna AS (2023) Peroneal nerve repair with cross-bridge ladder technique: parallel end-to-side neurorrhaphies. J Brachial Plex Peripher Nerve Inj 18(1):e21–e26. https://doi.org/10.1055/s-0043-1768996. eCollection 2023 Jan
2. Duscher D, Wenny R, Entenfellner J, Weninger P, Hirtler L (2014) Cutaneous innervation of the ankle: an anatomical study showing danger zones for ankle surgery. Clin Anat 27(4):653–658. https://doi.org/10.1002/ca.22347. Epub 2013 Dec 17
3. Hassanpour E, Yavari M, Karbalaeikhani A, Saremi H (2014) Nerve stripper-assisted sural nerve harvest. J Neurol Surg A Cent Eur Neurosurg 75(2):161–164. https://doi.org/10.1055/s--0032-1330117. Epub 2013 Feb 8
4. Joseph AW, Nagappan K, Joseph SS (2022) Endoscopic technique for sural nerve graft harvest with novel device. Facial Plast Surg Aesthet Med 24(2):124–125. https://doi.org/10.1089/fpsam.2021.0341. Epub 2022 Jan 18

29 Superficial Peroneal Nerve: Nervus Fibularis Superficialis

M. Rosa Morro-Martí, Amer Mustafa-Gondolbeu, Guillermo Tarnawski-Español, Pablo Martínez-Collado, and Manuel Llusa-Pérez

Indications

- Intraneural ganglion cyst from the proximal tibiofibular joint
- Compression neuropathies: at the entrance of the lateral compartment in the proximal leg or at the intermuscular septum or fascia between the anterior and lateral compartments
- Traumatic lesions of the common peroneal nerve, especially in forced varus of the knee (Platt syndrome) or lacerations
- Iatrogenic lesions after distal fibular osteosynthesis or fasciotomies for chronic compartment syndrome
- Tumors such as schwannomas (Fig. 29.1) and neurofibromas
- Neuritis

Supplementary Information The online version contains supplementary material available at https://doi.org/10.1007/978-3-031-73931-6_29.

M. R. Morro-Martí · P. Martínez-Collado · M. Llusa-Pérez (✉)
Department of Human Anatomy, University of Barcelona Medical School, Barcelona, Spain

Department of Orthopaedic Surgery and Traumatology, Vall d'Hebron Hospital, Barcelona, Spain
e-mail: mrmorro@ub.edu; mllusa@ub.edu

A. Mustafa-Gondolbeu
Department of Human Anatomy, University of Lleida Medical School, Lleida, Spain

Department of Orthopaedic Surgery and Traumatology, Arnau de Vilanova Hospital, Lleida, Spain

G. Tarnawski-Español
Department of Human Anatomy, University of Barcelona Medical School, Barcelona, Spain

Department of Orthopaedic Surgery and Traumatology, Fraternidad Muprespa Habana Hospital, Madrid, Spain

A. S. Hanna (ed.), *Nerves: Anatomy, Exposures, and Techniques*, https://doi.org/10.1007/978-3-031-73931-6_29

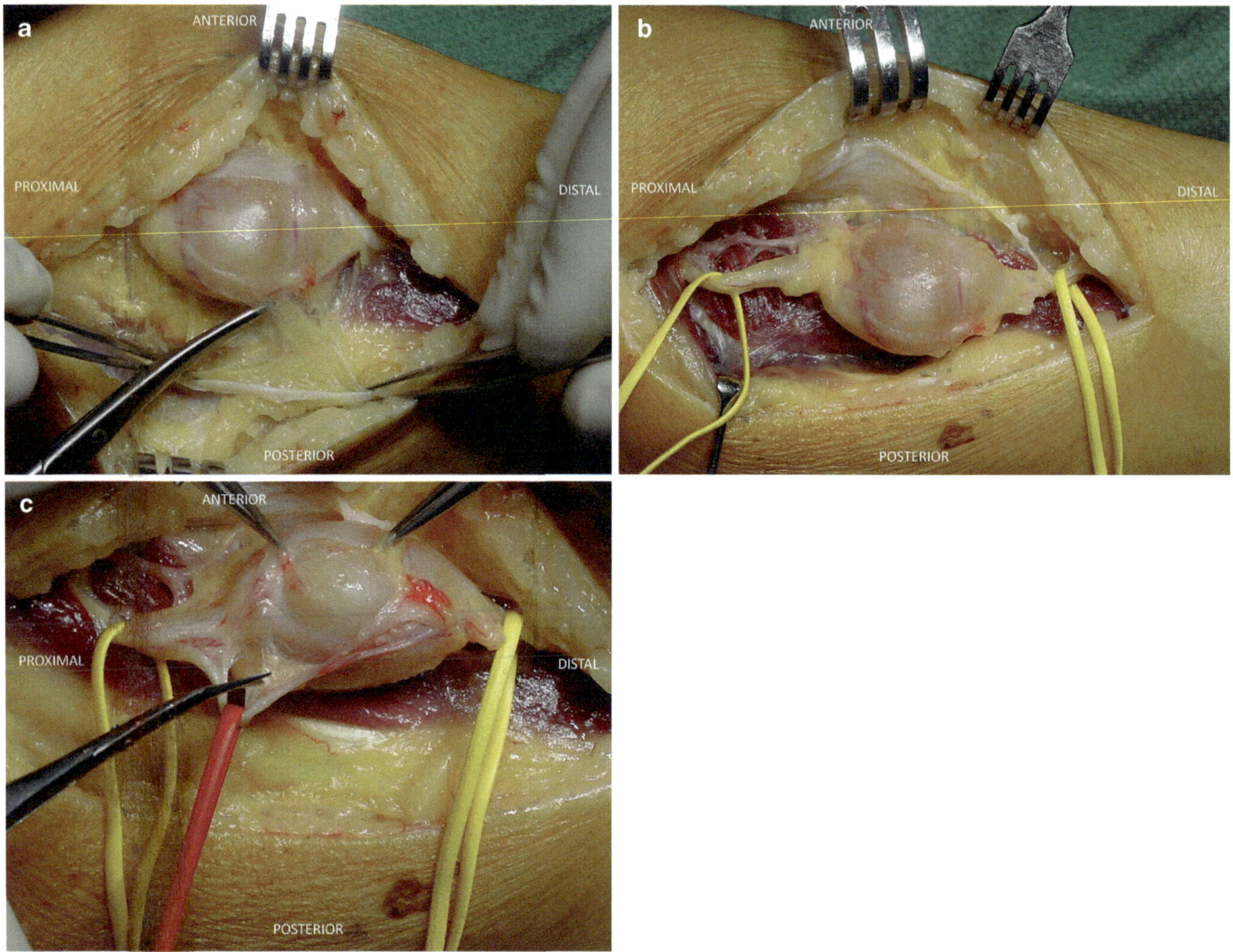

Fig. 29.1 Schwannoma of the superficial peroneal nerve at the mid-third of the leg. (**a**) Surgical exposure showing the tumor. (**b**) Isolation of the superficial peroneal nerve proximal and distal to the schwannoma (*yellow loops*), at the mid-third of the leg before perforating the fascia. (**c**) Resection of the schwannoma by entering the capsule and preserving the normal fascicles (*red loop*)

Surgical Anatomy

The common peroneal nerve courses toward the neck of the fibula behind the biceps femoris tendon. Before reaching and winding around the fibular neck, it gives off the lateral sural cutaneous nerve and the ramus communicans fibularis (Fig. 29.2) which will then form the sural nerve with the medial sural cutaneous nerve (branch of the tibial nerve). The common peroneal nerve at the level of the neck of the fibula passes under the peroneus longus arch of origin, where it gives off its first branch (proximal tibiofibular branch) and bifurcates into the superficial and deep peroneal nerves [1–3] (Fig. 29.3).

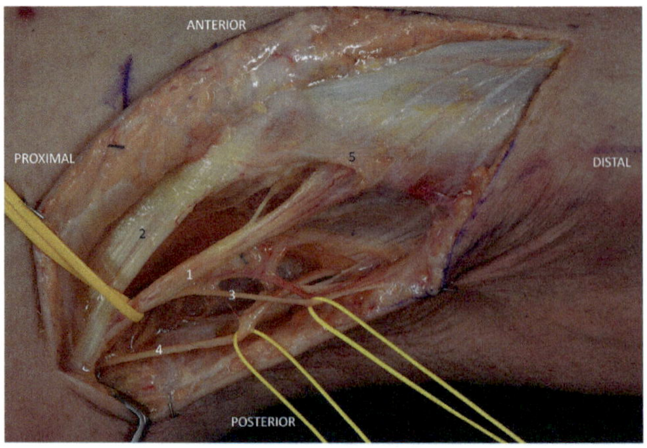

Fig. 29.2 Approach in an anatomical specimen to the common fibular nerve (*1*) at the knee. It is found just posterior to the biceps femoris tendon (*2*) and around the neck of the fibula. Identification of the lateral sural cutaneous nerve (*3*) and the ramus communicans fibularis (*4*) coming off the common fibular nerve and marked with yellow rubber bands. *5* peroneus longus arch

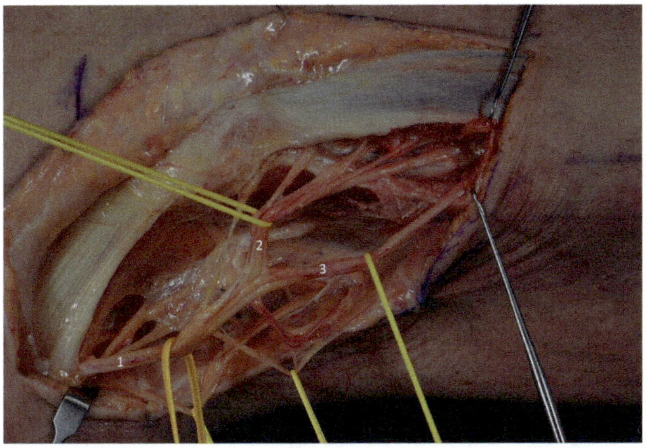

Fig. 29.3 Wider dissection of the common fibular nerve (*1*) and its branches in an anatomical specimen. The deep peroneal nerve (*2*) and its muscular branches entering the anterior compartment of the leg and the superficial peroneal nerve (*3*) in a more posterior position

The superficial peroneal nerve is located in the lateral compartment of the leg, which innervates, through muscular branches, the peroneus longus and brevis (Fig. 29.3). In the distal third of the leg, it perforates the fascia and is located superficially, dividing into two branches, the medial dorsal cutaneous nerve and the intermediate dorsal cutaneous nerve [4, 5] (Fig. 29.4).

The deep peroneal nerve penetrates the anterior compartment of the leg.

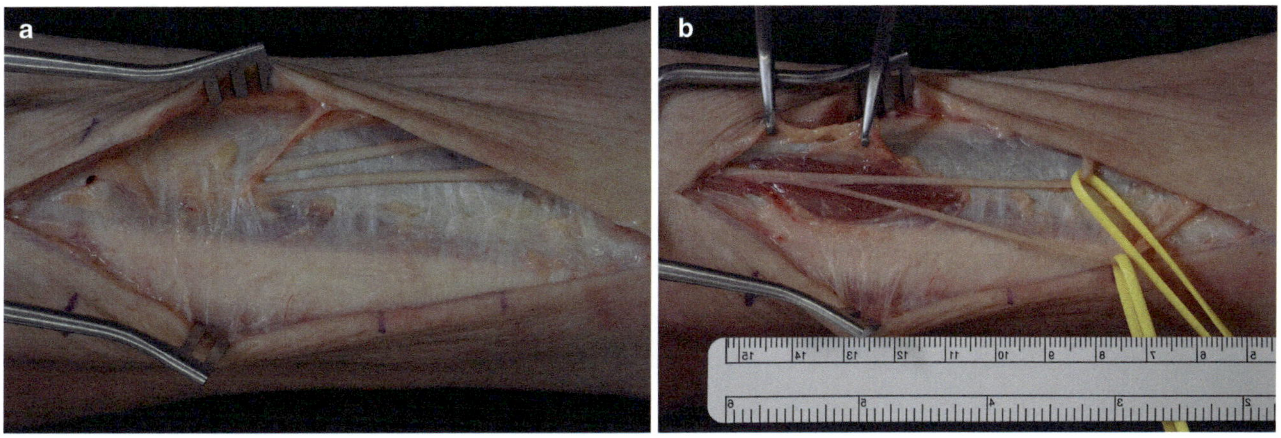

Fig. 29.4 Approach to the superficial peroneal nerve at the mid-third of the leg in an anatomical specimen. (**a**) Identification of the nerve over the deep fascia. (**b**) The deep fascia has been opened, and the nerve, followed proximally in the lateral compartment of the leg, is found between the peroneus longus and brevis muscles

Exposure

Approach to the Proximal Portion of the Nervus Fibularis Superficialis

1. Position: supine with a sandbag under the buttock of the affected limb, and the knee flexed 90° on the table or lateral decubitus on the nonsurgical side.
2. Incision: long-S-shaped incision following the course of the nerve at the level of the lateral aspect of the knee and leg, in the lateral compartment (Fig. 29.5).
3. The skin flaps are dissected through the subcutaneous fat tissue and the underlying fascia, avoiding the lateral sural cutaneous nerve and ramus communicans fibularis.
4. The nervus fibularis communis is identified at the posterior border of the biceps tendon and followed distally to the posterior border of the head of the fibula (Fig. 29.2).
5. Once it is localized, it is followed distally, cutting the fascia of the fibularis longus muscle in line with the pathway of the nerve (frequent compression site) (Fig. 29.3).
6. At this point, the nerve divides into the superficialis and profundus branches. The nervus fibularis superficialis can be followed in the lateral compartment, dissecting between the fibularis longus and brevis muscles. The nervus fibularis profundus perforates the anterior intermuscular septum to enter the anterior compartment of the leg.

Approach to the Distal Portion of the Nervus Fibularis Superficialis

To localize the distal subcutaneous branches of the superficial peroneal nerve, there is a useful clinical maneuver flexing and inverting the foot and flexing the fourth toe to tense the cutaneous branch of the dorsal intermediate cutaneous nerve that you see and can follow up to the distal leg (Figs. 29.6, 29.7, and 29.8).

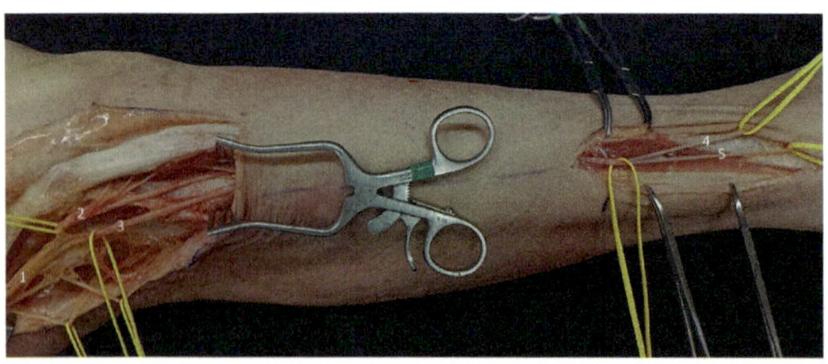

Fig. 29.5 General vision of the two approaches to the superficial fibular nerve at the knee and proximal third of the leg and in the mid-third of the leg in an anatomical specimen. *1* common peroneal nerve, *2* deep peroneal nerve, *3* superficial peroneal nerve, *4* medial and *5* intermediate dorsal cutaneous nerves

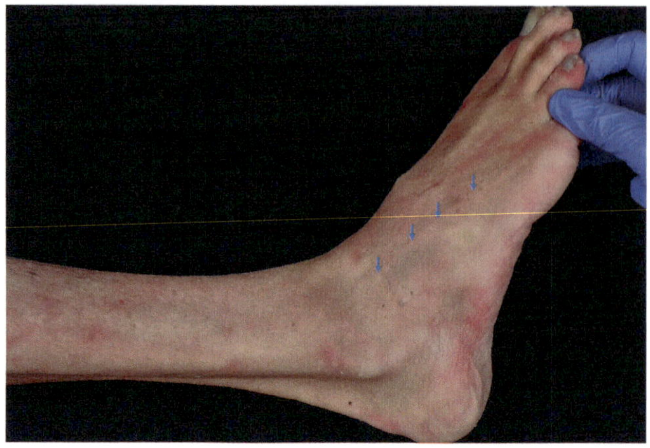

Fig. 29.6 Clinical maneuver of flexion of the fourth and/or fifth toe and flexion and inversion of the foot to tense the distal portion of the superficial peroneal nerve over the deep fascia. The dorsal intermediate cutaneous nerve can be seen and palpated through the skin (*blue arrows*)

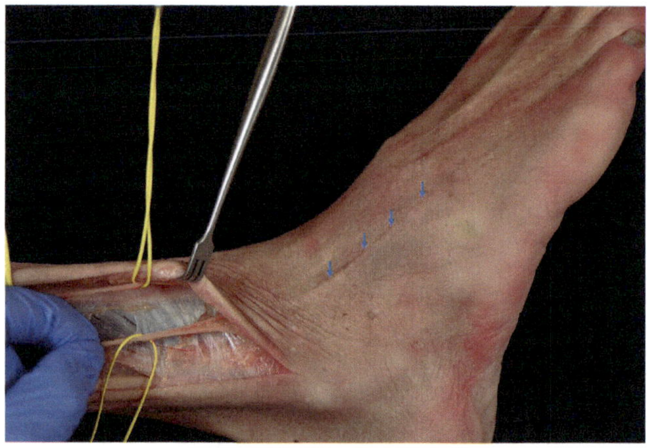

Fig. 29.7 Anatomical demonstration of the identification of the intermediate dorsal cutaneous nerve (*blue arrows*) by tensioning it by pulling it proximally

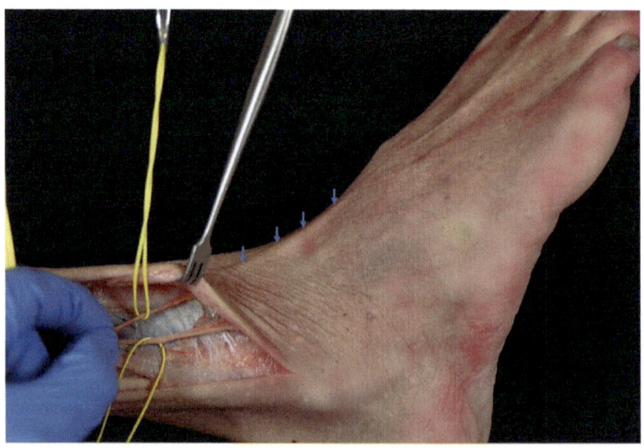

Fig. 29.8 Anatomical demonstration of the identification of the medial dorsal cutaneous nerve (*blue arrows*) by tensioning it by pulling it proximally

1. Position: supine with a sandbag under the buttock of the affected limb or lateral decubitus.
2. Incision: two fingerbreadths lateral to the shin of the tibia over the region 10 cm proximal to the lateral malleolus (Fig. 29.4b). The anatomy and relations of this nerve are variable, not only in location but also in number (in some cases, the two distal branches appear divided at this level).
3. The cutaneous branches of the nerve are usually found in the subcutaneous tissue over the fascia which must be followed proximally until they pierce the fascia (Fig. 29.4).
4. The anterior intermuscular septum is the reference to look for the exit of these branches. In occasions, it is easier to find the nerve by opening the lateral compartment and looking for it as it goes toward the anterior intermuscular septum (Fig. 29.9).

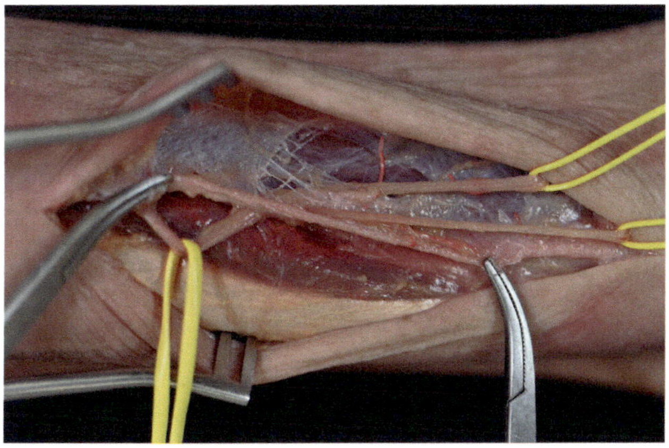

Fig. 29.9 Dissection of the superficial peroneal nerve and its distal cutaneous branches (*yellow loops*) perforating the deep fascia of the leg and, occasionally, the anterior intermuscular septum (*held by two Mosquito forceps*)

Complications

– Because of the superficial location of the nerve in the subcutaneous tissue, neuropathic pain can occur because of fibrosis.

References

1. Llusa M, Merí A, Ruano D (2008) Surgical atlas of the musculoskeletal system. AAOS, Rosemont
2. Tubbs RS, Loukas M, Hanna AS, Oskouian RJ (2019) Surgical anatomy of the lumbar plexus. Thieme, New York
3. Hanna AS (2015) Anatomy and exposures of spinal nerves. Springer, Cham
4. Solomon LB, Ferris L, Tedman R, Henneberg M (2001) Surgical anatomy of the sural and superficial fibular nerves with an emphasis of the approach to the lateral malleolus. J Anat 199:717–723. https://doi.org/10.1046/j.1469-7580.2001.19960717.x
5. Apaydin N, Basarir K, Loukas M, Tubbs RS, Uz A, Kinik H (2008) Compartmental anatomy of the superficial fibular nerve with an emphasis on fascia release operations of the leg. Surg Radiol Anat 30:47–52. https://doi.org/10.1007/s00276-007-0284-3

Obturator Nerve

30

Amgad S. Hanna and Mark E. Ehlers

Surgical Anatomy

The obturator nerve arises from the anterior division of L2–L4 ventral rami. It courses medial to the psoas major muscle, along the sidewall of the pelvis, with the iliac vessels. It exits the pelvis through the obturator canal, accompanied by the obturator artery, in the upper part of the obturator foramen, where it divides into anterior and posterior divisions. The anterior division passes above the obturator externus and then in between the adductor brevis posteriorly and pectineus and the adductor longus anteriorly. The posterior division passes through the obturator externus and then between the adductor brevis and the adductor magnus. The anterior division supplies the adductor longus, adductor brevis, and gracilis muscles. The posterior division supplies the obturator externus and the adductor part of adductor magnus. They also have articular branches and cutaneous branches that supply the medial aspect of the thigh. The nerve occasionally supplies the pectineus.

Clinical Significance

The gracilis branch is very important when harvesting the gracilis muscle for a free transfer with its vascular pedicle for brachial plexus injuries [1].

Anterior obturator neurectomy and adductor myotomy are used to treat spasticity of the adductor muscles, especially in children with cerebral palsy [2]. Intrapelvic obturator neurectomy can also be performed.

Supplementary Information The online version contains supplementary material available at https://doi.org/10.1007/978-3-031-73931-6_30.

A. S. Hanna (✉)
Department of Neurosurgery, University of Wisconsin School of Medicine and Public Health, Madison, WI, USA

M. E. Ehlers
Urology, Aurora Health Care Medical Group, Milwaukee, WI, USA
e-mail: mehlers@wisc.edu

The obturator nerve can be used as a donor for nerve transfers for femoral nerve palsy [3–5] and for urinary bladder reinnervation [6].

Exposure

Intrapelvic (Fig. 30.1; see also Fig. 23.3)

1. Open or laparoscopic.
2. General surgeon for access.
3. Horizontal Pfannenstiel incision can be used, or inferior midline.

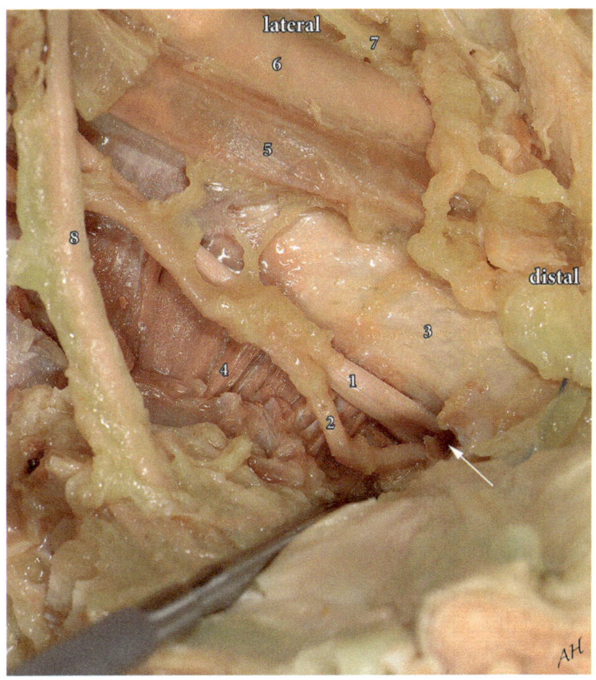

Fig. 30.1 Intrapelvic exposure of the left obturator nerve (*1*); the nerve exits the pelvis through the obturator canal (*arrow*) after it divides into anterior and posterior divisions, *2* obturator artery, *3* superior pubic ramus, *4* obturator internus, *5* external iliac vein, *6* external iliac artery, *7* genital branch of the genitofemoral nerve, *8* ureter

A. S. Hanna (ed.), *Nerves: Anatomy, Exposures, and Techniques*, https://doi.org/10.1007/978-3-031-73931-6_30

4. Once the abdomen is entered, the nerve is identified along the sidewall of the pelvis, medial to the psoas and external iliac vessels. Electrical stimulation is used for confirmation, with recordings from the adductor muscles.
5. If neurectomy is the goal, a segment of the nerve is then resected.

In the Thigh

1. Position: supine, with the hip abducted and externally rotated.

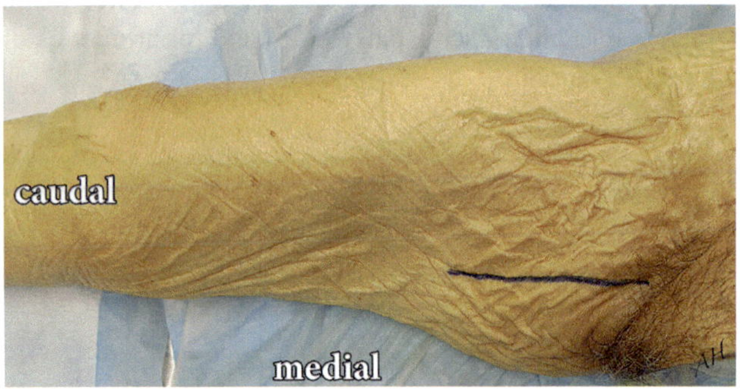

Fig. 30.2 Obturator nerve exposure in the right thigh. Incision is made along the adductor longus

2. Incision is made along the adductor longus tendon up to the pubic tubercle (Fig. 30.2).
3. The superficial and deep fasciae are opened.
4. The adductor longus and pectineus are identified.
5. The adductor longus can be resected first if myectomy is part of the procedure. The anterior division of the obturator nerve can then be found anterior to the adductor brevis.
6. If no myectomy is performed, the plane between the adductor longus and pectineus is entered (Fig. 30.3a). These two muscles are separated, and the anterior division of the obturator nerve is found deep to them (Fig. 30.3b), superficial to the adductor brevis. The author finds it easier to identify the gracilis branch medially then follow it proximally.
7. To find the posterior division, the adductor brevis can be retracted, and the nerve is found between the adductor brevis and magnus (Fig. 30.4).
8. The plane between the adductor longus and gracilis can be entered to isolate the gracilis branch of the anterior division as well as the gracilis main vascular pedicle (Fig. 30.5).

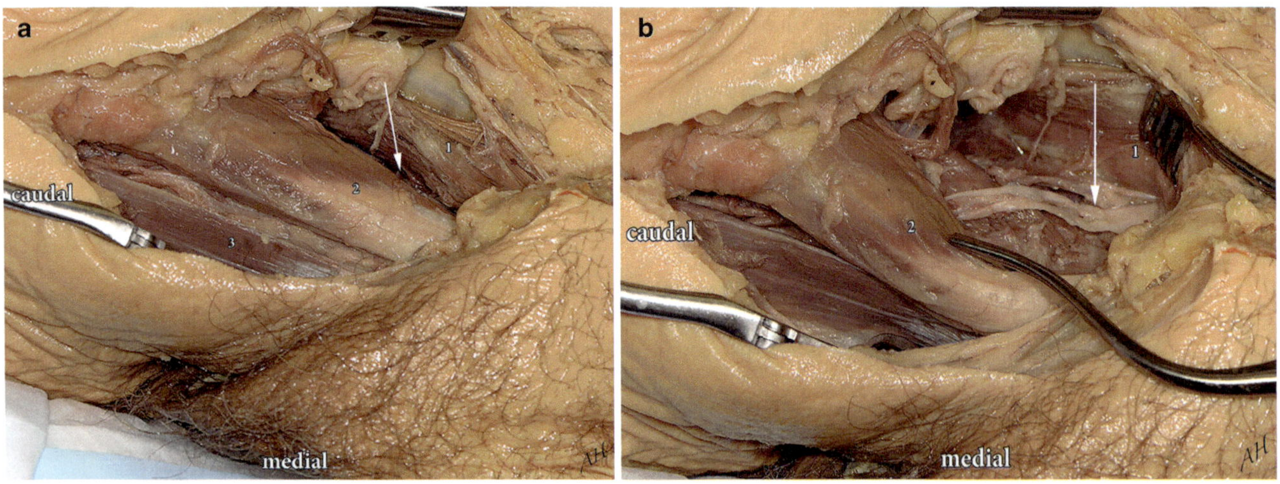

Fig. 30.3 (**a**) The plane (*arrow*) between the pectineus (*1*) and adductor longus (*2*) is entered to find the anterior division of the obturator nerve. *3* gracilis. (**b**) Once the pectineus (*1*) and adductor longus (*2*) are separated, the anterior division of the obturator nerve (*arrow*) can be found

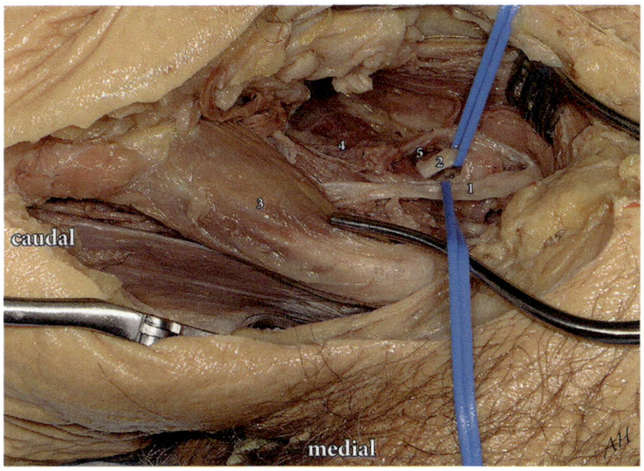

Fig. 30.4 The anterior division of the right obturator nerve (*1*) is observed between the adductor longus (*3*) and adductor brevis (*4*). The posterior division (*2*) is between the adductor brevis (*4*) and adductor magnus (*5*)

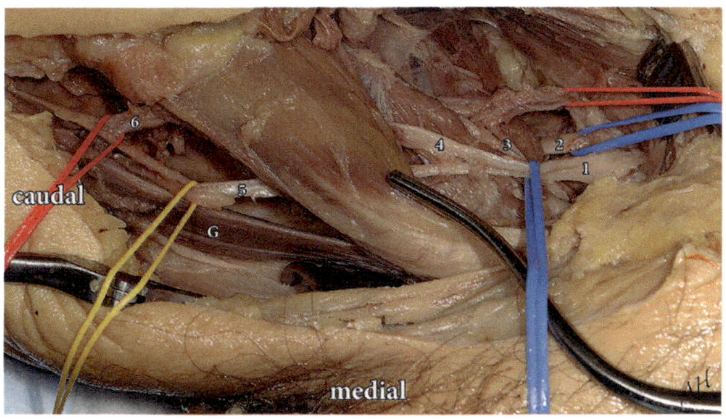

Fig. 30.5 The gracilis (*G*) neurovascular pedicle is dissected. *1* anterior division, *2* posterior division of the obturator nerve. Branches of the anterior division: *3* to adductor brevis, *4* to adductor longus, and *5* to gracilis. *6* gracilis vascular pedicle

References

1. Doi K, Sakai K, Kuwata N, Ihara K, Kawai S (1995) Double free-muscle transfer to restore prehension following complete brachial plexus avulsion. J Hand Surg Am 20(3):408–414. https://doi.org/10.1016/S0363-5023(05)80097-8
2. Snela S, Rydzak B (2002) The value of the adductor tenotomy with obturator neurectomy in the treatment of the hips at cerebral palsy children. Early clinical and radiological examination results. Orthop Traumatol Rehabil 4(1):11–14
3. Campbell AA, Eckhauser FE, Belzberg A, Campbell JN (2010) Obturator nerve transfer as an option for femoral nerve repair: case report. Neurosurgery 66(6 Suppl Operative):ons375. https://doi.org/10.1227/01.NEU.0000369649.31232.B0
4. Meng D, Zhou J, Lin Y, Xie Z, Chen H, Yu R, Lin H, Hou C (2018) Transfer of obturator nerve for femoral nerve injury: an experiment study in rats. Acta Neurochir (Wien) 160(7):1385–1391. https://doi.org/10.1007/s00701-018-3565-1. Epub 2018 May 28
5. Cao Y, Li Y, Zhang Y, Li S, Jiang J, Gu Y, Xu L (2021) Contralateral obturator nerve transfer for femoral nerve restoration: a case report. Br J Neurosurg 35(1):35–39. https://doi.org/10.1080/02688697.2020.1749983. Epub 2020 Apr 16. PMID: 32297522.
6. Johnston BR, Bazarek S, Sten M, et al (2022) Restoring bladder function using motor and sensory nerve transfers: a cadaveric feasibility study. J Neurosurg Spine 38(2):258–264. https://doi.org/10.3171/2022.8.SPINE22291

Ilioinguinal and Iliohypogastric Nerves

31

Amgad S. Hanna

Surgical Anatomy

The ilioinguinal nerve arises from the ventral ramus of L1, and iliohypogastric from T12 and L1. They emerge from the lateral aspect of the psoas muscle cranial to the lateral femoral cutaneous nerve. They course in the retroperitoneum ventral to quadratus lumborum and then pierce the transversus abdominis at the lateral part of the iliac crest to course between the transversus abdominis and internal oblique muscles. More anteriorly, they pierce the internal oblique to lie between this muscle and the external oblique. The ilioinguinal nerve supplies the skin of the medial groin, medial upper thigh, upper scrotum, and root of penis (mons pubis and labium majus in females) as well as the abdominal wall muscles. The iliohypogastric nerve supplies the area of the abdominal wall cranial to this. There are anatomical variabilities in the size and territory of these two nerves.

Clinical Significance

These two nerves can be injured during hernia repair, whether open or laparoscopic, with or without mesh placement. They can also be injured with lower abdominal incisions for other reasons like Cesarean section or female pelvic pathologies [1]. This may cause severe debilitating pain. If refractory to medical management, proximal neurectomy is a good surgical option [2]. Other percutaneous ablation options include radiofrequency, microwave, or cryoablation [3]. The genitofemoral nerve (L1, L2) is another nerve that can cause groin pain when injured. It is usually difficult to determine which nerve is the culprit in causing groin pain. Diagnostic ultrasound-guided nerve blocks can help differentiate [4] and guide subsequent therapies.

Supplementary Information The online version contains supplementary material available at https://doi.org/10.1007/978-3-031-73931-6_31.

A. S. Hanna (✉)
Department of Neurosurgery, University of Wisconsin School of Medicine and Public Health, Madison, WI, USA

Exposure

1. Position: supine, with or without a hip bump.
2. Ultrasound assistance could be used to find the nerve.
3. Incision should be parallel to and just above the anterior part of the iliac crest. It should extend anteriorly above the inguinal ligament (Fig. 31.1).

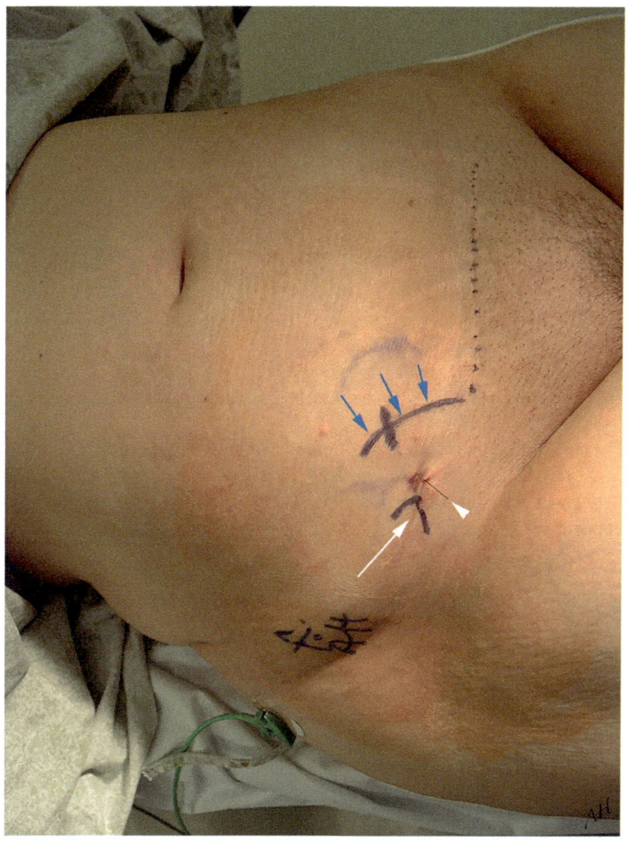

Fig. 31.1 This patient had a painful scar from previous Cesarean section (*dotted line*). She is positioned supine for exposure and transection of the right ilioinguinal nerve. The incision (*blue arrows*) is made parallel to and above the inguinal ligament. *White arrow* anterior superior iliac spine (ASIS), *arrowhead* guidewire placed using preoperative ultrasound for localization

A. S. Hanna (ed.), *Nerves: Anatomy, Exposures, and Techniques*, https://doi.org/10.1007/978-3-031-73931-6_31

4. The superficial fatty layer (Camper's fascia) and deep fibrous layer (Scarpa's fascia) are opened.
5. The external oblique muscle is opened along its fibers. Medially, the nerve can be found between the external and internal oblique muscles (Fig. 31.2).
6. The internal oblique is opened along its fibers. Self-retaining retractors are placed.
7. Laterally, the nerve is found between the internal oblique and the transversus abdominis muscles (Fig. 31.3), coursing parallel to the iliac crest, usually with the deep circumflex iliac vessels.
8. Scar tissue can be released, or a segment of the nerve can be transected, as indicated.
9. Of note, the iliohypogastric nerve can be in close proximity to the ilioinguinal nerve. If transection is planned, both nerves should be targeted.

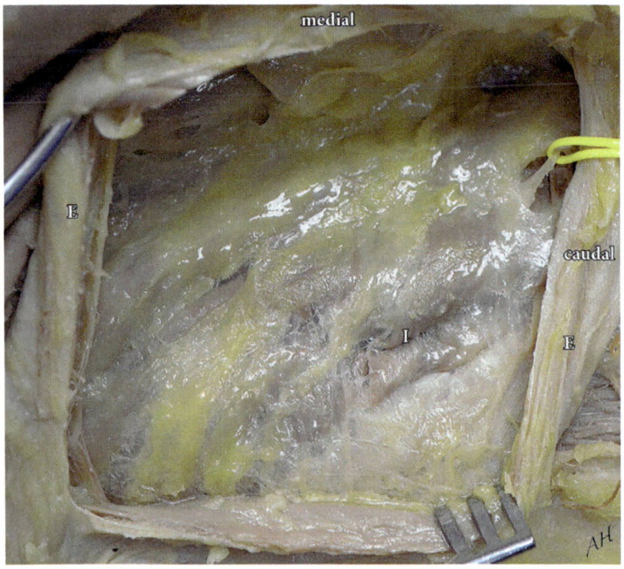

Fig. 31.2 In a cadaveric dissection, the right external oblique aponeurosis (*E*) is opened, revealing the ilioinguinal nerve (*yellow loop*) between it and the internal oblique (*I*) toward the medial part of the exposure

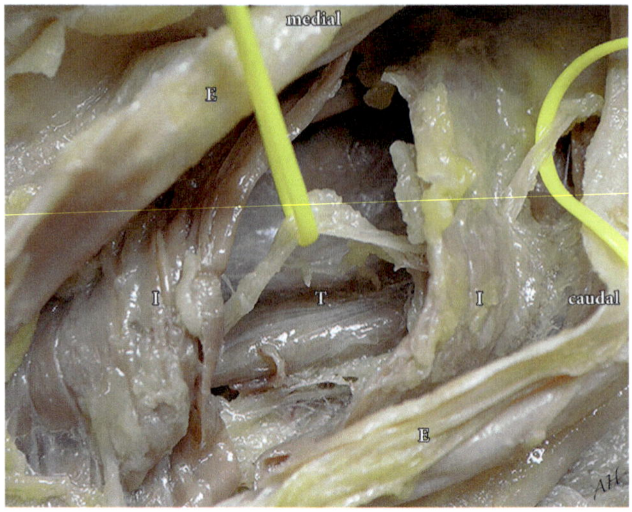

Fig. 31.3 More laterally, the ilioinguinal nerve (*yellow loop*) is found between the internal oblique (*I*) and transversus abdominis muscles (*T*). *E* external oblique

References

1. Stulz P, Pfeiffer KM (1982) Peripheral nerve injuries resulting from common surgical procedures in the lower portion of the abdomen. Arch Surg 117(3):324–327. https://doi.org/10.1001/archsurg.1982.01380270042009
2. Kim DH, Murovic JA, Tiel RL, Kline DG (2005) Surgical management of 33 ilioinguinal and iliohypogastric neuralgias at Louisiana State University Health Sciences Center. Neurosurgery 56(5):1013–1020
3. Daniels SP, Xu HS, Hanna A, Greenberg JA, Lee KS (2021) Ultrasound-guided microwave ablation in the treatment of inguinal neuralgia. Skelet Radiol 50(3):475–483. https://doi.org/10.1007/s00256-020-03618-2. Epub 2020 Sep 30
4. Lee KS, Sin JM, Patil PP, Hanna AS, Greenberg JA, Zea RD et al (2019) Ultrasound-guided microwave ablation for the management of inguinal neuralgia: a preliminary study with 1-year follow-up. J Vasc Interv Radiol 30(2):242–248. https://doi.org/10.1016/j.jvir.2018.10.031

Part V

Surgical Techniques

Nerve Trauma

32

Amgad S. Hanna and Thomas M. Staniszewski

Grading of Nerve Injuries

Seddon's Classification 1942 (Terms by Henry Cohen) [1]

- Neurapraxia: conduction block with minimal anatomical disruption
- Axonotmesis: axonal disruption
- Neurotmesis: complete nerve discontinuity

Sunderland's Classification 1951 [2]

- Grade I: neurapraxia
- Grade II: axonotmesis, nerve sheaths intact
- Grade III: axonotmesis, endoneurial disruption
- Grade IV: axonotmesis, perineurial disruption
- Grade V: neurotmesis

Timing of Nerve Repair

1. Sharp injuries usually result in neurotmesis and require immediate repair.
2. Blunt injuries, such as stretch or compression injuries, as well as civilian gunshot wounds usually result in an incomplete disruption of the nerve. They are either graded as axonotmesis or neurapraxia. These should be treated conservatively for potential spontaneous recovery. Surgery is indicated if they do not recover by 3–6 months.
3. Open crush injuries with damaged nerve endings are tagged initially. Repair is delayed for about 3 weeks. To tag a nerve, use colored nonabsorbable sutures like Prolene or Nylon and hemoclips (radio-opaque) with slight tension to avoid retraction.

Suturing

1. Magnification is recommended using a microscope or loupes.
2. Suture size varies from 5/0 to 9/0 depending on the size of the nerve. Traditionally non-absorbable sutures are used, more recently we showed similar results with monofilament vicryl sutures [3].
3. Avoid tension. To gain length, one may circumferentially dissect the nerve proximally and distally for better mobilization.
4. Minimize manipulation of the fascicles; as much as possible, use fine forceps to hold the nerve sheaths.
5. Trim the nerve endings to see sprouting fascicles, with some bleeding. Frozen section could be used to confirm suturing to viable nerve endings.
6. Use the minimum number of interrupted sutures to coapt the ends, typically two, 180° from each other. Flat (square) knots are preferred, usually three to four knots. The knots are tied tight enough to coapt the ends but not too tight to avoid crushing or misalignment of the nerve endings. Sutures need NOT be watertight.
7. May use a tube wrap and/or fibrin glue to reinforce the suture line.

Supplementary Information The online version contains supplementary material available at https://doi.org/10.1007/978-3-031-73931-6_32.

A. S. Hanna (✉)
Department of Neurosurgery, University of Wisconsin School of Medicine and Public Health, Madison, WI, USA

T. M. Staniszewski
Department of Neurological Surgery, University of Wisconsin School of Medicine and Public Health, Madison, WI, USA
e-mail: staniszewski@neurosurgery.wisc.edu

A. S. Hanna (ed.), *Nerves: Anatomy, Exposures, and Techniques*, https://doi.org/10.1007/978-3-031-73931-6_32

Direct Repair

1. Direct repair should always be attempted as long as it is not done under tension.
2. Limb flexion or shortening can be used on occasions to overcome a gap, with slow progressive extension over time, preferably with ultrasound monitoring.
3. Attempt to match fascicles, by their sizes and/or the vessels in the nerve sheaths.
4. Suture technique described above.

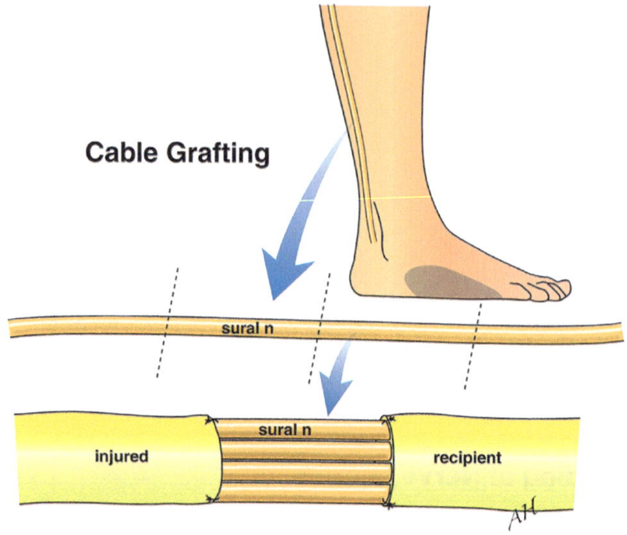

Fig. 32.1 Technique of cable grafting. A donor nerve (*sural n*) is harvested from the outer aspect of the leg anterior to the Achilles tendon. Several segments of nerve are cut (*dashed lines*) to match the length and diameter desired for the injured recipient nerve. This usually results in an area of sensory loss on the outer aspect of the dorsum of the foot (*shaded area*). (Copyright Amgad Hanna, published with permission)

Grafting (Figs. 32.1 and 32.2)

1. If direct repair is not possible, a nerve graft is used to bridge the gap.
2. Donors: autografts—sural nerve (see Chap. 28), superficial radial nerve, or other sensory, and occasionally redundant motor nerves. Allografts are also available.
3. Ensure that the proximal stump is healthy by inspecting it, trimming as needed, and functional by using neuromonitoring with somatosensory-evoked potentials and/or motor-evoked potentials.

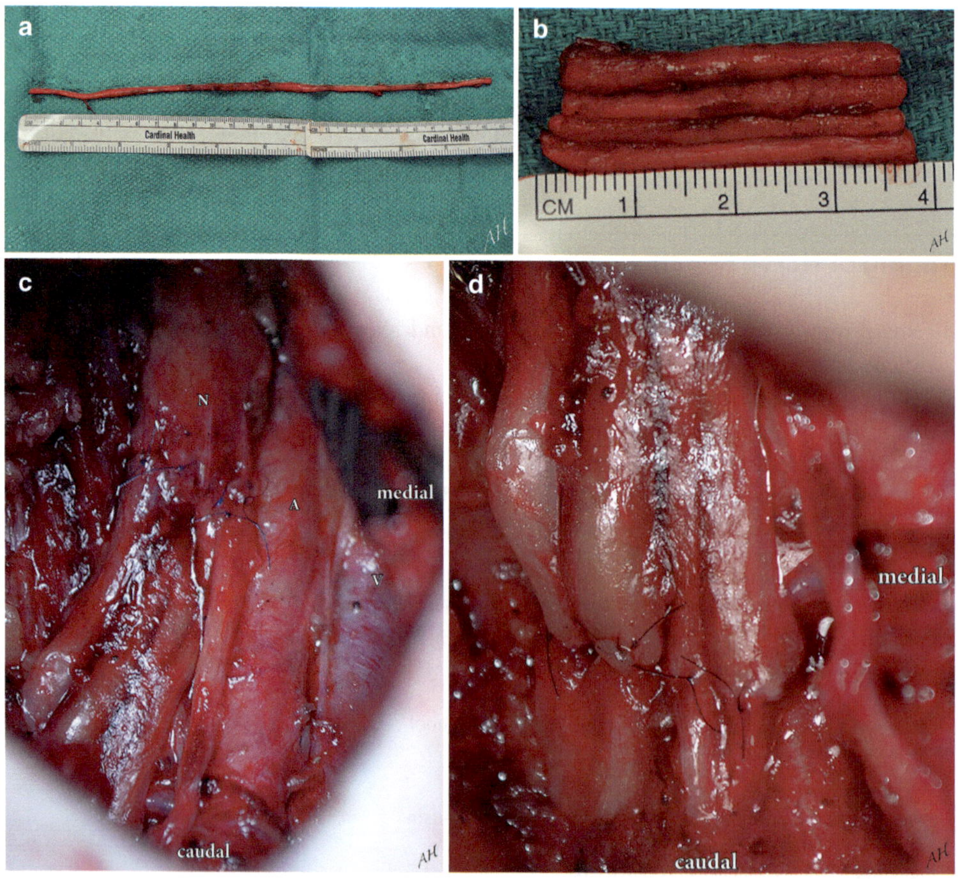

Fig. 32.2 A case of iatrogenic femoral nerve injury repaired acutely. (**a**) Sural nerve harvest. (**b**) Four cables are used to match the size of the femoral nerve. (**c**) Proximal suture line with 5-0 Prolene. *V* femoral vein, *A* femoral artery, *N* femoral nerve, proximal stump. (**d**) Distal suture line

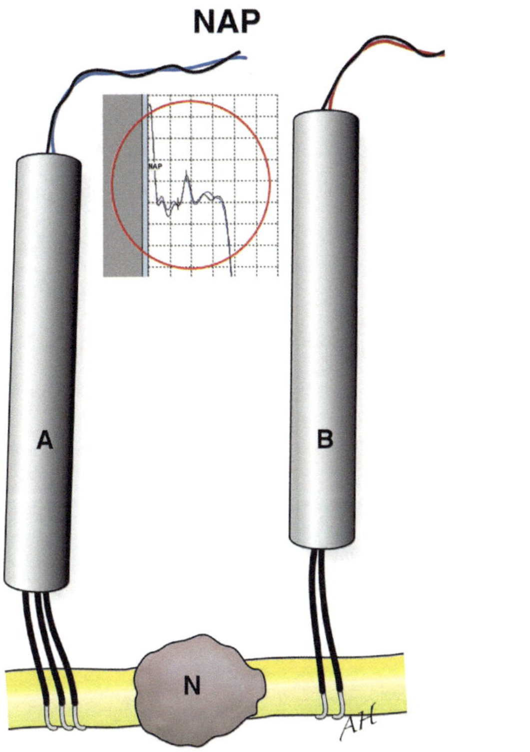

Fig. 32.3 Neuroma in continuity (*N*). This can be tested for nerve action potentials (*NAP*). Stimulating (*A*) and receiving (*B*) electrodes are placed on either side of the neuroma. Graph showing positive NAPs. The presence of NAPs signifies the presence of viable axons through the neuroma. (Copyright Amgad Hanna, published with permission)

4. Suture technique described above.
5. Nerve action potentials (NAPs) can be used to test a neuroma in continuity, intraoperatively, for the presence of functional axons (Fig. 32.3) [4]. Placing a wet sponge in between the two electrodes on the nerve may improve recordings [5].

Nerve Transfers

Nerve transfers: Take a branch or a fascicle from a normal donor nerve to re-innervate a paralyzed muscle (Fig. 32.4). Advantages: short distance to target, exposure away from injured/scarred area, and growing axons have to cross only one suture line. Rarely, if there is a gap between the donor and recipient nerves, an interposition graft can be used, but this lowers the chances of regeneration. In case the recipient nerve has residual function, it is not transected, and the donor nerve is sutured end-to-side, by opening a slit in the epineurium (sometimes also perineurium) of the recipient nerve.

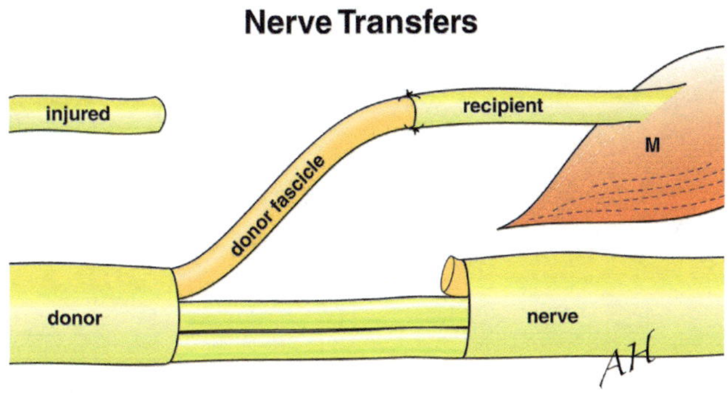

Fig. 32.4 Technique of nerve transfers. A fascicle is selected from a donor nerve and cut distally. The nonfunctional recipient nerve is cut proximally and sutured to the donor fascicle. This technique has the advantage of being close to the target muscle (*M*), away from the zone of injury, and having the regenerating axons cross one suture line only, allowing a shorter recovery time. (Copyright Amgad Hanna, published with permission)

Individual chapters are dedicated to different nerve transfers; here, we describe nerve transfer for elbow flexion and radial to axillary nerve transfer.

Nerve Transfer for Elbow Flexion (Oberlin) (Figs. 32.5 and 32.6) [6]

- The patient is positioned supine with the arm abducted on a hand table. Incision is made in the inner aspect of the arm along the neurovascular bundle.
- The musculocutaneous nerve and its branches are identified between the biceps and brachialis. Single transfer targets the biceps branch, and double transfer targets both biceps and brachialis branches.
- The ulnar nerve can be found posterior to the brachial artery, while the median nerve is anterior to it. Either or both nerves can be used as donors, ulnar typically better tolerated.
- Interfascicular dissection allows identification of fascicles that can be used as donors. Triggered EMG allows selection of fascicles with wrist function rather than hand function. The epineurium is opened using fine forceps and micro-scissors or tenotomy scissors. Careful dissection allows separation of the donor fascicle over a short distance (to avoid disruption of cross-bridging fibers).
- Donors are cut distally and recipients proximally. Coaptation is done under an operating microscope using 9-0 sutures. The suture sites can be reinforced by wrap tubes and/or fibrin glue.

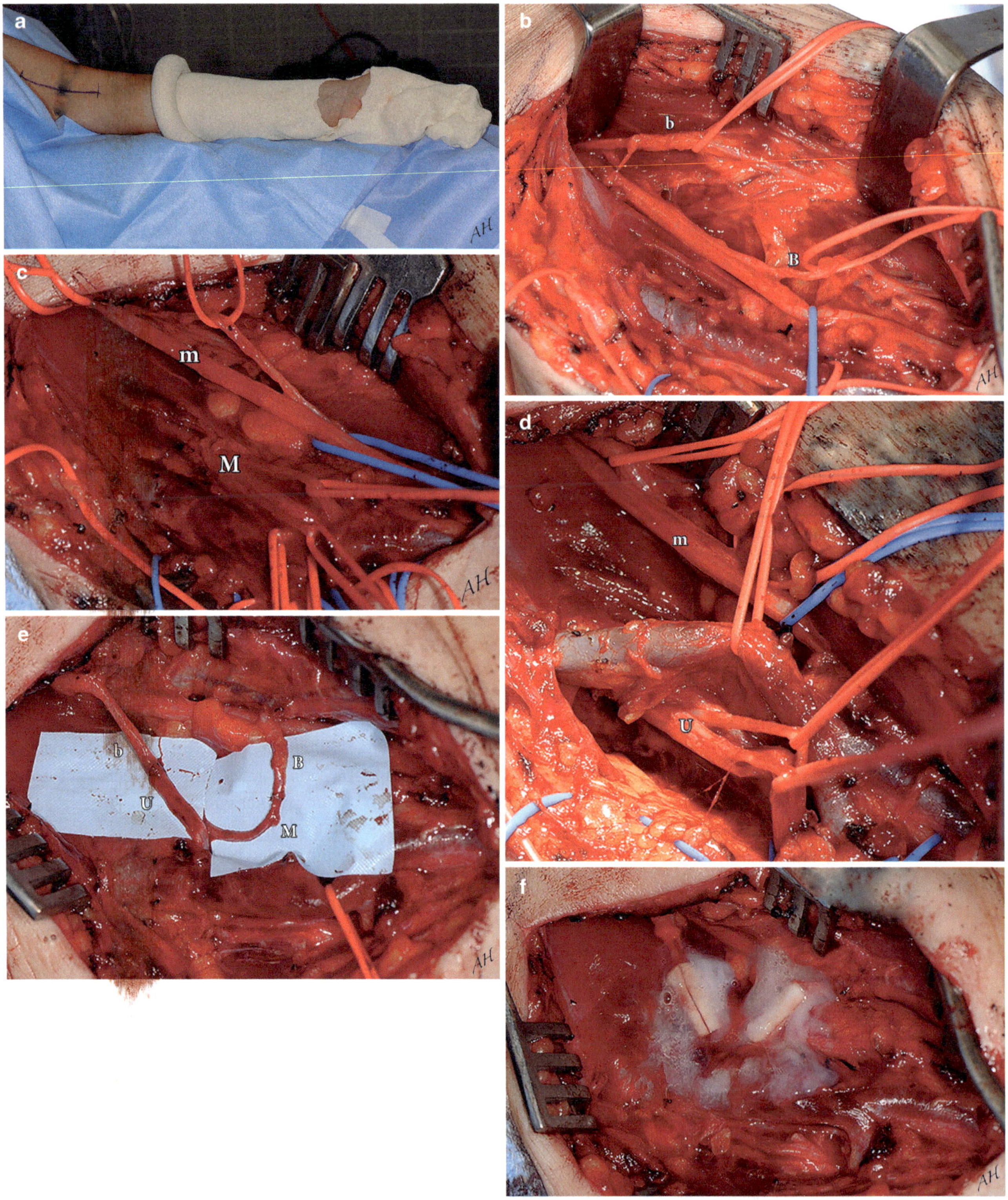

Fig. 32.5 Double fascicular nerve transfer for elbow flexion. (**a**) The patient is positioned supine with the arm abducted. (**b**) The musculocutaneous nerve is exposed with its branches to the biceps brachii (*b*) and brachialis (*B*). These are the targets. (**c**) Interfascicular dissection of the median nerve (*M*) allows identification of fascicles that can be used as donors. Triggered EMG allows the selection of fascicles with wrist function (flexor carpi radialis) rather than hand function. *m* musculocutaneous nerve. (**d**) The process is repeated with the ulnar nerve (*U*), identifying flexor carpi ulnaris branches. *m* musculocutaneous nerve. (**e**) Donors are cut distally and recipients proximally. An ulnar fascicle (*U*) is transferred to the biceps brachii branch (*b*), and a median fascicle (*M*) is transferred to the brachialis branch (*B*). (**f**) The suture sites can be supplemented with wrap tubes and fibrin glue

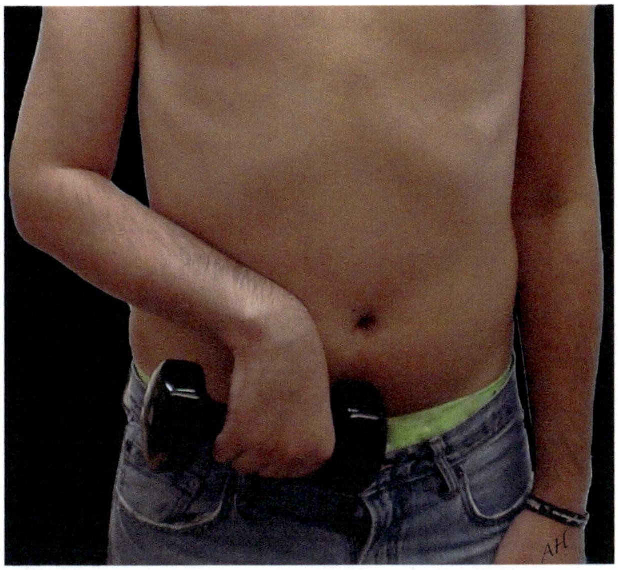

Fig. 32.6 One year after double transfer for elbow flexion, another patient is able to lift 8 pounds. Note that initially flexing the wrist helps with elbow flexion, due to the original function of the donor nerves

Radial to Axillary Nerve Transfer (Somsak) (Leechavengvongs) (Fig. 32.7) [7]

- The patient is positioned supine with a shoulder bump, lateral on a beanbag, or prone, depending on what other procedures are to be performed in the same setting. Incision is made along the posterior border of deltoid and between the long and lateral heads of triceps, in the direction of the olecranon.
- At the posterior border of the deltoid, the cutaneous branch of the axillary nerve (superior lateral brachial cutaneous nerve) can be identified and followed proximally to find the posterior division of the axillary nerve. The deltoid is retracted anteriorly, and the posterior division of the axillary nerve is followed proximally until the main trunk of the axillary nerve is found in the quadrangular space. The anterior division is deep and wraps around the humerus. This is the target.
- There is a white raphe that separates the lateral and long heads of the triceps. These two heads of the triceps are separated, and the radial nerve is found deep in that space.
- The radial nerve can be followed up toward the lower triangular space. In this location, it is separated from the axillary nerve by the teres major tendon.
- Using electrical stimulation, a triceps branch of adequate diameter and length is selected and cut distally to use as a donor. This is then reflected up in a U-turn fashion to meet the axillary nerve. Additional length could be achieved by dissecting the branch from the radial nerve as proximal as possible and occasionally releasing part of the teres major tendon.
- The anterior division of the axillary nerve is cut proximally and sutured to the selected triceps branch.

Tube Repair

Occasionally, for short gaps, especially in digital nerves, a tube is used to bridge the gap. The nerve endings are sutured to the ends of the tube.

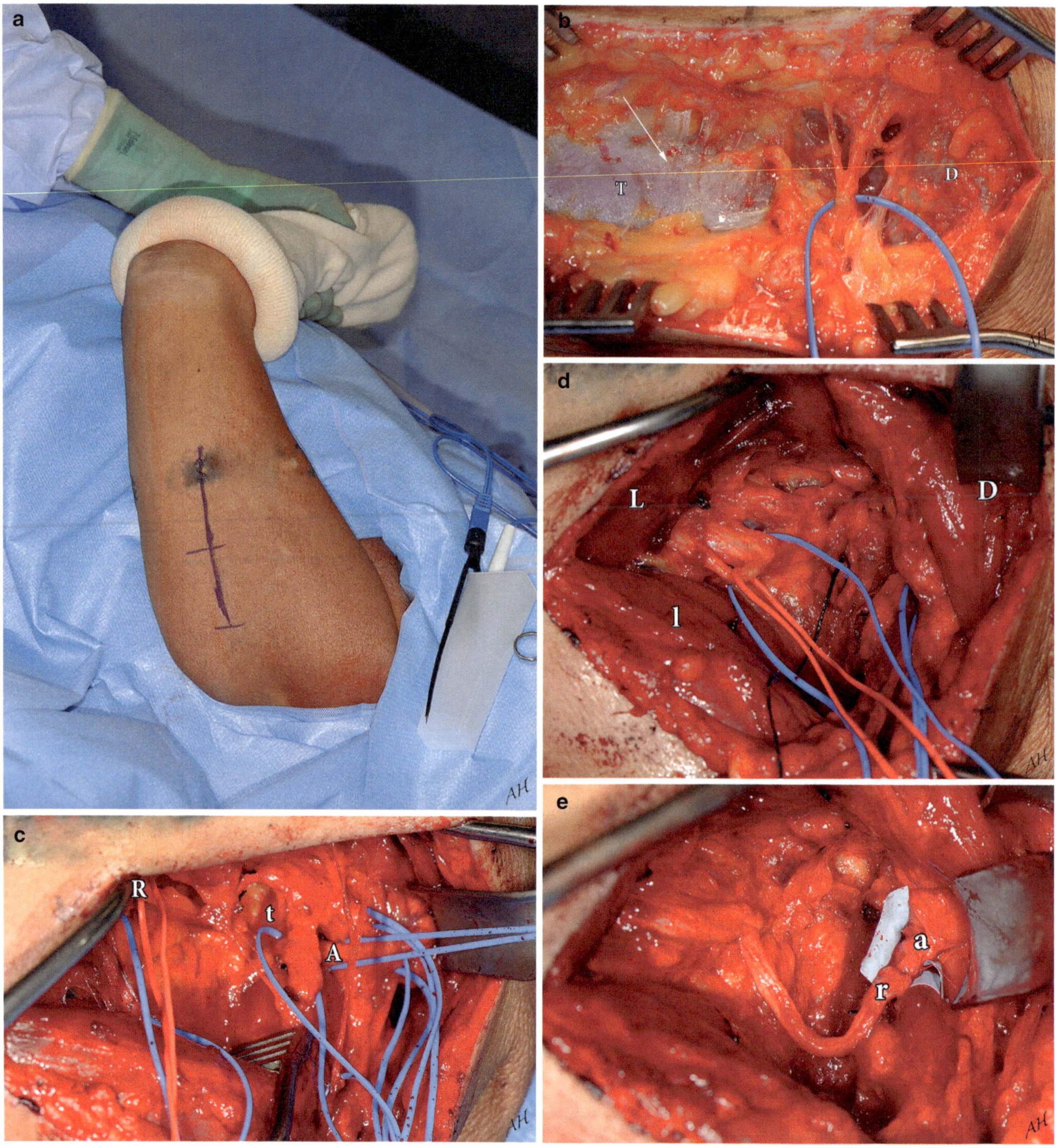

Fig. 32.7 Radial to axillary nerve transfer. (**a**) The patient is positioned supine with a shoulder bump, lateral on a beanbag, or prone. (**b**) At the posterior border of the deltoid (*D*), the cutaneous branch of the axillary nerve (superior lateral brachial cutaneous nerve) can be identified (*blue loop*) and followed proximally to find the posterior division of the axillary nerve. Note the white raphe (*arrow*) between the lateral and long heads of the triceps (*T*). This is the plane of the radial nerve. (**c**) The deltoid is retracted anteriorly, and the axillary nerve (*A*) is found in the quadrangular space. The radial nerve (*R*) is observed more distally in the lower triangular space. The teres major tendon (*t*) separates the two nerves. (**d**) The radial nerve is found between the lateral (*L*) and long (*l*) heads of the triceps. A triceps branch (*red loop*) is selected and cut distally to use as a donor. *D* deltoid. (**e**) The anterior division of the axillary nerve (*a*) is cut proximally and sutured to a triceps branch of the radial nerve (*r*)

References

1. Seddon HJ (1942) A classification of nerve injuries. Br Med J 4260:237–239. https://doi.org/10.1136/bmj.2.4260.237
2. Sunderland S (1951) A classification of peripheral nerve injuries producing loss of function. Brain 74:491–516
3. Hanna AS, Mickelson E, Omar AH, et al (2024) Comparison of nylon, vicryl, and fibrin glue for nerve grafting in rats. Neurol Res 46(10):972–981. https://doi.org/10.1080/01616412.2024.2376307. Epub 2024 Jul 15.
4. Robert EG, Happel LT, Kline DG (2009) Intraoperative nerve action potential recordings: technical considerations, problems, and pitfalls. Neurosurgery 65(4 Suppl):A97–A104. https://doi.org/10.1227/01.NEU.0000347473.67188.75
5. Wu G, Belzberg A, Nance J, Gutierrez-Hernandez S, Ritzl EK, Ringkamp M (2020) Solutions to the technical challenges embedded in the current methods for intraoperative peripheral nerve action potential recordings. J Neurosurg 133:884–893. https://doi.org/10.3171/2019.5.JNS19146. Epub 2019 Aug 16.
6. Oberlin C, Béal D, Leechavengvongs S, Salon A, Dauge MC, Sarcy JJ (1994) Nerve transfer to biceps muscle using a part of ulnar nerve for C5-C6 avulsion of the brachial plexus: Anatomical study and report of four cases. J Hand Surg Am 19A(2):232–237. https://doi.org/10.1016/0363-5023(94)90011-6
7. Leechavengvongs S, Witoonchart K, Uerpairojkit C, Thuvasethakul P (2003) Nerve transfer to deltoid muscle using the nerve to the long head of the triceps, part II: a report of 7 cases. J Hand Surg Am 28(4):633–638. https://doi.org/10.1016/s0363-5023(03)00199-0

Neonatal Obstetrical Brachial Plexus Injury

33

Lars W. Meisner, Joyce A. Koueik, Michael L. Bentz, and Bermans J. Iskandar

Diagnosis

Neonatal obstetrical brachial plexus injuries (OBPI) occur in 0.4–4 per 1000 births and are caused by separation of the neck and shoulder during birth, often in association with shoulder dystocia or macrosomia. An infant with an OBPI can present with paralysis or weakness of the arm, forearm, and/or hand muscles. Most OBPI involve the upper plexus, or Erb-Duchenne, in which injury occurs to the C5 and C6 nerves/upper trunk in which the arm is positioned in an extended, adducted, and internally rotated position. However, the injury may also extend to C7/middle trunk, C8, and T1/lower trunk, leading to a complete or near-complete brachial plexopathy and a flail arm. Early diagnosis and management can significantly improve outcomes.

Supplementary Information The online version contains supplementary material available at https://doi.org/10.1007/978-3-031-73931-6_33.

L. W. Meisner · J. A. Koueik
Department of Neurological Surgery, University of Wisconsin Hospitals and Clinics, Madison, Wisconsin, USA
e-mail: meisner@neurosurgery.wisc.edu; koueik@neurosurgery.wisc.edu

M. L. Bentz
Division of Plastic and Reconstructive Surgery, Department of Surgery, University of Wisconsin-Madison, Madison, WI, USA
e-mail: bentz@surgery.wisc.edu

B. J. Iskandar (✉)
Department of Neurosurgery, University of Wisconsin Hospitals and Clinics, Madison, WI, USA
e-mail: iskandar@neurosurgery.wisc.edu

Type of Repair and Surgical Technique

The primary goal of surgical intervention is reinnervation of shoulder abduction and elbow flexion. Less commonly, reinnervation to restore hand function is pursued. The type of reinnervation depends on the severity and location of the neuroma:

- The more common *upper plexus injury* with intact lower plexus is treated with nerve transfers from within the plexus (e.g., medial pectoral nerve, ulnar nerve, median nerve, and/or radial nerve).
- A *complete plexus injury* with no functional nerves requires reaching for donor nerves outside the brachial plexus (e.g., spinal accessory nerve, C4 nerve root, phrenic nerve, intercostal nerves, and/or contralateral C7).

There is still a role for exploring the zone of injury and attempting graft repair, especially in postganglionic (nonavulsion) injuries. This can improve function but may also help with pain by resecting the neuroma. In recent years and in many centers, nerve grafting and repair at the level of the neuroma have been replaced by distal nerve transfers, in which fascicles from neighboring functional nerves (e.g., ulnar nerve) are used to innervate dysfunctional nerves (e.g., musculocutaneous nerve). Advantages of distal nerve transfers include

- A shorter distance for axons to grow between the end of the donor nerve (or transfer site), and the target muscle presumably leads to faster recovery and decreased risk of muscle atrophy.
- Surgery on intact distal nerves in the arm instead of that at the level of the injury is simpler, as it avoids a complex neuroma with abnormal anatomy (Table 33.1).

A popular repair technique with excellent functional outcomes to restore shoulder abduction in an upper plexopathy is the double nerve transfer, in which the spinal accessory

A. S. Hanna (ed.), *Nerves: Anatomy, Exposures, and Techniques*, https://doi.org/10.1007/978-3-031-73931-6_33

Table 33.1 Surgical methods to reinnervate shoulder abduction and elbow flexion after an OBPI

Nerve transfer techniques	Functional deficit correction
Complete plexopathy	
Spinal accessory nerve to suprascapular nerve	Shoulder abduction and external rotation
Intercostal nerves to musculocutaneous nerve	Elbow flexion
Phrenic nerve to musculocutaneous nerve	Elbow flexion
Contralateral C7	Multiple targets (upper or lower trunk)
Upper plexopathy	
Any of the above, and/or	
Medial head of the triceps branch of the radial nerve to axillary nerve	Shoulder abduction
Medial pectoral nerve to the musculocutaneous nerve	Elbow flexion
Ulnar and/or median nerve fascicle transfer to musculocutaneous nerve	Elbow flexion

nerve is used to reinnervate the suprascapular nerve, and the medial head of triceps branch of the radial nerve is used to reinnervate the axillary nerve [1]. A useful technique to restore elbow flexion in an upper plexopathy is the double fascicular nerve transfer, in which an ulnar nerve fascicle is used to reinnervate the biceps branch of the musculocutaneous nerve, and a median nerve fascicle is used to reinnervate the brachialis branch of musculocutaneous nerve; however, some authors have reported that a single transfer is just as good as a double transfer. The representative surgical technique illustrated in this chapter is the posterior spinal accessory to suprascapular nerve transfer. Other transfers are addressed in other chapters.

Prognosis and Timing of Repair

Prognosis is estimated using various grading systems [2], all of which show that the probability of *spontaneous recovery* exceeds 90% in lower grade injuries and falls below 40% in higher grade injuries. When spontaneous recovery does not occur or is insufficient, surgery is offered. *Surgical success* ranges from 76 to 88%, depending mainly on the type and location of injury and the timing of repair [3].

The type of injury (i.e., avulsion vs. stretch, complete vs. partial) is important for both prognosis and the timing of repair.

- *A total plexopathy* associated with Horner's syndrome and scapular winging indicating nerve root avulsion will not recover spontaneously and should be repaired early (i.e., within weeks instead of months). Although it is generally acknowledged that the severity of a complete injury and the need to reach outside the brachial plexus for donor nerves lead to poorer outcomes than a partial injury, the results are nonetheless favorable [4].
- *A partial plexopathy* portends a better functional outcome long-term than a complete plexopathy. In addition, most agree that the absence of spontaneous recovery of anti-gravity function in shoulder abduction and elbow flexion within 3–6 months of the injury prompts surgical repair because the longer the muscles and neuromuscular junctions are inactive, the more atrophy sets in, which leads to less favorable functional outcomes [5]. More specifically, biceps brachii function is an excellent indicator of recovery because its function cannot be duplicated by other muscles. However, owing to the lack of rigorous comparative studies, the exact timing of surgery within 6 months post-injury (post-delivery) is controversial. While many centers, including ours, offer surgery at 6 months post-injury based on the data that further spontaneous recovery can occur in the 4th and 5th month, others advise surgery at 3 months post-injury based on improved results reported by small studies [6].

Finally, if repair is delayed, or if there is residual long-term functional limitation despite nerve transfer, function can be further improved years later using a variety of *orthopedic techniques* including tenodesis, capsulodesis, osteotomy, arthrodesis, and occasionally, microsurgical free tissue transfer [7].

Spinal Accessory to Suprascapular Nerve Transfer Via Posterior Approach

1. Position is prone with arms adducted. The acromion and dorsal midline are marked, and a line is drawn along the superior scapular border between the two marks. The spinal accessory nerve is located approximately 40% of the distance from midline to acromion along this line, approximately at the superior angle of the scapula. The suprascapular nerve is located in the suprascapular notch, found halfway between the superior angle of the scapula and the acromion (Fig. 33.1). This point also corresponds to the medial aspect of the coracoid process anteriorly.

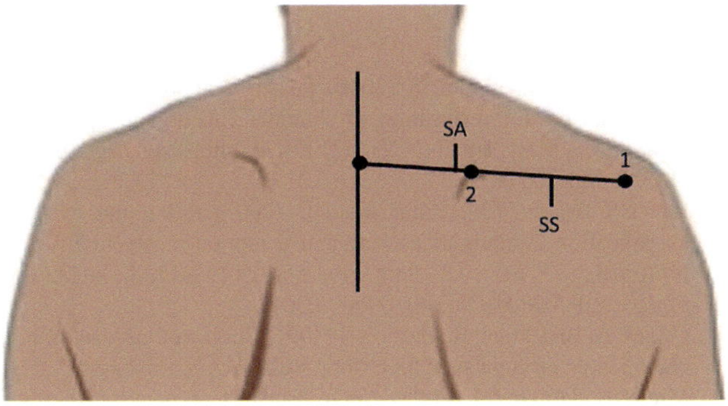

Fig. 33.1 The distal spinal accessory nerve (*SA*) is found 40% of the distance from the dorsal midline to the acromion (*1*) along the superior scapular border. Halfway between to superior scapular angle (*2*) and the acromion is the suprascapular notch (*SS*), in which the suprascapular nerve is located

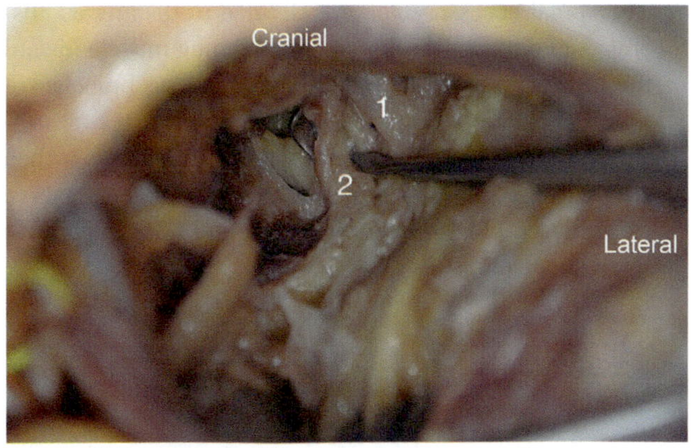

Fig. 33.3 The suprascapular artery (*1*) is typically superficial to the suprascapular ligament (*2*). The surgical tool is within the suprascapular notch with the nerve deep to it

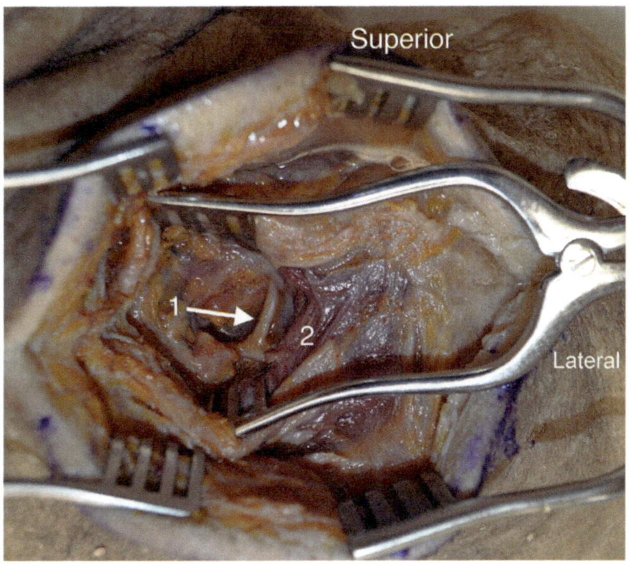

Fig. 33.2 Cadaver dissection showing the distal spinal accessory nerve (*1*), which is found entering the deep surface of the trapezius (*2*) and running in a superolateral to inferomedial direction

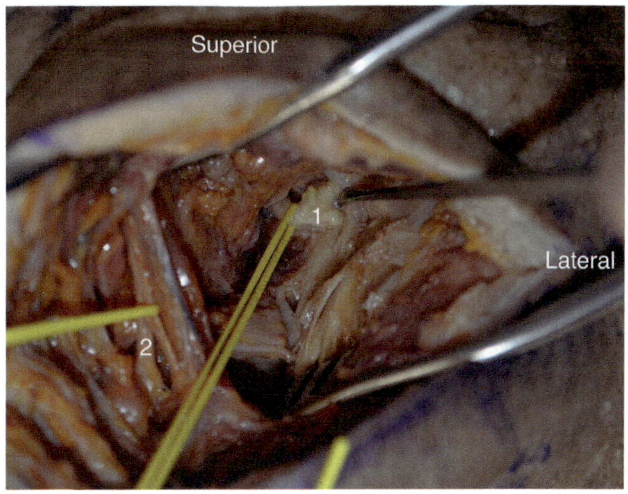

Fig. 33.4 The suprascapular nerve (*1*), seen only after sharp dissection of the overlying ligament, runs within the suprascapular notch. Between the spinal accessory nerve (*2*) and the suprascapular nerve is an intervening band of trapezius muscle and small vessels

2. A horizontal incision along the line described above is made encompassing the expected locations of the spinal accessory and suprascapular nerves.
3. The fibers of the trapezius are separated parallel to their course. The spinal accessory nerve is found running in a superolateral to inferomedial direction as it enters the deep surface of the trapezius muscle (Fig. 33.2). Surrounded by adipose tissue, the nerve is the easiest to locate with the aid of a nerve stimulator. Of note, there is a fascial layer separating the trapezius from its nerve supply; therefore it is advisable to stimulate through the fascia to open it in the correct place.
4. The superior border of the scapula is palpated, and the dissection is carried through or above the supraspinatus muscle, taking care to avoid injury to the suprascapular artery, which typically courses superficial to the ligament forming the roof of the scapular notch (Fig. 33.3). In difficult dissections, a Doppler probe can be used to locate the suprascapular artery, which is a good landmark for the ligament and the nerve deep to it.
5. The ligament and notch are palpated and exposed bluntly prior to the sharp division of the ligament. The ligament feels softer to palpation than the hard bony upper border of the scapula. Once the ligament is divided, the suprascapular nerve is identified as it passes through the suprascapular notch (Fig. 33.4).
6. The suprascapular nerve is dissected as proximally as possible and divided to reduce tension on the transfer.

7. The spinal accessory nerve is divided as distally as possible and tunneled through the intervening muscle toward the suprascapular nerve. Additional trapezius branches of the spinal accessory nerve are left undisrupted.
8. The proximal end of the spinal accessory nerve is then sutured to the distal segment of the suprascapular nerve using interrupted 9-0 nylon with the aid of the operative microscope (Fig. 33.5).

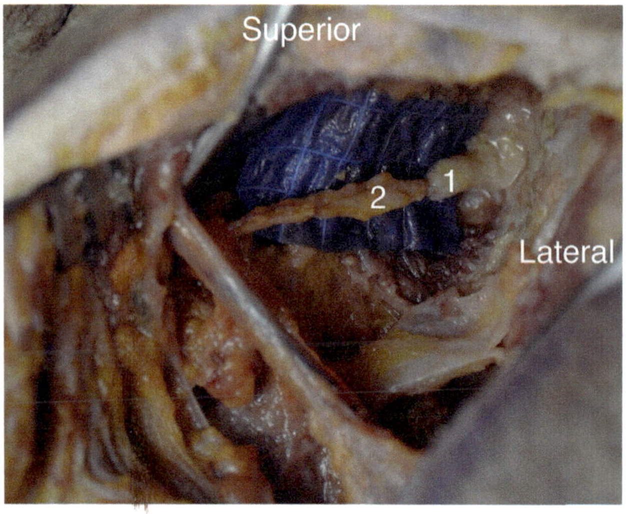

Fig. 33.5 The suprascapular nerve (*1*) is dissected and divided as proximally as possible, while the spinal accessory nerve (*2*) is dissected as distally as possible, divided, and tunneled under the intervening band of muscles and vessels. The nerves are sutured with 9-0 nylon under the operative microscope

References

1. Colbert SH, Mackinnon S (2006) Posterior approach for double nerve transfer for restoration of shoulder function in upper brachial plexus palsy. Hand (N Y) 1(2):71–77. https://doi.org/10.1007/s11552-006-9004-4
2. Bae DS, Waters PM, Zurakowski D (2003) Reliability of three classification systems measuring active motion in brachial plexus birth palsy. J Bone Jt Surg Am 85(9):1733–1738. https://doi.org/10.2106/00004623-200309000-00012
3. Gilbert A, Brockman R, Carlioz H (1991) Surgical treatment of brachial plexus birth palsy. Clin Orthop Relat Res 264:39–47
4. Midha R, Drake JM (2005) Nerve transfers in severe obstetrical brachial plexus palsy. Semin Plast Surg 19(1):75–85. https://doi.org/10.1055/s-2005-867114
5. Smith BW, Daunter AK, Yang LJ, Wilson TJ (2018) An update on the management of neonatal brachial plexus palsy-replacing old paradigms: a review. JAMA Pediatr 172(6):585–591. https://doi.org/10.1001/jamapediatrics.2018.0124
6. Pondaag W, Malessy MJ (2014) The evidence for nerve repair in obstetric brachial plexus palsy revisited. Biomed Res Int 2014:434619. https://doi.org/10.1155/2014/434619. Epub 2014 Jan 16
7. Vekris MD, Lykissas MG, Beris AE, Manoudis G, Vekris AD, Soucacos PN (2008) Management of obstetrical brachial plexus palsy with early plexus microreconstruction and late muscle transfers. Microsurgery 28(4):252–261. https://doi.org/10.1002/micr.20493

End-to-Side Neurorrhaphy

34

Fausto Viterbo, Balduino F. M. Neto, and Lucas V. Magnani

Introduction

The treatment of nerve injuries involves, among other treatments, the use of nerve grafts. Classically, end-to-end neurorrhaphy with or without grafts seemed to be the most acceptable option. However, this type of suture often causes damage to the donor nerve, since it needs to be sectioned, which may sacrifice its motor and/or sensory function.

To avoid this, Viterbo et al. [1–3], created the end-to-side neurorrhaphy without sectioning any part of the donor nerve, demonstrated the growth of axons, and opened new possibilities for treating nerve injuries.

Tips

Although its objective is not to harm the donor nerve axons, like all nerve surgery we can have neurapraxia which generates a physiological and not anatomical loss of function.

In nerves smaller than 1.5 mm, there is no need to remove the epineurium. In larger nerves, such as the femoral nerve used in penile reinnervation surgery (see Chap. 59) [4], the epineurium and perineurium are thicker; therefore, we must remove the epineurium and perineurium windows before coaptation. In these cases, there may be temporary damage to the donor nerve, compromising sensory and/or motor functions, for about 3–6 months.

F. Viterbo (✉)
Plastic Surgery, University of the State of São Paulo (UNESP), São Paulo, Brazil
e-mail: fv@faustoviterbo.com.br

B. F. M. Neto
Botucatu School of Medicine, HC-FMB, UNESP, São Paulo, Brazil

L. V. Magnani
School of Medicine of Botucatu, São Paulo State University, UNESP, São Paulo, Brazil
e-mail: lucas.v.magnani@unesp.br

With the end-to-side technique, as opposed to end-to-end neurorrhaphy, pressure on the suture is welcome, and there must be compression of the receptor nerve on the axon of the donor nerve, as observed in experimental studies [5].

Surgical Techniques

In the experience of the senior author, several ways are accepted in the execution of end-to-side neurorrhaphy. These include the following.

Direct Suture with the Epineurium Window (Fig. 34.1)

This technique is performed with at least four cardinal suture points, being especially useful for nerves with a caliber greater than 1.5 mm [6].

Direct Suturing Without the Epineurium Window (Figs. 34.2 and 34.3)

This is performed with at least two suture points; eventually, one or more sutures can be added to obtain a tight coaptation in nerves smaller than 1.5 mm and in deeper locations.

Embracing Technique [5] (Figs. 34.4 and 34.5)

In this technique, the distal stump of the recipient nerve is placed close to the donor nerve, and the suture needle passes in the receptor nerve, apprehending its epineurium and perineurium. Then, the suture thread passes under the donor nerve, surrounding it, and the needle will grasp the point that would correspond to 180° in relation to the first needle entrance in the distal stump of the recipient nerve, also grasp-

A. S. Hanna (ed.), *Nerves: Anatomy, Exposures, and Techniques*, https://doi.org/10.1007/978-3-031-73931-6_34

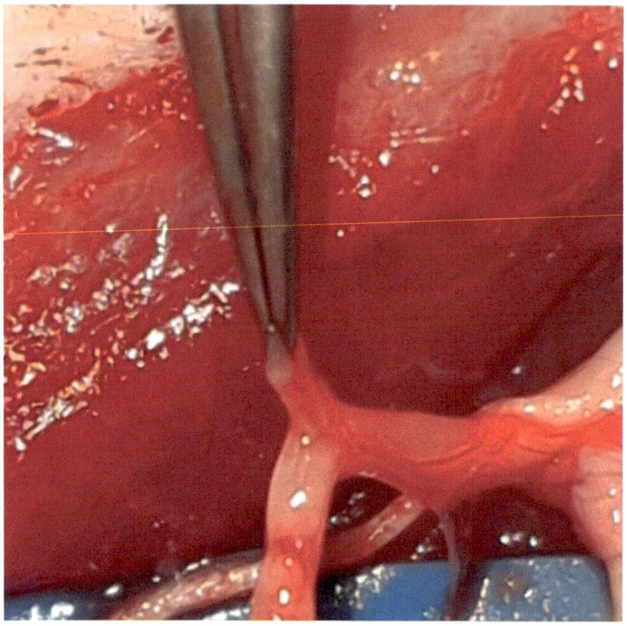

Fig. 34.1 Epineurium window performed in the tibial nerve in rat

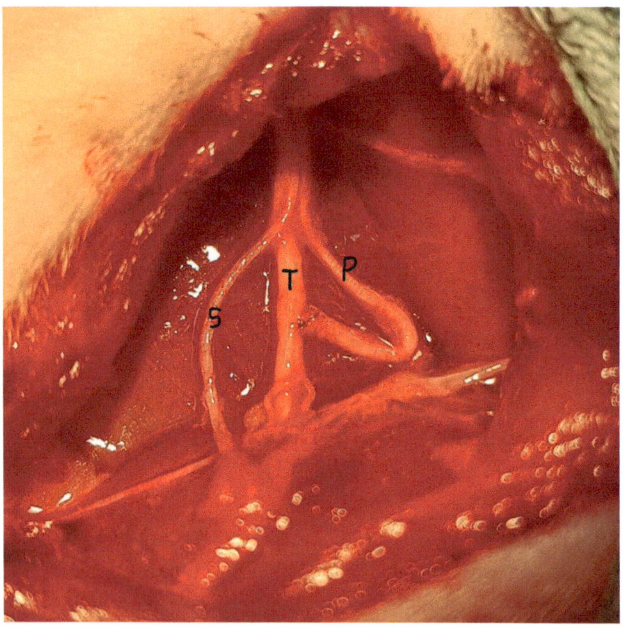

Fig. 34.2 End-to-side neurorrhaphy without epineurium window performed between the common peroneal (*P*) and the tibial (*T*) nerves in rat. *S* sural nerve

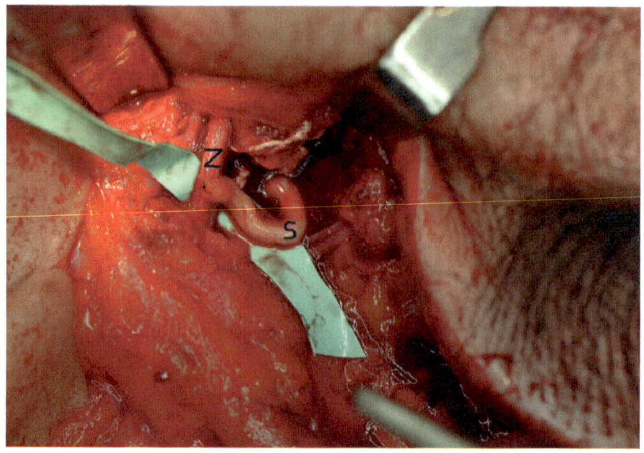

Fig. 34.3 End-to-side neurorrhaphy without epineurium window performed between a sural nerve graft (*S*) and the zygomatic branch (*Z*) of the facial nerve in a patient

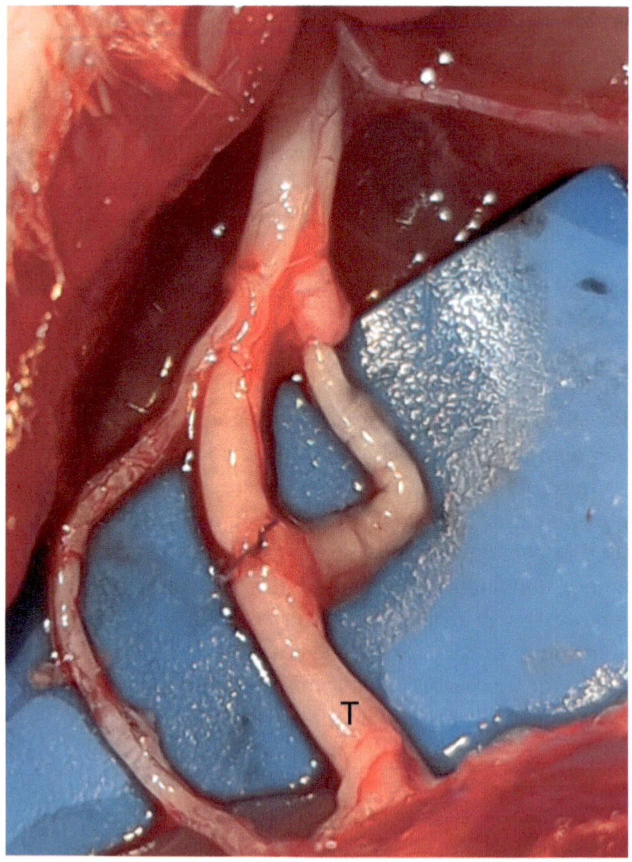

Fig. 34.4 Embracing neurorrhaphy performed between the common peroneal and the tibial (*T*) nerve in rat

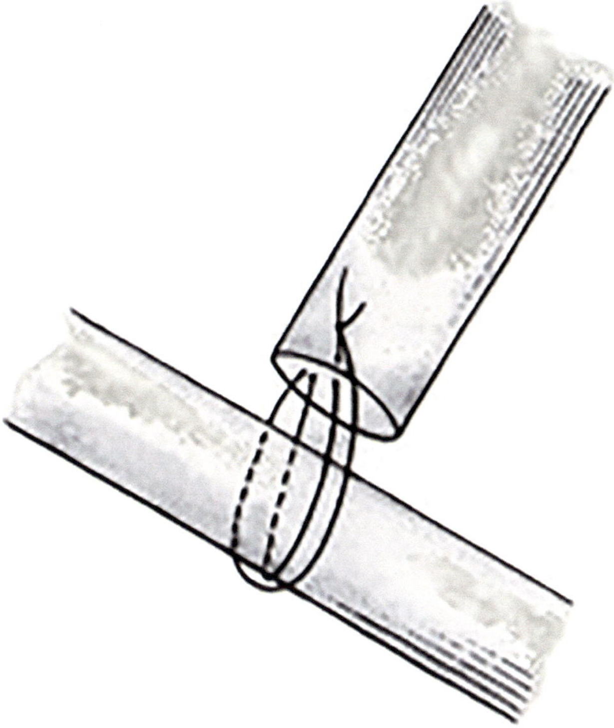

Fig. 34.5 Schematic representation of embracing neurorrhaphy

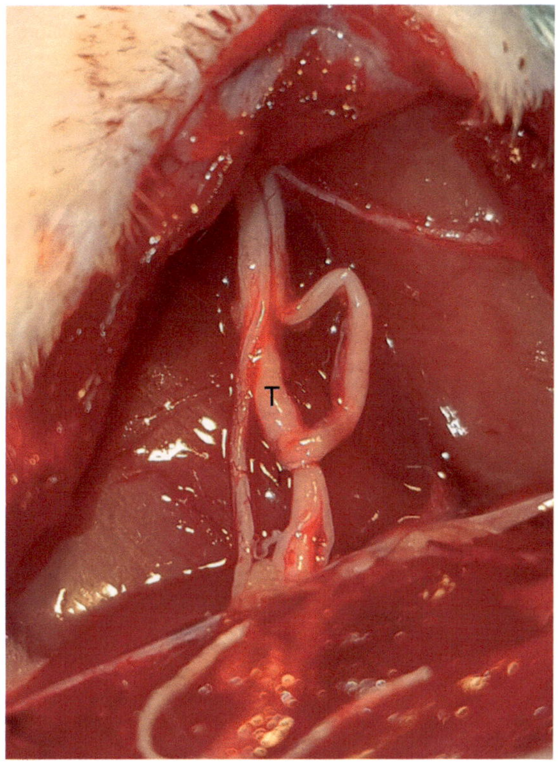

Fig. 34.6 Onlay suturing technique performed between the common peroneal and the tibial (*T*) nerve in rat

ing the epineurium and perineurium. The stitch contours the donor nerve again, returning to the stitch initially passed, to be finally tied off. This causes an approximation of the distal stump of the receptor nerve with a little pressure. There is no damage to the donor nerve. It is essential to seek a firm contact pressure between the nerves but not so strong as to cause a stenosis on the donor nerve. It is especially useful for small nerves (<1.5 mm) and hard-to-reach places.

Onlay Suturing Technique (Fig. 34.6)

This is especially useful for small nerves, where it is difficult to apply sutures directly to the donor nerve. The suture is applied on two opposite sides of the recipient nerve, directly into the tissue below, and surrounding the donor nerve, paying attention to the fact that there must be tight contact under pressure between the two nerves.

References

1. Viterbo F, Trindade JC, Hoshino K, Mazzoni A (1994) Two end-to-side neurorrhaphies and nerve graft with removal of the epineural sheath: experimental study in rats. Br J Plast Surg 47(2):75–80
2. Viterbo F, Teixeira E, Hoshino K, Padovani CR (1998) End-to-side neurorrhaphy with and without perineurium. Sao Paulo Med J (Revista Paulista de Medicina) 116(5):1808–1814
3. Viterbo F, Trindade JC, Hoshino K, Mazzoni NA (1992) Latero-terminal neurorrhaphy without removal of the epineural sheath. Experimental study in rats. Revista Paulista de Medicina 110(6):267–275
4. Souza Trindade JC, Viterbo F, Petean Trindade A, Fávaro WJ, Trindade-Filho JCS (2017) Long-term follow-up of treatment of erectile dysfunction after radical prostatectomy using nerve grafts and end-to-side somatic-autonomic neurorraphy: a new technique. BJU Int 119(6):948–954
5. Viterbo F, Salvio AG, Griva BL, Maciel FO (2012) The embracing end-to-side neurorrhaphy in rats. Acta Cirurgica Brasileira 27(3):260–265
6. Viterbo F, Trindade JC, Hoshimo K, Mazzoni NA (1994) End-to-side neurorrhaphy with removal of epineural sheath: an experimental study in rats. Plast Reconstr Surg 94(7):1038–1047. https://doi.org/10.1097/00006534-199412000-00019

Radial Nerve Motor Branch to Anterior Interosseous Nerve Transfer

35

Lars W. Meisner, Daniel J. Burkett, Shady Elmaraghi, Brian H. Gander, and Amgad S. Hanna

Indications

Etiologies of anterior interosseous nerve (AIN) palsy include fracture to the humerus, radius, or ulna, lacerations, penetrating injuries, or neuralgic amyotrophy (Parsonage–Turner syndrome). Patients present with difficulty grasping small objects between the thumb and index finger. Isolated AIN injuries do not present with associated cutaneous sensory loss. Physical examination will reveal inability to flex at the interphalangeal joint of the thumb (flexor pollicis longus [FPL] palsy) and distal interphalangeal joints of index and sometimes middle finger (lateral half of flexor digitorum profundus [FDP] palsy). The "pinch grip" test can be utilized to evaluate for AIN palsy. As the patient attempts to forcefully pinch the tips of the thumb and index finger into an OK sign (Fig. 35.1a), the pulps touch rather than the tips (Fig. 35.1b).

Electrodiagnostic studies can also be useful, primarily assessing the FPL and pronator quadratus (PQ) functions since FDP receives dual innervation with the ulnar nerve. Imaging using MRI or high-resolution ultrasound is recommended. If no cause is identified or in blunt injuries, expectant management is appropriate for 8–12 weeks. Inflammatory conditions could resolve spontaneously with time. If weakness persists, surgical management is indicated. This can vary from simple nerve decompression to interfascicular decompression, to nerve transfer. In this chapter, we describe nerve transfer from extensor carpi radialis brevis (ECRB) to AIN [1, 2]. Cases that present late or fail nerve transfer can be considered for tendon transfers (Chap. 43) [3].

Supplementary Information The online version contains supplementary material available at https://doi.org/10.1007/978-3-031-73931-6_35.

L. W. Meisner · A. S. Hanna (✉)
Department of Neurosurgery, University of Wisconsin School of Medicine and Public Health, Madison, WI, USA

D. J. Burkett
Department of Neurosurgery, SSM Health—Dean Medical Group, Madison, WI, USA
e-mail: daniel.burkett@ssmhealth.com

S. Elmaraghi
Department of Plastic Surgery, Vanderbilt Health, Nashville, TN, USA
e-mail: shady.elmaraghi@outlook.com

B. H. Gander
Division of Plastic and Reconstructive Surgery, Department of Surgery, University of Wisconsin Hospitals and Clinics, Madison, WI, USA
e-mail: gander@surgery.wisc.edu

A. S. Hanna (ed.), *Nerves: Anatomy, Exposures, and Techniques*, https://doi.org/10.1007/978-3-031-73931-6_35

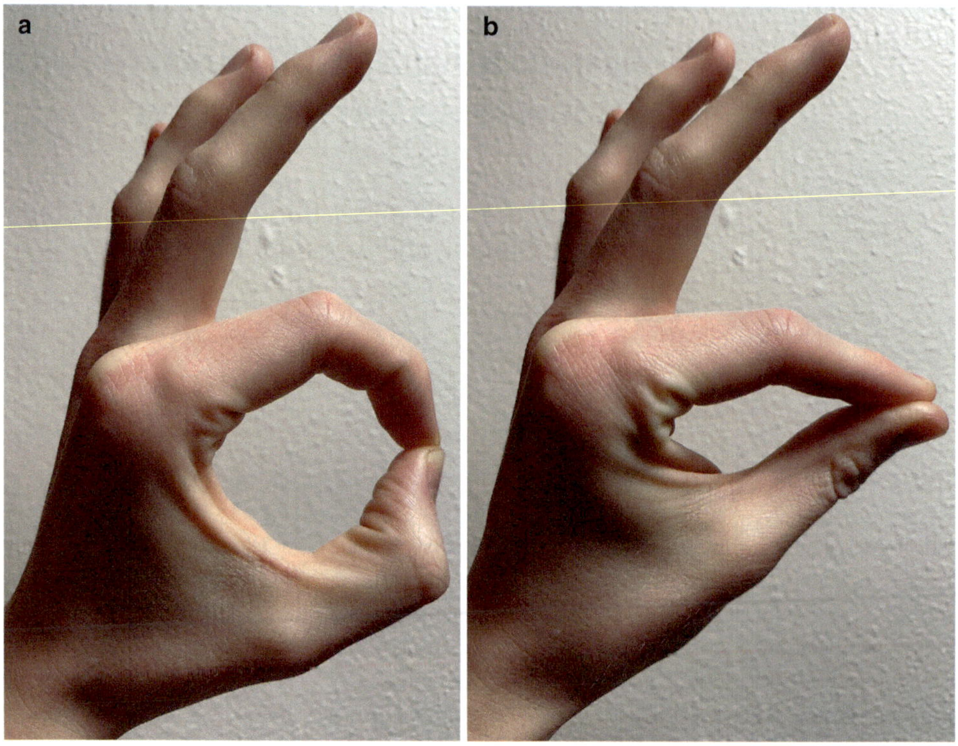

Fig. 35.1 "Pinch sign"; the subject attempts to forcefully pinch the tips of the thumb and index finger into an OK sign (**a**); in cases of AIN palsy, the pulps touch rather than the tips (**b**)

Surgical Technique

1. Position: supine, with the arm extended on an arm board with a tourniquet.
2. Incision: "Lazy-S" just distal to the elbow crease in the forearm (Fig. 35.2a).
3. Using a combination of blunt dissection and electrocautery, the lateral antebrachial cutaneous nerve and the cephalic vein are identified (Fig. 35.2b).
4. Dissection is carried down to the bicipital aponeurosis (lacertus fibrosus), which is then divided to identify the median nerve and brachial artery (Fig. 35.3a).
5. The dissection is continued distally between the two heads of the pronator teres to identify the AIN, which runs deeply and radially from the median nerve (Fig. 35.3b). Lack of recovery should be confirmed by the absence of response on intraoperative stimulation.
6. The radial nerve is then explored laterally. The radial vessels are retracted medially, and the vascular perforators are carefully cauterized or clipped/ligated and cut.

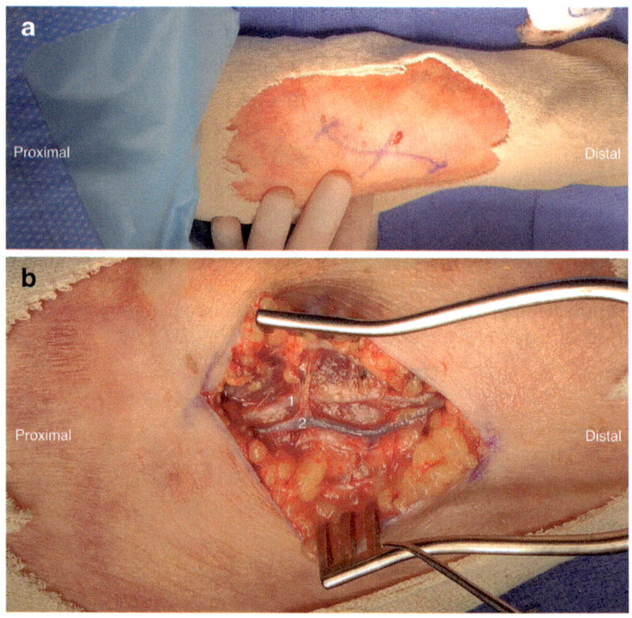

Fig. 35.2 (**a**) The patient is positioned supine, with the left arm extended on an arm board. A "Lazy-S" incision is made just distal to the elbow crease in the forearm. (**b**) The dissection is carried down to identify the lateral antebrachial cutaneous nerve (*1*) and the cephalic vein (*2*)

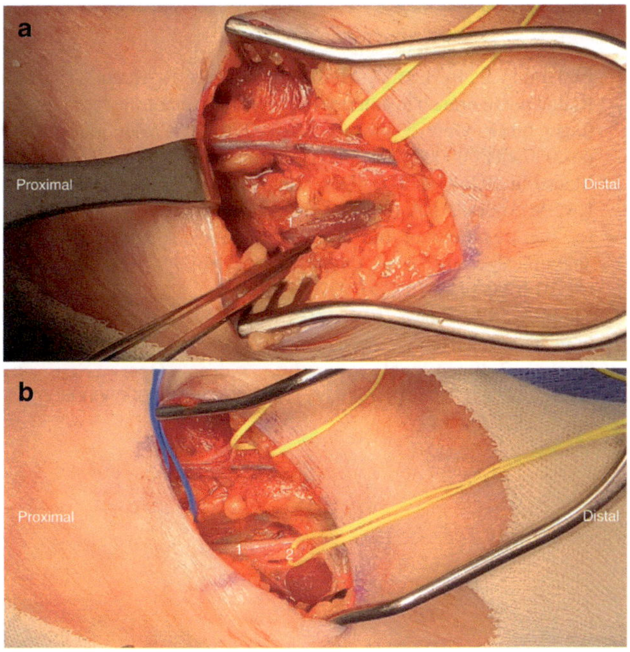

Fig. 35.3 (**a**) The lacertus fibrosus is then divided to identify the median nerve (*1*), running between the two heads of the pronator teres. (**b**) The dissection is continued distally to identify the anterior interosseous nerve (*2*). *1* median nerve

7. The brachioradialis is elevated, allowing identification of the radial sensory nerve and the deep radial nerve.
8. The nerve to the ECRB is then identified arising from the deep radial nerve (Fig. 35.4).
9. Intraoperative nerve stimulation should produce wrist extension, confirming the ECRB is a good functional donor. This is then traced, first distally to its branching point and then proximally with interfascicular dissection to gain further length.
10. The nerve to the ECRB is then cut at its most distal site (Fig. 35.5a). The AIN is then cut as proximal as possible (Fig. 35.5b).

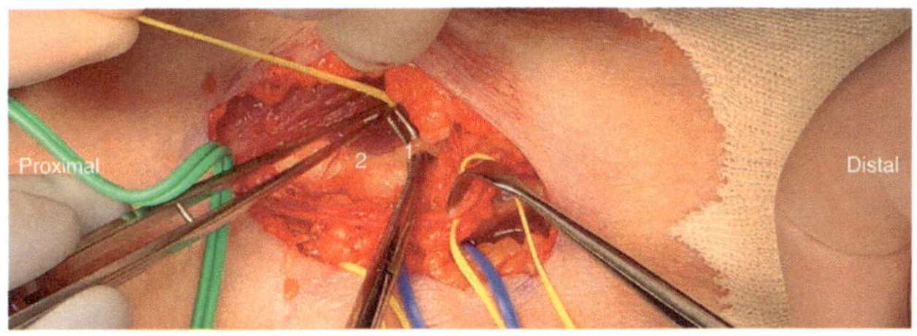

Fig. 35.4 Laterally, the nerve to the ECRB (*1*) is identified arising from the deep radial nerve (*2*) deep and medial to brachioradialis

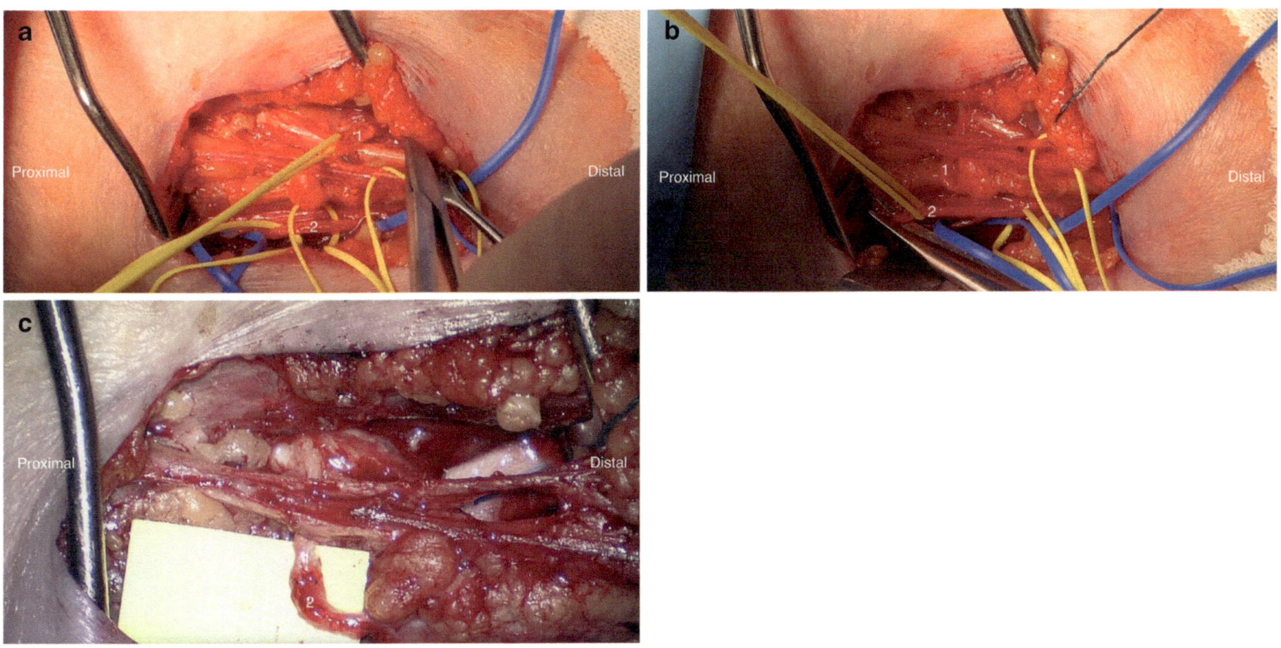

Fig. 35.5 (**a**) The nerve to the ECRB (*1*) is cut at its most distal site. (**b**) The AIN (*2*) is cut as proximal as possible. (**c**) The nerve ends are approximated in the midline of the forearm and sutured end-to-end using 9-0 Nylon (or Vicryl), under the operative microscope. *1* ECRB, *2* AIN

11. The nerve ends are approximated and sutured end-to-end with 9-0 sutures (traditionally Nylon but more recently we have been using monofilament Vicryl) under an operative microscope (Fig. 35.5c). A nerve tube and/or fibrin glue can then be used to protect the sutured ends.

Complications

1. Vascular injuries
2. Iatrogenic nerve injury
3. Wound infection
4. Failure of recovery; should consider tendon transfers (see Chap. 43)

References

1. Elmaraghi S, Burkett D, Meisner L, Gander B, Hanna A (2022) Radial nerve branch to anterior interosseous nerve transfer to restore finger pinch. Oper Neurosurg 22(6):e276. https://doi.org/10.1227/ons.0000000000000170. Epub 2022 Apr 14
2. Matavelli FC, Gobbi L, Dos Santos MPS, Caetano EB, Vieira LA, de Andrade RA (2019) Transfer of the radial nerve branches for the treatment of the anterior interosseous nerve lesion: an anatomical study. Acta Ortop Bras 27(6):298–303. https://doi.org/10.1590/1413-785220192706226097
3. Miranda SP, Zager EL (2022) Commentary: Radial nerve branch to anterior interosseous nerve transfer to restore finger pinch: 2-dimensional operative video. Oper Neurosurg 22(6):e277–e278. https://doi.org/10.1227/ons.0000000000000241. Epub 2022 Apr 14

Median Nerve Motor Branch to Posterior Interosseous Nerve Transfer

36

Pradeep K. Attaluri, Shady Elmaraghi, Robert E. George, Thomas M. Staniszewski, and Amgad S. Hanna

Indications

A full history, brachial plexus physical examination, and electrodiagnostic studies are essential to establish a diagnosis and achieve successful outcomes. The mechanism of injury, chronicity of injury, location, and serial physical examinations to evaluate for spontaneous radial nerve regeneration are necessary. Additionally, examination of the donor nerve, in this case the median nerve, is also especially important to evaluate. Patients with a Sunderland Type IV or V axonal injury with no spontaneous regeneration by 3 months post-injury are candidates for this nerve transfer in order to restore wrist and finger extension [1]. The target recipient is the posterior interosseous nerve (PIN), and the donor is a median nerve motor branch. Options are either pronator teres (PT) or flexor digitorum superficialis (FDS) branches. However, it is preferable to save the PT for potential tendon transfer, which could be performed at the same time as the nerve transfer or at a later date [2].

Surgical Anatomy

The radial nerve, as it relates to the forearm, emerges after piercing the lateral intermuscular septum and runs between the brachialis and brachioradialis. It divides 2 cm distal to the elbow into the superficial radial sensory branch (SRN) and the deep radial nerve. Prominent vessels, known as the "Leash of Henry," cross the deep radial nerve. Prior to giving off the PIN branch, there are branches to the brachioradialis (BR), extensor carpi radialis longus (ECRL), and extensor carpi radialis brevis (ECRB) [3]. The PIN then emerges distal to the supinator branches, passes under the supinator muscle, and gives off branches to the extensor digitorum communis (EDC), extensor carpi ulnaris (ECU), extensor digiti quinti (EDQ), extensor pollicis longus (EPL), extensor pollicis brevis (EPB), abductor pollicis longus (APL), and extensor indicis proprius (EIP) as it travels distally.

The median nerve, as it enters to the forearm, passes posterior to the lacertus fibrosus to lie medial to the brachial artery. In the antecubital fossa, the median nerve gives off motor branches to the PT (1–4 branches), flexor carpi radialis (FCR), palmaris longus (PL), and FDS. Then, the median nerve passes between the two heads of the PT [3]. The median nerve continues posterior to the fibrous arch of the FDS (sublime bridge). The anterior interosseous nerve (AIN) arises from the dorsoradial surface of the median nerve proper, approximately 5–8 cm distal to the medial epicondyle. The AIN travels between the FDS and flexor digitorum profundus (FDP), giving off multiple motor branches, and then passes between and supplies the flexor pollicis longus (FPL) and the lateral half of FDP, then deep to the pronator quadratus (PQ), supplying it prior to entering the wrist joint.

Supplementary Information The online version contains supplementary material available at https://doi.org/10.1007/978-3-031-73931-6_36.

P. K. Attaluri
Division of Plastic Surgery, Department of Surgery, University of Wisconsin-Madison, Madison, WI, USA
e-mail: pattaluri@uwhealth.org

S. Elmaraghi
Department of Plastic Surgery, Vanderbilt Health, Nashville, TN, USA
e-mail: shady.elmaraghi@outlook.com

R. E. George
Division of Plastic and Reconstructive Surgery, Department of Surgery, University of Wisconsin-Madison, Madison, WI, USA
e-mail: rgeorge@uwhealth.org

T. M. Staniszewski
Department of Neurological Surgery, University of Wisconsin School of Medicine and Public Health, Madison, WI, USA
e-mail: staniszewski@neurosurgery.wisc.edu

A. S. Hanna (✉)
Department of Neurosurgery, University of Wisconsin School of Medicine and Public Health, Madison, WI, USA

A. S. Hanna (ed.), *Nerves: Anatomy, Exposures, and Techniques*, https://doi.org/10.1007/978-3-031-73931-6_36

Surgical Technique

1. The patient is positioned supine, with the affected arm abducted on an arm table. It is important to communicate with anesthesia to avoid long-acting paralytics, as nerve stimulation will be used through the case. An upper arm tourniquet is placed; with an understanding, this will have to be released prior to nerve stimulation.
2. Mark incision as shown (Fig. 36.1). A lazy-S incision is used on the volar forearm to allow access to both median and radial nerve branches.
3. Make the incision using a 15-blade. Continue with tenotomy dissection through the subcutaneous tissue to the fascia, with special attention paid to the lateral antebrachial cutaneous (LABC) nerve which runs parallel to the cephalic vein (Fig. 36.2).

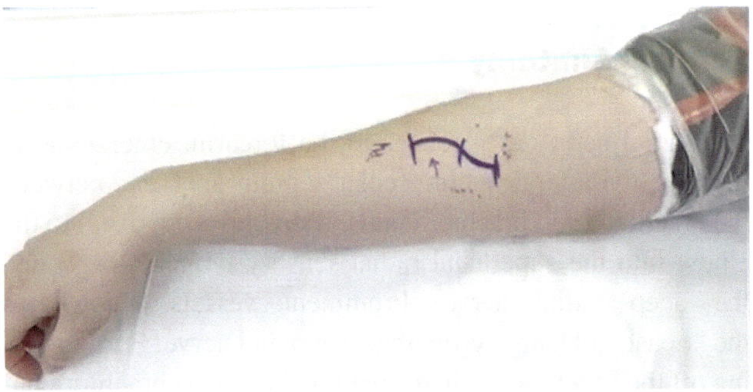

Fig. 36.1 Incision over the volar proximal forearm to expose both radial and median nerves

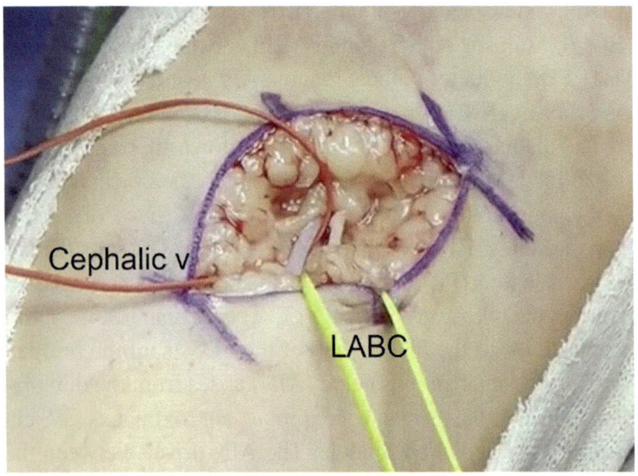

Fig. 36.2 After making the incision, it is important to protect the lateral antebrachial cutaneous nerve (LABC, *yellow vessel loop*) and the cephalic vein (*red vessel loop*)

4. We will then release the bicipital aponeurosis (lacertus fibrosus) to gain access to the median nerve (Fig. 36.3).
5. The median nerve branches can be best identified by separating the two heads of pronator teres and opening the sublime bridge (Fig. 36.4).
6. At this point, nerve stimulation will be used. So, depending on the tourniquet time, it might be necessary to release the tourniquet to allow for a response
   (a) The PT nerve branch will be the most superficial and proximal branch of the median nerve.
   (b) The FDS nerve branch will lie on the ulnar aspect of the median nerve, just distal to the FCR and PL branches.
7. Dissect the FDS branch as distal as possible and use a vessel loop to tag these nerves (Fig. 36.4).
8. Now, we will gain exposure of our recipient PIN through the same incision.
9. Identify the radial sensory nerve posterior to the BR muscle and follow this proximally to the main radial nerve. This is then followed distally to identify the deep radial nerve (Fig. 36.5).
10. Release the tendinous leading edge of the ECRB and release the tendinous leading edge of the supinator muscle (Fröhse arcade) to fully decompress and gain length on the PIN.
11. Now, we will divide the branch to FDS distally and the PIN as proximal as possible to ensure adequate length.
12. Using 9-0 suture (traditionally Nylon, more recently we use monofilament Vicryl) and microscope, coapt the FDS nerve to the PIN (Fig. 36.6). May reinforce the repair with fibrin glue and/or tubes.
13. Ensure meticulous hemostasis in the wound and close the incision using 3-0 monocryl in a deep dermal fashion and 4-0 monocryl in a running subcuticular fashion.
14. Splint immobilization followed by aggressive cortical re-training with occupational therapy is crucial to success.

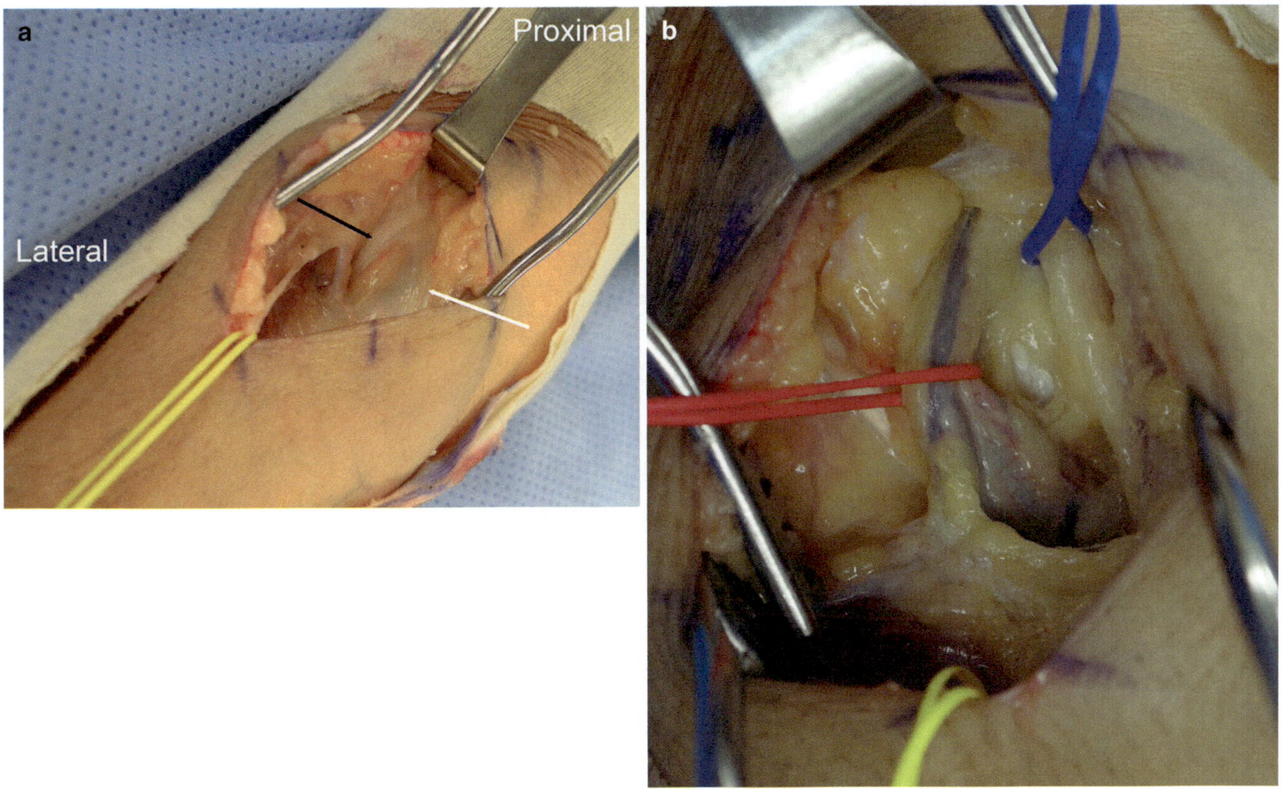

Fig. 36.3 (**a**) The bicipital aponeurosis (lacertus fibrosus, *white arrow*) is observed medially, while the biceps tendon (*black arrow*) is lateral. (**b**) Once the bicipital aponeurosis is opened, the median nerve (*blue loop*) and the brachial vessels (*red loop*) are visualized

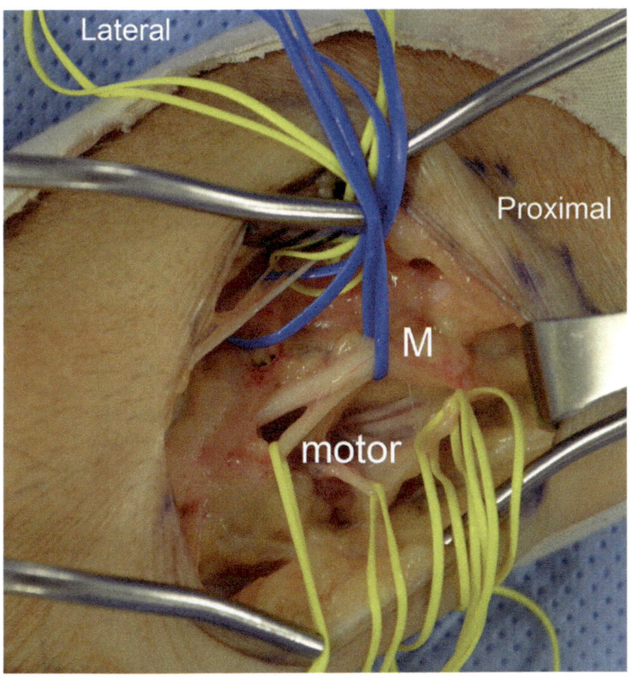

Fig. 36.4 The median nerve (M) and its motor branches are isolated. Using a nerve stimulator, a good donor branch is selected: PT or FDS

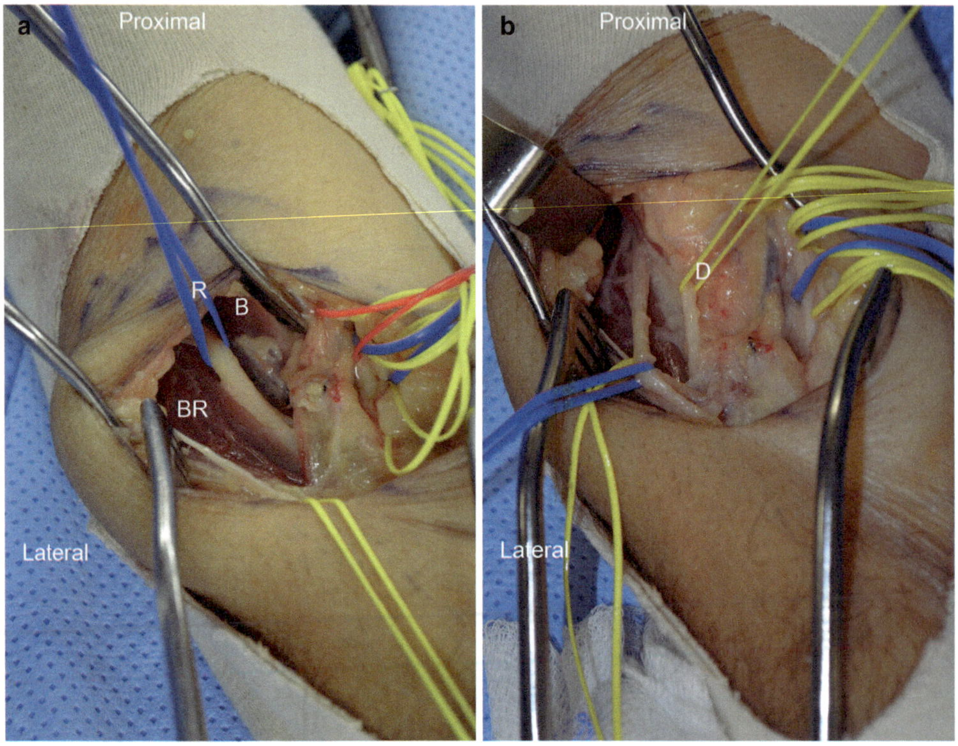

Fig. 36.5 (**a**) The radial nerve (*R, blue loop*) is found between the brachioradialis (*BR*) laterally and the brachialis (*B*) medially. (**b**) The deep radial nerve (*D*) is isolated and prepared for coaptation

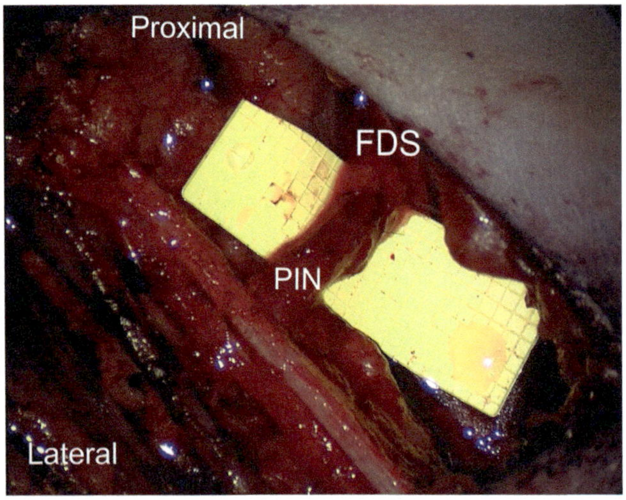

Fig. 36.6 FDS (cut distally) to PIN (cut proximally) coaptation under an operative microscope. *FDS* flexor digitorum superficialis branch, *PIN* posterior interosseous nerve

Complications

1. Hematoma
2. Wound infection
3. Wound dehiscence
4. Temporary weakness of finger flexion
5. Injury to LABC, superficial radial nerve, or radial vessels
6. Failure of recovery, in which case tendon transfers should be considered (Chap. 43)

References

1. Ray WZ, Mackinnon SE (2011) Clinical outcomes following median to radial nerve transfers. J Hand Surg Am 36(2):201–208. https://doi.org/10.1016/j.jhsa.2010.09.034. Epub 2010 Dec 18
2. Brown JM, Tung THH, Mackinnon SE (2010) Median to radial nerve transfer to restore wrist and finger extension: technical nuances. Neurosurgery 66(3 Suppl Operative):75–83. https://doi.org/10.1227/01.NEU.0000354364.13224.C8
3. Mackinnon SE, Roque B, Tung TH (2007) Median to radial nerve transfer for treatment of radial nerve palsy. Case report. J Neurosurg 107(3):666–671. https://doi.org/10.3171/JNS-07/09/0666

Anterior Interosseous Nerve to Ulnar Motor Nerve Transfer

37

Simon G. Ammanuel, Thomas M. Staniszewski, and Amgad S. Hanna

Indications

- End-to-end, severe ulnar neuropathy of various causes resulting in ulnar claw hand: metacarpophalangeal (MCP) joint hyperextension and interphalangeal (IP) joint flexion in the medial two fingers (Fig. 37.1). Etiologies include trauma to the ulnar nerve or brachial plexus (lower trunk/ medial cord) [1, 2].
- End-to-side, used to reinforce a proximal repair of the ulnar nerve or in cases of severe ulnar neuropathy (baby-sitting, supercharge) [3].

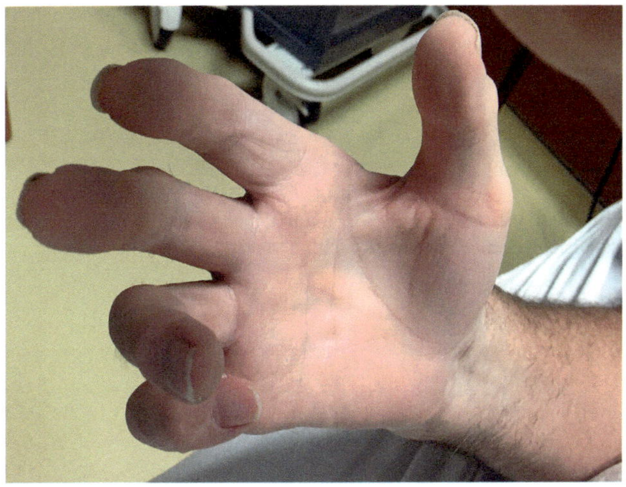

Fig. 37.1 Ulnar claw hand: The patient is unable to extend the medial two fingers at the IP joints

Surgical Technique

1. The patient is placed in a supine position, with the arm abducted and supinated. Tourniquet is typically used.
2. An incision is made lateral to the flexor carpi ulnaris tendon and pisiform, splitting the distance between ulnar and median nerves. Incision extends to the hand lateral to the hypothenar eminence, crossing the wrist obliquely or in a zigzag fashion (Fig. 37.2).
3. The flexor carpi ulnaris tendon is retracted medially to allow visualization of the neurovascular bundle (Fig. 37.3). The ulnar nerve is dissected free, it's medial to the artery.
4. Using blunt and sharp dissection, Guyon's canal is unroofed. This will expose the superficial and deep terminal branches of the ulnar nerve (Fig. 37.4). Detachment of the hypothenar arch will allow the release of the deep motor branch of the ulnar nerve.

Supplementary Information The online version contains supplementary material available at https://doi.org/10.1007/978-3-031-73931-6_37.

S. G. Ammanuel
Department of Neurological Surgery, University of Wisconsin Hospitals and Clinics, Madison, WI, USA
e-mail: SAmmanuel@uwhealth.org

T. M. Staniszewski
Department of Neurological Surgery, University of Wisconsin School of Medicine and Public Health, Madison, WI, USA
e-mail: staniszewski@neurosurgery.wisc.edu

A. S. Hanna (✉)
Department of Neurosurgery, University of Wisconsin School of Medicine and Public Health, Madison, WI, USA

A. S. Hanna (ed.), *Nerves: Anatomy, Exposures, and Techniques*, https://doi.org/10.1007/978-3-031-73931-6_37

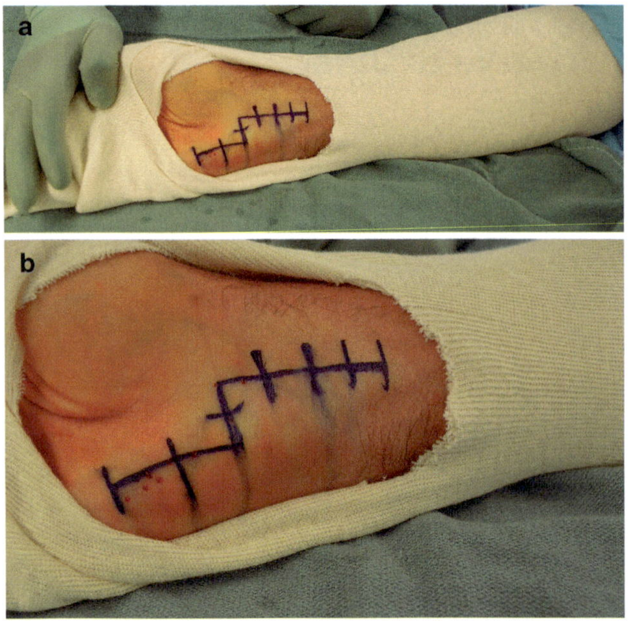

Fig. 37.2 Incision for right AIN to ulnar motor nerve transfer, splitting the distance between median and ulnar nerves

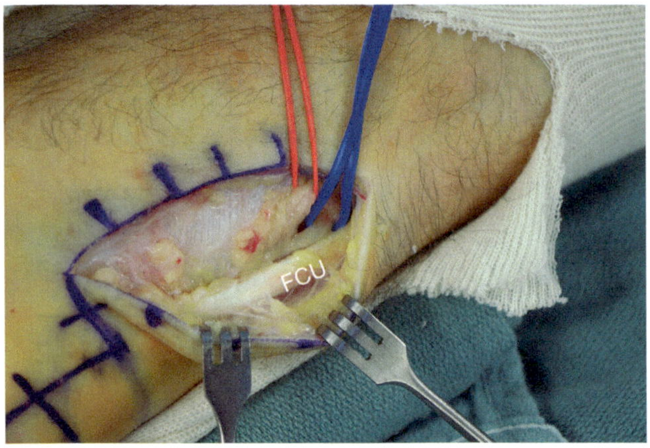

Fig. 37.3 The ulnar nerve (*blue loop*) and ulnar artery (*red loop*) are found lateral to the flexor carpi ulnaris (*FCU*) tendon

5. More proximally, the long flexor tendons are retracted laterally to expose the pronator quadratus. The neurovascular bundle including the anterior interosseous nerve (AIN) is identified proximal to the pronator quadratus. A nerve stimulator is used to identify AIN (Fig. 37.5a). One may have to deflate the tourniquet to get a good response.

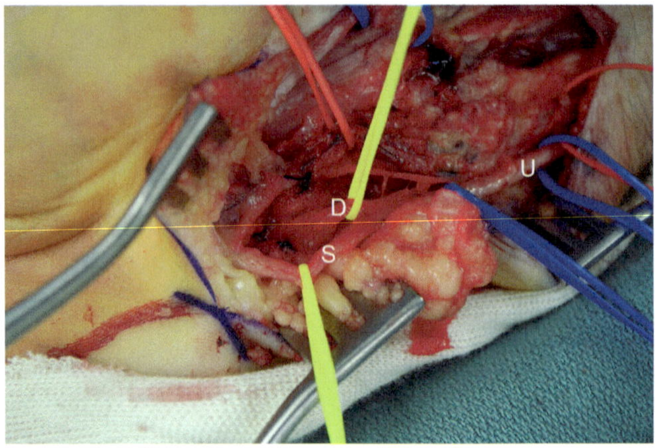

Fig. 37.4 The ulnar nerve (*U*) splits into superficial (*S*) and deep (*D*) components, distally

6. Once the nerve is identified, it is dissected free and followed deep to the pronator quadratus, until almost midportion of the muscle where it starts giving off muscular branches (Fig. 37.5b).
7. The ulnar motor branch is dissected off the main sensory branch from distal to proximal, skipping short segments to protect the interfascicular connections. In the forearm, the motor component lies between the ulnar nerve's main sensory portion and the ulnar nerve's dorsal cutaneous branch (Fig. 37.6).
8. The AIN is transected distally at the midportion of the pronator quadratus and then mobilized medially toward the ulnar nerve. The microscope is brought into the operative field.
9. End-to-end transfer (Fig. 37.7): The motor branch of the ulnar nerve is transected proximally and then aligned with the AIN donor. Using a 9-0 monofilament suture, we perform simple interrupted sutures, we usually two, between the two nerve endings.
10. End-to-side transfer: We create a small perineurial window in the ulnar motor branch laterally, which is coapted with the cut end of the AIN. Simple interrupted sutures are placed between the AIN end and the edges of the perineurial window. This coaptation needs to be tighter than end-to-end.
11. Before suturing the ends together, mobilize the hand and wrist to ensure the nerve transfer is tension-free. Once the nerve transfer is completed, the suture line can be reinforced by nerve tubes and/or fibrin glue, and the wound is irrigated and closed in layers in a standard fashion. A wrist splint is placed for 3 weeks.

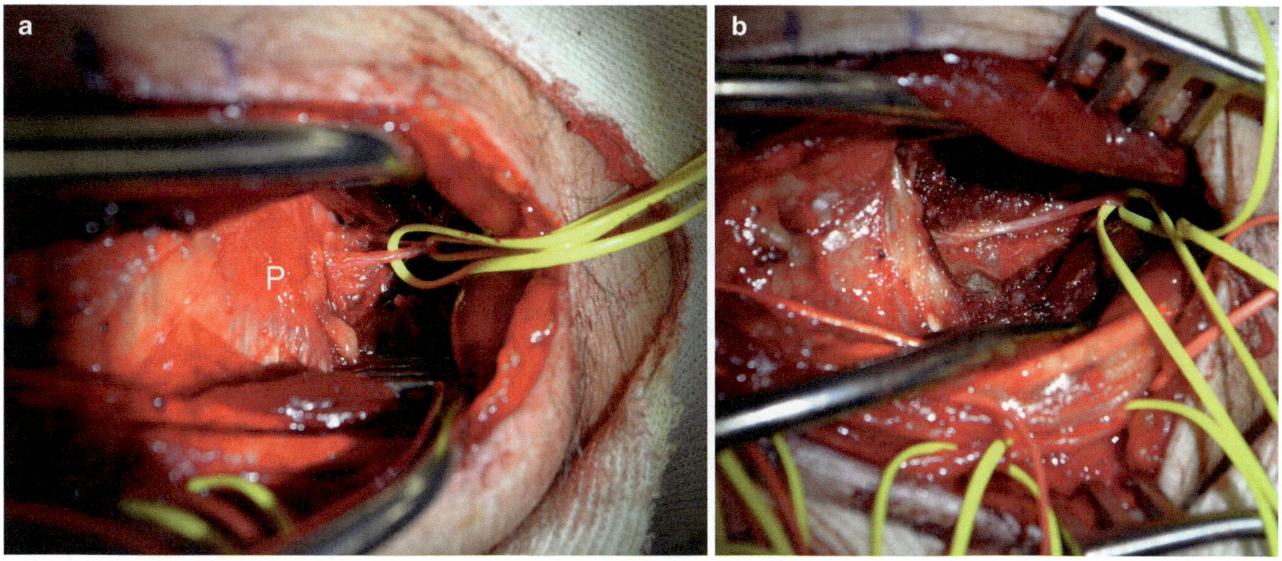

Fig. 37.5 (**a**) The AIN (*yellow loop*) is seen entering pronator quadratus (*P*). Note that *P* is the only transverse muscle in this area. (**b**) The nerve is followed distally under the muscle until it starts branching

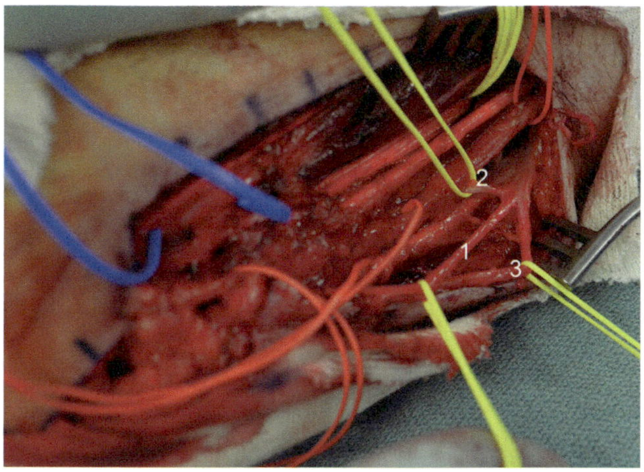

Fig. 37.6 The motor component of the ulnar nerve (*1*) is found between the main sensory (*2*) and dorsal cutaneous branch (*3*)

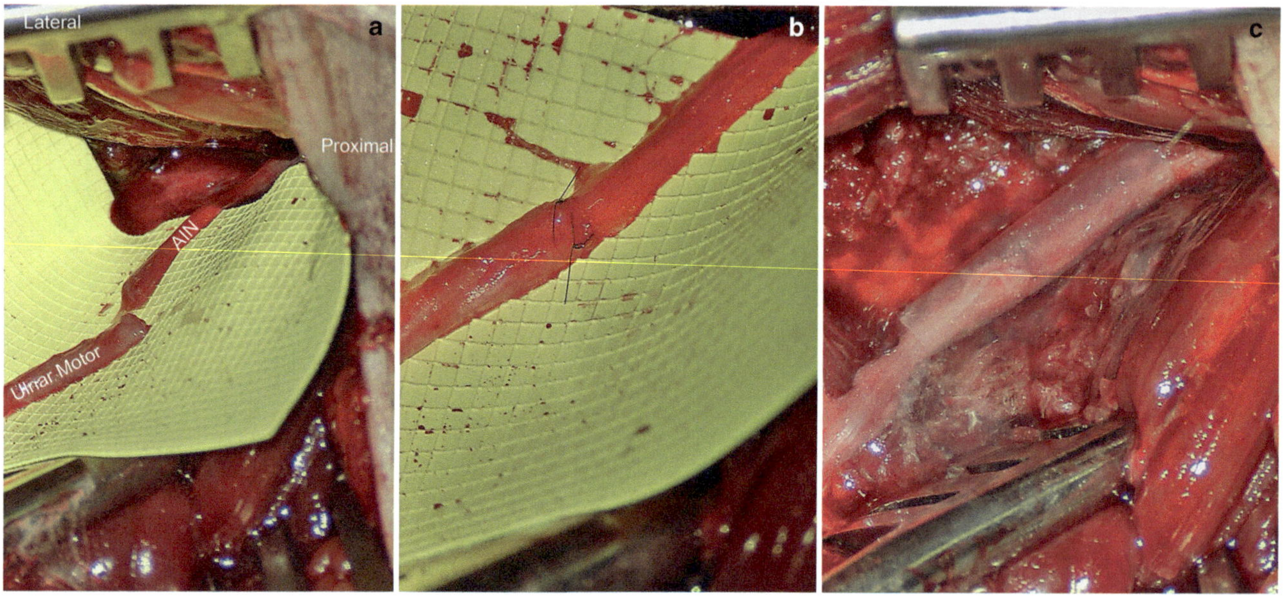

Fig. 37.7 End-to-end coaptation of AIN to ulnar motor nerve. (**a**) Apposition of the nerve ends. (**b**) Two interrupted sutures are placed under an operative microscope. (**c**) The neurorrhaphy is reinforced with a nerve tube and/or fibrin glue

Complications

1. Failure to improve clawing of the hand. Tendon transfers should be considered (Chap. 43)
2. Weakness in pronation of the forearm
3. Vascular injury, in particular, ulnar artery
4. Wound infection and dehiscence

References

1. Brown JM, Yee A, Mackinnon SE (2009) Distal median to ulnar nerve transfers to restore ulnar motor and sensory function within the hand: technical nuances. Neurosurgery 65(5):966–977. https://doi.org/10.1227/01.NEU.0000358951.64043.73
2. Novak CB, Mackinnon SE (2002) Distal anterior interosseous nerve transfer to the deep motor branch of the ulnar nerve for reconstruction of high ulnar nerve injuries. J Reconstruct Microsurg 18(6):459–464. https://doi.org/10.1055/s-2002-33326
3. Thakkar M, Rose A, King W, Engelman K, Bednarz B (2022) Anterior interosseous nerve to ulnar nerve transfer: a systematic review. JPRAS Open 32:195–210. https://doi.org/10.1016/j.jpra.2022.02.007

Intercostal to Musculocutaneous Nerve Transfer

38

Rebecca D. Funk, Jacob W. Sveum, and A. Neil Salyapongse

Indications

Restoration of elbow flexion is a primary goal in nerve transfers for brachial plexus injury with a focus on reinnervation of the biceps and/or brachialis muscles. As intercostal nerves are extraplexus and their rates of success as donor nerves are somewhat less reliable than intraplexus nerve transfers, they should be primarily used to address complete brachial plexus injuries (avulsion) [1]. Rib fractures are not an absolute contraindication for intercostal nerve harvest, though additional care should be taken during dissection in these cases to avoid iatrogenic injury [2]. At the caudal aspect of the rib, the neurovascular arrangement from cranial to caudal is vein, artery, and nerve (VAN), respectively.

Surgical Technique

Positioning

The patient is positioned supine, with the affected arm abducted on an arm table. A folded blanket or small bump to elevate the shoulder and chest wall can facilitate exposure.

Supplementary Information The online version contains supplementary material available at https://doi.org/10.1007/978-3-031-73931-6_38.

R. D. Funk
Department of Orthopedics and Rehabilitation, University of Wisconsin, Madison, WI, USA
e-mail: RFunk@uwhealth.org

J. W. Sveum
Department of Neurosurgery, University of Wisconsin School of Medicine and Public Health, Madison, WI, USA
e-mail: jsveum@wisc.edu

A. N. Salyapongse (✉)
Madison Surgery Center, Department of Orthopedics, University of Wisconsin School of Medicine and Public Health, Madison, WI, USA
e-mail: ASalyapongse@uwhealth.org

Intercostal Nerve Harvest

1. Design an incision starting in the anterior axillary line near the axilla and extending caudally and slightly anteriorly. At the level of the sixth intercostal space, the incision may be curved toward the sternum to gain enough length anteriorly.
2. Incise the skin sharply and dissect through the superficial and deep fasciae until the investing muscle fascia over the serratus anterior and pectoralis is reached.
3. Elevate the pectoralis major muscle with cautery until the natural plane deep to the muscle is entered.
4. Blunt dissection deep to the pectoralis major can be performed, with care taken to identify pectoral nerves and perforating intercostal vessels which will occur more laterally, the more caudally the dissection progresses.
5. The most caudal origins of the pectoralis major may be divided using electrocautery, revealing the pectoralis minor, the origin of which serves as an important landmark to identify the 3rd–5th ribs.
6. Identify target ribs (typically 3rd–6th) and dissect off serratus anterior from anterior to posterior away from the ribs using monopolar cautery.
7. The intercostal nerve may be identified either through a transmuscular or subperiosteal approach:
   (a) *Transmuscular approach*
      - Beginning near the anterior axillary line, divide the external intercostal muscle just caudal to the rib with either monopolar or bipolar electrocautery. The external intercostal muscle fibers will sweep from cephalad and lateral toward the inferior rib medially (Fig. 38.1).
      - The internal intercostal muscle fibers will be identifiable running in the opposite direction to the external intercostal fibers. Divide these immediately caudal to the rib using a fine hemostat to lift the muscle and bipolar cautery to divide the muscle and minimize bleeding.

A. S. Hanna (ed.), *Nerves: Anatomy, Exposures, and Techniques*, https://doi.org/10.1007/978-3-031-73931-6_38

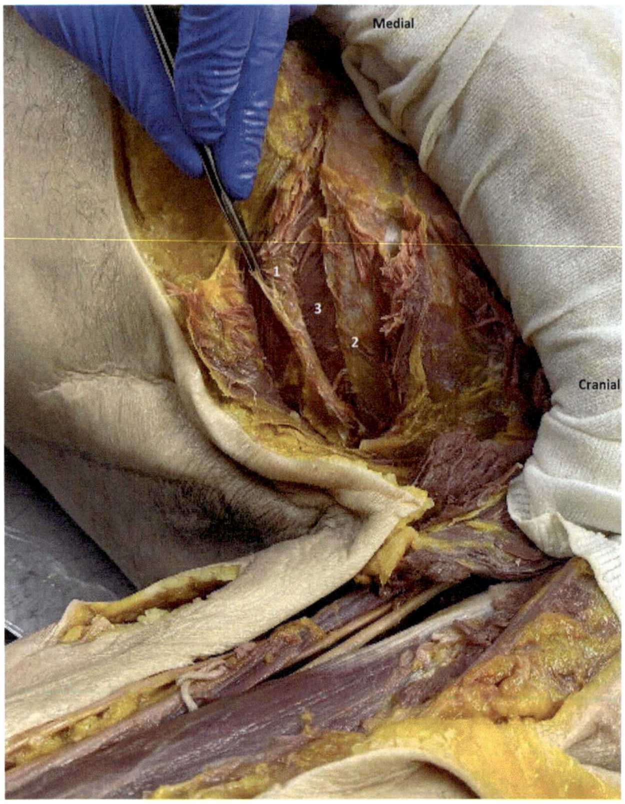

Fig. 38.1 After dissection of serratus off-target ribs, identify the external intercostal muscles (*1*) and sharply incise off the inferior aspect of the target rib (*2*) to expose the internal intercostal muscles (*3*)

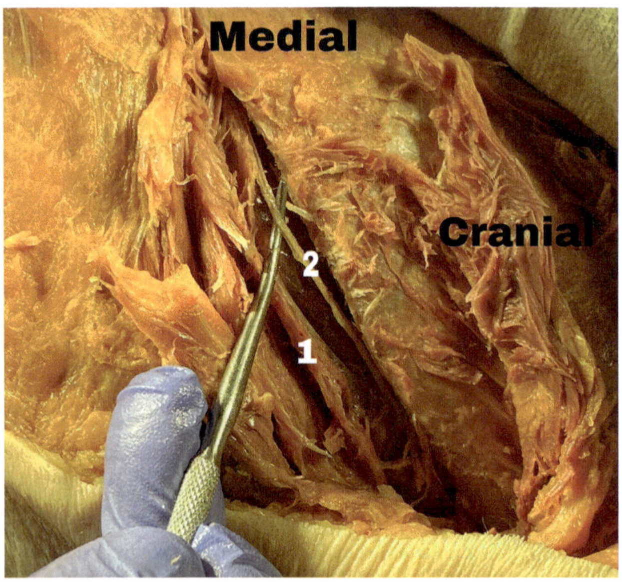

Fig. 38.2 Maintaining hemostasis with bipolar, dissect the internal intercostal muscles (*1*) off the inferior aspect of the target rib to expose the intercostal nerve (*2*) running along the caudal aspect of the rib

- The intercostal nerve can be identified running at the caudal margin of the rib (Fig. 38.2) between the internal intercostal and innermost intercostal. As the nerve progresses anteriorly, its course will continue to run slightly farther caudally.
- Use a nerve stimulator to confirm the motor fibers. The cutaneous branches of the intercostals, especially lateral cutaneous, may be harvested for sensory reconstruction of the median nerve.
- Pass a vessel loop around the nerve to facilitate dissection from the anterior axillary line toward the sternum. A small accessory branch will often be encountered and may be divided.
- Continue dissection anteriorly until an adequate length has been obtained.
- Posterior dissection follows a similar approach up to the mid-axillary line.
- Do not divide the nerve distally/anteriorly until the recipient nerve has been prepared.
- Harvest up to four levels of nerves as necessary for the number of recipient nerves (i.e., three intercostal nerves for the musculocutaneous alone vs. two each for a simultaneous musculocutaneous and obturator nerve stump of a gracilis transfer).

(b) *Subperiosteal approach*
- Sharply open periosteum at the caudal margin of the rib with a #15 blade.
- Using a periosteal elevator (typically a #9), gently elevate in a subperiosteal plane the soft tissues from the concavity of the inferior and deep surface of the rib.
- A Ragnell retractor is used by an assistant to retract the rib margin cranially. Carefully incise the thick periosteum, roughly 3–4 mm cranial to the free caudal edge of the rib to identify the neurovascular bundle.
- Identify the intercostal nerve as the most caudal structure in the neurovascular bundle, gently free it from the vessels, and pass a vessel loop around the nerve.
- Anterior and posterior dissection should proceed as per the transmuscular approach, with the difference that the periosteal flap will be sequentially divided rather than the muscles, and more rib retraction is usually necessary.
- As the dissection proceeds anteriorly, transition across the periosteal flap margin and into the muscles may be required to expose the increasingly caudal course of the nerve.

Musculocutaneous Nerve Preparation

1. The incision for exposure of the musculocutaneous nerve will depend on other necessary exposures. If the infraclavicular brachial plexus has been exposed, then continuation of the incision onto the medial arm provides excellent access (see also Chap. 8 for infraclavicular brachial plexus dissection details). If the brachial plexus is not being explored, then the incision should be designed along the medial arm.
2. Identify the neurovascular bundle in the medial arm through palpation of the brachial artery.
3. Design an incision from the axilla over the proximal third of the arm directly over the brachial artery.
4. Dissect through the subcutaneous tissue with monopolar cautery until the fascia investing the anterior compartment muscles and the neurovascular bundle is reached.
5. Identify and protect the medial brachial cutaneous nerve (may be used as a graft as needed). Medial antebrachial cutaneous nerve may also be identified here.
6. Carefully open the fascia overlying the neurovascular bundle.
7. Identify and protect the basilic vein, retracting this caudally and revealing the brachial artery and venae comitantes.
8. Retract the brachial artery posteriorly, exposing the interval between the brachialis (deep) and the biceps (superficial).
9. Bluntly dissect with scissors or hemostat laterally in this plane, identifying the musculocutaneous nerve as it courses between the two muscles.
10. Pass a vessel loop around the nerve to facilitate dissection.
11. Follow the nerve proximally to where it enters the coracobrachialis.
12. Divide the coracobrachialis superficial to the nerve and continue dissection proximally to the "M" of the lower plexus (Fig. 38.3): musculocutaneous, median, and ulnar nerves.
13. Sharply incise the most proximal portion of the musculocutaneous nerve to provide a clean end for subsequent end-to-end neurorrhaphy.

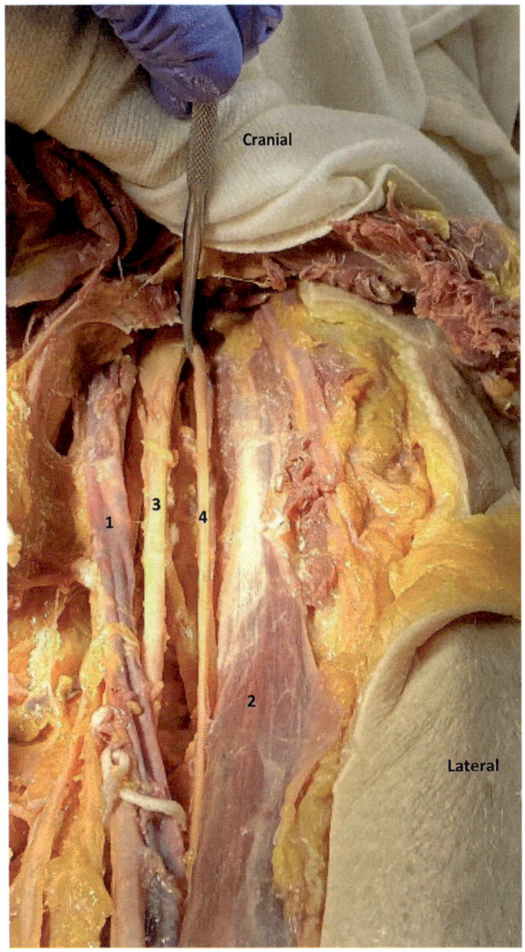

Fig. 38.3 In the arm, after delineation and dissection of the neurovascular bundle, the overlying fascia is opened, and the vessels (*1*) are retracted medially to expose the plane between the biceps (*2*) and brachialis. This allows visualization of the proximal aspect of the median (*3*) and musculocutaneous (*4*) nerves

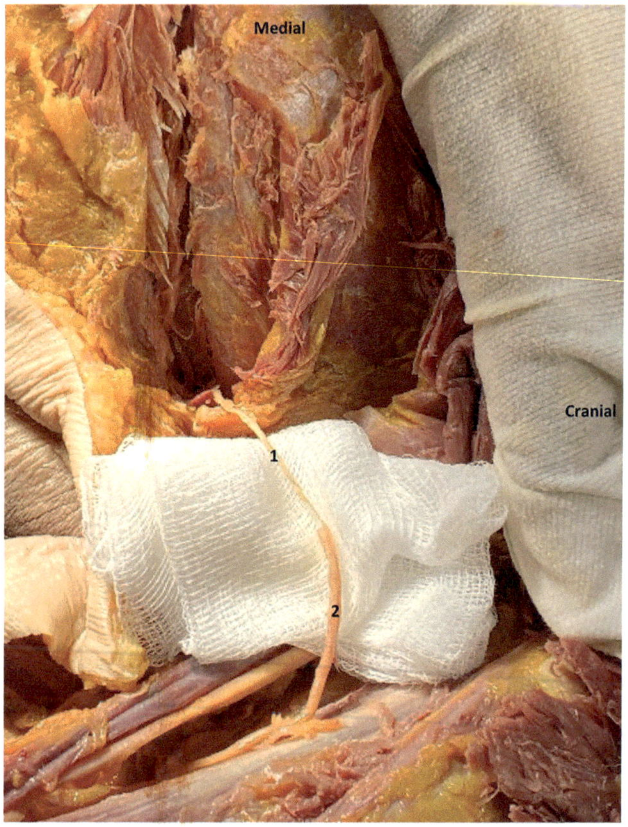

Fig. 38.4 Target intercostal nerves (*1*) are incised medially and brought cephalad and lateral for neurorrhaphy with the proximal aspect of prepared musculocutaneous nerve (*2*)

Neurorrhaphy

1. Incise the medial aspect of exposed intercostal nerves (typically three branches) and bring them laterally and cephalad to suture them to the prepared proximal end of the musculocutaneous nerve (Fig. 38.4). Care must be taken to repair the appropriate motor segments of the intercostal nerves to the central motor fascicle of the musculocutaneous nerve.
2. Coaptation of the nerves may be performed under loupe or microscope magnification.
3. For coaptation, 9-0 Nylon (or Vicryl) epineurial or perineurial sutures are used.
4. May reinforce the neurorrhaphy with a nerve conduit and/or fibrin sealant.
5. Close the wound in a layered fashion.

Postoperative Management

1. Maintain the shoulder in minimal abduction with a sling.
2. If combined with a free innervated muscle transfer, consider a specific sling that incorporates a foam wedge to slightly abduct the arm from the body and avoid pressure on the vascular anastomoses.
3. At 3 weeks, the sling may be removed and physical therapy for the arm and shoulder resumed.

Complications

Traumatic brachial plexus injuries are commonly associated with rib fractures, secondary to the often-high energy mechanism. Although harvesting of intercostal nerves with concomitant rib fractures does not necessarily increase the rate of complications, it does increase the complexity of dissection and the likelihood of fracture-related intercostal nerve damage. Careful consideration must be given to intercostal nerve harvest with known concurrent phrenic nerve palsy to avoid associated respiratory distress. After nerve transfer, patients may notice firing of the elbow flexors with the respiratory cycle as well as coughing, or sneezing, though this has been shown to diminish over time.

The most common complication associated with intercostal nerve harvest is pneumothorax from the violation of pleura. This can be safely addressed with the intraoperative placement of a small feeding tube deep to the parietal pleura secured with absorbable sutures to be pulled later with the resolution of the pneumothorax. Postoperative follow-up chest X-ray is warranted to monitor the pneumothorax [3].

References

1. Xiao C, Lao J, Wang T, Zhao X, Liu J, Gu Y (2014) Intercostal nerve transfer to neurotize the musculocutaneous nerve after traumatic brachial plexus avulsion: a comparison of two, three, and four nerve transfers. J Reconstr Microsurg 30(5):297–304. https://doi.org/10.1055/s-0033-1361840. Epub 2014 Mar 28
2. Forli A, Bouyer M, Aribert M, Curvale C, Delord M, Corcella D, Moutet F (2017) Upper limb nerve transfers: a review. Transferts nerveux au membre supérieur: mise au point. Hand Surg Rehabil 36(3):151–172. https://doi.org/10.1016/j.hansur.2016.11.007. Epub 2017 May 3
3. Samardzić M, Rasulić L, Grujicić D, Milicić B (2000) Results of nerve transfers to the musculocutaneous and axillary nerves. Neurosurgery 46(1):93–103

Sensory Nerve Transfers

39

Shady Elmaraghi, Pradeep K. Attaluri, Robert E. George, and Brian H. Gander

Principles of Sensory Nerve Transfers

An important concern when performing any nerve transfer is avoidance of significantly downgrading function, and so donor nerve selection must be carefully considered. In the case of sensory nerve transfers, multiple strategies can be utilized to minimize sensory disturbances in the donor nerve distribution. Donor selection should be targeting nerves that have redundancy in their sensory distribution (i.e., dorsal branch of the ulnar nerve [DBUN], dorsal sensory branches to the digits), considering donors that provide sensation to low-contact areas (i.e., third webspace branch of the median), or utilizing end-to-side nerve transfers [1]. Sensory axons have been shown to sprout across end-to-side coaptations as long as a perineurial window is created, but it is important to note that end-to-side nerve transfers rarely produce greater than protective sensation, leading some authors to suggest only using them in noncritical areas, while other authors have reported unsatisfactory results and have abandoned those procedures completely [2, 3].

Supplementary Information The online version contains supplementary material available at https://doi.org/10.1007/978-3-031-73931-6_39.

S. Elmaraghi
Department of Plastic Surgery, Vanderbilt Health, Nashville, TN, USA
e-mail: shady.elmaraghi@outlook.com

P. K. Attaluri
Division of Plastic Surgery, Department of Surgery, University of Wisconsin-Madison, Madison, WI, USA
e-mail: pattaluri@uwhealth.org

R. E. George · B. H. Gander (✉)
Division of Plastic and Reconstructive Surgery, Department of Surgery, University of Wisconsin-Madison, Madison, WI, USA
e-mail: rgeorge@uwhealth.org; gander@surgery.wisc.edu

Before considering sensory nerve transfers, careful testing of the proposed donor and recipient distributions should be performed. Goals of the procedure should be discussed with the patient, and expectations set, as sensory recovery beyond protective sensation is rarely achieved. Bertelli and Ghizoni advocate Semmes–Weinstein monofilament testing of the donor and recipient distributions, only considering donor nerves from distributions with perception of a 2.00 g monofilament, indicative of protective sensation. An inability to feel pressure exerted by a 4.00 g monofilament was considered a loss of protective sensation [4].

Complications of Sensory Nerve Transfers

Multiple authors have expressed caution in using branches of the radial sensory nerve, especially at or proximal to the wrist, as donors in sensory nerve transfers due to the risk of painful neuromas [1]. In addition, authors have reported issues with inappropriate localization after sensory nerve transfers, which may be improved by sensory re-education. Bertelli and Ghizoni reported a 25% rate of referred localization (localizing stimuli to the donor nerve distribution rather than the recipient distribution) after very distal nerve transfers for the restoration of fingertip sensation—although they add that no patients complained of paresthesia or even noticed this until it was pointed out during testing [5].

Sensory Restoration of the Median Nerve

Sensory restoration of the median nerve is primarily focused on restoring sensation to the thumb and index fingers for improvement in prehensile dexterity. Although median nerve injuries may cause paresthesia or anesthesia in the palm, they only lead to wounds on the digits, and so the focus of sensory restoration should be on restoring sensation to the distal digits [1].

A. S. Hanna (ed.), *Nerves: Anatomy, Exposures, and Techniques*, https://doi.org/10.1007/978-3-031-73931-6_39

DBUN to Median Nerve

1. The patient is placed in a supine position with the arm out on an arm table. A tourniquet may be used if intraoperative nerve stimulation is not planned. If this is planned, tourniquet time should be limited to less than 30 min.
2. A 10 cm incision is made on the radial edge of the flexor carpi ulnaris (FCU) to the proximal wrist crease and connected to a carpal tunnel incision with a diagonal incision at the distal wrist crease (Fig. 39.1).
3. The ulnar nerve is identified proximally, deep to the FCU, medial to the ulnar artery. This is traced distally to identify the takeoff of the DBUN, which is followed until it begins branching significantly. Several large branches can be followed if length is needed.
4. The DBUN is separated proximally from the main ulnar nerve to gain length.
5. A standard open carpal tunnel release is then performed, and the median nerve is identified and traced proximally into the previous wound.
6. The recurrent motor branch of the median nerve to the thumb is identified and dissected proximally from the sensory component of the median nerve.
7. Care is taken to also isolate the palmar cutaneous branch of the median nerve to increase the axonal count to the digits.
8. The DBUN is then divided as distally as possible—if length is needed, this can be done after the branching point at the wrist (Fig. 39.2).
9. The DBUN is passed under the FCU tendon to the point of proximal dissection of the median sensory fascicles.
10. These fascicles are divided from the median nerve proper, as proximally as possible to avoid tension on the coaptation.
11. The nerves are coapted using a 9-0 nylon suture and reinforced with fibrin glue before closure (Fig. 39.3).

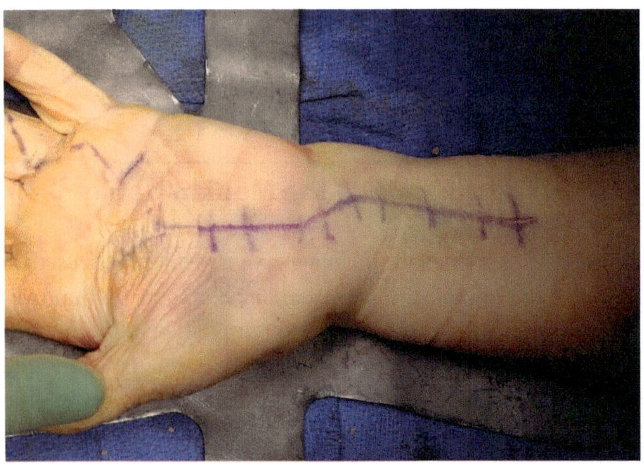

Fig. 39.1 Incision design

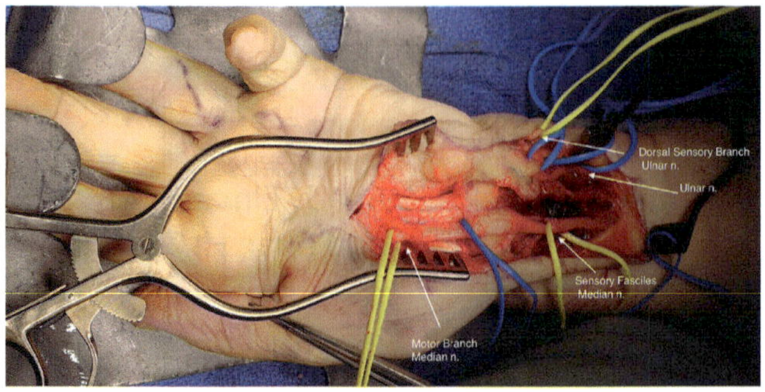

Fig. 39.2 Median and ulnar nerves before division

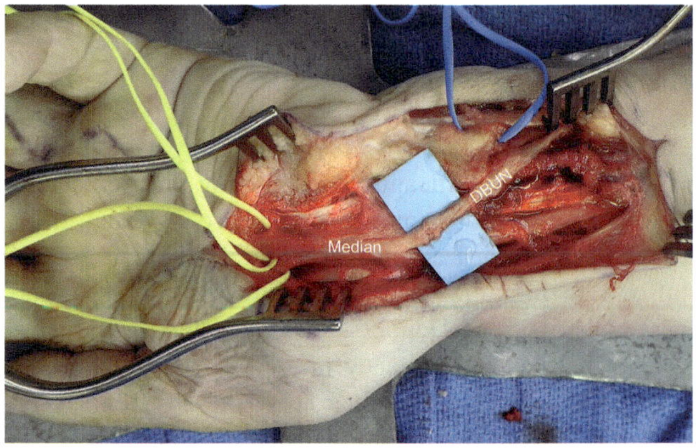

Fig. 39.3 Coaptation of DBUN to the sensory fascicles of the median nerve

Radial Sensory to Common Digital Nerve

1. A standard open carpal tunnel incision is designed over the proximal palm and extended to the metacarpophalangeal crease of the index finger in a Brunner fashion to identify the common digital branches of the median nerve (Fig. 39.4).
2. An incision is designed on the dorsal skin from the base of the first webspace along the ulnar border of the first metacarpal to identify the distal radial sensory nerve (Fig. 39.5).
3. Care is taken to protect the superficial palmar arch in the midpalm, along the axis of Kaplan's cardinal line (Fig. 39.6).
4. Dorsally, skin flaps are raised radially and ulnarly, taking care to avoid injury to the distal branches of the radial nerve which are found immediately subcutaneously (Fig. 39.7).
5. Length can be obtained on the median nerve branch by interfascicular dissection proximal to the carpal tunnel.
6. Once an adequate length is achieved, the fascicles of the common digital branch are divided and then transposed dorsally through a subcutaneous tunnel in the first webspace.
7. The nerves are coapted on the dorsal hand with 9-0 nylon suture.

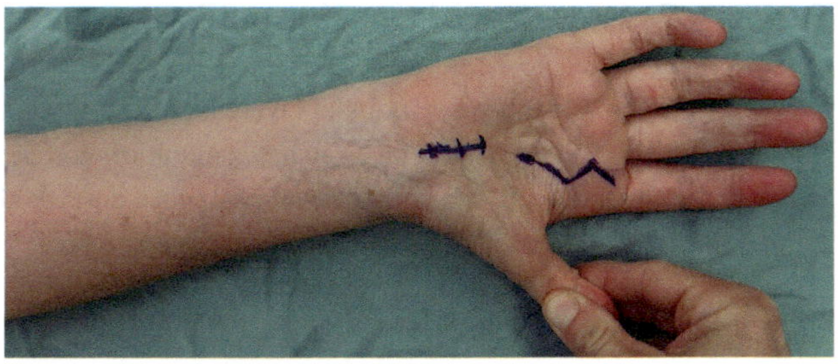

Fig. 39.4 Volar incisions for identification of the median nerve and common digital branches

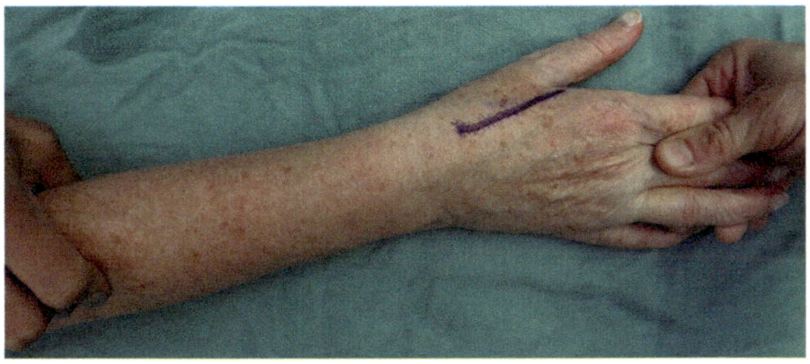

Fig. 39.5 Dorsal incision for identification of distal radial sensory branches

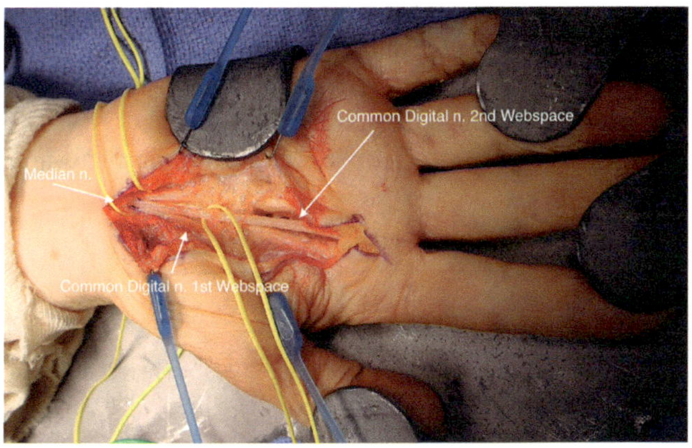

Fig. 39.6 Identification of the common digital nerve to the first webspace

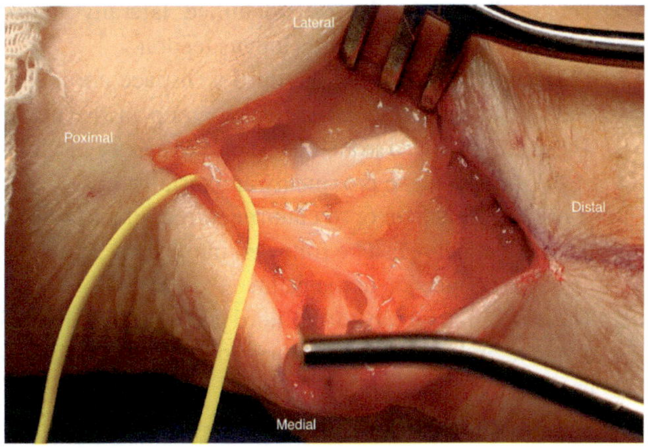

Fig. 39.7 Identification of the distal radial sensory nerve on the dorsum of the hand

Sensory Restoration of the Ulnar Nerve

Sensory restoration of the ulnar nerve is primarily focused on providing protective sensation to the medial side of the hand and the small finger. The most commonly described transfers are those of the common digital nerve to the third webspace to the ulnar sensory branch after the take-off of the dorsal branch of the ulnar nerve and those which use the lateral antebrachial cutaneous (LABC) nerve as donors.

Common Digital Nerve to Third Webspace to Ulnar Sensory Nerve Transfer

1. A longitudinal incision is designed over the FCU in the medial forearm. This extends in a zigzag fashion starting several centimeters proximal to the proximal wrist crease and connected to an incision slightly ulnar to a standard open carpal tunnel incision in the palm (just radial to the hook of the hamate).
2. Guyon's canal is opened to identify the ulnar neurovascular bundle. The ulnar vessels are swept laterally to fully expose the ulnar nerve.
3. The motor component can be identified by releasing the hypothenar muscular attachment to the hook of the hamate. This may be needed to confirm the targeted sensory fascicles of the ulnar nerve.
4. Dissection is continued proximally in the forearm, following the ulnar nerve deep to the FCU tendon.
5. The sensory component is followed and should continue as the radial superficial fascicles in the forearm.

6. The median nerve is then identified laterally in the wound, deep to the palmaris longus tendon.
7. The sensory fascicles to the third webspace are identified as the most medial fascicular group in the nerve. These are separated from the rest of the sensory fascicles of the median nerve proximally and distally.
8. If needed for length or to confirm correct identification, the median nerve can be followed into the carpal tunnel through the incision in the palm.
9. The fascicular group to the third webspace is divided distally, and the ulnar sensory component is divided proximally.
10. Coaptation is performed using 9-0 nylon suture in the distal forearm.

Sensory Restoration of the Radial Nerve

It is important to distinguish between anesthesia or diminished sensation in the radial sensory distribution and causalgia or paresthesia due to radial nerve injury, as these present distinct pathological entities with different therapeutic considerations. Sensory restoration of the radial nerve is much less commonly described or pursued as the functional disturbance of radial sensory denervation is much less apparent than in the case of median and ulnar nerves. In addition, the dorsal hand is rarely a contact surface, and its sensation is not critical in prehensile activities.

Radial Sensory to Median End-to-Side

1. A 10 cm incision is designed on the radial aspect of the mid-to-distal forearm.
2. Dissection is carried out proximally between the flexor carpi radialis (FCR) and the brachioradialis (BR) muscle bellies to identify the radial sensory branch, which will be seen coursing deep to the brachioradialis tendon. This is followed proximally to its takeoff and divided proximally for length.
3. The median nerve is identified more distally in the wound, coursing deep and ulnar to the FCR tendon, and followed proximally.
4. The epineurium is incised on the ulnovolar portion of the median nerve corresponding to the fascicular group to the third webspace.
5. A small neurotomy is performed in this fascicular group to promote axonal sprouting.
6. The distal stump of the radial nerve is brought medially and coapted to the ulnovolar portion of the median nerve in an end-to-side fashion.

Sensory Restoration of the Plantar Foot

Lower extremity sensory nerve transfers were first described in the early 1980s and have recently regained attention for the treatment of diabetic neuropathy. Agarwal et al. have described saphenous to tibial nerve transfer with promising results [6].

1. Incision is designed anterior to the medial malleolus, and the saphenous nerve runs with the saphenous vein, which is palpable in many patients.
2. The nerve is dissected proximally for approximately 7 cm or as much a length as needed for a tension-free coaptation
3. A separate incision is made posterior to the medial malleolus to identify the posterior tibial neurovascular bundle.
4. The tibial nerve is identified just posterior to the vascular bundle in the tarsal tunnel; this is followed proximally and distally.
5. Intraoperative nerve stimulation is used to identify the sensory fascicles of the tibial nerve, and intraneural dissection is performed to separate them from the motor fascicles.
6. A subcutaneous tunnel is made for the passage of the saphenous nerve posteriorly for coaptation.
7. Sensory fascicles of the tibial nerve are divided proximally after adequate intraneural dissection.
8. The saphenous nerve is divided distally and transferred posteriorly through the subcutaneous tunnel.
9. End-to-end coaptation is performed using the microsurgical technique.

References

1. Boyd KU, Nimigan AS, Mackinnon SE (2011) Nerve reconstruction in the hand and upper extremity. Clin Plast Surg 38(4):643–660. https://doi.org/10.1016/j.cps.2011.07.008
2. Brown JM, Mackinnon SE (2008) Nerve transfers in the forearm and hand. Hand Clin 24(4):319–340. https://doi.org/10.1016/j.hcl.2008.08.002
3. Bertelli JA, Ghizoni MF (2003) Nerve repair by end-to-side coaptation or fascicular transfer: a clinical study. J Reconstr Microsurg 19(5):313–318. https://doi.org/10.1055/s-2003-42499
4. Bertelli JA (2012) Distal sensory nerve transfers in lower-type injuries of the brachial plexus. J Hand Surg Am 37(6):1194–1199. https://doi.org/10.1016/j.jhsa.2012.02.047. Epub 2012 Apr 24
5. Bertelli JA, Ghizoni MF (2011) Very distal sensory nerve transfers in high median nerve lesions. J Hand Surg 36(3):387–393. https://doi.org/10.1016/j.jhsa.2010.11.049. Epub 2011 Feb 4
6. Agarwal P, Sharma D, Nebhani D, Kukrele R, Kukrele P (2021) Saphenous nerve to posterior tibial nerve transfer: a new approach to restore sensations of sole in diabetic sensory polyneuropathy. J Plast Reconstr Aesthet Surg 74(9):2110–2119. https://doi.org/10.1016/j.bjps.2021.01.012. Epub 2021 5

Contralateral C7 Transfer for Brachial Plexus Injuries

40

Ann R. Schwentker, Liann C. Casey, and Kevin J. Little

Indications

In cases where there are insufficient nerve donors on the injured side, the use of a contralateral C7 (cC7) has been described for reconstruction of the brachial plexus [1]. Long subcutaneous nerve grafts give poor results. Use of ipsilateral vascularized ulnar nerve graft has been used in adults [2]. For children, dissection of a retropharyngeal tunnel allows short nerve grafts to be used for reconstruction and decreases the time to reinnervation [3]. In very young children, independent function without the need for mirror movement may be achieved [4]. Because of the risks, retropharyngeal cross C7 transfer is best reserved for severe injuries with four or five nerve root avulsions (preganglionic injury resulting in a flail arm) where ipsilateral donor nerves are severely lacking. The middle trunk contains fewer motor axons than the other trunks, and in cases where c5 is intact, use of grafts from C5 to the lower trunk and cC7 to the upper trunk is preferred (Fig. 40.1). In cases where five roots are avulsed, cC7 to the lower trunk can provide a usable grasp. Spinal accessory can be transferred to the suprascapular nerve to provide external rotation and up to 90° of abduction, and intercostals are used for the musculocutaneous nerve to provide elbow flexion.

Supplementary Information The online version contains supplementary material available at https://doi.org/10.1007/978-3-031-73931-6_40.

A. R. Schwentker (✉)
University of Cincinnati, Cincinnati Children's Hospital Medical Center, Cincinnati, OH, USA
e-mail: Ann.schwentker@cchmc.org

L. C. Casey
University of Cincinnati, Cincinnati, OH, USA
e-mail: caseyln@ucmail.uc.edu

K. J. Little
Cincinnati Children's Hospital Medical Center, Cincinnati, OH, USA
e-mail: Kevin.little@cchmc.org

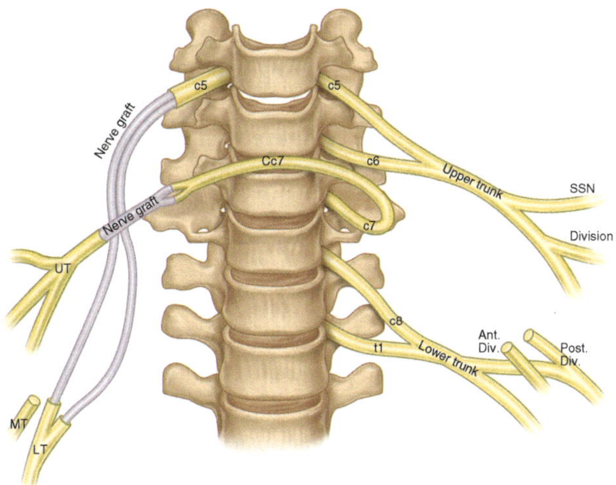

Fig. 40.1 Contralateral C7 transfer to the upper trunk via nerve grafts. Neuroma at C5 has been resected with sural nerve grafts from C5 to the lower trunk. The middle trunk is left unreconstructed and can serve as a nerve graft material

Surgical Technique

1. Position: supine with a shoulder roll, both arms and the entire neck prepped and draped. The head is turned side to side during the procedure to facilitate exposure.
2. Dissection of the injured plexus is performed to determine the nature of the injury.
3. Dissection of the uninjured plexus is then performed to identify all spinal nerves, trunks, and divisions.
4. Beginning at the C6 tubercle, blunt dissection across the longus colli muscles allows safe passage across the neck behind the esophagus in a relatively avascular plane. The plane of dissection is behind the anterior scalene muscles to protect the phrenic nerves. Sharp dissection is avoided.
5. A Penrose drain is passed through the tunnel and used to retract the neck structures anteriorly.

A. S. Hanna (ed.), *Nerves: Anatomy, Exposures, and Techniques*, https://doi.org/10.1007/978-3-031-73931-6_40

6. The uninjured plexus is stimulated to ensure that the structures are all accurately identified.
7. The anterior and posterior divisions of the middle trunk are divided as far distally as possible, being certain not to injure the lower trunk contribution to the posterior cord.
8. Division of the C7 contribution to the long thoracic nerve will also be required to allow cC7 to reach as far as possible.
9. A red rubber catheter with the end cut off is passed through the neck and used to gently suction cC7 through the tunnel.
10. The injured upper or lower trunk is cut back to the uninjured nerve under a microscope magnification.
11. Sural nerve grafts or ipsilateral middle trunk can be used to bridge the gap (typically 2–5 cm) between cC7 and the recipient plexus, targeting either the lower trunk or upper trunk.
12. Neurorrhaphy can be completed with fibrin glue in children. Sutures are preferred in adults.

Complications

1. Damage to one or both phrenic nerves. In infants, phrenic nerve paresis often presents as failure to thrive and requires nasogastric tube feeding until the child recovers. Bilateral phrenic nerve injury can require prolonged ventilator support.
2. Esophageal leak can lead to infection and potential mediastinitis.
3. Injury to the normal plexus resulting in permanent deficits. Temporary triceps weakness lasting less than 3 weeks occurs in less than half of infants. Minor sensory deficits are less common in children than adults.
4. Thoracic duct injury or lymphatic leak.
5. Pneumothorax during dissection of T1.
6. Bleeding due to vascular injury.
7. Wound infection is extremely uncommon.

References

1. Gu YD, Zhang GM, Chen DS, Cheng XM, Zhang LY, Yan JG et al (1991) Cervical nerve root transfer from contralateral normal side for treatment of brachial plexus root avulsions. Chin Med J (Engl) 104(3):208–211
2. Chen L, Gu YD (1994) An experimental study of contralateral c7 root transfer with vascularized nerve grafting to treat brachial plexus root avulsion. J Hand Surg Br 19(1):60–66. https://doi.org/10.1016/0266-7681(94)90051-5
3. Mcguiness CN, Kay SP (2002) The prespinal route in contralateral c7 nerve root transfer for brachial plexus avulsion injuries. J Hand Surg Br 27(2):159–160. https://doi.org/10.1054/jhsb.2001.0665
4. Vu AT, Sparkman DM, van Belle CJ, Yakuboff KP, Schwentker AR (2018) Retropharyngeal contralateral c7 nerve transfer to the lower trunk for brachial plexus birth injury: technique and results. J Hand Surg Am 43(5):417–424. https://doi.org/10.1016/j.jhsa.2017.12.001. Epub 2018 Feb 3

Free Functioning Muscle Transfer in Brachial Plexus Reconstruction

41

Nicole A. Zelenski and Alexander Y. Shin

Introduction of the Concept of Free Functioning Muscle Transfer

Rationale

A free functioning muscle transfer (FFMT) is a muscle that has been removed from its native location with its nerve and vascular pedicle and transferred to another location in the body for the purpose of restoring motor function. The vascular pedicle is anastomosed to a donor artery and vein to restore perfusion. Similarly, the motor nerve of the transferred muscle is coapted to a donor motor nerve. The donor nerve axons grow into the FFMT nerve and ultimately reinnervate the muscle.

Indications

A FFMT has been used to reanimate/reconstruct a number of functions, including finger flexion after Volkmann's ischemic contracture [1], facial expression in Bell's palsy [2], and elbow flexion in brachial plexus injuries (BPI) [3]. FFMTs were first described for brachial plexus reconstruction by Ikuta et al., who used a gracilis muscle to restore elbow flexion in a 10-year-old child with chronic BPI [3]. FFMT can be used for reconstruction of BPI in both the acute [4, 5] and chronic setting [6–8]. It is commonly used in chronic BPI that present late and are outside the window where primary nerve surgery can provide acceptable recovery. After chronic denervation or time from injury greater than 9–12 months, primary nerve surgery is not typically successful, and the use of an FFMT provides an alternative treatment option in these cases. A FFMT transferred from another site provides a muscle that can be innervated by a functioning extraplexal nerve to restore function. Typically, FFMTs are used to restore elbow flexion in the chronic setting but can also be used to restore elbow extension, wrist/finger extension, or finger flexion.

FFMTs have been applied in acute pan plexus injuries to restore rudimentary grasp [4, 5] and elbow flexion [9, 10]. A muscle with a proximally located neurovascular pedicle with a distal long tendon, such as gracilis, is ideal for FFMT in brachial plexus reconstructions.

Contraindications

For a FFMT to restore a function, several requirements must be met. The first is a supple limb with a clean and relatively scar-free recipient bed. Elbow or hand contracture is a contraindication and must be addressed prior to reconstruction. Surgical release followed by extensive therapy may be necessary to prepare a limb for receipt of a FFMT. The extremity must also have a recipient site with a suitably located and uninjured artery, nerve, and vein to be used for coaptations. In brachial plexus reconstruction, the thoracoacromial artery is a reliable donor artery and cephalic vein is a reliable donor vein. Vascular injuries to the thoracoacromial artery or subclavian artery system have demonstrated inferior outcomes after gracilis FFMT [11]. This is likely due to the awkward inset of the flap when other donor vessels, such as the thoracodorsal artery, are used. The FFMT is ideally attached proximally on the acromion and clavicle; thus, anastomosis to a vessel other than the thoracoacromial trunk precludes this ideal inset and may negatively affect outcomes [11]. The donor nerve ideally should be uninjured by trauma, demonstrate

Supplementary Information The online version contains supplementary material available at https://doi.org/10.1007/978-3-031-73931-6_41.

N. A. Zelenski
Department of Orthopaedics, Emory University School of Medicine, Atlanta, GA, USA
e-mail: nicole.ann.zelenski@emory.edu

A. Y. Shin (✉)
Mayo Clinic, Division of Hand Surgery, Department of Orthopaedic Surgery, Rochester, MN, USA
e-mail: shin.alexander@mayo.edu

A. S. Hanna (ed.), *Nerves: Anatomy, Exposures, and Techniques*, https://doi.org/10.1007/978-3-031-73931-6_41

normal motor function, and be expendable without decreasing a necessary function to the patient. Spinal accessory, intercostals, and long thoracic nerves can be used. Nerve grafts should be avoided if possible, as this negatively affects outcomes.

FFMT Choices

A number of muscles can be used for reconstruction after BPI and include the gracilis, latissimus dorsi, adductor longus, and rectus femoris. The gracilis is the most commonly used FFMT [12]. Although the rectus femoris and latissimus dorsi have excellent strength due to the large cross-sectional area with strong contractile force, the excursion, bulk, and lack of tendon at both ends make application difficult. Although the gracilis has considerably less cross-sectional area than the rectus femoris, latissimus, or biceps muscle that it is intended to replace, it is superior in excursion and has excellent proximal and distal tendons for attachment. The gracilis configuration makes it ideal for elbow flexion as well as finger flexion. Other advantages to gracilis for FFMT include the proximal position of its neurovascular pedicle, which permits rapid reinnervation from the donor nerve, and its long length and shape facilitate its subcutaneous passage into the forearm to reanimate the wrist and hand [12].

Evaluation of Patient, Preoperative Testing, Prerequisites for Use

FFMT is one of the most complex techniques in brachial plexus reconstruction. The following should be evaluated prior to surgery.

Passive Range of Motion

Full passive range of motion across the joint to be reanimated is essential. If stiffness is present, physical therapy should first be considered. If physical therapy fails, surgical release may be indicated. Patients with avulsion injury may develop a hand with a stiff and edematous intrinsic-minus posture with fixed finger metacarpophalangeal joint extension. These patients require restoration of supple joints and may later require positioning of metacarpophalangeal joints in a flexed posture by tenodesis, capsulodesis, or arthrodesis to optimize outcomes of finger flexion.

Vascular Assessment of the Donor Artery

A good artery is mandatory for anastomosis of the FFMT, and assessment should be performed prior to surgery. Vascular injuries are common in adult BPI, occurring in >10% of patients [2]. The rate is >30% in the American population with pan plexus injuries. Generally, it is our practice to use the thoracoacromial artery if the FFMT is transferred for brachial plexus reconstructions. Avulsion of the subclavian or axillary vessels is generally a contraindication for FFMT because patency of the thoracoacromial or thoracodorsal vessels is needed for the FFMT anastomosis. Additionally, concomitant vascular injury has been associated with worse functional outcome following reconstructive surgery of adult traumatic BPI [11]. Computerized tomographic angiography (CTA) or digital subtraction angiography (DSA) can be useful to assess upper extremity vascularity and donor vessels.

Donor Nerve

There must be an uninjured, expendable motor nerve in close proximity to the neurovascular pedicle of the transferred muscle. In most brachial plexus cases, this will be an extraplexal nerve (spinal accessory nerve or intercostal nerves). Other nerves can be used as well, including contralateral C7 or intraplexal donors such as a fascicle of an intact ulnar nerve or long thoracic nerve [13]. Electrodiagnostic studies can help rule out nerves that have been injured but often must be specifically requested to be evaluated. Ultimately, intraoperative stimulation of the nerve is required to determine the viability of the donor nerve.

Stable Wound Bed

A stable wound bed free of scars is required for transfer. Although some FFMT such as gracilis can be transferred in its fascial sheath, a well-vascularized bed is a requisite for tendon gliding. Similarly, there must be adequate skin coverage to cover the muscle after transfer. Skin grafting on a FFMT may lead to adhesions and decrease excursion of the muscle. Although a small skin paddle can be harvested with the gracilis, larger skin paddles extending beyond the proximal 1/3 of the muscle can lead to venous congestion if not harvested with additional venous outflow [14].

Anatomy of the Gracilis

The gracilis muscle is located in the medial thigh and originates from the lower half of the symphysis pubis and medial portion of the inferior pubic ramus by a thin aponeurosis. The muscle is flat and courses distally until it ends in a round tendon that inserts onto the medial surface of the proximal tibia after passing posterior to the medial femoral condyle

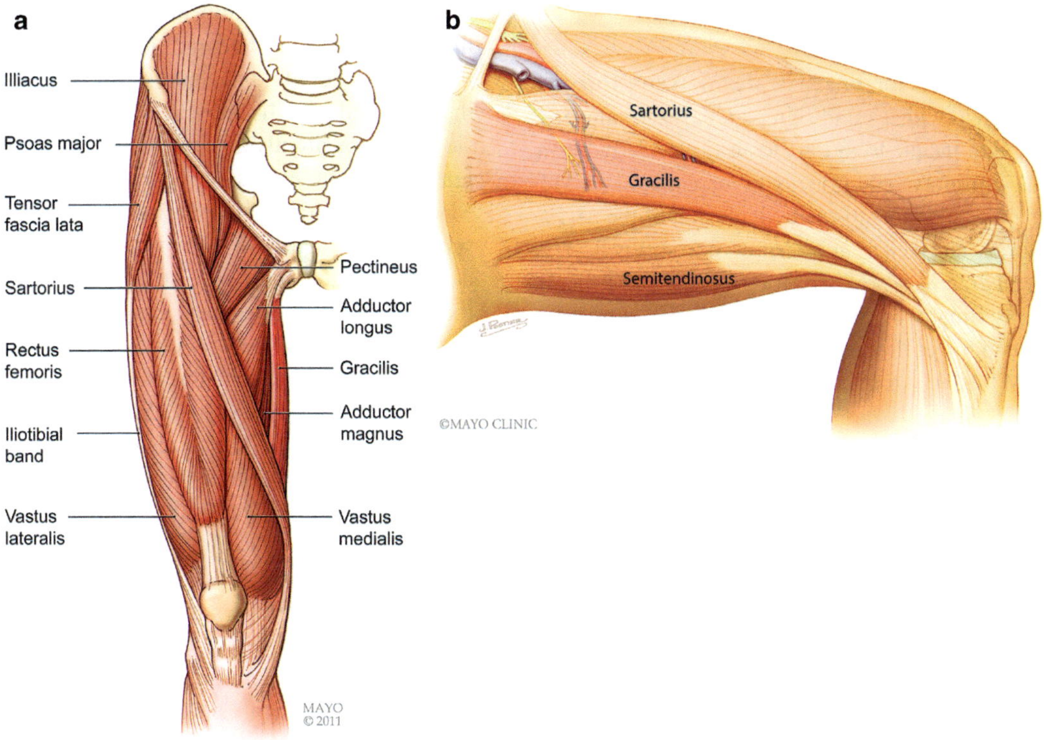

Fig. 41.1 Anatomy. The gracilis muscle is situated in the medial thigh and is the most superficial of the adductor muscle group. Used with permission of Mayo Foundation for Medical Education and Research. All rights reserved [16]

(Fig. 41.1). It acts as one of four adductors and both flexes and medially rotates the leg. The gracilis muscle measures approximately 5–6 cm in width, 24–30 cm in length, and has an additional 10–12 cm of tendon. The muscle is thin and flat proximally (approximately 2–5 cm in thickness), becomes round in the middle, and tapers to the size of the gracilis tendon distally.

Regarding its blood supply, the gracilis is a type II muscle (one dominant pedicle and minor pedicle(s)) per the Mathes and Nahai's classification [15]. The larger dominant vascular pedicle is the medial femoral circumflex artery and is capable of sustaining the circulation of the muscle even after division of the minor pedicles. The dominant vascular pedicle can originate from the profunda femoris artery or the medial circumflex femoral vessels [12]. In this exposure, the pedicle courses beneath the adductor longus muscle and superficial to the adductor magnus muscle, giving off branches to these muscles along its course, which must be carefully ligated during dissection. The length of the pedicle is 6–8 cm from the profunda femoris and has a diameter of approximately 1.6–1.8 mm.

The veins of the gracilis muscle are the venae comitantes of the medial circumflex artery. The entire muscle and proximal half of the cutaneous territory are drained by the venae comitantes into the deep veins associated with the profunda femoris artery. The proximal veins of the pedicle have a lumen diameter of 1.5–2.5 mm. The size of the skin paddle is limited by the cutaneous drainage of the venae comitantes, and large skin paddle over distal muscle should be avoided.

The motor nerve of the gracilis muscle is from the anterior branch of the obturator nerve. The nerve enters the muscle separately and superior to the major vascular pedicle by approximately 2–3 cm. The motor nerve is dissected proximally between the adductor longus and magnus to increase length. The motor nerve gives off branches to the adductor muscles throughout its course, and an interfascicular dissection should be performed to increase length of the nerve.

The vascularization of the medial thigh skin is variable and is not entirely from musculocutaneous perforating vessels from the gracilis. The reliable island of skin based off the medial femoral circumflex relies on small perforating musculocutaneous arteries that are distributed mostly over the proximal portion of the muscle [16]. The skin paddle typically measures up to 8 × 24 cm and is usually designed over the proximal two-thirds of the muscle to ensure inclusion of both perforating arteries as well as adequate venous drainage [10, 16]. To improve the survival of the skin flap, it is best to include the fascia surrounding the gracilis [10].

Surgical Technique

1. The gracilis FFMT for brachial plexus reconstruction may be designed with a small skin paddle for monitoring or a larger skin paddle to aid in closure in a scarred or a contracted extremity. The gracilis myocutaneous FFMT requires careful planning to ensure inclusion of the perforating arteries and veins and ensure skin survival. The contralateral gracilis is preferred for gracilis FFMT that is anchored proximally on the clavicle/acromion to be used for biceps and finger flexion reconstruction, as the vessels of the FFMT have direct course to the thoracoacromial artery.
2. The harvest is started distally at the knee over the pes anserinus. The tibial plateau is marked, and a longitudinal skin incision is made approximately 4 cm distal to the plateau on the medial face of the tibia (Fig. 41.2a). The gracilis tendon can be palpated and is the most superior tendinous insertion. The sartorius fascia is incised, taking care not to penetrate the tendons beneath. The most proximal tendon is the tendon from the gracilis muscle and is dissected until umbilical tape can be placed circumferentially around the tendon (Fig. 41.2b). A 4 cm incision is made in the distal thigh while pulling the distal tendon which tents the skin in the distal medial thigh (Fig. 41.2c). The myotendinous portion of the gracilis is identified. The entire gracilis can be pulled to confirm continuity with the tendon located in the proximal tibia. All soft tissue attachments are divided subcutaneously as well as circumferentially around the distal muscle under the skin bridge until the tendon glides smoothly.
3. Once the tendinous portion has been identified and freed, traction is applied causing the entire muscle to "bowstring," outlining the specific area of cutaneous territory overlying the muscle (Fig. 41.2d). This skin can be incorporated into the musculocutaneous flap if required. At this point, we recommend using a handheld sterile Doppler to identify and mark skin perforators overlying the proximal gracilis muscle. An elliptical shaped incision is drawn slightly anterior to the anterior border of the gracilis muscle, including the identified skin perforators. Since the perorating vessels arise through the anterior septum, it is important to include this area in the paddle design for better survival. This is a slight modification of the original technique where the paddle was placed more posteriorly (Fig. 41.2e).
4. The proximal thigh incision is made along the anterior border of the skin paddle, and dissection is carried toward the adductor longus. The fascia of the adductor longus is incised and the fascial edge sewn to the skin paddle (Fig. 41.3a and b). The fascia of the adductor longus is retracted to expose the obturator nerve and medial femoral circumflex artery, which are dissected proximally. The adductor longus can be retracted medially and superiorly to give gentle traction on the perforators to this muscle for ligation. Once perforators to the adductor longus are ligated, the pedicles are dissected to the profunda femoris (Fig. 41.3c). The obturator nerve is identified as entering the deep surface of the gracilis obliquely to the vascular pedicle and can be stimulated with a nerve stimulator to verify contraction (Fig. 41.3d). A vessel loop is placed around the nerve, and dissection should be carried as far proximal as possible. To increase length of nerve, the branches to the adductor muscles are meticulously dissected in an interfascicular fashion from the gracilis motor branch before cutting it. A nerve pedicle of 8–12 cm can be obtained; it is imperative to have a long nerve pedicle for a proper insert. The gracilis muscle fascia should not be penetrated, and muscle should not be visible (Fig. 41.3e).

Fig. 41.2 Distal harvest. (**a**) When a full length gracilis is needed, the harvest begins distally, where the gracilis tendon at the pes anserinus can be identified (*b*). *a* distal thigh incision overlying musculotendinous junction of gracilis, *c* distal pole of the patella, *d* tibial tuberosity. (**b**) At the pes anserinus, the gracilis tendon is the most proximal tendinous insertion while the distal tendon is the semitendinosus tendon. Once the superficial overlying sartorius fascia is divided, umbilical tape is placed around the superior gracilis tendon, and the multiple soft tissue attachments to the gracilis tendon are divided. (**c**) The gracilis tendon can be pulled, causing the distal muscle to "bowstring," and an incision can be drawn over the musculotendinous junction (*a*). *b* incision over pes anserinus (**d**) Multiple soft tissue attachments are released between the two tendons, and traction can be applied to the muscle/tendon, causing the entire muscle extending to the pubic symphysis to "bowstring," outlining the area of cutaneous territory overlying the muscle that may be incorporated into the musculocutaneous flap if required. (**e**) A sterile Doppler can be used to identify and mark skin perforators overlying the proximal gracilis muscle and an elliptical shaped incision drawn slightly anterior to the anterior border of the gracilis muscle, including the identified skin perforators. Since the perorating vessels arise through the anterior septum, it is important to include this area in the paddle design. The surgical marking (*a*) indicates a classic area of skin paddle centered over the gracilis muscle. Yellow circle (*b*) indicates new anterior location of skin paddle. Used with permission of Mayo Foundation for Medical Education and Research. All rights reserved [16]

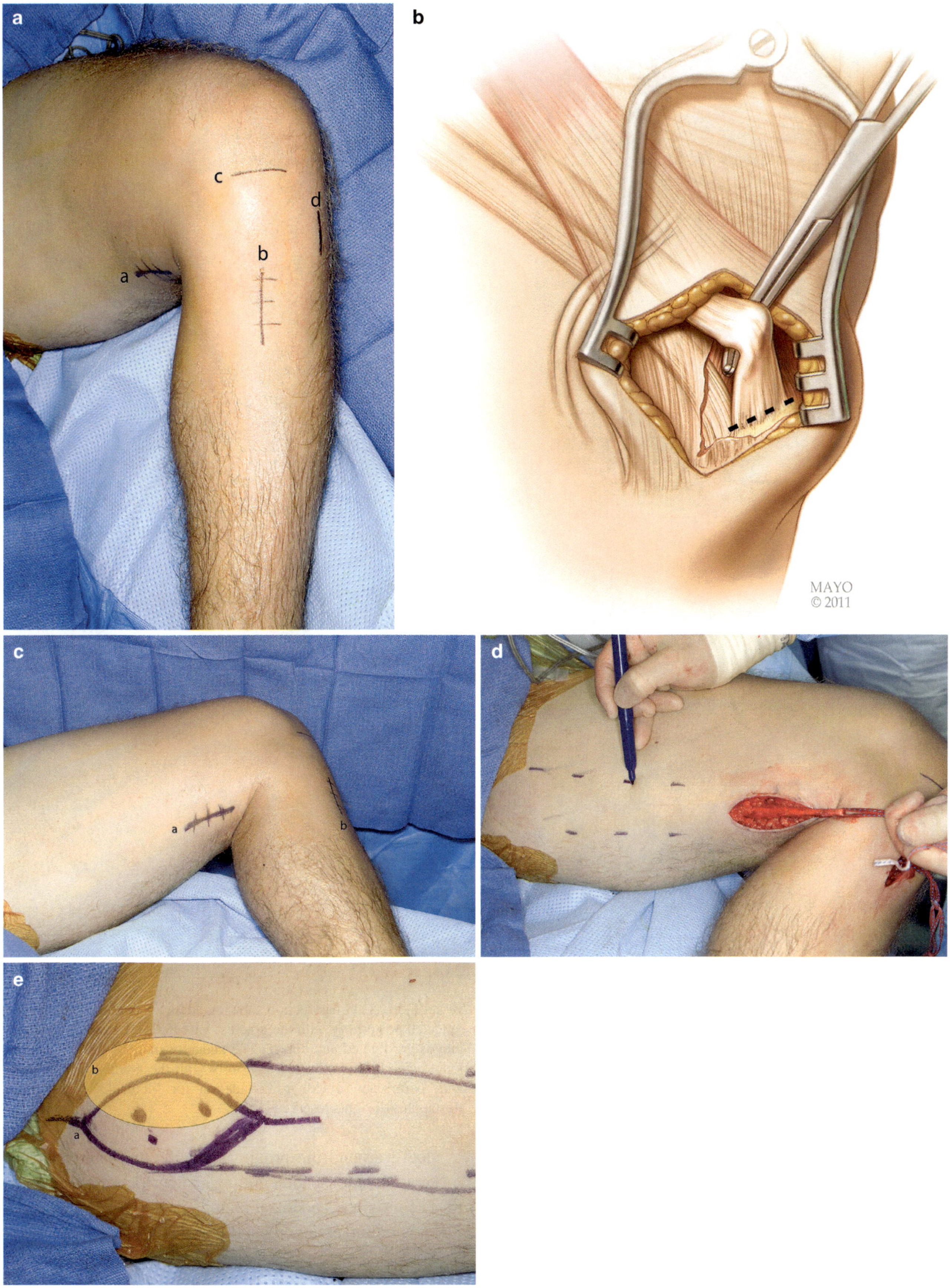
MAYO
© 2011

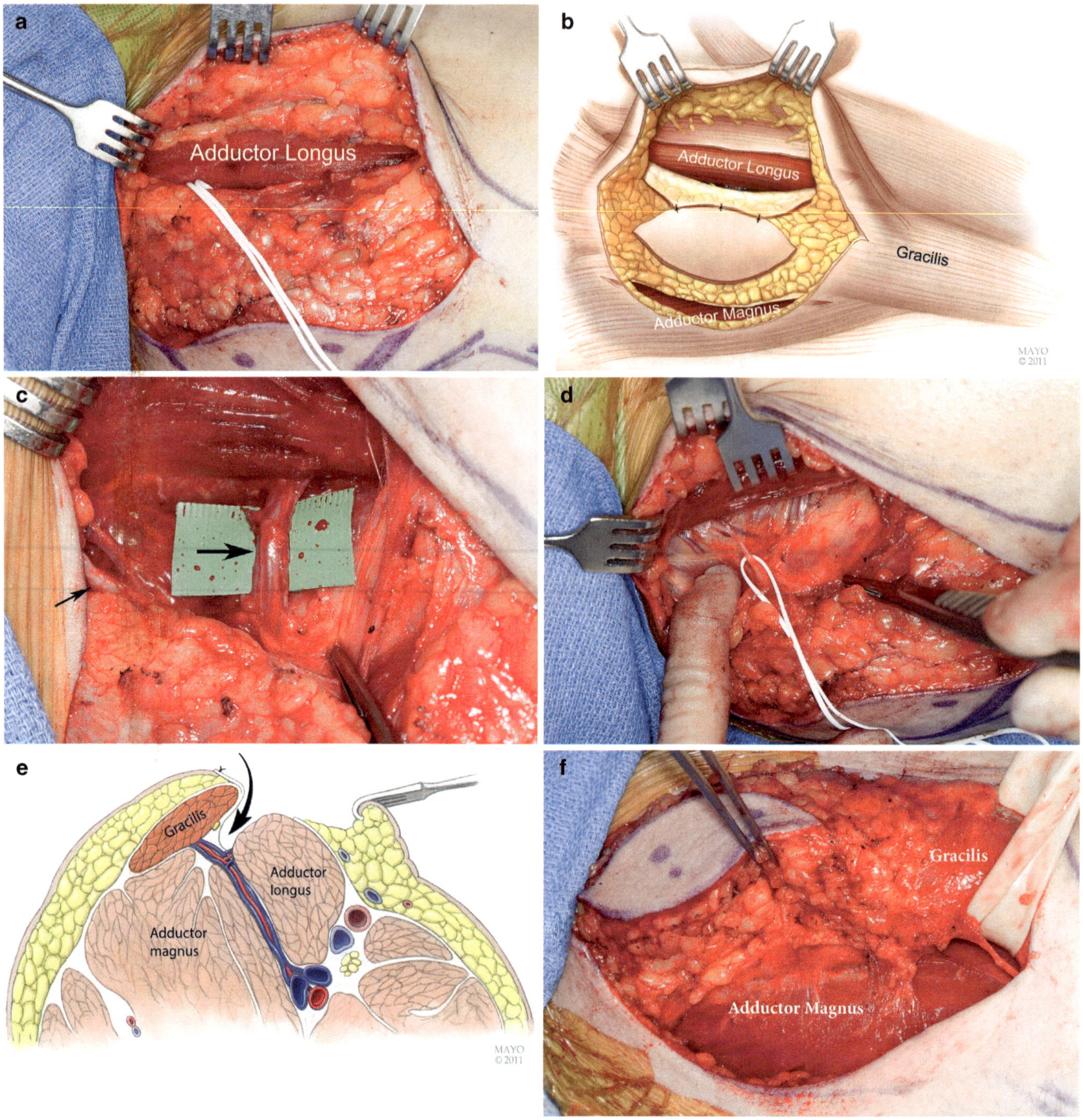

Fig. 41.3 Proximal dissection. (**a**) The fascia of the adductor longus is incised longitudinally and (**b**) The fascial edge is sewn to the skin paddle. The interval between the adductor longus and gracilis is developed. (**c**) The obturator nerve (*small arrow*) and the dominant proximal artery and venae comitantes (*large arrow*) are identified. (**d**) The adductor longus is retracted and the obturator branch to gracilis is isolated with a vessel loop. (**e**) Cross-section showing adductor longus fascia cut and reflected posteriorly with the gracilis. Vascular perforators to adductor longus are ligated and cut. (**f**) The adductor magnus fascia is incised longitudinally and reflected anteriorly with the gracilis muscle. Used with permission of Mayo Foundation for Medical Education and Research. All rights reserved [16]

5. The posterior skin paddle incision is made and dissection carried down to the level of the adductor magnus muscle. The adductor magnus fascia is incised longitudinally and reflected with the gracilis muscle (Fig. 41.3f). A fascial sleeve around the proximal gracilis and skin paddle is kept intact for tendon gliding and perforator protection.
6. The proximal and distal thigh incisions can be connected by blunt finger dissection in the areolar plane. The second

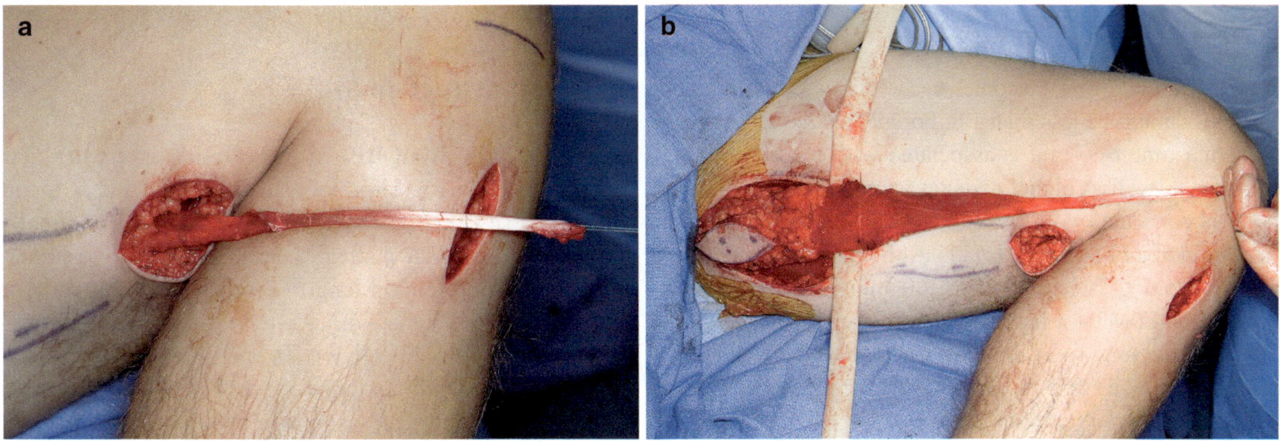

Fig. 41.4 Final steps. (**a**) The distal tendon of the gracilis is then detached from the pes anserinus and passed first into the distal thigh incision. (**b**) The gracilis muscle is then gently delivered out of the proximal thigh incision. Used with permission of Mayo Foundation for Medical Education and Research. All rights reserved [16]

(minor) pedicle can often be felt and can be ligated. The distal tendon is finally detached from the pes anserinus and passed into the distal thigh incision and then out of the proximal thigh incision (Fig. 41.4a). The entire gracilis muscle and tendon can be delivered out of the proximal incision (Fig. 41.4b).

7. At this point, the gracilis is attached only by the proximal tendinous origin at the pubic tubercle and the vascular pedicle. The proximal attachment is tendinous laterally and muscular medially. The tendon is dissected off the adductor longus tendon, and using an angled electrocautery tip, the gracilis tendon is detached from the public rami. The flap harvest is now complete. A papaverine-soaked sponge is placed over the vessels until the recipient site has been prepared. The skin paddle can be temporarily stapled to the anterior skin incision to prevent tension on the pedicle until the FFMT is ready to be transferred.
8. The flap should be inset on the distal clavicle/acromion. Prior to removal of the gracilis from the leg, the upper extremity is prepared. The donor vessels are identified and dissected free; the donor nerve is dissected and placed near the donor vessels. In a patient who has a complete BPI, the pectoralis major tendon is released to allow for a straight course of the gracilis muscle. In a partial injury, if pectoralis major is functional, it is not released. Transosseous sutures are placed through the acromion, and suture anchors are placed in the distal clavicle to secure the proximal tendon of the gracilis. Subcutaneous tunnels are fashioned, and the distal tendon insertion is prepared. Occasionally, the gracilis distal tendon needs to be prolonged. Harvest of the flexor carpi radialis or the semitendinosus tendon is performed, and the tendon graft is Pulvertaft woven into the distal gracilis tendon prior to transfer. The microscope is set up, the gracilis vascular pedicle is clamped and disconnected, and the gracilis is ready for transfer. After removal from the leg, the proximal tendon should be secured to the acromion and clavicle using the previously placed sutures. The gracilis vessels are placed at the same level as the thoracoacromial artery. Re-establishment of vascular flow within 60 min of ischemia time is ideal. After the vascular anastomoses are complete, the donor motor nerve can be coapted to the obturator branch of the gracilis. Finally, tensioning of the gracilis is performed. The flap is tensioned such that the elbow is maintained in 30° of flexion at rest. The distal tendon is woven into the biceps tendon for elbow flexion and possibly the flexor digitorum profundus (FDP) for finger flexion.

Tips/Tricks

Long Obturator Nerve Harvest, Long Intercostal or XI Harvest

It is of utmost importance to obtain primary coaptation of the obturator nerve to the motor neurotizer in the upper extremity. A nerve graft can drastically decrease functional outcomes and should be avoided. To do this, a very long obturator nerve must be harvested during the gracilis harvest. An interfascicular dissection excluding the adductor motor branches can be used to obtain a long obturator nerve graft with the gracilis. Similarly, spinal accessary as well as intercostal nerves should be harvested as distally as possible to increase excursion.

Short Ischemia Time

In order to maximize outcomes, ischemia time in functional muscles should be less than 1 h. For all free tissue transfers, ischemia time >60 min is associated with total and partial flap loss as well as higher revision rates [17]. Ischemia time >4 h is correlated with a complete lack of functional reinnervation of a FFMT muscle [17]. Although there is no direct data indicating ischemia time <60 min improves muscle strength in FFMT for brachial plexopathy, significantly longer ischemia time was found in patients who had bad results (MRC grade < 3) than those with MRC grade > 3 in gracilis FFMT transferred for elbow flexion [18].

Anatomical Landmarks

Use of the distal-first harvest technique described in this chapter allows for easy identification of the gracilis tendon and, by proxy, the muscle for harvest. If starting proximally, it can be difficult to distinguish the gracilis muscle from the adductor longus or sartorius in the medial thigh. With the knee at 90° and the hip abducted (i.e., figure of 4 position), the adductor longus is the most prominent and superficial muscle in the medial thigh. As such, it is often thought to be gracilis, and placement of the skin paddle over this muscle can be disastrous. The gracilis muscle can be marked prior to surgery by connecting the line from the pubic symphysis to the pes insertion. The gracilis muscle can be confirmed by firm palpation and "grabbing" of the muscle thought to be gracilis in the proximal thigh. This should stimulate contraction of the muscle visible at the knee, distal to the articulation of the femur and tibia. If the contraction ends proximal to the knee, it is likely the adductor longus muscle.

Team Approach

Several surgical teams are used to accomplish a single stage reconstruction in a timely fashion. The first team explores the brachial plexus, performs and interprets intraoperative neuromonitoring, and prepares the spinal accessory nerve. A second team prepares the gracilis muscle including the preparation of the recipient arm. If possible, a third team prepares the intercostal motor and sensory nerves, triceps and biceps motor nerves, and thoracoacromial vessels. Sural or radial sensory grafts are harvested by any available team. Typically, the entire procedure can be performed in 6–7 h with a three-team approach.

Expected Outcomes

Late Reconstruction

When the time from BPI to presentation is greater than 9–12 months, a FFMT is indicated. The gracilis is favorable in these situations because of the reliable, proximally based neurovascular pedicle that allows for early reinnervation and long tendon length. Proximally, the gracilis is secured to the clavicle, while distally, the gracilis tendon is woven into the biceps tendon. In one series, 79% of gracilis FFMT for elbow flexion alone achieved at least grade 4 strength [19]. A larger systematic review of patients with chronic BPI examining gracilis, rectus femoris, or latissimus FFMT found a mean success rate (MRC grade > 3) of 65% [20].

Double FFMT in Acute BPI

Doi et al. described a double gracilis transfer to provide elbow flexion and extension, hand sensibility, as well as grasp and release [21]. In the first stage, reconstruction of the shoulder is combined with a gracilis FFMT innervated by spinal accessory nerve to produced elbow flexion and finger extension. In the second procedure, a few weeks later, the other gracilis is transferred and neurotized to motor intercostal nerves and anastomosed to the finger flexor tendons to create elbow extension and finger flexion. The sensory intercostal nerves are neurotized to the lateral cord contribution of the median nerve for hand sensation. Doi reported good outcomes with the double gracilis FFMT procedure. Mean elbow power achieved with a double FFMT was MRC grade 3.9, and mean passive arc of motion was 112° [21, 22]. Satbhai et al. described higher improvement in the Disabilities of the Arm, Shoulder, and Hand (DASH) score compared to the single FFMT group; however, there was no significant correlation found between improvement in DASH and any other measured factor (age, shoulder range of motion, elbow range of motion, elbow flexion power, finger active movement) [22]. Despite this reported success with the Doi procedure, it is a daunting undertaking for both surgeon and patient and can have significant social and economic demands. Additionally, other groups have not had such promising results as Doi et al. In 2004, Barrie et al. reported worse elbow flexion strength in patients who had dual reconstruction than those who only underwent one gracilis FFMT for elbow flexion [23].

The Mayo Single FFMT in Acute BPI

Due to the relatively poor outcomes of the Doi procedure, the Mayo group made modifications of the gracilis FFMT originally described by Doi et al. A single gracilis FFMT is performed to restore both elbow flexion and finger flexion (Fig. 41.5). The gracilis is secured proximally to the clavicle with suture anchors as previously described. The muscle is tunneled into the forearm beneath the biceps tendon and lacertus to create a pulley effect. The vascular anastomosis is preferentially performed end-to-end to the thoracoacromial trunk, and the neurorrhaphy is completed with two intercostals or spinal accessory nerve. Triceps reanimation is necessary for independent finger flexion. Regardless of goals of hand function, the gracilis is inserted into the FDP tendons using a FCR autograft. Triceps reinnervation is typically accomplished by spinal accessory to triceps transfer with an interposition sural nerve graft. Second-stage surgery is usually necessary, consisting of wrist, first carpometacarpal, and thumb interphalangeal joint arthrodesis. These improve hand function, hand control, and appearance [21]. The main advantage of this technique is the ability to perform the entire reconstruction in a single stage. Barrie et al. described average elbow flexion strength of at least MRC grade 4 in 80% of patients after single-stage procedure. Additionally, it is our clinical experience that approximately 1 in 4 patients gain functional use of their hand that is useful for daily activities with a single stage reconstruction (unpublished data).

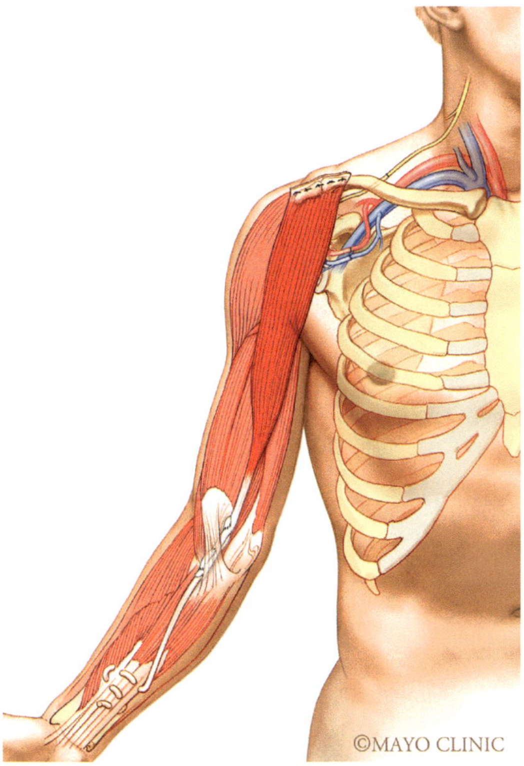

Fig. 41.5 Proximally, the gracilis is secured to the clavicle, while distally, the gracilis tendon is elongated with an FCR autograft and woven into the flexor digitorum profundus tendon. The nerve to gracilis is connected to the spinal accessory nerve (shown here) or intercostal nerves. The vascular pedicle is anastomosed to the thoracoacromial artery and cephalic vein. Used with permission of Mayo Foundation for Medical Education and Research. All rights reserved [16]

Summary

Free functioning muscle transfer is a powerful tool in upper extremity reconstruction for BPI when other options are not available. It can be used in chronic BPI after the time for nerve recovery has passed or in acute pan plexus injuries. Patient selection, an experienced surgical team, and excellent postoperative rehabilitation are keys to success.

References

1. Stevanovic M, Sharpe F (2014) Functional free muscle transfer for upper extremity reconstruction. Plast Reconstr Surg 134(2):257e–274e. https://doi.org/10.1097/PRS.0000000000000405
2. Sturm JT, Perry JF (1987) Brachial plexus injuries from blunt trauma—a harbinger of vascular and thoracic injury. Ann Emerg Med 16(4):404–406. https://doi.org/10.1016/s0196-0644(87)80359-1
3. Ikuta Y, Yoshioka K, Tsuge K (1979) Free muscle graft as applied to brachial plexus injury-case report and experimental study. Ann Acad Med Singap 8(4):454–458
4. Doi K, Muramatsu K, Hattori Y, Otsuka K, Tan SH, Nanda V et al (2000) Restoration of prehension with the double free muscle technique following complete avulsion of the brachial plexus. Indications and long-term results. J Bone Joint Surg Am 82(5):652–666
5. Shin AY, Spinner RJ, Steinmann SP, Bishop AT (2005) Adult traumatic brachial plexus injuries. J Am Acad Orthop Surg 13(6):382–396. https://doi.org/10.5435/00124635-200510000-00003
6. Giuffre JL, Kakar S, Bishop AT, Spinner RJ, Shin AY (2010) Current concepts of the treatment of adult brachial plexus injuries. J Hand Surg Am 35(4):678–688. https://doi.org/10.1016/j.jhsa.2010.01.021
7. Doi K, Kuwata N, Muramatsu K, Hottori Y, Kawai S (1999) Double muscle transfer for upper extremity reconstruction following complete avulsion of the brachial plexus. Hand Clin 15(4):757–767
8. Akasaka Y, Hara T, Takahashi M (1990) Restoration of elbow flexion and wrist extension in brachial plexus paralyses by means of free muscle transplantation innervated by intercostal nerve. Ann Chir Main Memb Super 9(5):341–350. https://doi.org/10.1016/s0753-9053(05)80507-1
9. Maldonado AA, Kircher MF, Spinner RJ, Bishop AT, Shin AY (2017) Free functioning gracilis muscle transfer with and without simultaneous intercostal nerve transfer to musculocutaneous nerve for restoration of ebow flexion after traumatic adult brachial pan-plexus injury. J Hand Surg Am 42(4):293.e1–293.e7. https://doi.org/10.1016/j.jhsa.2017.01.014. Epub 2017 Feb 27
10. Maldonado AA, Kircher MF, Spinner RJ, Bishop AT, Shin AY (2016) Free functioning gracilis muscle transfer versus intercostal nerve transfer to musculocutaneous nerve for restoration of

elbow flexion after traumatic adult brachial pan-plexus injury. Plast Reconstr Surg 138(3):483e–488e. https://doi.org/10.1097/PRS.0000000000002471
11. Huang AE, Noland SS, Spinner RJ, Bishop AT, Shin AY (2020) Outcomes of reconstructive surgery in traumatic brachial plexus injury with concomitant vascular injury. World Neurosurg 135:e350–e357. https://doi.org/10.1016/j.wneu.2019.11.166. Epub 2019 Dec 16
12. Spinner RJ, Shin AY, Elhassan BT, Bishop AT (2016) Traumatic brachial plexus injury. In: Wolfe SW, Hotchkiss RN, Pederson WC, Scott H, Kozin MD, Cohen MS (eds) Green's operative hand surgery. Elsevier, Philadelphia, PA, pp 1146–1207
13. Soldado F, Bertelli J (2013) Free gracilis transfer reinnervated by the nerve to the supinator for the reconstruction of finger and thumb extension in longstanding C7-T1 brachial plexus root avulsion. J Hand Surg Am 38(5):941–946. https://doi.org/10.1016/j.jhsa.2013.02.009. Epub 2013 Apr 6
14. McCraw JB, Dibbell DG (1977) Experimental definition of independent myocutaneous vascular territories. Plast Reconst Surg 60(2):212–220. https://doi.org/10.1097/00006534-197708000-00007
15. Doi K, Hattori Y, Tan S-H, Dhawan V (2002) Basic science behind functioning free muscle transplantation. Clin Plast Surg 29(4):483–495, v-vi. https://doi.org/10.1016/s0094-1298(02)00020-2
16. Giuffre JL, Bishop AT, Shin AY (2012) Harvest of an entire gracilis muscle and tendon for use in functional muscle transfer: a novel technique. J Reconstr Microsurg 28(5):349–358. https://doi.org/10.1055/s-0032-1313767. Epub 2012 May 15
17. Kuzon WM Jr, McKee NH, Fish JS, Pynn BR, Rosenblatt JD (1988) The effect of intraoperative ischemia on the recovery of contractile function after free muscle transfer. J Hand Surg Am 13(2):263–273. https://doi.org/10.1016/s0363-5023(88)80062-5
18. Martins-Filho FVF, do Carmo Iwase F, Silva GB, Cho AB, Wei TH, de Rezende MR, Mattar R Jr, Iamaguchi RB (2021) Do technical components of microanastomoses influence the functional outcome of free gracilis muscle transfer for elbow flexion in traumatic brachial plexus injury? Orthop Traumatol Surg Res 107(2):102827. https://doi.org/10.1016/j.otsr.2021.102827. Epub 2021 Jan 28
19. Xu WD, Lu JZ, Qiu YQ, Jiang S, Xu L, Xu JG et al (2008) Hand prehension recovery after brachial plexus avulsion injury by performing a full-length phrenic nerve transfer via endoscopic thoracic surgery. J Neurosurg 108(6):1215–1219. https://doi.org/10.3171/JNS/2008/108/6/1215
20. Oliver JD, Beal C, Graham EM, Santosa KB, Hu MS (2020) Functioning free muscle transfer for brachial plexus injury: a systematic review and pooled analysis comparing functional outcomes of intercostal nerve and spinal accessory nerve grafts. J Reconstr Microsurg 36(8):567–571. https://doi.org/10.1055/s--0040-1713147. Epub 2020 Jun 11
21. Doi K (2008) Management of total paralysis of the brachial plexus by the double free-muscle transfer technique. J Hand Surg Eur Vol 33(3):240–251. https://doi.org/10.1177/1753193408090140
22. Satbhai NG, Doi K, Hattori Y, Sakamoto S (2016) Functional outcome and quality of life after traumatic total brachial plexus injury treated by nerve transfer or single/double free muscle transfers. Bone Joint J 98-B(2):209–217. https://doi.org/10.1302/0301-620X.98B2.35101
23. Barrie KA, Steinmann SP, Shin AY, Spinner RJ, Bishop AT (2004) Gracilis free muscle transfer for restoration of function after complete brachial plexus avulsion. Neurosurg Focus 16(5):E8. https://doi.org/10.3171/foc.2004.16.5.9

Lower Extremity Nerve Transfers

42

Niles J. Batdorf, Luke T. Juckett, and Amy M. Moore

Surgical Principles

Patients need a complete physical examination before surgery to assess donor and recipient function. Surgery is not offered unless there is a known permanent nerve injury (oncologic resection) or enough time (3–6 months) has elapsed after a trauma without significant recovery or where recovery has plateaued. Electromyography (EMG) is useful to confirm clinical findings and to ensure a lack of spontaneous recovery. The donor nerve must be strong and expendable. The concept of "donor distal, recipient proximal" is followed to avoid tension at the coaptation site. This means dissection and transection are performed distally on the donor and proximally on the recipient to allow for a tension-free coaptation. Nerve grafts are to be avoided whenever possible, and nerves need to be coapted without tension after accounting for joint movement. The coaptation is performed with 9–0 nylon and fibrin glue under loupe magnification or an operating microscope.

Supplementary Information The online version contains supplementary material available at https://doi.org/10.1007/978-3-031-73931-6_42.

N. J. Batdorf
Plastic and Reconstructive Surgery Department, The Ohio State University, Columbus, OH, USA
e-mail: niles.batdorf@osumc.edu

L. T. Juckett
Department of Plastic and Reconstructive Surgery, Maxillofacial and Oral Health, University of Virginia, Charlottesville, VA, USA
e-mail: luke.juckett@osumc.edu, eyr7tv@uvahealth.org

A. M. Moore (✉)
Plastic and Reconstructive Surgery Department, The Ohio State University Wexner Medical Center, Columbus, OH, USA
e-mail: amy.m.moore@osumc.edu

Surgical Techniques

Restoration of Gluteal Nerve Function

1. The patient is positioned prone (Fig. 42.1a), and an incision is made over the superolateral buttock and the gluteus maximus is exposed.
2. The gluteus maximus muscle is split obliquely along its fibers (Fig. 42.1b).
3. The superior gluteal nerve is favored over the inferior gluteal nerve due to its importance in hip stability [2]. The superior gluteal nerve innervates the gluteus medius, minimus, and the tensor fasciae latae, while the inferior gluteal nerve innervates the gluteus maximus. The superior gluteal nerve passes cranial to the piriformis muscle, then between gluteus medius and minimus [1]. The nerve will be cut as proximal as possible.
4. The sciatic nerve is found exiting caudal to the piriformis muscle as it descends towards the posterior thigh over the gemelli and obturator internus.
5. The sciatic nerve is dissected free from surrounding tissue, and an epineurotomy is performed to allow for an internal neurolysis [1].
6. A handheld nerve stimulator is then used to identify the strongest expendable donor fascicle. It is then vessel looped, pulled away from other fascicles, and the remaining sciatic fascicles are stimulated to ensure there are remaining redundant fascicles to avoid a donor deficit (Fig. 42.1c).
7. The selected donor fascicle is cut as distal as possible, then transferred end-to-end (ETE) to the cut end of the superior gluteal nerve connected to the gluteus medius or end-to-side (ETS) depending on the clinical situation (Fig. 42.1d).

A. S. Hanna (ed.), *Nerves: Anatomy, Exposures, and Techniques*, https://doi.org/10.1007/978-3-031-73931-6_42

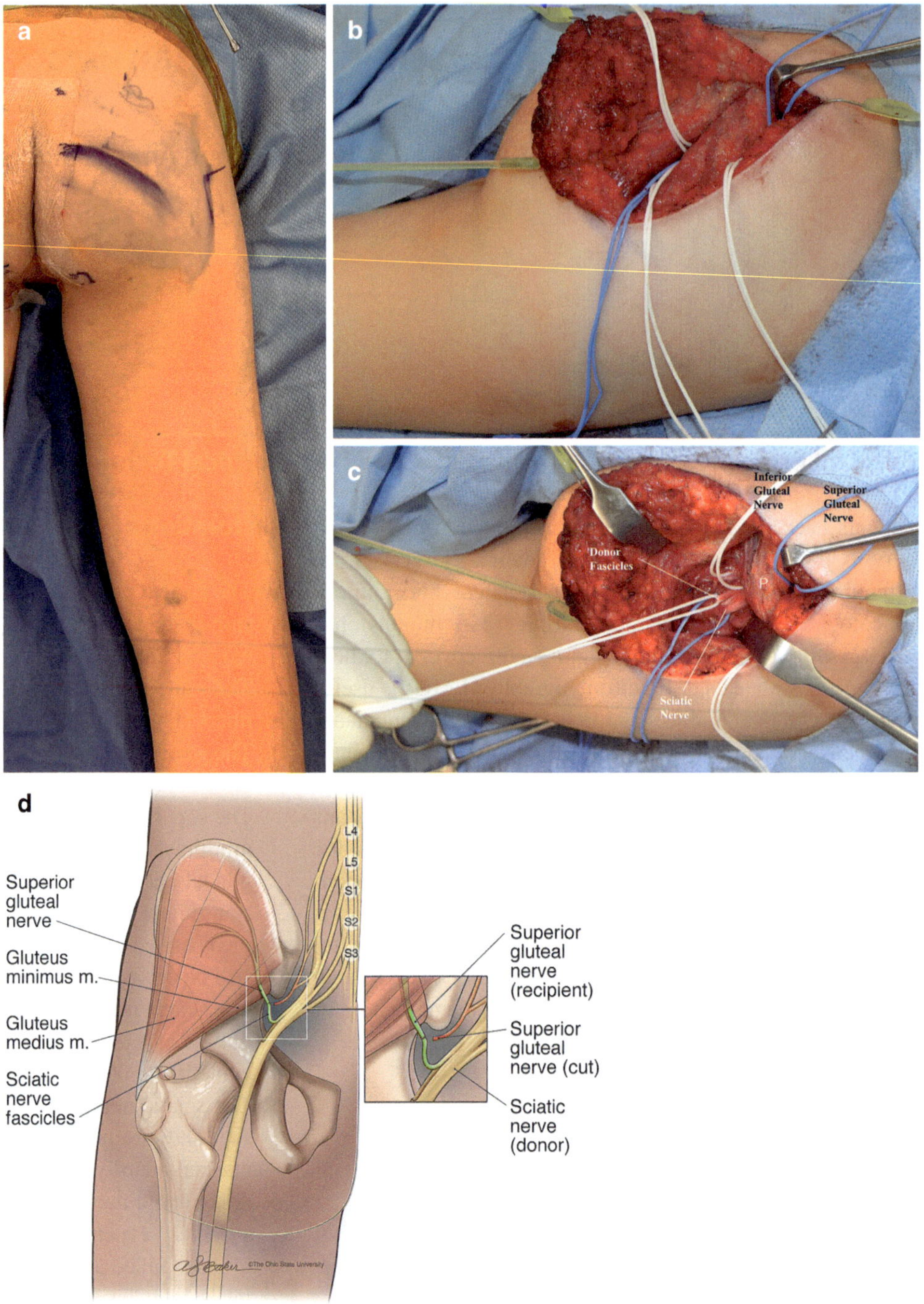

Fig. 42.1 Sciatic to superior gluteal nerve transfer. (**a**) A curvilinear buttock incision is performed to expose the gluteus maximus. (**b**) The gluteus maximus is split in line, with its fibers being careful to maintain meticulous hemostasis. (**c**) Exposure of the sciatic and superior gluteal nerves. (**d**) Schematic demonstrating final configuration of transfer of expendable sciatic donor fascicles to the superior gluteal nerve. *P* piriformis. Reproduced with the permission from The Ohio State University. All rights reserved [1]

Restoration of Femoral Nerve Function

Femoral nerve function can be restored through use of sciatic fascicles, nerve to sartorius, anterior division of the obturator nerve, or thoracoabdominal intercostal nerves.

Sciatic Fascicular Transfer to the Femoral Nerve

1. In prone position, dissection is carried down between the biceps femoris and the semitendinosus in the proximal thigh.

2. Internal neurolysis of the sciatic nerve is performed, and donor fascicles are identified and encircled with a vessel loop.
3. If two nerve transfers are being performed using the sciatic nerve as the donor, the tibial is used for one transfer and the peroneal for the other (e.g., tibial fascicles to superior gluteal nerve and peroneal fascicles to femoral) [1].
4. Provisional closure of posterior thigh incision is performed and covered with an adhesive dressing.
5. Patient is then repositioned supine, and femoral nerve exposed lateral to the femoral artery and caudal to the inguinal ligament.
6. Function of femoral nerve branches is assessed using a handheld nerve stimulator after neurolysis.
7. A subcutaneous tunnel is created between the femoral nerve and sciatic incisions after flexing and abducting the hip (Fig. 42.2a) [1].
8. The vastus medialis and intermedius are utilized as recipient nerves due to their length before entering their

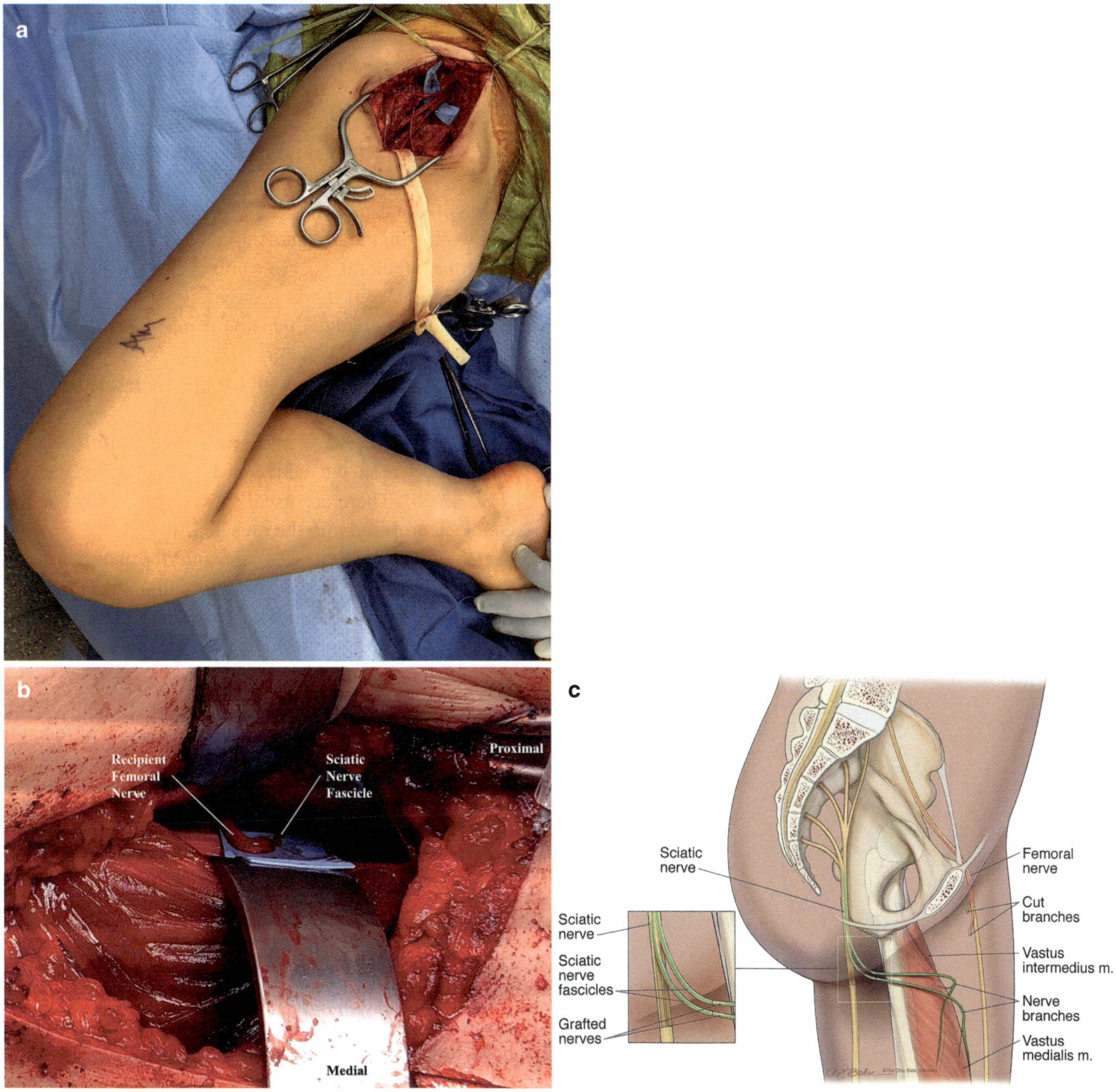

Fig. 42.2 Sciatic to femoral nerve transfer. (**a**) Anterior incision for dissection of the femoral nerve. Neurolysis of the vastus medialis and intermedius nerves is carried as far as possible proximally to gain extra length for the transfer. (**b**) The recipient femoral nerve branches are passed through a tunnel and coapted to the donor sciatic fascicles through a posterior incision. (**c**) Schematic demonstrating final configuration of transfer of expendable sciatic donor fascicles to reinnervate branches of the femoral nerve. Reproduced with the permission from The Ohio State University. All rights reserved [1]

respective muscles (Fig. 42.2b). They are tunneled back toward the sciatic nerve donor fascicles, the extra length obtained in these nerves allows for coaptation without a nerve graft (Fig. 42.2c) [1].

Nerve to Sartorius Transfer to the Femoral Nerve in the Case of Partial Femoral Nerve Injury

In partial femoral nerve injuries, the nerve branch to sartorius may be working and can be used as a donor for restoring quadriceps function. Multiple nerves can be divided distally as they enter the proximal sartorius muscle if they are stimulating strongly and can then be transferred to any of the non-functional quadriceps motor nerves (Fig. 42.3) [1].

Thoracoabdominal Intercostal Nerve Transfer to the Femoral Nerve

1. If there are no available donors in the lower extremity, a lower paramedian incision is made in the abdomen.
2. The anterior rectus sheath is incised, retracting the rectus muscle medially, which allows visualization of its segmental innervation from the intercostal nerves (Fig. 42.4a) [1].

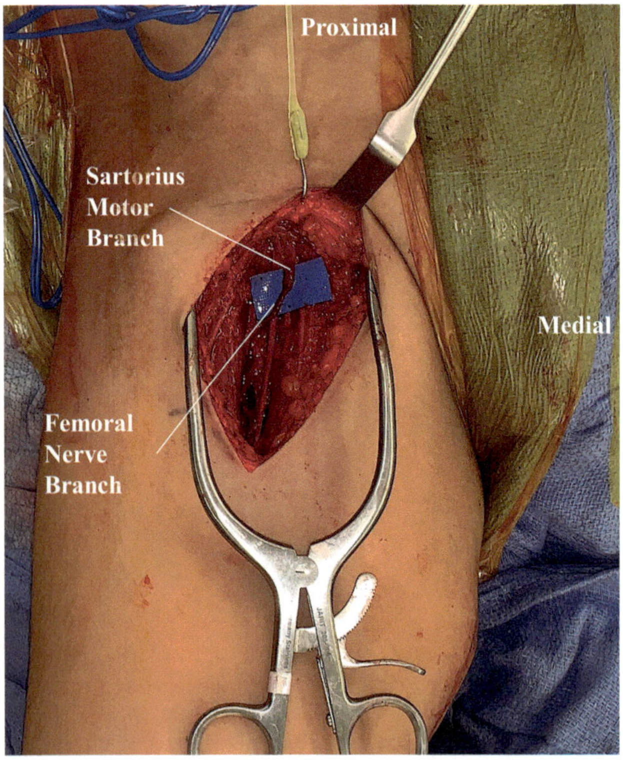

Fig. 42.3 Sartorius to femoral nerve transfer

3. Two to three lower intercostal nerves are dissected free and divided as they enter the muscle (Fig. 42.4b).
4. A sural or saphenous nerve graft is needed for this transfer to the femoral nerve (Fig. 42.4c). It is harvested in a standard fashion from the posterolateral leg [1]. More than one cable is usually needed.
5. After coaptation to the intercostal donors, the nerve graft(s) is (are) passed through a subcutaneous tunnel (Fig. 42.4d) and coapted to the femoral nerve branch recipient(s) without tension (Fig. 42.4e).
6. The average length of the autograft is 8–10 cm. The increased length of graft can contribute to decreased regeneration over time, thus limiting the effectiveness of the transfer in patients who present late or in older adults with slower regeneration rates.

Obturator to Femoral Nerve Transfer

1. A longitudinal incision is made over the femoral nerve below the inguinal ligament as previously described, and the femoral nerve branches are neurolyzed (Fig. 42.5a).
2. A separate longitudinal incision is made just posterior to the adductor longus tendon.
3. Dissection is carried through the muscle fascia medial to the adductor longus.
4. The obturator nerve to the gracilis is identified in the interval between the adductor longus and the gracilis (Fig. 42.5b). There are usually two larger branches that can be neurolyzed into the muscle [3].
5. The three motor branches of the anterior obturator nerve (adductor longus, brevis, and gracilis) are found on the anterior surface of adductor brevis. The posterior branch of the obturator nerve to adductor magnus is preserved.
6. Anteriorly, for the femoral nerve exposure, dissection is performed lateral to the femoral vessels. Lack of function of the femoral nerve branches is confirmed using a handheld nerve stimulator. Target recipients are dissected as proximal as possible and transected.
7. The anterior branch of the obturator nerve supplies the gracilis, adductor longus, and adductor brevis. One to three of the branches are dissected distally and then transected depending on the need.
8. The donor nerves are then transposed laterally, and nerve coaptations are performed as previously described.
9. The lower limb is taken through full range of motion in order to ascertain that the transfer is tension-free.

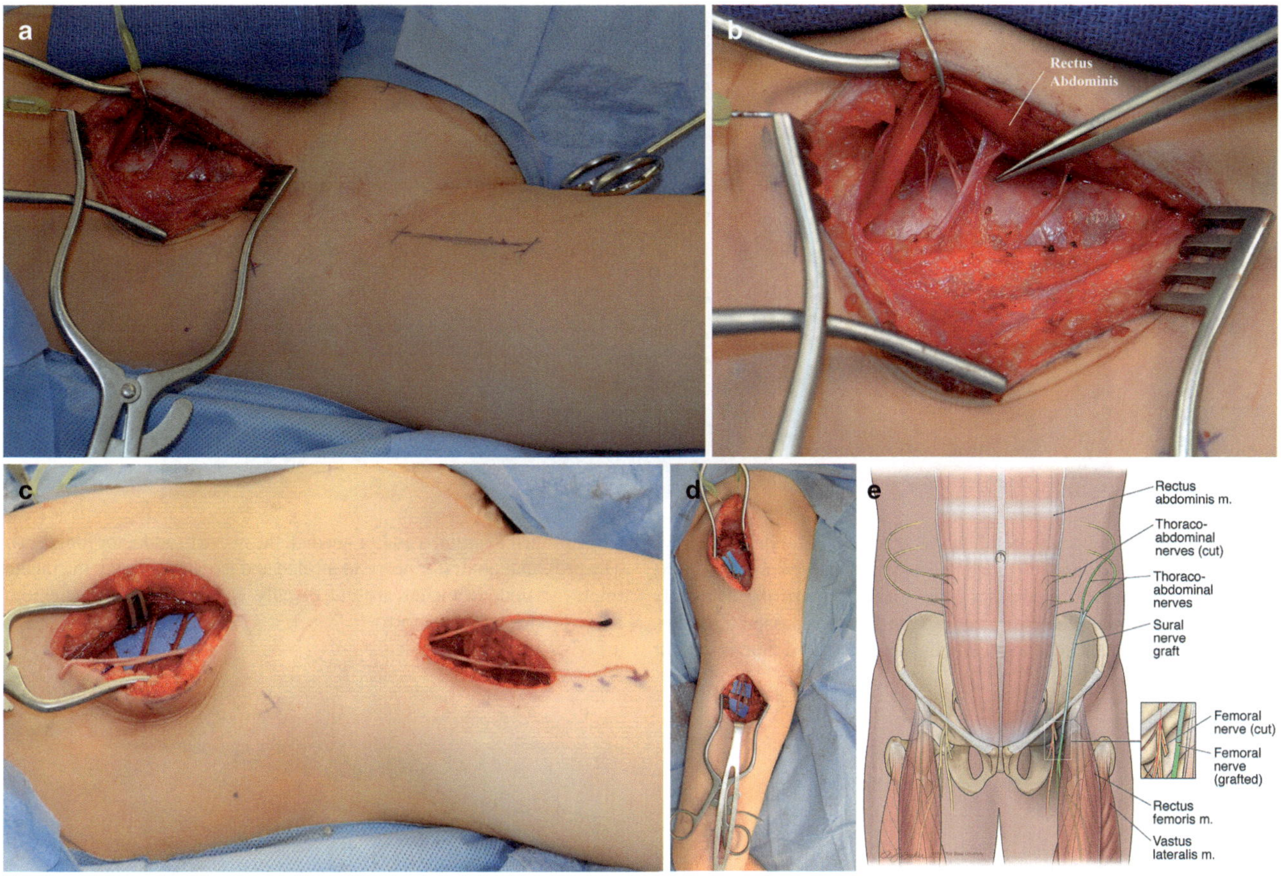

Fig. 42.4 Intercostal to femoral nerve transfer. (**a**) The anterior rectus sheath is incised, and several nerve fascicles are dissected free from underneath the rectus muscle. (**b**) Motor nerves can be seen entering the rectus muscle. (**c**) Dissection of the femoral nerve has been performed. A tunnel has been created subcutaneously between the femoral nerve incision and the abdominal incision. Sural nerve grafts have been passed through the tunnel. (**d**) Completed nerve coaptations from thoracoabdominal donors to femoral nerve branch recipients with sural nerve grafts. (**e**) Schematic representing final configuration of donor thoracoabdominal nerve transfer to recipient femoral nerve branches. Reproduced with the permission from The Ohio State University. All rights reserved [1]

Vastus Lateralis and Medialis Branches to Medial and Lateral Gastrocnemius Branches of the Tibial Nerve

1. In prone position, a long curvilinear incision is made through the popliteal fossa.
2. The sciatic nerve is exposed proximally and the tibial, peroneal, and sural nerves distally.
3. Tibial nerve motor branches entering the medial and lateral gastrocnemius muscles are neurolyzed proximally as far as possible above the popliteal crease (Fig. 42.6a).
4. The sural nerve is harvested from the ipsilateral leg in anticipation of nerve grafting to the vastus lateralis branch. Previous description used the contralateral sural nerve to maintain an intact sural nerve for potential sensory reinnervation distally. This is no longer performed because efficacy was not proven.
5. The medial and lateral gastrocnemius branches are divided as far proximal as possible (Fig. 42.6b) and then tagged with a Prolene suture and connected to a Weck-Cel® (McKesson Medical-Surgical, Irving, TX, USA) spear that has had the sponge removed to aid in rapid retrieval through anterior incisions. They are then passed anteriorly in subcutaneous tunnels towards the distal vastus medialis and lateralis, respectively. The skin is marked anteriorly over the Weck-Cel® spears to help identify the nerves once supine.
6. The incisions are closed, and the patient is then positioned supine.
7. An anterolateral incision is made on the medial border of vastus lateralis, and a plane is developed between the rectus femoris and vastus lateralis.
8. The tagged motor nerve to lateral gastrocnemius should be encountered in the tunnel created during the first stage of the operation. After sharply releasing the investing muscle fascia, a handheld nerve stimulator is used to find distal motor branches entering the vastus lateralis. Two or three branches (usually found 15 cm proximal to

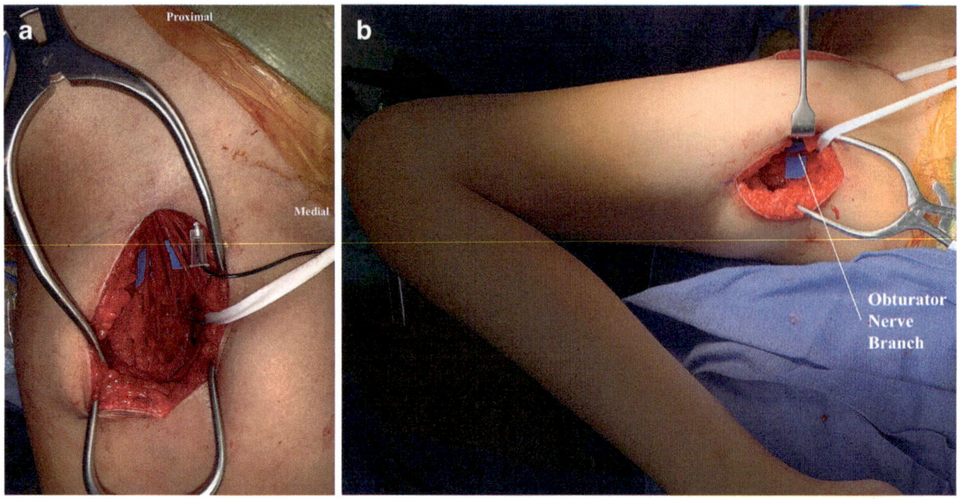

Fig. 42.5 Obturator to femoral nerve transfer. (**a**) Femoral nerve branches are exposed and tested using a handheld nerve stimulator. The vastus intermedius and medialis are the longest nerves if sufficiently neurolyzed proximally. They are cut proximally, then passed through a tunnel underneath the adductor longus towards the donor obturator nerve branch to gracilis and, if needed, the nerve to adductor longus. (**b**) The proximal obturator nerve identified and isolated through the medial thigh incision. Branches are cut distally and coapted to the femoral nerve branches end-to-end

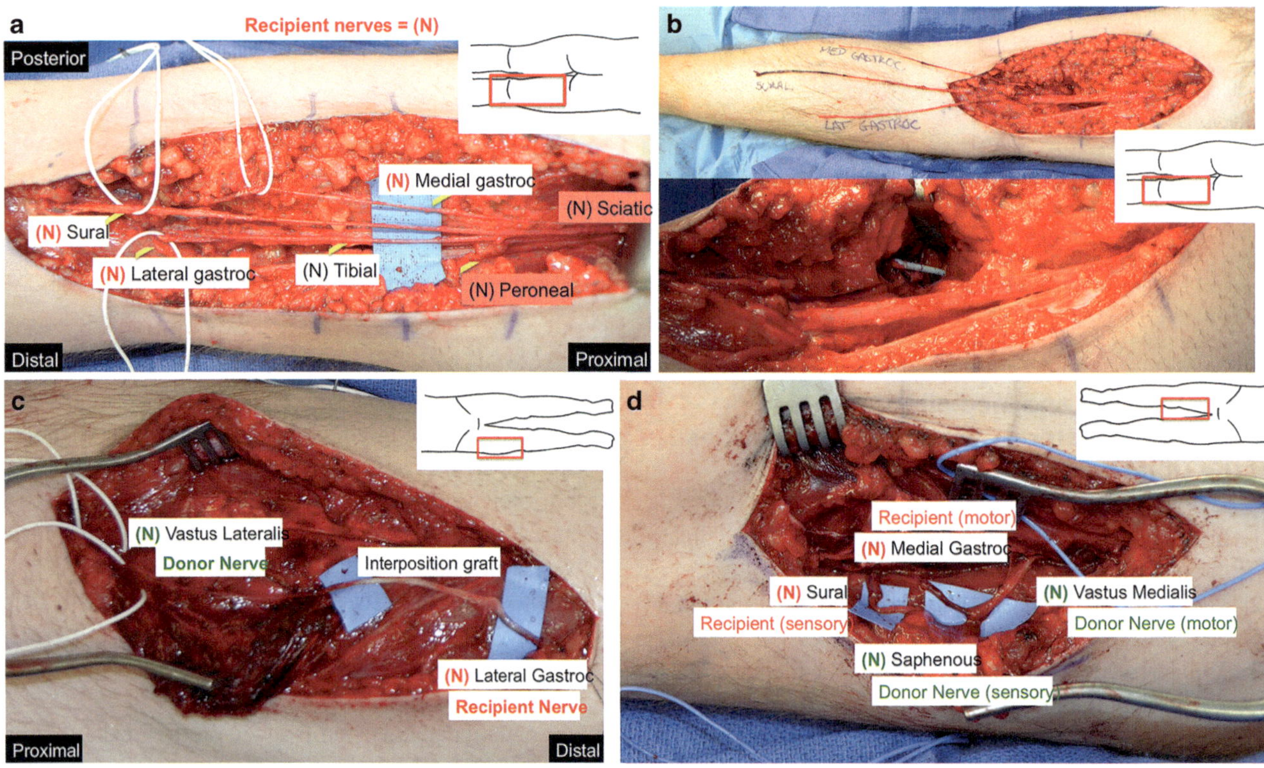

Fig. 42.6 Femoral to tibial nerve transfer. (**a**) Prone. Neurolysis of the right tibial nerve branches to the medial gastrocnemius (*gastroc*), sural, and lateral gastrocnemius nerves. (**b**) Proximal neurolysis and division of the recipient tibial nerve branches (*upper*). The nerves are divided proximally and reflected caudally for illustration. Soft tissue tunnels are created to pass the nerves to the anterior thigh (*lower*). (**c**) Supine. A lateral incision is used to coapt the terminal branches of the vastus lateralis nerve to the lateral gastrocnemius nerve through an interpositional nerve graft (sural nerve). (**d**) Through a medial incision, the terminal branches to the vastus medialis nerve and the saphenous nerve are directly coapted to the nerve to the medial gastrocnemius and sural nerves, respectively. Currently, we do not recommend the sensory nerve transfer, and the ipsilateral sural nerve is used as a graft instead. Published with permission from Journal of Neurosurgery. All rights reserved [4]

the patella) are dissected until they enter the muscle and divided distally. They are then dissected proximally to gain extra length [4].

9. These branches are then coapted using an intercalary sural nerve graft to the lateral gastrocnemius motor nerve in a tension-free manner after freely moving the knee (Fig. 42.6c).
10. An anteromedial incision is made just proximal to medial femoral condyle.
11. The tagged medial gastrocnemius branch should be encountered within the dissection. After incising the muscle fascia of the posterior border of vastus medialis, the saphenous nerve is encountered and protected. About two or three terminal femoral motor branches are encountered while dissecting on the undersurface of the muscle as they pass into the muscle (about 10.7 cm proximal to the patella) [4].
12. These nerve branches are divided as distal as possible and coapted to the nerve to the medial gastrocnemius muscle (Fig. 42.6d). This can be performed without a nerve graft.

Partial Tibial Nerve Transfer to Tibialis Anterior Motor Branch

1. In supine position, a lateral incision is made from the fibular head distally for approximately 12 cm.
2. The common peroneal nerve is dissected from the fibular neck distally as it divides into deep and superficial branches.
3. A fat stripe demarcates the interval between the soleus and peroneus longus muscles.
4. The deep peroneal nerve is traced distally after incising the fat stripe and elevating the soleus off the fibula.
5. The peroneal nerve is seen as it divides into its articular, deep, and superficial branches, and the tibial nerve and posterior tibial artery are encountered medial and posterior to the fibula (Fig. 42.7a) [5].
6. Motor branches to the tibialis anterior are identified and can arise from the articular and deep branches of the peroneal nerve.
7. Motor branches to the tibialis anterior are dissected proximally and divided after sufficient length is obtained.
8. A longitudinal epineurotomy of the tibial nerve is performed, and branches to flexor hallucis longus or flexor digitorum longus are selected, and an internal neurolysis is performed to isolate these branches after confirming them with a handheld nerve stimulator. They are neurolyzed and divided distally after sufficient length is obtained [5].
9. The interosseous membrane is divided in order to directly transfer the motor nerve to the tibialis anterior from the anterior compartment directly to the donor tibial nerve branches in the deep posterior compartment (Fig. 42.7b).
10. The nerve coaptation is completed in the deep posterior compartment in the usual fashion (Fig. 42.7c).
11. The outcomes of this nerve transfer can be variable given the non-synergistic nature of the transfer, the mechanism of trauma, and the limited recovery of one muscle for ankle dorsiflexion [6]. Often, ankle-foot arthroses are required for ambulation over distances.

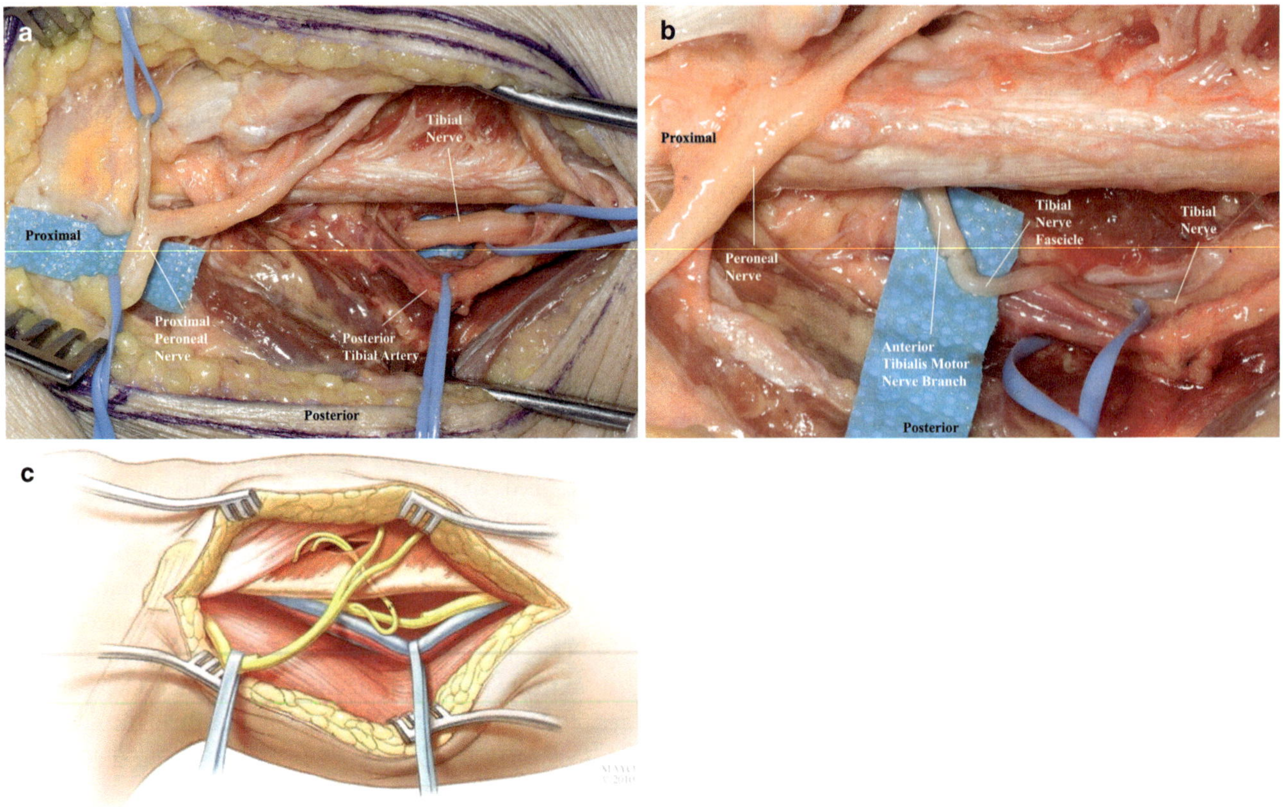

Fig. 42.7 Tibial to peroneal nerve transfer. (**a**) The peroneal nerve is seen coursing over the fibula while the tibial nerve is looped more distally. The posterior tibial artery is also looped and retracted. Used with permission of Wolters Kluwer Health, Inc.—Clinical Orthopaedics and Related Research [5]. (**b**) The peroneal branch to tibialis anterior has been transected proximally, then passed posteriorly through the interosseous membrane. The expendable donor fascicles from the tibial nerve have been divided distally and are turned to meet the recipient fascicles. (**c**) Final schematic showing transfer of donor tibial fascicles to recipient peroneal nerve branch to tibialis anterior." Used with permission of Mayo Foundation for Medical Education and Research. All rights reserved [5]

References

1. Moore AM, Bettlach CR, Tung TT, West JM, Russo SA (2021) Lower extremity nerve transfers in acute flaccid myelitis patients: a case series. Plast Reconstr Surg Glob Open 9(7):e3699. https://doi.org/10.1097/GOX.0000000000003699. eCollection 2021 July
2. Craig A (2013) Entrapment neuropathies of the lower extremity. PM R 5(5 Suppl):S31–S40. https://doi.org/10.1016/j.pmrj.2013.03.029. Epub 2013 Mar 28
3. Peters BR, Ha AY, Moore AM, Tung TH (2022) Nerve transfers for femoral nerve palsy: an updated approach and surgical technique. J Neurosurg 136(3):856–866. https://doi.org/10.3171/2021.2.JNS203463. Print 2022 Mar 1
4. Moore AM, Krauss EM, Parikh RP, Franco MJ, Tung TH (2018) Femoral nerve transfers for restoring tibial nerve function: an anatomical study and clinical correlation: a report of 2 cases. J Neurosurg 129(4):1024–1033. https://doi.org/10.3171/2017.5.JNS163076. Epub 2017 Nov 3
5. Giuffre JL, Bishop AT, Spinner RJ, Levy BA, Shin AY (2012) Partial tibial nerve transfer to the tibialis anterior motor branch to treat peroneal nerve injury after knee trauma. Clin Orthop Relat Res 470(3):779–790. https://doi.org/10.1007/s11999-011-1924-9
6. Head LK, Hicks K, Wolff G, Boyd KU (2019) Clinical outcomes of nerve transfers in peroneal nerve palsy: a systematic review and meta-analysis. J Reconstr Microsurg 35(1):57–65. https://doi.org/10.1055/s-0038-1667047. Epub 2018 Aug 22

Tendon Transfers for Upper Limb Nerve Injuries

43

Thomas G. Knoedler, Akram M. Eraky,
and A. Neil Salyapongse

Abbreviations

ADQ	Abductor digiti quinti
APB	Abductor pollicis brevis
APL	Abductor pollicis longus
BR	Brachioradialis
ECRB	Extensor carpi radialis brevis
ECRL	Extensor carpi radialis longus
EDC	Extensor digitorum communis
EIP	Extensor indicis proprius
EPB	Extensor pollicis brevis
EPL	Extensor pollicis longus
FCR	Flexor carpi radialis
FCU	Flexor carpi ulnaris
FDP	Flexor digitorum profundus
FDS	Flexor digitorum superficialis
FPL	Flexor pollicis longus
IP	Interphalangeal
MCP	Metacarpophalangeal
PIP	Proximal interphalangeal
PL	Palmaris longus
PT	Pronator teres
WALANT	Wide-awake, local anesthesia, no tourniquet

Supplementary Information The online version contains supplementary material available at https://doi.org/10.1007/978-3-031-73931-6_43.

T. G. Knoedler
Department of Orthopaedic Surgery, Lewis Katz School of Medicine at Temple University, Philadelphia, PA, USA
e-mail: TKnoedler@uwhealth.org

A. M. Eraky
Department of Neurosurgery, University of Wisconsin School of Medicine and Public Health, Madison, WI, USA
e-mail: eraky@mcw.edu

A. N. Salyapongse (✉)
Madison Surgery Center, Department of Orthopedics, University of Wisconsin School of Medicine and Public Health, Madison, WI, USA
e-mail: ASalyapongse@uwhealth.org

Introduction

Tendon transfers are an option to regain hand function in the setting of nerve injury. Radial nerve injuries are the most common upper limb deficit, followed by median, then ulnar. Generally, a transfer may be considered in the setting of functional motor deficit when nerve repair and/or transfer are not feasible, such as late clinical presentation, prior failed nerve transfer, or when no reasonable nerve donor exists.

There are several requirements for a successful tendon transfer. First, an adequate scaffold, including bony stability and healed soft tissue, is necessary. In addition, to prevent scarring from limiting excursion, transfers require virgin tissue in which to pass tendons. Joints must be supple, because a tendon transfer will never be able to move a joint beyond its passive range of motion. Finally, protective sensation is important, as a lack of sensation will limit the functionality of the limb [1–3].

General Principles

1. Anesthesia choice may be regional block (axillary or supraclavicular) or general via endotracheal tube or laryngeal mask. Exceptions are the very distal, isolated transfers involving only one or two tendons, which can be performed under wide-awake, local anesthesia, no tourniquet (WALANT) [3].
2. For all upper extremity transfers, the patient should be positioned supine with the arm resting on a hand table.
3. Utilization of an upper arm tourniquet is recommended for all procedures except for the WALANT.
4. Joining the donor and recipient tendons may be accomplished through a variety of techniques. Pulvertaft weaves with three or more passes have been the most commonly employed; however, side-to-side junctures with either multiple (often 6) figure-of-eight sutures or a running, locking suture technique are also effective choices [3].

A. S. Hanna (ed.), *Nerves: Anatomy, Exposures, and Techniques*, https://doi.org/10.1007/978-3-031-73931-6_43

Radial Nerve Deficits [3]

Radial nerve sensory deficits typically do not cause a significant functional deficit. Radial motor deficits, on the other hand, can be quite debilitating, leaving the wrist in a flexed position which limits power grip, and preventing finger and thumb extension, which are critical for grasping objects.

The goals of tendon transfers for radial nerve deficits include restoring wrist extension, finger extension at the metacarpophalangeal (MCP) joints, thumb extension, and thumb abduction.

Pronator Teres (PT) to Extensor Carpi Radialis Brevis (ECRB)

- Two incisions are typically necessary: a volar longitudinal incision along the radial aspect of the mid-shaft of the radius for harvest of the pronator teres tendon (Fig. 43.1a) and a dorsal incision over the radial wrist extensors proximal to the first compartment musculotendinous junction (Fig. 43.1b).

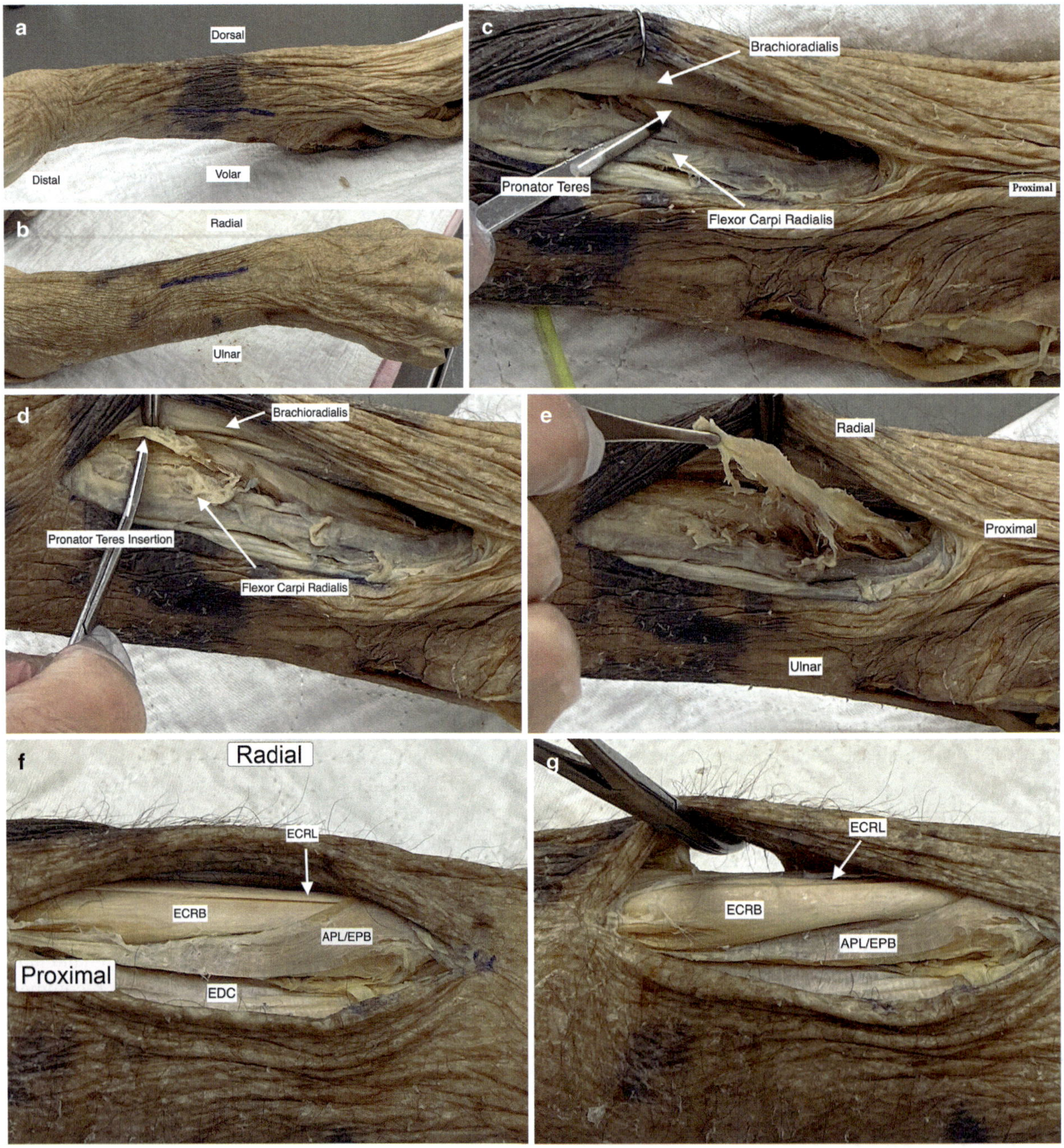

Fig. 43.1 (**a**) Volar, radial incision for pronator teres harvest. (**b**) Dorsal Incision overlying the first compartment musculotendinous junction. (**c**) Exposure of pronator teres. (**d**) Distal release of pronator teres. (**e**) Proximal release of pronator trees. (**f**) Dorsal exposure of ECRL and ECRB musculotendinous junctions. (**g**) Tunnel beneath brachioradialis and superficial radial nerve. (**h**) The pronator teres is passed through the subcutaneous tunnel. (**i**) Pronator teres transferred dorsally to connect to ERB

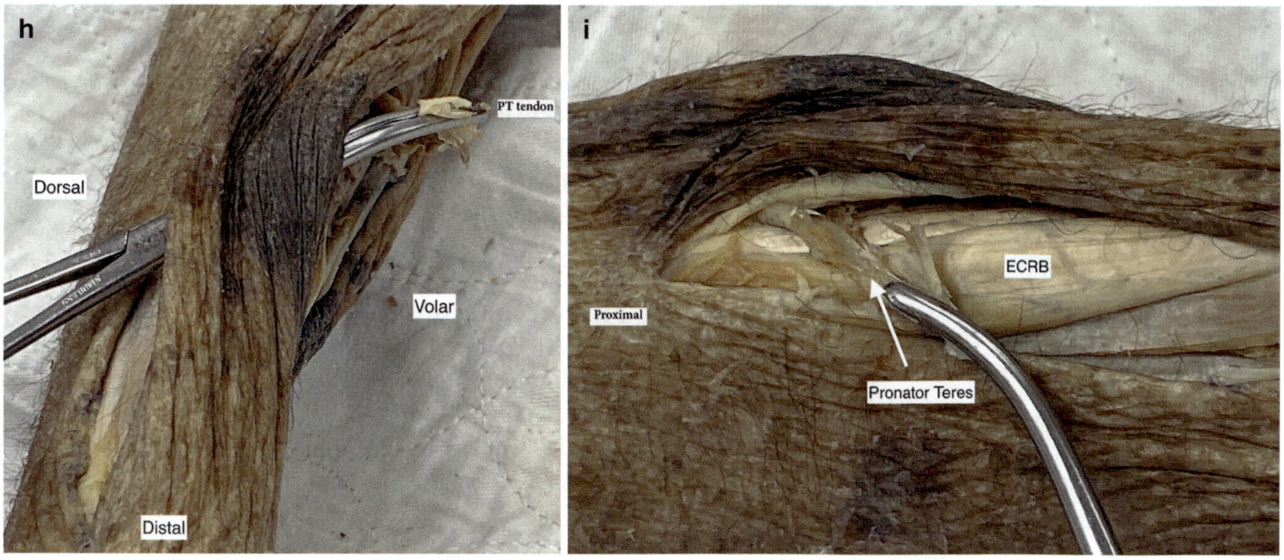

Fig. 43.1 (continued)

- Volarly, blunt dissection is carried down to the interval between the brachioradialis (BR) and flexor carpi radialis (FCR) while looking for and protecting the superficial radial nerve as the dissection proceeds distally and dorsally along the radius.
- This interval is developed to expose the pronator teres (Fig. 43.1c).
- The pronator teres is released distally with a strip of periosteum to lengthen the insertion (Fig. 43.1d).
- The muscle is partially released proximally to improve its excursion (Fig. 43.1e).
- Through the dorsal incision, the musculotendinous junctions of the extensor carpi radialis longus (ECRL, more radial tendon) and the ECRB are exposed (Fig. 43.1f).
- A tunnel is created deep to the BR (Fig. 43.1g) and superficial radial nerve, and the pronator teres is passed through the tunnel to the dorsal aspect of the forearm (Fig. 43.1h and i).
- The pronator teres is attached to the ECRB with a Pulvertaft weave.

Flexor Carpi Radialis (FCR) to Extensor Digitorum Communis (EDC)

1. Skin incision #1: 5 cm volar longitudinal incision overlying the distal extent of the FCR.
2. The FCR is exposed, protecting the radial artery and median nerve (Fig. 43.2a).
3. Skin incision #2: 3 cm dorsal longitudinal incision centered between the radius and ulna, just proximal to the extensor retinaculum.
4. The EDC is identified.
5. The FCR is divided as distally as possible with the wrist in flexion to maximize harvest length.
6. A tunnel is created around the radial border of the wrist with care being taken to remain immediately superficial to the investing fascia of the muscles and tendons and deep to the superficial radial nerve.
7. The FCR tendon is passed dorsally into the incision used to expose the EDC.
8. The EDC tendons may be divided at the musculocutaneous junction or left intact. Leaving the EDC intact will allow weaving the FCR into the group of tendons en masse. Dividing the EDC tendons allows individual tensioning of the finger extension by weaving each EDC into the FCR (Fig. 43.2b).
9. The fingers are placed into extension, and EDC tendons are attached to the FCR with a Pulvertaft weave.

Flexor Carpi Ulnaris (FCU) to ECRB

This is uncommonly used except in the setting of a combined median and radial nerve injuries.

1. Skin incision #1: longitudinal incision overlying FCU just proximal to the pisiform.
2. Blunt dissection is carried down to the FCU (Fig. 43.3a). The tendon is isolated while protecting the ulnar neurovascular bundle, which lies radial and deep to the tendon (Fig. 43.3b). A Penrose drain is placed around the tendon, and the FCU muscle belly is mobilized.
3. FCU is divided just proximal to the pisiform. The tendon is passed through a subcutaneous tunnel, on the ulnar side, to the dorsum of the forearm (Fig. 43.3c).

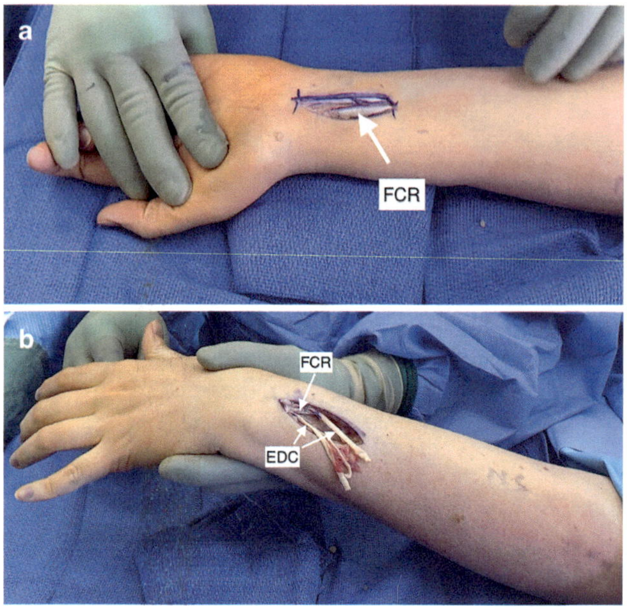

Fig. 43.2 (**a**) Exposure of FCR. (**b**) The FCR is attached to the EDC with a Pulvertaft weave

4. Skin incision #2: longitudinal dorsal incision over ECRB musculotendinous junction (Fig. 43.3d).
5. The ECRB tendon is divided proximally and passed ulnarly either superficial or deep to the EDC toward the FCU tendon.
6. With the wrist in full extension, the ECRB and FCU are joined with a Pulvertaft weave (Fig. 43.3e).

Flexor Digitorum Superficialis (FDS) to EDC

1. Skin incision #1: 1 cm longitudinal incisions overlying the A1 pulleys (Fig. 43.4a).
2. FDS tendons are localized and isolated (Fig. 43.4b).
3. Fingers are flexed to allow for additional length, and the tendons are transected at the level of the chiasm (Fig. 43.4c).
4. FDS tendons are drawn back to the level of the distal forearm (Fig. 43.4d).
5. Skin incision: dorsal incision overlying extensor retinaculum.

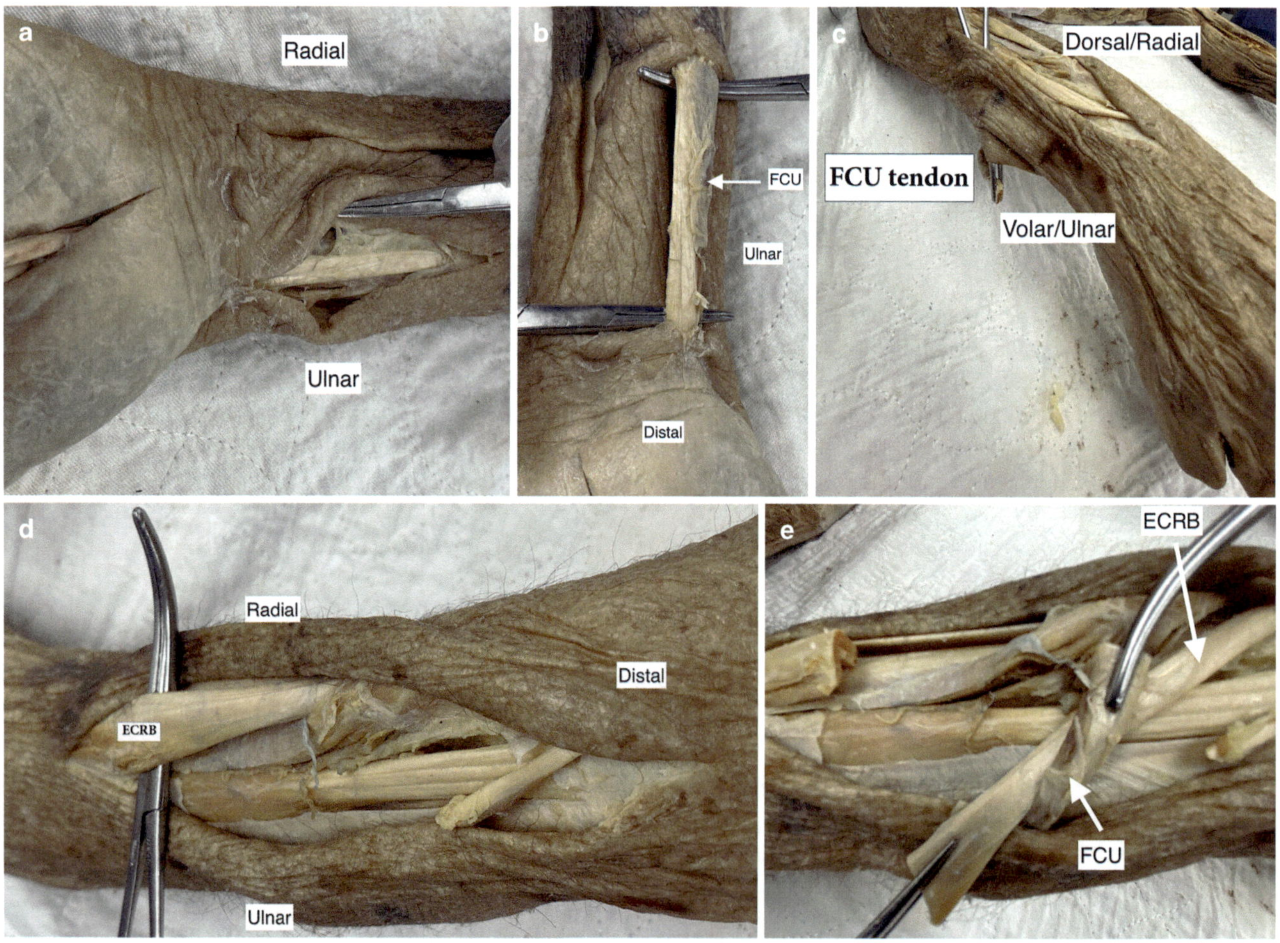

Fig. 43.3 (**a**) FCU exposed while protecting the neurovascular bundle, which is radial and deep. (**b**) The FCU is dissected to allow for excursion. (**c**) The FCU is cut at the pisiform insertion and passed through a subcutaneous tunnel from volar to dorsal. (**d**) The ECRB is exposed at the musculotendinous junction. (**e**) The ECRB and FCU are joined together via Pulvertaft weave

6. The fourth compartment is entered, and extensor indicis proprius (EIP) and EDC are identified.
7. A tunnel is created to the radial border of the wrist, superficial to the fascia and deep to the cutaneous nerve branches (Fig. 43.4e).
8. FDS tendons are passed through the tunnel (Fig. 43.4f and g) to the level of the EDC tendons (Fig. 43.4h and i).
9. The EDC tendons are divided proximally and drawn into the wound.
10. The wrist is positioned in full extension with the metacarpophalangeal (MCP) joints in slight hyperextension. FDS is attached to the extensor tendons with a Pulvertaft weave.

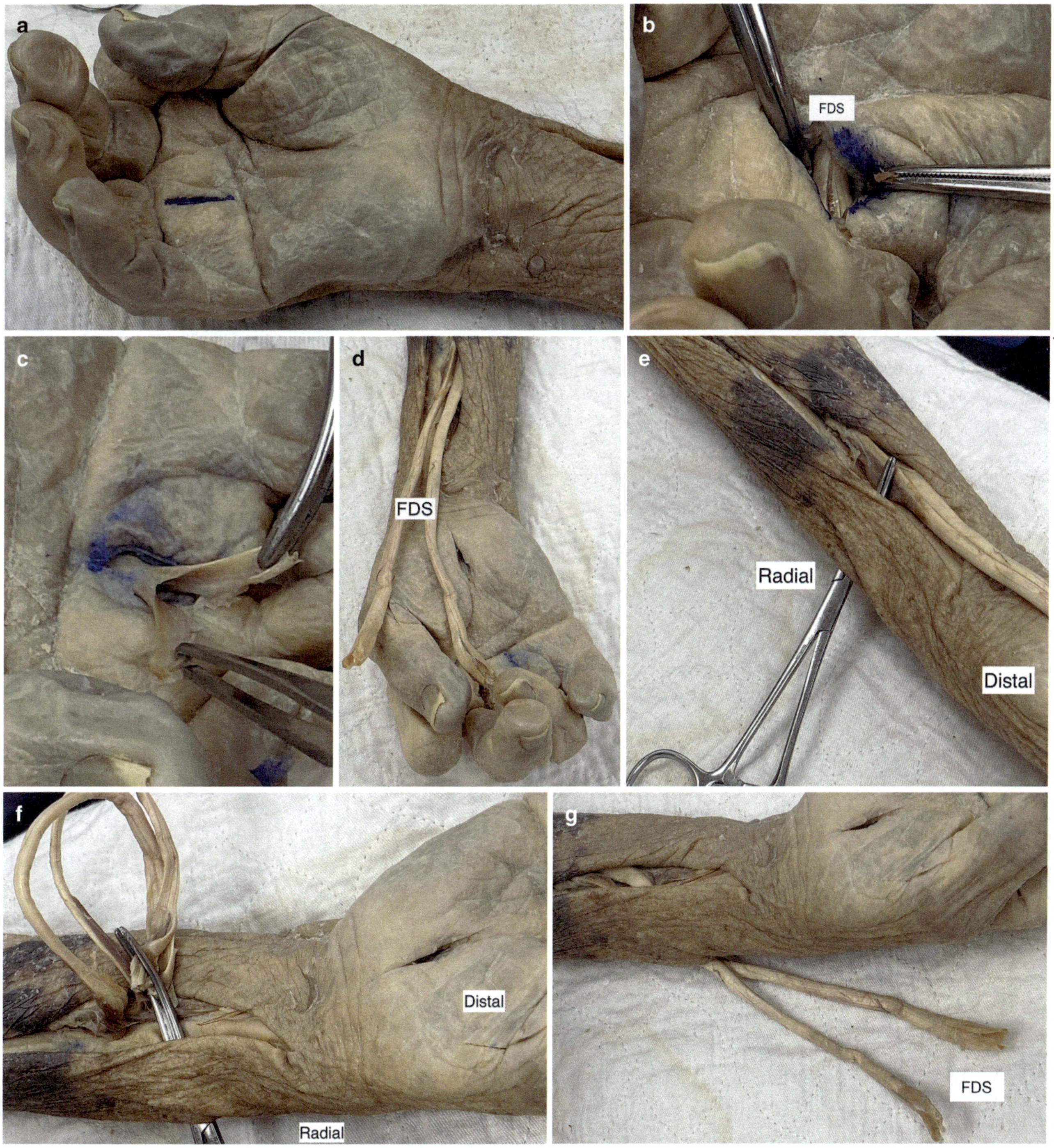

Fig. 43.4 (**a**) Skin incision centered over the ring finger A1 pulley. (**b**) Exposure of FDS tendons. (**c**) The FDS has been cut at the level of the chiasm. (**d**) FDS tendons have been drawn back through the proximal incision. (**e**) A Kelly clamp lies in a subcutaneous tunnel on the radial border of the forearm, passing from dorsal to volar. (**f**) The FDS tendons are grasped volarly with the Kelly. (**g**) FDS passed through the subcutaneous tunnel to the dorsal aspect of the forearm. (**h**) FDS pulled through the dorsal incision. (**i**) FDS tendons are brought to the level of the EDC

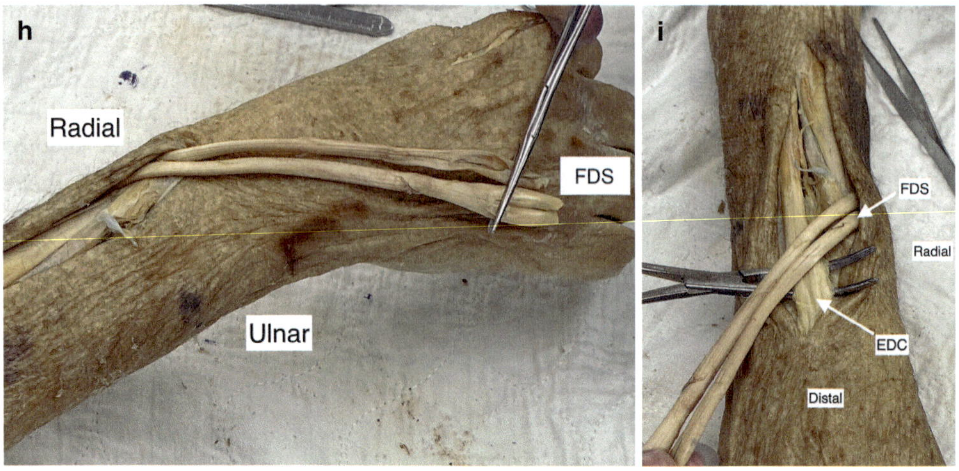

Fig. 43.4 (continued)

Palmaris Longus (PL) to Extensor Pollicis Longus (EPL) (Video 43.1)

Prior to surgery make sure the patient has a palmaris longus (the muscle can be absent), by asking the patient to touch the thumb to the little finger.

1. The patient is positioned supine with a hand table.
2. Skin incision #1: longitudinal incision overlying the palmaris longus.
3. The palmaris is divided at its junction with the palmar fascia.
4. The palmaris is freed to the mid-forearm, protecting the median nerve.
5. Skin incision #2: 1 cm dorsal incision overlying the snuffbox.
6. EPL is transected proximally at the musculotendinous junction.
7. A tunnel is created superficial to the investing fascia and deep to the radial sensory nerve branches.
8. The palmaris tendon is routed to the dorsal incision to the level of the EPL tendon.
9. The thumb is positioned in full extension and abduction with slight wrist palmar flexion to bring the two tendon edges together (Fig. 43.5).
10. A Pulvertaft weave is performed.
11. Tension is evaluated with the tenodesis effect.

FDS to Additional Finger Extensors: EPL/EIP/Abductor Pollicis Longus (APL)

1. Harvest of the FDS proceeds as per the steps for transfer to the EDC.

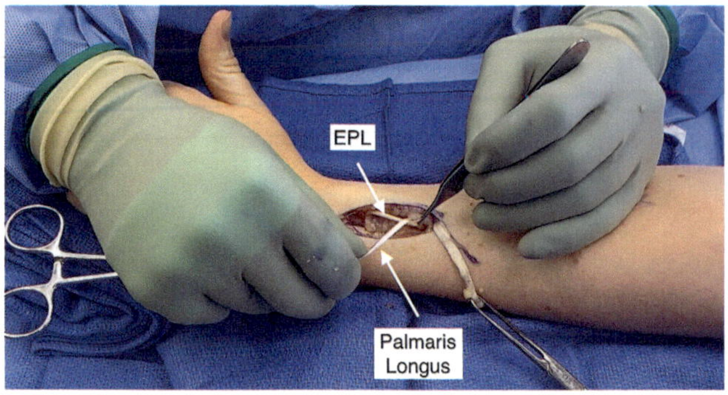

Fig. 43.5 The palmaris longus tendon (held by hand) has been passed dorsally and crosses the EPL tendon (held in Adson pickup). The Allis clamp is holding the FCR tendon prepared for transfer to the EDC

2. Skin incisions: centered over the dorsal wrist over the radial wrist extensors; palpation of the first compartment musculature can help identify the incision.
3. EPL may be identified as in the palmaris transfer (Fig. 43.6a and b).
4. EIP can be found deep and radial within the fourth compartment; the tendon will have the most distal muscle belly of the five tendons within this compartment.
5. APL can be identified by following the palpable first compartment musculature distally and excluding the extensor pollicis brevis (EPB) tendon. Identification of the EPB may be anatomical (the more dorsal and ulnar tendon) and mechanical through traction on the tendon and observation of extension of the thumb MCP joint.
6. Junction of the FDS to the target tendon should be performed under tenodesis of the wrist to set the tension.

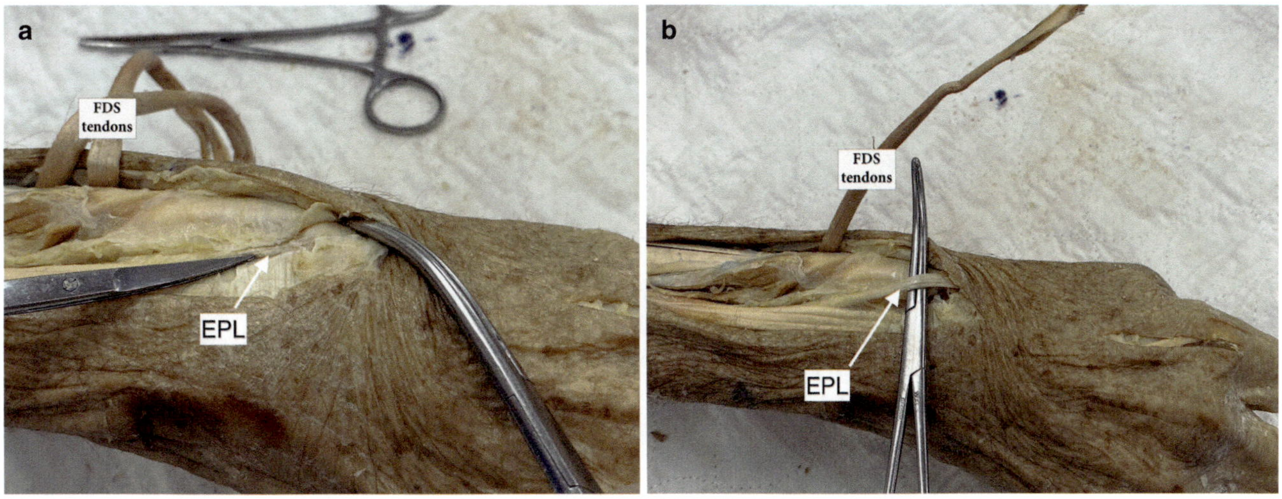

Fig. 43.6 (**a**) Proximally, the two FDS tendons (ring and middle) are seen. They have been routed around the radial side of the wrist. The small scissor points to EPL. (**b**) The EPL is identified for transfer. Only one FDS tendon is seen at the top of the image

Median Nerve Deficits [3]

The median nerve provides sensation to an area of the hand, which is critical for fine motor skills. Loss of median nerve sensation may temper the utility of even a technically successful tendon transfer, as patients may either struggle in situations where they are unable to visually accommodate, or they may simply choose to bypass the affected hand. Laying forth expectations for function in the setting of impaired sensation is important in the preoperative decision-making process.

Median nerve motor deficits are classified as either high or low depending on whether the lesion is proximal or distal to the anterior interosseous nerve (AIN). In low median nerve palsies, the goal of surgery is to restore thumb opposition. In high median nerve palsies, there are additional deficits in pronation, finger flexion, and thumb flexion with denervation to the pronator teres, FCR, FDS, and the flexor digitorum profundus (FDP) to the index and middle fingers [1, 3].

Low Median

FDS to Abductor Pollicis Brevis (APB) and MCP Joint

1. Skin incision #1: 2 cm longitudinal incision on the radial aspect of the base of the proximal phalanx of the thumb at the junction of the glabrous skin.
2. Blunt dissection is carried down through the subcutaneous tissues while protecting the radial digital nerve palmarly and the superficial radial nerve dorsally.
3. The APB tendon is exposed.
4. Skin incision #2: 1 cm longitudinal incision over the A1 pulley of the ring finger (Fig. 43.7a).
5. Blunt dissection is carried down to the A1 pulley. The FDS and FDP are identified, and the FDS is gently mobilized (Fig. 43.7b).
6. Skin incision #3: 1.5 cm longitudinal incision just distal and ulnar to the carpal tunnel (Fig. 43.7c).
7. A 1.5 cm diameter window is excised from the superficial palmar fascia. The fascia is preserved radially to act as a pulley.
8. The FDS tendon is then identified deep to the fascial window and proximal to the superficial palmar arch.
9. The finger is flexed to deliver the FDS chiasm proximally into the wound. The FDS tendon is then divided in the incision near the A1 pulley, 1 cm distal to the chiasm.
10. The tendon is then drawn into the incision in the palm (Fig. 43.7d).
11. A subcutaneous tunnel is created between the palm and thumb incisions (Fig. 43.7e), and the tendon is passed to the base of the thumb (Fig. 43.7f and g).
12. The tendon is then attached by a Pulvertaft weave to the fascial confluence near the MCP joint.

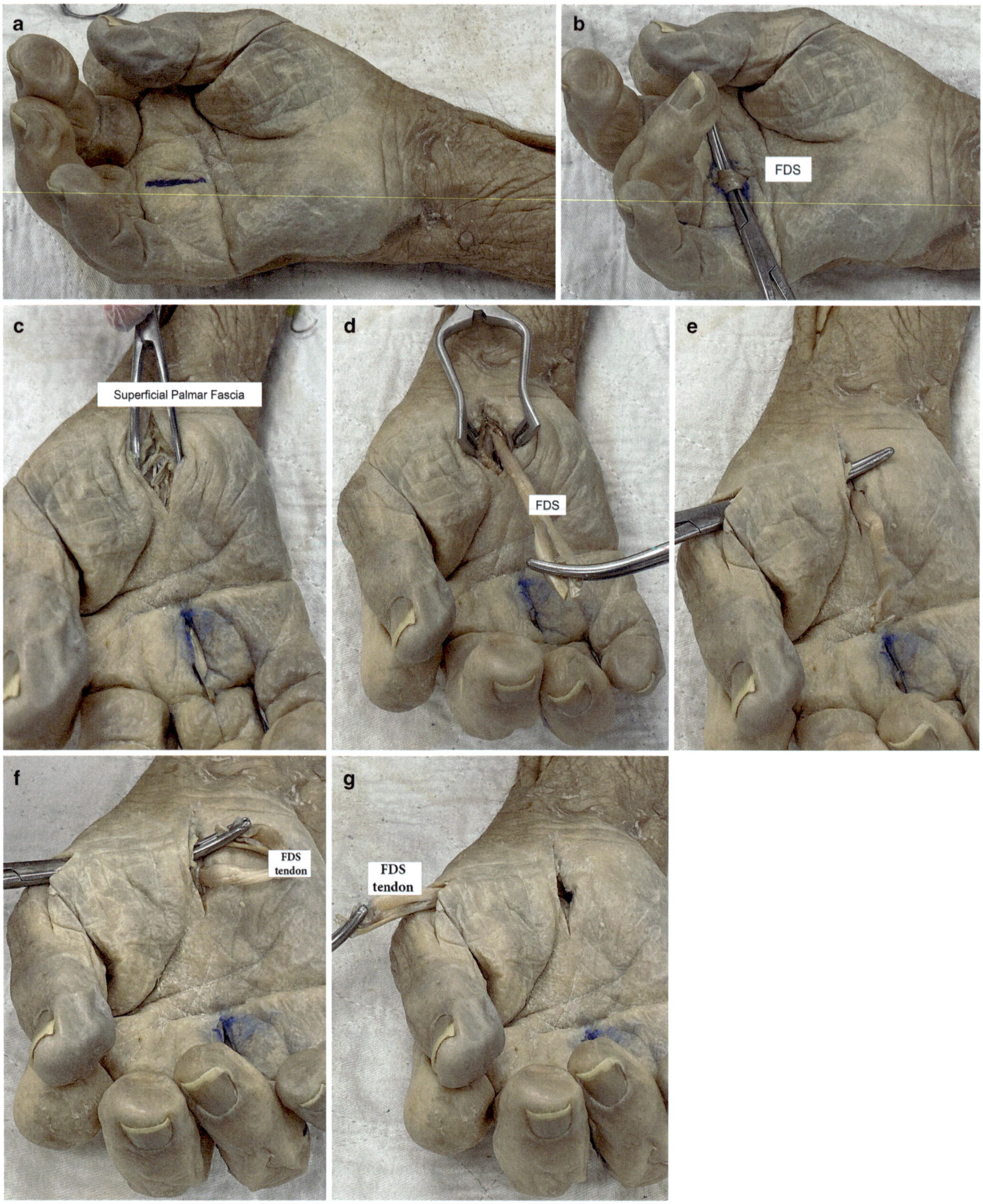

Fig. 43.7 (**a**) Incision overlying the ring finger A1 pulley. (**b**) FDS is exposed and mobilized. (**c**) The superficial palmar fascia is identified then a window opening is made through it. (**d**) FDS is cut distally and drawn proximally through the palmar incision. (**e**) A hemostat is used to create a subcutaneous tunnel from the palmar incision to the APB insertion site. (**f**) FDS is grasped through the tunnel. (**g**) FDS has now been passed towards the APB insertion site

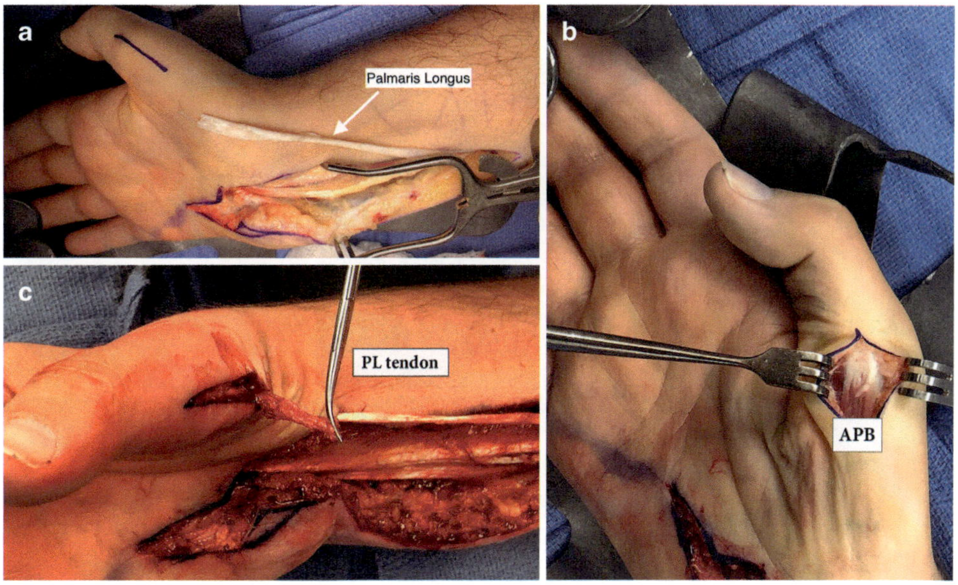

Fig. 43.8 (**a**) The palmaris longus has been identified and released from the palmar fascia It is shown here passing towards the base of the thumb. Note, the incision here is longer than usual, because this particular case also included an AIN transfer. (**b**) The APB insertion is shown here on the radial border of the base of the thumb proximal phalanx and the metacarpophalangeal joint capsule. (**c**) The palmaris longus has been passed through a subcutaneous tunnel to the base of the thumb

PL Abductorplasty

1. Preoperatively, the presence of the PL is confirmed by having the patient touch the thumb and small finger with the wrist flexed.
2. Incision #1: longitudinal incision centered over the PL extending from the distal wrist crease to the proximal palmar crease.
3. PL tendon is dissected proximal to distal. PL is released distally with a 1 cm^2 patch of the superficial palmar fascia (Fig. 43.8a).
4. Incision #2: small longitudinal incision over the thumb MCP joint exposing the APB (Fig. 43.8b).
5. A subcutaneous tunnel is created from the palmar incision to the radial incision, and the tendon is passed (Fig. 43.8c).
6. The thumb is placed in abduction and pronation/opposition, and the palmaris is attached to the APB with a Pulvertaft weave.

Abductor Digiti Quinti (ADQ) to APB

1. Skin incision: zigzag incision starting from the ulnar border of the small finger proximal phalanx along the radial border of the hypothenar eminence to the pisiform.
2. The ADQ is separated from the flexor digiti minimi, protecting the sensory nerve to the small finger.
3. The ADQ is released distally along with a portion of the lateral band to increase length.
4. The ADQ is dissected proximally to the pisiform while protecting the neurovascular bundle, which is deep and radial.
5. A subcutaneous tunnel is created to the base of the thumb.
6. The ADQ is attached to the base of the thumb.

EIP to APB (Video 43.2)

1. Skin incision #1: dorsal longitudinal incision 2–3 cm over the index finger MCP. The EIP will be the ulnar and deeper of two tendons to the index finger (EDC tendon is more radial and superficial). The EIP is isolated and freed. The extensor hood is incised to gain more length (Fig. 43.9a) The tendon is released distally and the extensor hood repaired.
2. Skin incision #2: longitudinal 2–3 cm incision on the dorsal forearm ulnar to Lister's tubercle overlying the fourth compartment, and just proximal to the extensor retinaculum.
3. Blunt dissection is carried down through subcutaneous tissue to fascia overlying the fourth compartment.
4. EIP muscle belly is identified deep to the EDC tendons (Fig. 43.9b), and the tendon is drawn through the proximal incision.
5. A subcutaneous tunnel is created superficial to the muscle fascia toward the ulnar styloid, care being taken to remain deep to the dorsal branch of ulnar nerve (DBUN).
6. Skin incision #3: 1 cm incision overlying ulnar styloid.
7. Blunt dissection is carried down to the level of fascia overlying extensor carpi ulnaris (ECU).

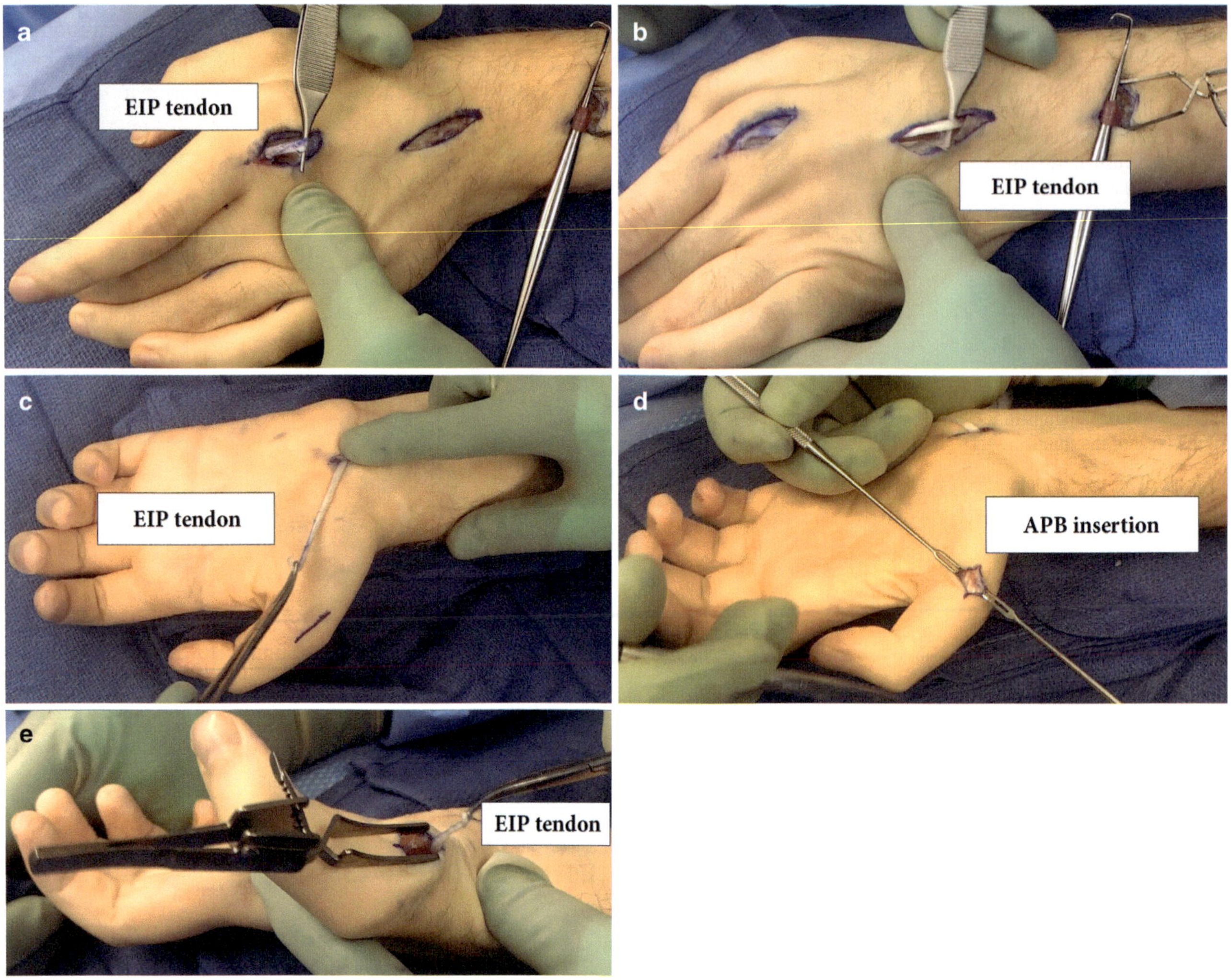

Fig. 43.9 (**a**) The EIP is shown here lying under an Adson pickup. (**b**) The EIP tendon lies under an Adson pickup. The EIP muscle belly lies under the Ragnell retractor (Integra). (**c**) The EIP tendon is cut distally and passed ulnarly through the volar incision just proximal to the carpal tunnel. (**d**) The APB insertion is shown between the two skin hook retractors. (**e**) The EIP has been passed to the APB base and is shown here grasped by a hemostat

8. The tendon is passed to the ulnar incision.
9. Skin incision #4: volar incision in line with palmaris longus just proximal to carpal tunnel.
10. The tendon is passed through the volar incision (Fig. 43.9c).
11. Skin incision #5: curvilinear incision at junction of dorsal and glabrous skin of thumb over MCP joint.
12. Dissection is carried down to level of APB insertion (Fig. 43.9d).
13. A subcutaneous tunnel is created from carpal tunnel incision to APB insertion.
14. The tendon is passed from the ulnar incision to the carpal tunnel and then to the APB base (Fig. 43.9e).
15. The thumb is placed in full palmar abduction and pronation, and the tendon is secured with a Pulvertaft weave.

High Median

BR to Flexor Pollicis Longus (FPL)

1. Skin incision: longitudinal radial incision from radial styloid to musculotendinous junction of BR (Fig. 43.10a).
2. Blunt dissection is carried down, and the BR is exposed while protecting the superficial radial nerve.
3. The BR is mobilized proximally (Fig. 43.10b).
4. The FPL is identified deep to the FCR (Fig. 43.10c).
5. The BR is released from its distal insertion. The BR and FPL are attached using a Pulvertaft weave. Tension is adjusted until there is lateral pinch with wrist extension (Fig. 43.10d).

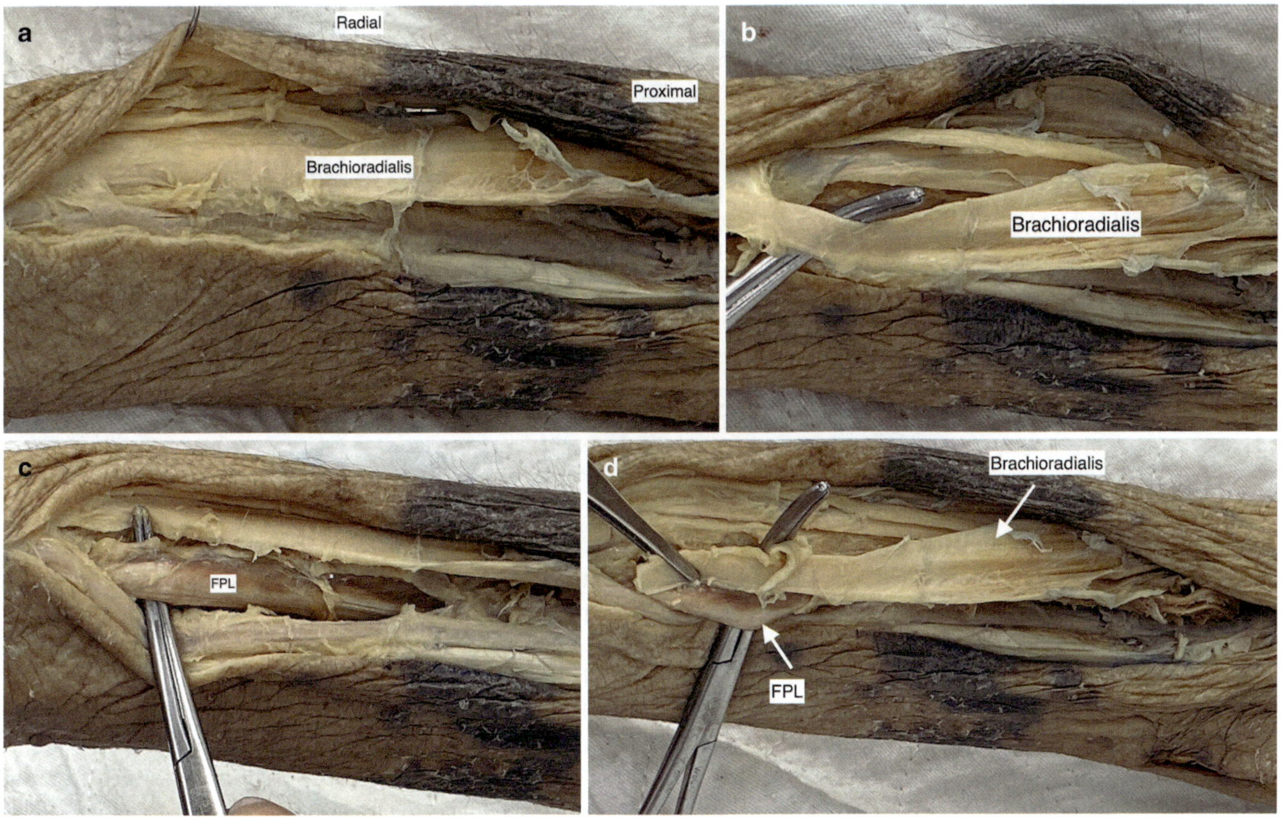

Fig. 43.10 (**a**) Volar exposure of a right forearm. The brachioradialis is exposed. (**b**) BR is elevated with a hemostat. (**c**) The FPL (lifted by the hemostat) is identified deep to the FCR. (**d**) BR and FPL are shown tensioned together

Side-to-Side Weave of FDP Index/Long (Median Innervated) into the Ring/Small (Ulnar Innervated)

1. Skin incision: volar longitudinal beginning at the distal wrist crease in the midline and extending approximately 10 cm proximally.
2. The palmaris longus tendon is identified for potential harvest.
3. Using gentle, blunt dissection, the FDS and median nerve are mobilized ulnarly.
4. The FPL is identified radially and excluded from the weave.
5. The FDP tendons to the index, middle, ring, and small are identified via traction and observation of finger flexion, including the distal interphalangeal joints.
6. While maintaining the fingers in a normal resting cascade (progressively increased flexion from radial to ulnar digits), the four tendons are joined with either multiple, large permanent braided sutures (2-0, figure-of-eight) or the palmaris tendon is harvested and joined to the FDP tendons by weaving the palmaris through the four FDP in a Pulvertaft fashion.

Ulnar Nerve Deficits [3]

The ulnar nerve supplies the ulnar border of the hand as well as the small and ring fingers. It gives motor supply to the FCU, FDP to the ring and small fingers, as well as the majority of hand intrinsic muscles, including the hypothenar muscles, interossei, lumbricals to the small and ring finger, and thumb adductor. Sensation is provided to the medial one and a half fingers and ulnar aspect of the hand.

Ulnar nerve deficits may result in the characteristic ulnar claw hand, with MCP extension, and interphalangeal (IP) joint flexion of the small and ring fingers. It may also limit thumb adduction [1, 3].

The goals of surgery are to correct clawing, improve thumb pinch, and restore normal finger flexion.

Passive Techniques

In the setting of low ulnar palsies, the chief deficits are loss of coordination in the hand and a "claw" posture of the ulnar-sided digits. When the patient demonstrates adequate extension of the proximal interphalangeal joints of the fingers with

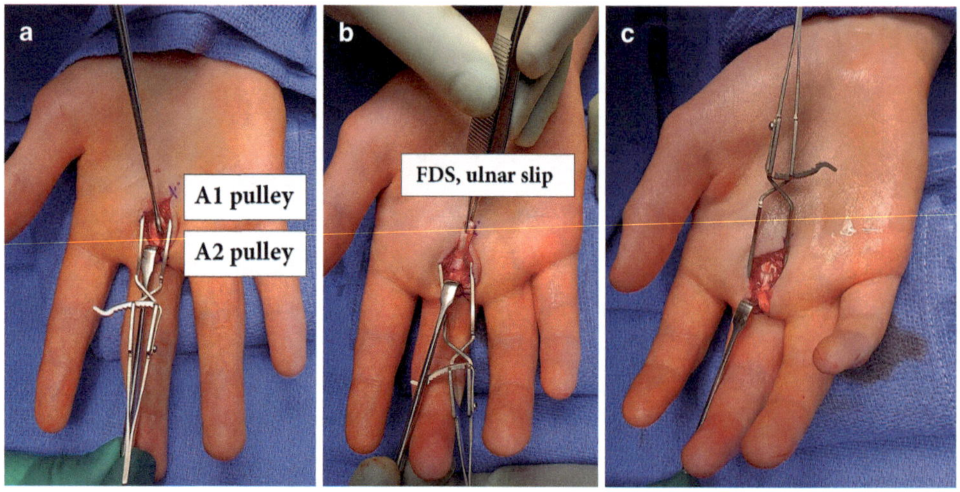

Fig. 43.11 (**a**) The middle finger A1 pulley is shown at the tip of the probe. (**b**) The Ulnar slip of the FDS has been released and pulled back under the A1 pulley. (**c**) The Ulnar slip of the FDS has been passed over the A1 pulley and sutured to the A1 pulley and the radial slip of the FDS

the metacarpophalangeal joints blocked in mild flexion, a formal tendon transfer may not be necessary. In this setting, procedures that take advantage of tenodesis effects may suffice to correct clawing.

Zancolli Lasso (Video 43.3)

1. If possible, the procedure is performed awake with local anesthesia.
2. Incision: 2 cm longitudinal incision centered over the A1 pulley.
3. Blunt dissection is carried down to expose the A1 and A2 pulleys as well as the FDS proximal to the A1 pulley (Fig. 43.11a).
4. The A2 pulley is incised to create a 0.5 cm window.
5. The ulnar slip of FDS is released distally and pulled back proximally under the A1 pulley (Fig. 43.11b).
6. The ulnar slip is then passed superficial to the A1 pulley and sutured to the A1 pulley and the remaining FDS distal to the A1 pulley (Fig. 43.11c). By limiting the length of the FDS from the A1 pulley to the insertion on the middle phalanx, the degree of extension at the metacarpophalangeal (MP) joint is limited, thereby allowing the central slip contribution to dynamically extend the finger at PIP.
7. The hand is taken through a range of motion, and tension is adjusted as needed.

Sling Tenodesis

1. Requires the presence of a donor tendon, typically palmaris longus or plantaris.
2. The procedure begins with a harvest of the palmaris (refer to PL transfer technique above) or plantaris (refer to ECRL to lateral bands technique below).
3. Midlateral incisions over the radial border of the small finger and the ulnar border of the ring finger proximal phalanges are created.
4. A dorsal, longitudinal incision is created over the interval between the metacarpal heads.
5. Blunt dissection through the dorsal incision allows identification of the palmar, inter-metacarpal plate.
6. Blunt dissection with a hemostat is performed from the phalangeal incision to the dorsal incision, with one tunnel passing palmar to the intermetacarpal plate and the second passing dorsal.
7. The tendon graft is passed from distal to proximal, then grasped on the opposite side of the intermetacarpal plate and drawn distally into the other digit.
8. With the metacarpophalangeal joints flexed to 50–60 degrees and the interphalangeal joints straight, the two ends of the tendon graft are joined to the lateral bands with a single figure-of-eight suture.
9. Tension of the tenodesis is checked with passive (or active if done under WALANT) motion. As the fingers move into extension, the graft tension should tighten, pulling on the lateral bands and extending the interphalangeal joints.

Active Techniques

Dynamic transfers can be used to restore active ulnar innervated muscle function, including thumb adduction or MCP flexion with PIP joint extension (intrinsic plus positioning).

ECRL to Radial Lateral Bands with Plantaris Autograft (Video 43.4)

1. The patient is positioned supine with a hand table. The arm and ipsilateral leg are prepped and draped.
2. Skin incision #1: 2 cm longitudinal incision overlying the base of the second metacarpal.

3. Dissection is carried down and the ECRL is identified at its insertion (Fig. 43.12a).
4. Skin incision #2: 2 cm longitudinal incision over the dorsum of the forearm centered between the radius and ulna, just proximal to the distal radioulnar joint.
5. Dissection is carried down, and the ECRL is identified.
6. The ECRL is released distally at its insertion and pulled back through the proximal incision.
7. Skin incision #3: 4 cm incision at the proximal 1/3 of the leg along the medial aspect. The gastrocnemius is palpated, and the incision is placed along the anterior border of the muscle.
8. Dissection is carried down to the investing fascia of the posterior compartment. The compartment is entered, and a plane developed between the gastrocnemius and the soleus (Fig. 43.12b).
9. The plantaris is identified and isolated.
10. Skin incision #4: 3 cm longitudinal incision at the insertion of the plantaris into the Achilles tendon. This can be palpated by plantaris excursion proximally.
11. The plantaris is isolated proximally and distally and released at both ends.
12. The plantaris tendon is divided into the number of fingers to be treated and woven into the ECRL with enough excursion to reach the PIP of all the intended target fingers (Fig. 43.12c).
13. Skin incision #5: 1 cm midlateral incision overlying radial aspect of proximal phalanx of target fingers.
14. The radial lateral bands are identified (Fig. 43.12d).
15. A subcutaneous tunnel is created starting at the lateral bands, passing palmar to the intermetacarpal plate, then slightly more dorsal toward the proximal incision (Fig. 43.12e).
16. The plantaris bands are passed through the tunnel to the radial lateral bands (Fig. 43.12f).
17. The fingers are placed into intrinsic plus position (MCP flexed, IP joints extended) and the plantaris is attached to the radial lateral band using a series of figure-of-eight sutures.
18. Sedation is reduced and the patient is allowed to take the hand through range of motion. Tension is adjusted as needed.

EIP to Adductor Pollicis

1. Skin incisions: a 2–3 cm longitudinal incision over the dorsal index metacarpophalangeal joint and a 3 cm incision over the dorsoulnar aspect of the thumb metacarpophalangeal joint.
2. EIP is identified as the deeper and more ulnar of the two tendons at the index MCP joint (Fig. 43.13a).
3. The EIP is harvested with a small extension onto the conjoined extensor tendon over the proximal third of the proximal phalanx (Fig. 43.13b).
4. The adductor pollicis insertion is identified on the proximal phalanx/extensor hood of the thumb (Fig. 43.13c).
5. A tunnel is created with blunt dissection using a right-angle clamp immediately adjacent to the neck of the index metacarpal and extended toward the adductor insertion (Fig. 43.13d)
6. The EIP is passed (on the ulnar side) deep to the index metacarpal neck and drawn radially toward the adductor insertion.
7. The tendons are joined via Pulvertaft weave or side-to-side suturing (Fig. 43.13e).

FDS to Lateral Band

1. Skin incision #1: a longitudinal or chevron incision in the palm centered over the radial aspect of the flexor tendons.
2. Blunt dissection is carried down to the tendons. Neurovascular structures are protected.
3. The sheath is opened over FDS and FDP (as in Fig. 43.4a and b).
4. Skin incision #2: mid-lateral radial sided incision overlying the proximal phalanx of the small and ring fingers (Fig. 43.14a). One FDS may be split into its two halves to transfer to the lateral bands of two adjacent digits.
5. Blunt dissection is carried down. The neurovascular bundle is protected and reflected palmarly. The lateral band and the extensor mechanism are identified and dissected free from the underlying bone. They are traced back proximally (Fig. 43.14b).
6. The FDS to the ring finger is identified, the finger is flexed, and the FDS is divided distally to allow for maximal length (as in Fig. 43.4c).
7. The FDS tendon is passed palmar to intermetacarpal plate, then slightly more dorsal toward incision overlying lateral band (Fig. 43.14c).
8. The small and ring fingers are placed into intrinsic plus position (MCP flexed, IP joints extended), and the FDS is sutured to the lateral band using a series of figure-of-eight sutures (Fig. 43.14d).
9. Sedation is reduced, and the patient is allowed to take the hand through range of motion. Tension is adjusted as needed.

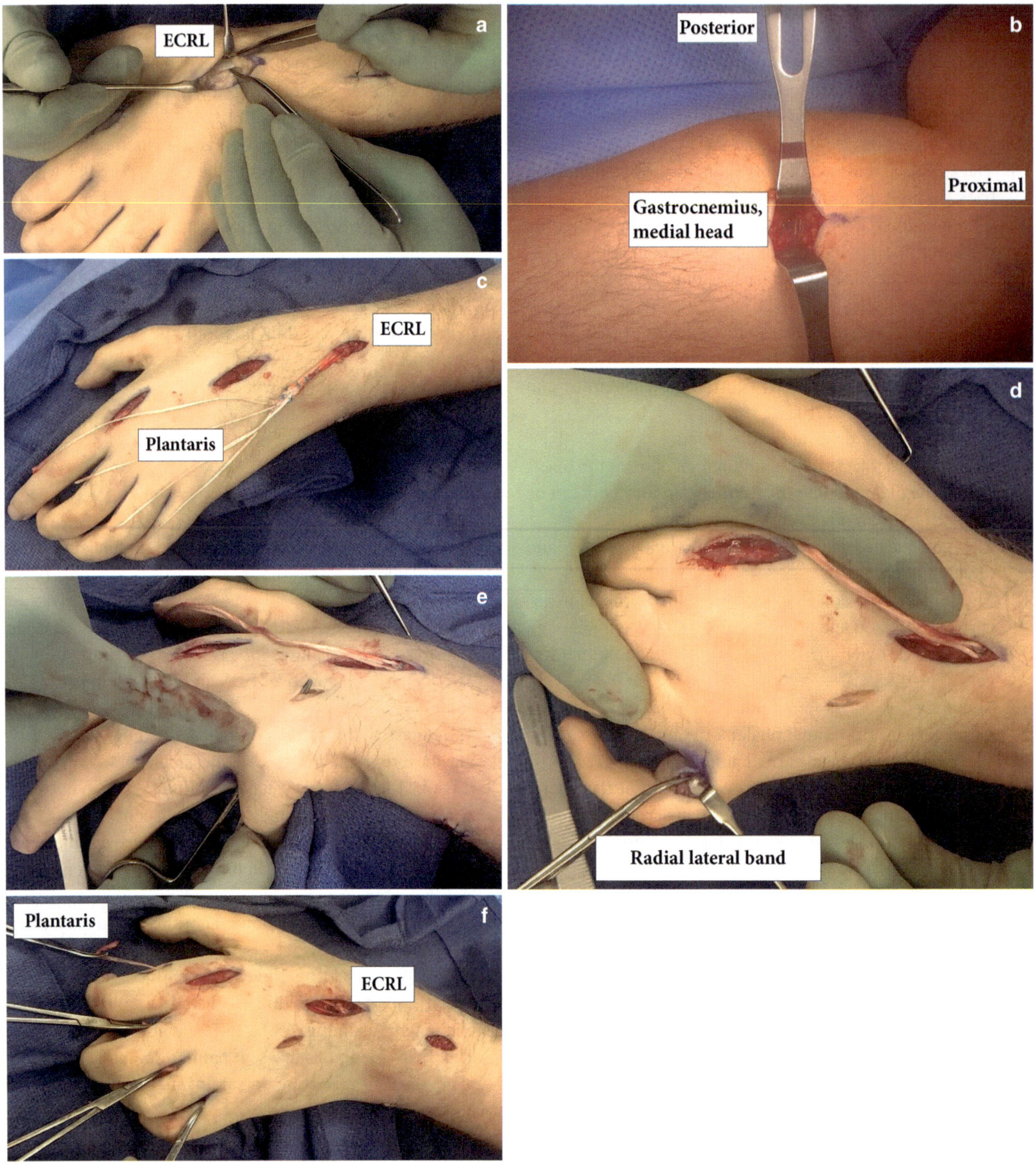

Fig. 43.12 (**a**) The ECRL is exposed near its insertion on the base of the second metacarpal. (**b**) A left leg is shown. Dissection has been carried down between gastrocnemius and soleus. (**c**) Limbs of the plantaris tendon have been woven into the ECRL, ensuring enough length to reach the insertion point of the radial lateral bands at the PIP joint. (**d**) The radial lateral band insertion for the small finger is exposed. (**e**) A hemostat has been passed from the radial lateral band insertion palmar to the intermetacarpal plate to the proximal incision. (**f**) The plantaris tendon autograft limbs have been passed in the path of the intrinsic muscles. They are shown here grasped by hemostats

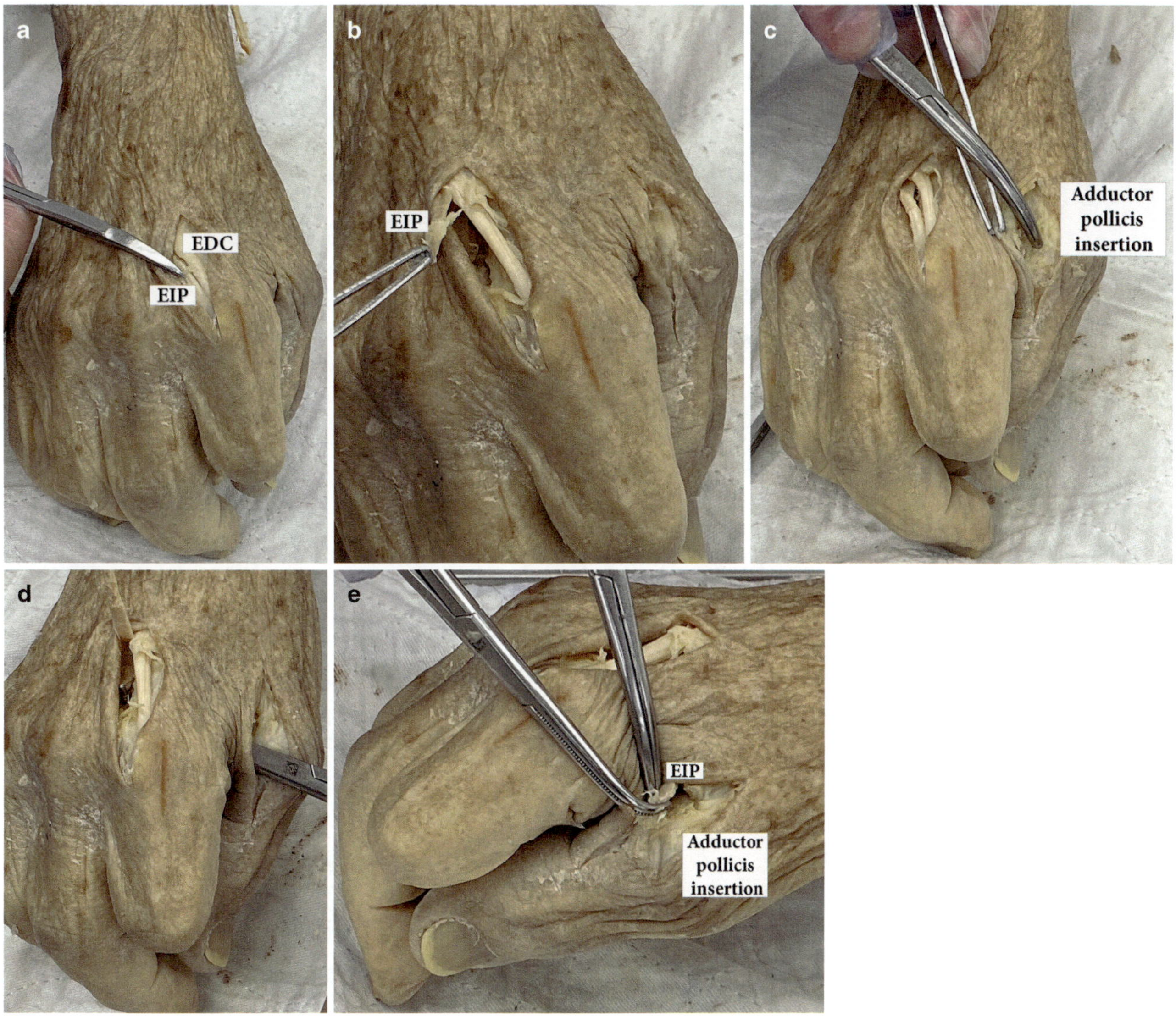

Fig. 43.13 (**a**) The EIP is deep and ulnar to the EDC to the index finger. (**b**) The EIP cut distally. (**c**) Insertion of the adductor pollicis on the ulnar aspect of the proximal phalanx of the thumb. (**d**) The right-angle clamp lies in the tunnel from the adductor insertion to the EIP slip volar to the second metacarpal neck. (**e**)The EIP tendon, held by the right-angle clamp, has been passed towards the adductor insertion

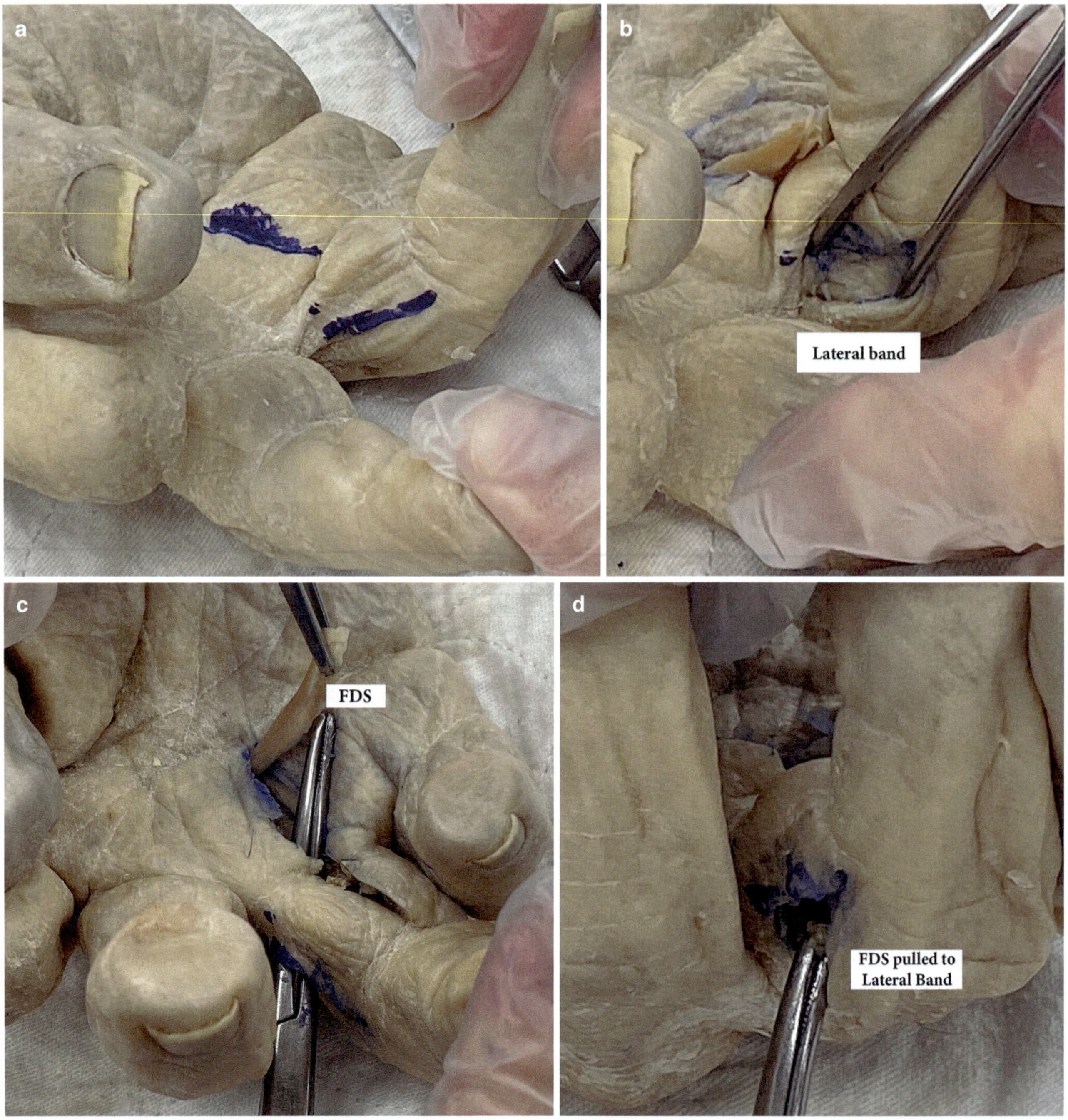

Fig. 43.14 (**a**) An incision is marked overlying the radial aspect of the ring finger. (**b**) The lateral bands to the ring finger lie between the prongs of the forceps. (**c**) The hemostat lies in the path of the intrinsic muscles from the radial lateral band to the FDS. (**d**) The FDS is grasped with the tip of the hemostat. It has been passed to the radial lateral band insertion

References

1. Loewenstein SN, Adkinson JM (2019) Tendon transfers for peripheral nerve palsies. Clin Plast Surg 46(3):307–315. https://doi.org/10.1016/j.cps.2019.02.004. Epub 2019 Apr 12
2. Livermore A, Tueting JL (2016) Biomechanics of tendon transfers. Hand Clin 32(3):291–302. https://doi.org/10.1016/j.hcl.2016.03.011. Epub 2016 Jun 3
3. Davis TRC (2017) Principles of tendon transfers of median, radial, and ulnar nerves. In: Wolfe SW, Pederson WC, Kozin SH, Cohen MS (eds) Green's operative hand surgery, 7th edn. Elsevier, Philadelphia, PA, pp 1023–1079

Tendon Transfers for Restoration of Shoulder Function

44

Abdulaziz F. Ahmed, Ryan Lohre, Karan Dua, and Bassem T. Elhassan

Indications

Muscle tendon transfers (MTTs) are effective procedures to restore shoulder function and reduce pain for various muscle-tendon or neurologic deficiencies around the shoulder. These deficiencies can include anterosuperior rotator cuff deficiency, posterosuperior rotator cuff deficiency, and deltoid deficiency or dysfunction. These deficiencies can occur through traumatic or degenerative changes, or through cervical (C5) radiculopathy, brachial plexopathy, or suprascapular or axillary nerve palsies.

A latissimus dorsi (LD) transfer and a lower trapezius tendon (LTT) transfer are typically indicated in persistent shoulder weakness in shoulder forward elevation and external rotation caused by irreparable posterosuperior rotator cuff tears involving both the supraspinatus and infraspinatus tendons with or without teres minor involvement. We prefer to perform an LTT transfer because of its synergistic contraction during external rotation and its similar line of pull to the deficient infraspinatus [1].

Both pectoralis major (PM) or LD transfer to the most proximal aspect of the lesser tuberosity of the proximal humerus are options to reconstruct anterosuperior rotator cuff deficiency leading to weakness in shoulder internal rotation and elevation. Anterosuperior cuff deficiency consists of subscapularis tendon deficiency with or without supraspinatus involvement. The PM has been considered the historical gold standard; however, it has mixed results and may be biomechanically unfavorable. Our preference is to perform a LD transfer, which has demonstrated clinical superiority when compared to PM transfer [2].

Pedicled LD transfer and pedicled PM transfer are the treatment options for deltoid dysfunction or paralysis and are concurrently performed with a reverse shoulder arthroplasty (RSA). We prefer to utilize a pedicled PM transfer to reconstruct the anterior deltoid [3].

Open Lower Trapezius for Restoration of Shoulder External Rotation and Elevation

Patient Positioning and Equipment

- Patient position: Beach chair position or lateral decubitus on standard operating room table.
- Allograft: Achilles tendon.
- Equipment: Open surgical instrumentation, electrocautery, oscillating saw, osteotomes.
- Implants: Multiple suture anchors and non-absorbable tape sutures, low profile locking plates.
- Immobilization: External rotation shoulder brace.

Surgical Technique

1. Lower trapezius tendon harvest: A 5-cm incision is made parallel and distal to the scapular spine. The incision should be from 2 cm medial to 3 cm lateral to the medial scapular border (Fig. 44.1). After incising the skin and subcutaneous tissue, a fat pad is identified at the most lateral part of the incision until the infraspinatus fascia is visualized. The

Supplementary Information The online version contains supplementary material available at https://doi.org/10.1007/978-3-031-73931-6_44.

A. F. Ahmed
Missouri Orthopaedic Institute, Department of Orthopaedic Surgery, University of Missouri School of Medicine, Columbia, MO, USA

R. Lohre
Department of Orthopaedic Surgery, Harvard Medical School, Massachusetts General Hospital, Boston, MA, USA

K. Dua
Department of Orthopaedic Surgery, New York-Presbytarian/Columbia University Irving Medical Center, New York, NY, USA

B. T. Elhassan (✉)
Department of Orthopaedic Surgery, Harvard Medical School, Massachusetts General Hospital, Boston, MA, USA
e-mail: belhassan@mgh.harvard.edu

A. S. Hanna (ed.), *Nerves: Anatomy, Exposures, and Techniques*, https://doi.org/10.1007/978-3-031-73931-6_44

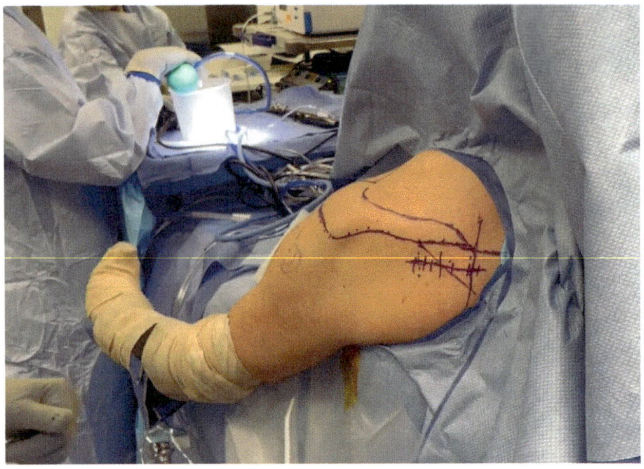

Fig. 44.1 Lower trapezius harvest incision is placed distal to the scapular spine from 1–2 cm medial to the medial scapular border to 3–4 cm lateral to the medial scapular border

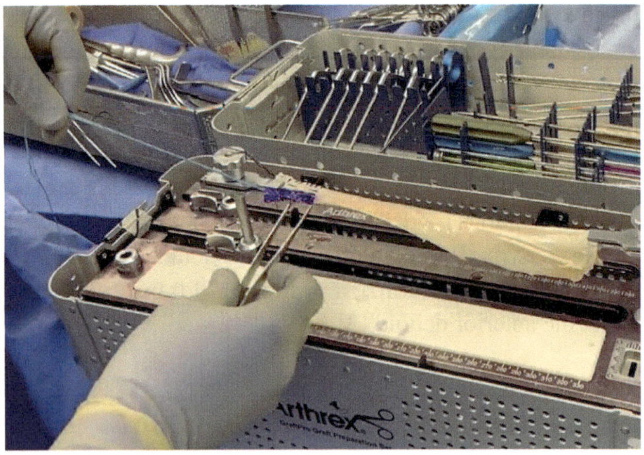

Fig. 44.2 The Achilles tendon allograft is prepped using a graft preparation set. The medial and lateral parts of the tendon are prepped with reinforced suture tapes in a Krackow pattern, resulting in four suture limbs

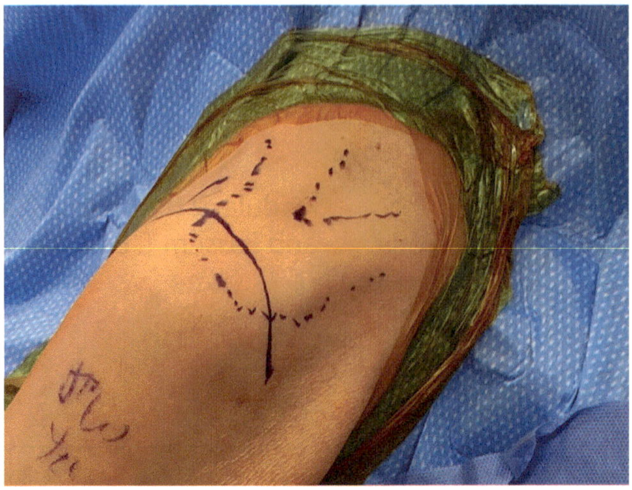

Fig. 44.3 Sabre incision for the acromial osteotomy approach to the glenohumeral joint. Notice that the incision is 1 cm medial to the lateral edge of the acromion

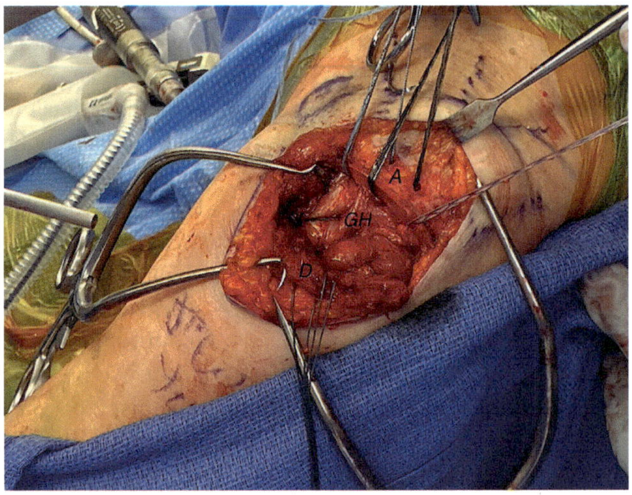

Fig. 44.4 The lateral 1 cm of the lateral acromion (*A*) has been osteotomized taking with it the middle deltoid (*D*). Afterwards, excellent exposure to the glenohumeral joint (*GH*) can be obtained

LTT is then identified inserting on the scapular spine and is released from its insertion from its most lateral insertion toward the most medial insertion on the scapular spine. The excursion of the tendon is maximized, releasing the soft tissue attachments inferior to the lower trapezius tendon. Video 44.1 demonstrates the LTT harvest.

2. Achilles allograft preparation: An allograft is required as the lower trapezius tendon is short and must be augmented to reach the greater tuberosity of the humerus. The allograft is prepared by placing non-absorbable suture tapes of different colors in a Krackow fashion on each side of the Achilles tendon narrow/calcaneal end (Fig. 44.2).
3. Shoulder exposure through an acromial osteotomy: A saber incision is made medial to the lateral border of the acromion (Fig. 44.3). The intervals between the anterior and middle deltoid, and the middle and posterior deltoid are developed. An electrical saw is used to perform a 5 mm thick lateral acromion osteotomy that is attached to the middle deltoid. The osteotomized acromion and middle deltoid are reflected laterally to provide excellent exposure of the glenohumeral joint (Fig. 44.4). The posterosuperior cuff footprint is debrided until bleeding bone is encountered.
4. Creation of a tunnel between the harvest incision and the glenohumeral joint: the tunnel must be deep to the posterior deltoid, and a grasping instrument is passed from the glenohumeral joint into the lower trapezius harvest incision. The allograft is then retrieved from the harvest incision into the glenohumeral joint, with the narrow end of the allograft pointing toward the joint.

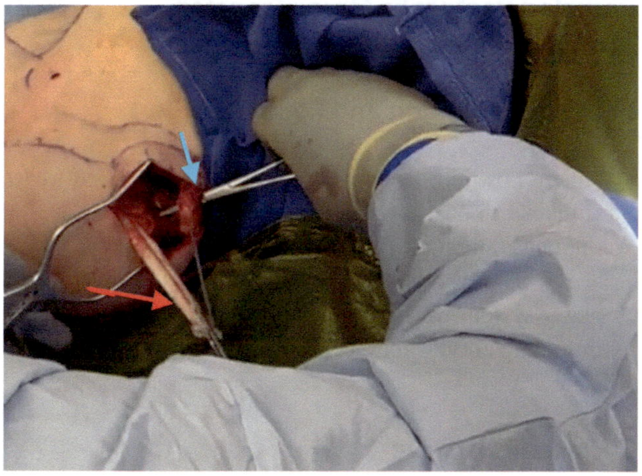

Fig. 44.5 A clamp has been introduced through the lower trapezius tendon (*blue arrow*) to weave it with Achilles tendon allograft in a Pulvertaft fashion. *Red arrow* broad end of the Achilles tendon allograft.

5. Allograft fixation: The medial sutures from the Achilles tendon are fixed to the anteromedial footprint of the supraspinatus with a 5.5 mm suture anchor, whereas the lateral suture is fixed to the anterior lateral footprint of the supraspinatus with another suture anchor. One can perform additional fixation by placing two more additional anchors. One anchor medial is placed to the allograft at the articular cartilage margin of the greater tuberosity. Sutures from the prior anchor are then draped over the allograft and fixed at the lateral margin of the greater tuberosity with another anchor in a lateral row/seatbelt fashion.
6. Lower trapezius to Achilles tendon allograft weave: The arm is placed in abduction and external rotation. The broad end of the Achilles allograft is then weaved into the lower trapezius tendon in a Pulvertaft fashion (Fig. 44.5).
7. The middle deltoid and acromial osteotomies are repaired back to the lateral acromion by using multiple suture tapes in a cow-hitch fashion.
8. Postoperative care: The patient is immobilized in an external rotation shoulder brace for a period of 8 weeks prior to beginning graduated motion.

Open Latissimus Transfer for Anterosuperior Rotator Cuff Deficiency for Restoration of Shoulder Internal Rotation and Elevation

Patient Positioning and Equipment

- Patient position: Beach chair with the head raised to 70° with an arm positioner.
- Allograft: Achilles tendon (optional).
- Equipment: Open surgical equipment including retractors, electrocautery.

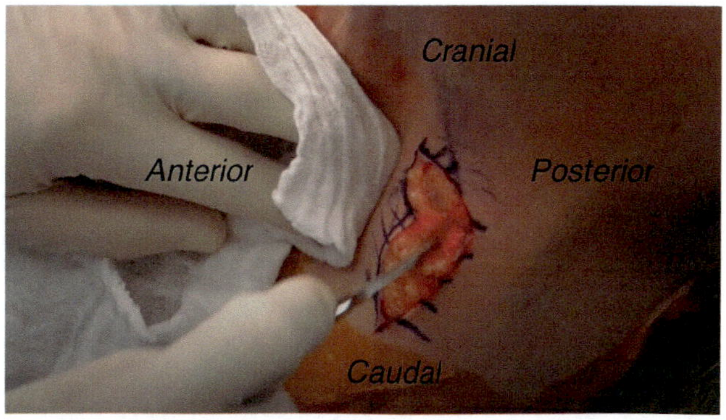

Fig. 44.6 Latissimus dorsi harvest through an axillary incision made at the posterior axillary fold

- Implants: Multiple suture anchors and non-absorbable tape sutures, tenodesis buttons.
- Immobilization: Shoulder immobilizer/sling with an abduction pillow.

Surgical Technique

1. A standard deltopectoral approach is utilized. The pectoralis major insertion on the proximal humerus is released at its proximal edge by 1–2 cm to facilitate exposure of the latissimus dorsi tendon.
2. The latissimus dorsi tendon is separated from the teres major tendon, and the bridging fascia is released. In up to 30% of cases, the latissimus dorsi tendon and the teres major will be conjoined, which would require meticulous dissection to separate them.
3. The latissimus dorsi tendon is then released from its insertion and tagged with a suture. To gain further excursion, the latissimus dorsi tendon is further released from bone and released from other surrounding soft tissue adhesions in a proximal-lateral to distal-medial direction.
4. If the latissimus dorsi continues to have inadequate excursion, one can harvest the tendon from the axillary incision (Fig. 44.6, Video 44.2). This requires an assistant to hold the arm in flexion and internal rotation; thereafter a 5-cm incision is made at the posterior axillary fold. Skin flaps are raised, and dissection is carried down until a muscular and a tendon structure are identified. The tendon represents the latissimus dorsi tendon, whereas the muscular structure is the teres major muscle. The latissimus dorsi is separated from the teres major, and the tendon is retrieved fully from the axillary incision to ensure all soft tissue tethers are released (Fig. 44.7). The tendon is retrieved into the glenohumeral joint with a long grasping instrument.

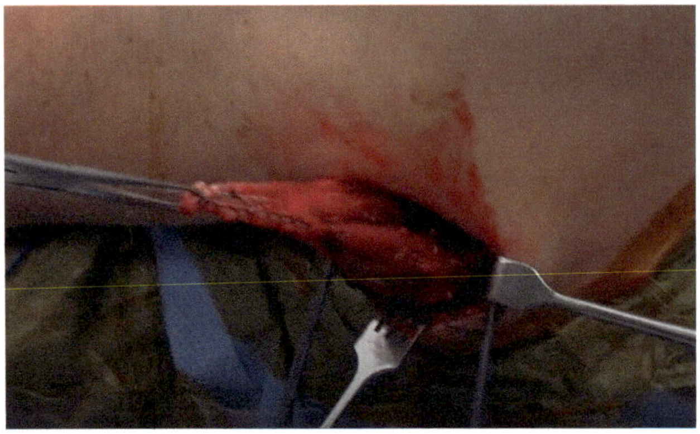

Fig. 44.7 The latissimus dorsi tendon has been harvested and pulled maximally through the axillary incision. This ensures that all potential soft tissue tethers are released and provides maximal excursion of the tendon. The arm is forward elevated maximally in the scapular plane

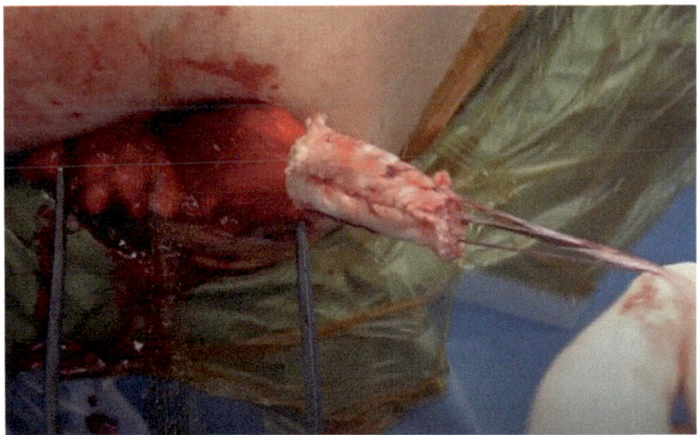

Fig. 44.8 If the latissimus dorsi tendon is frayed, it can be reinforced with the thick portion of the Achilles tendon allograft by combining the allograft with the latissimus tendon by using suture tapes in a Krackow fashion

5. If the latissimus dorsi tendon appears too thin or frayed, we do augment it with the narrow part of the Achilles tendon. This is done by suturing the Achilles narrow end to the latissimus dorsi tendon with medial and lateral suture tapes in Krackow fashion (Fig. 44.8).
6. The latissimus tendon is then reattached to the upper subscapularis footprint with the use of suture anchors. If the supraspinatus tendon is also deficient, the latissimus dorsi tendon is fixed more proximally at the anterior footprint of the supraspinatus across the bicipital groove.
7. The released pectoralis major tendon is then repaired to the proximal humerus with the use of suture buttons.
8. Postoperative care: The patient is immobilized in a shoulder immobilizer/sling with the arm in neutral to internal rotation.

Pedicled Pectoralis Major Transfer for Deltoid Deficiency

Patient Positioning and Equipment

- Patient position: beach chair with the head raised to 70° with an arm positioner.
- Implants: multiple suture-button fixation device and heavy non-absorbable sutures, reverse shoulder arthroplasty system.
- Immobilization: shoulder spica cast.

Surgical Technique

1. Draping should allow sufficient access to the sternum.
2. A large curvilinear incision is started from 2 cm proximal of the xyphoid process and medial to the sternocostal junction. The incision is extended to the sternoclavicular joint, extending just distal to the clavicle. The incision continues to extend laterally across the acromioclavicular joint and then proceeds to the anterolateral acromion before extending distally into a deltopectoral approach.
3. Deep dissection is performed along the incision, and large skin flaps are developed to visualize the entire pectoralis major. Three distinct parts of the pectoralis major are then identified: the clavicular origin, the upper sternal, and the lower sternal origins (Fig. 44.9, Video 44.3).
4. A plane is developed between the upper and lower halves of the pectoralis major sternal heads. Essentially, we would harvest the clavicular head and the upper part of the sternal head. The lower sternal part of the pectoralis muscle is left intact. The clavicular and upper sternal pectoralis muscle parts are detached from the clavicle and sternum. If the harvested clavicular and upper sternal heads are unable to be flipped laterally easily, then the insertion of the clavicular/upper sternal pectoralis muscle is released from the humerus to allow for proper orientation of the muscle (Fig. 44.10). The location of the neurovascular pedicle is identified on the undersurface of the muscle near the middle of the clavicle distal to the subclavius muscle (Fig. 44.11).
5. The transferred muscle is protected with a moist gauze, and a reverse shoulder arthroplasty is performed.
6. The atrophic anterior deltoid is excised. The anterolateral acromion and the anterior lateral clavicle are decorticated with a high-speed burr.

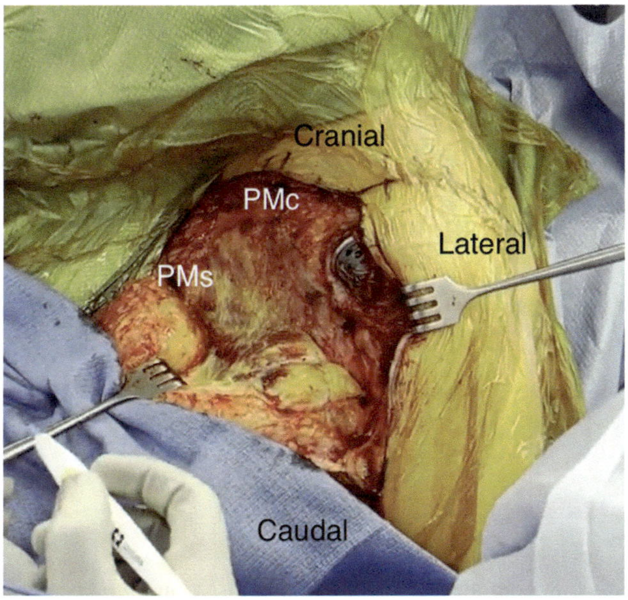

Fig. 44.9 An intraoperative photograph demonstrating an extensile approach exposing a prior failed hemiarthroplasty. This extensile approach allows a complete exposure of the pectoralis major at both its sternal and clavicular origins. *PMs* pectoralis major sternal head, *PMc* pectoralis major clavicular head

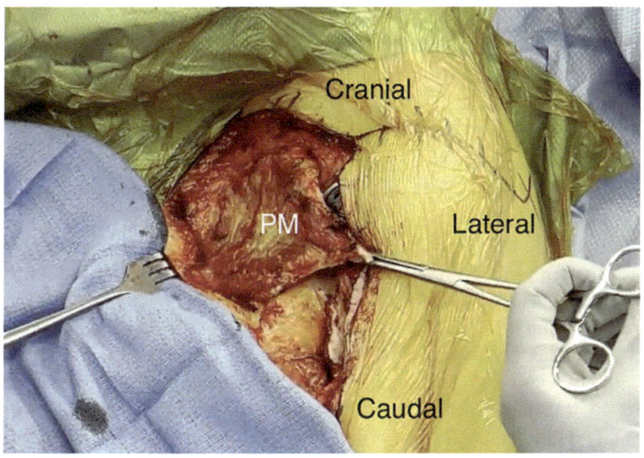

Fig. 44.10 The humeral insertions of upper sternal and clavicular portions of the pectoralis major (*PM*) are released from the humerus

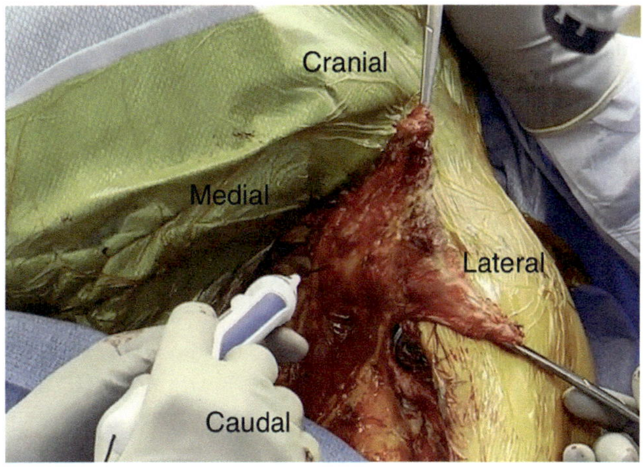

Fig. 44.11 The pectoralis major origins at the clavicle and the upper sternum are released to allow flipping of the pectoralis major laterally. The pedicle is located near the middle of the clavicle, just distal to the subclavius muscle. We further confirm the pedicle by stimulating the nerves with a nerve stimulator

7. Fixation of the transferred pedicled pectoralis major muscle:
   (a) The muscle is then rotated so that the most medial portion is lateral (Fig. 44.12). One must be cognizant to avoid pulling excessively on the muscle as this might tear the pedicle.
   (b) The new most medial clavicular origin of the pectoralis major (originally the most lateral clavicular origin of the pectoralis major) is fixed first with a suture button construct into the clavicle to avoid any tethering on the pedicle.
   (c) The remaining clavicular pectoralis muscle is then fixed to the anterior lateral third of the clavicle and anterolateral acromion by using suture button fixation.
   (d) We typically supplement fixation by using 7–8 suture buttons into the clavicle and anterolateral acromion.
   (e) The arm is placed in approximately 60° of flexion. The humeral insertion is attached again using suture buttons bicortically to the humeral shaft at the level of the prior deltoid insertion.
8. Postoperative care: a shoulder spica cast for a period of 8 weeks postoperatively. The arm remains in a flexed position of 45–60° with slight internal rotation.

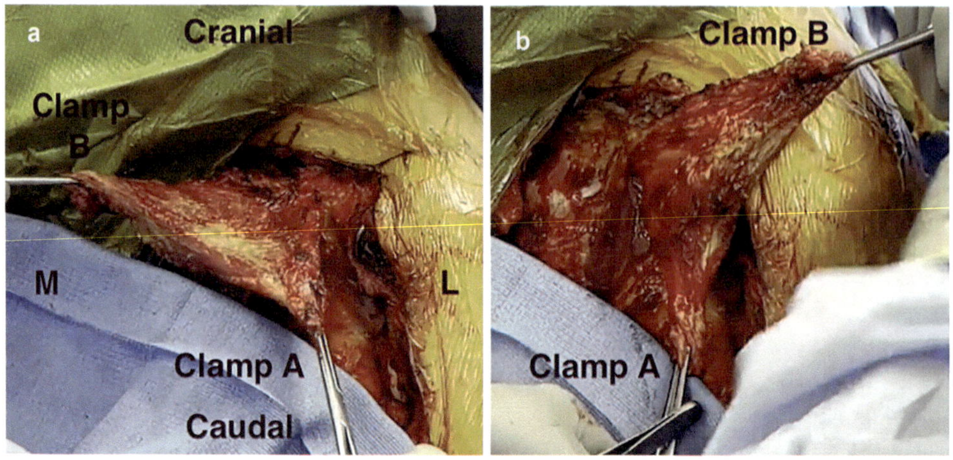

Fig. 44.12 (**a**) Anatomical orientation of the pectoralis major muscle. The distal clamp (A) is holding the humeral insertion and the medial clamp (B) is holding the upper edge of the sternal origin. (**b**) Orientation of the freed pectoralis major muscle, which is rotated (flipped). *M* medial, *L* lateral

Complications

- Hematoma: Drain placement might help reduce hematoma collection.
- Infection: This is related to the extensive soft tissue dissection, dead space, and the use of allograft. We routinely administer cefazolin and vancomycin intravenous antibiotics intraoperatively. We also soak the allograft in a vancomycin solution, and we administer vancomycin powder locally at the incision to reduce the risk of infection.
- Failure of tendon transfer: One must ensure that the appropriate immobilization method is utilized for each tendon transfer.
- Neurovascular injury:
  - The lower trapezius transfer: the spinal accessory nerve is found approximately 2 cm medial to the medial border of the scapula, and it is deep to the trapezius muscle.
  - The latissimus dorsi transfer: the radial nerve passes medial to the latissimus dorsi tendon.
  - The pectoralis major transfer: the lateral and medial pectoral nerves are found at an average distance of 8.5 cm medial to the humeral insertion of the pectoralis major and consistently medial to the pectoralis minor. The neurovascular pedicle of the pectoralis major is encountered near the middle of the clavicle, distal to the subclavius muscle near the subclavian artery and vein and brachial plexus.
- Shoulder stiffness.

References

1. Elhassan BT, Wagner ER, Werthel JD (2016) Outcome of lower trapezius transfer to reconstruct massive irreparable posterior-superior rotator cuff tear. J Shoulder Elbow Surg 25(8):1346–1353. https://doi.org/10.1016/j.jse.2015.12.006. Epub 2016 Mar 8
2. Elhassan BT, Wagner ER, Kany J (2020) Latissimus dorsi transfer for irreparable subscapularis tear. J Shoulder Elb Surg 29(10):2128–2134. https://doi.org/10.1016/j.jse.2020.02.019. Epub 2020 Jun 9
3. Elhassan BT, Wagner ER, Werthel JD, Lehanneur M, Lee J (2018) Outcome of reverse shoulder arthroplasty with pedicled pectoralis transfer in patients with deltoid paralysis. J Shoulder Elb Surg 27(1):96–103. https://doi.org/10.1016/j.jse.2017.07.007. Epub 2017 Sep 20

Secondary Glenohumeral Procedures in the Child with Brachial Plexus Birth Injury

45

Benjamin K. Gundlach, Eugene Park, Dan A. Zlotolow, and Scott H. Kozin

Indications

Open reduction of the glenohumeral joint is performed on children with brachial plexus birth injury (BPBI) who develop glenohumeral dysplasia and internal rotation contracture. The infant proximal humerus is largely unossified and is therefore poorly visualized on radiographs. Glenohumeral dysplasia is best diagnosed using MRI or ultrasound (US) (Fig. 45.1). Compared to an MRI, US has the primary benefit of not requiring anesthesia and can be easily performed in an outpatient setting, allowing for serial exams. US also allows for dynamic assessment of the glenohumeral joint during passive range of motion [1]. Internal rotation contracture is defined as passive external rotation less than the contralateral arm, with surgical reduction indicated when passive external rotation is less than 30°.

All images are Courtesy of Shriners Hospital for Children, Philadelphia.

Supplementary Information The online version contains supplementary material available at https://doi.org/10.1007/978-3-031-73931-6_45.

B. K. Gundlach
Boston Children's Hospital, Harvard Medical School, Department of Orthopedics, Boston, MA, USA

E. Park
Sidney Kimmel Medical College of Thomas Jefferson University, Shriners Hospital for Children, Philadelphia, PA, USA

D. A. Zlotolow
Sidney Kimmel Medical College of Thomas Jefferson University, Shriners Hospital for Children, Philadelphia, PA, USA

The Hospital for Special Surgery, New York, NY, USA

S. H. Kozin (✉)
Lewis Katz School of Medicine at Temple University, Sidney Kimmel Medical College at Thomas Jefferson University, Philadelphia, PA, USA

Shriners Hopsital for Children, Philadelphia, PA, USA
e-mail: skozin@shrinenet.org

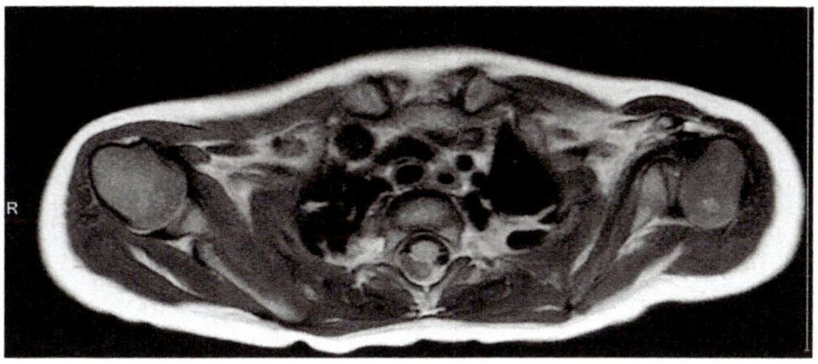

Fig. 45.1 An axial MRI demonstrating severe left glenohumeral dysplasia with posterior subluxation, compared to a normal right glenohumeral joint

The subscapularis has been implicated as a key deforming force of the glenohumeral joint in the BPBI patient. Due to its C5/6/7 innervation, the subscapularis is uniformly affected in BPBI, resulting in decreased strength and excursion. Therefore, most operations targeting glenohumeral dysplasia aim to reduce the effects of the subscapularis in some manner, be it tenotomy or submuscular slide off the scapula. Additionally, the upper third of the developing glenoid and coracoid base share a secondary ossification center. As such, glenoid retroversion is often accompanied by coracoid retroversion, with the coracoid occupying a more posterior and lateral space than normal and blocking humeral head reduction. Thus, we regularly perform coracoidectomy during open shoulder reductions [2].

Lastly, tendon transfer of the latissimus dorsi (LD) and/or the teres major (TM) is often performed concurrently to improve active external rotation and shoulder elevation. Tendon transfer should not be performed in children who lack strong active internal rotation (hand-to-navel ability on the modified Mallet scale), as the ability to reach midline can be lost in these children [3]. The LD especially is strongly innervated by the C7 root; therefore, we also recommend against tendon transfers in patients who sustained a BPBI involving C7 that have not regained midline strength of M4 or greater [4].

A. S. Hanna (ed.), *Nerves: Anatomy, Exposures, and Techniques*, https://doi.org/10.1007/978-3-031-73931-6_45

Shoulder Ultrasound

1. Position: Lateral decubitus with the injured extremity up, stabilized using a bean bag positioner.
2. Select an US probe that will allow for signal penetration to the depth of the child's shoulder. We prefer a linear 12 MHz probe.
3. The probe is placed posterior-superiorly and oriented along the horizontal axis of the glenohumeral joint to obtain an axial image.
4. The humeral head ossific nucleus, the labrum, the glenoid, and the scapular spine should be visualized together to confirm correct probe placement (Fig. 45.2).
5. Starting with the shoulder in maximal internal rotation, the shoulder is brought into neutral and then maximal external rotation (ER). In severe cases of internal rotation contracture, the shoulder cannot be externally rotated even to neutral.
6. In a mobile, reducible glenohumeral joint, as the humerus is externally rotated, the ossific nucleus of the humeral head will face the glenoid. As the humerus is placed into maximum external rotation, the ossific nucleus will become difficult to visualize as it "disappears" into the anterior aspect of the glenohumeral joint.
7. In a dysplastic glenohumeral joint, the ossific nucleus will be posteriorly translated compared to the axis of the scapula, the glenoid vault will be retroverted, and the alpha angle will be increased. In external rotation, the ossific nucleus will remain posteriorly displaced (Figs. 45.3 and 45.4).

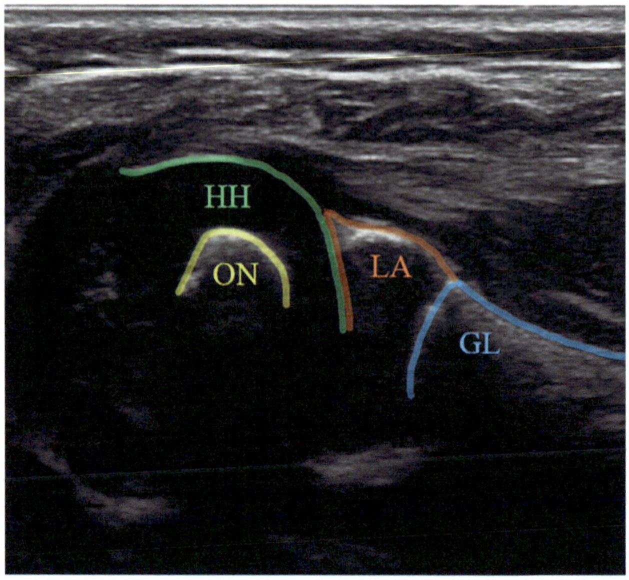

Fig. 45.2 A normal glenohumeral joint ultrasound with illustration overlaid to outline the humeral head (*HH*), the ossific nucleus (*ON*), labrum (*LA*), and glenoid (*GL*)

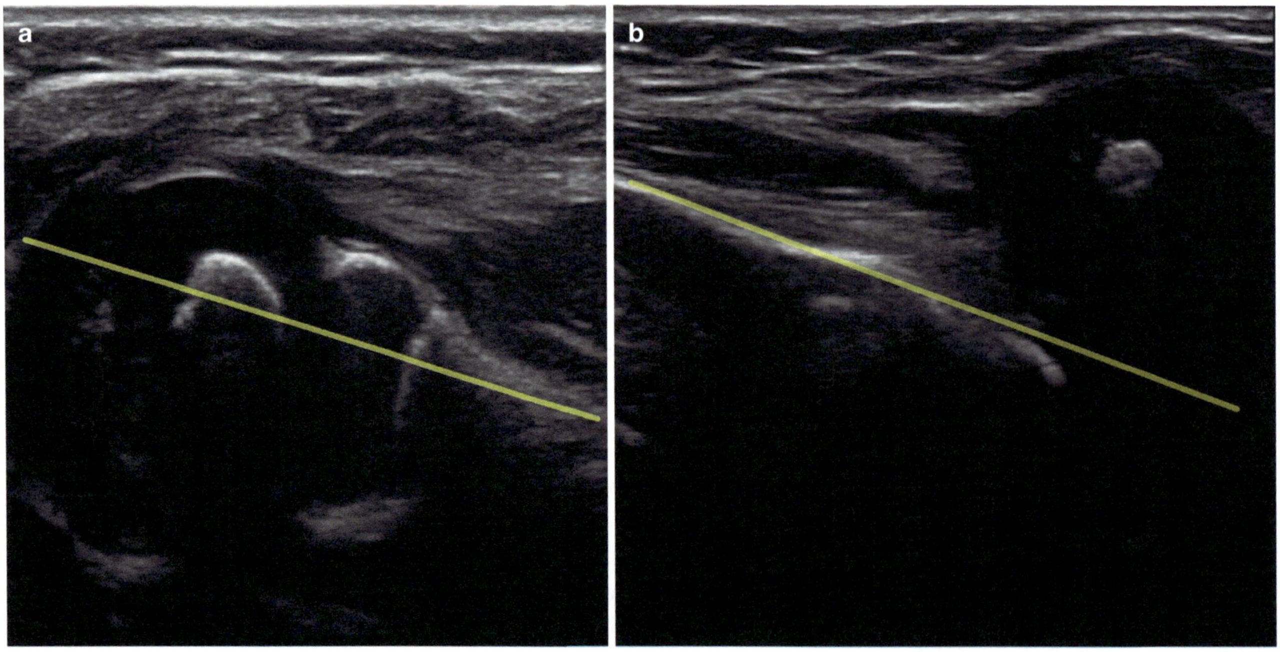

Fig. 45.3 (**a**) Normal glenohumeral joint ultrasound. The *yellow line* is drawn down the long axis of the scapula and bisects the humeral head. (**b**) Shoulder affected by severe glenohumeral dysplasia, with the humeral head markedly subluxated posterior to the scapular axis

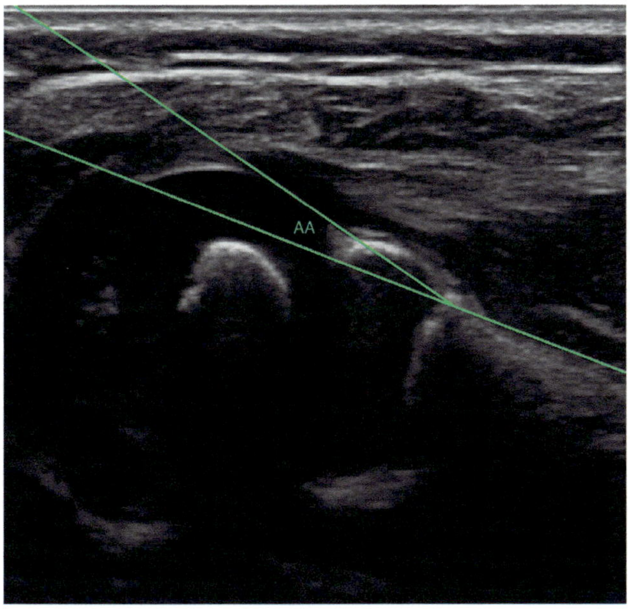

Fig. 45.4 The alpha angle (*AA*) is formed between the posterior scapular margin and a line starting at the posterior corner of the glenoid and running tangential to the humeral head

Open Shoulder Reduction Technique

1. Position: Lateral decubitus with the injured extremity up, stabilized using a bean-bag positioner. The surgeon stands anterior to the child.
2. An anterior deltopectoral incision is planned with the proximal extent overlying the coracoid process and extending just distal to the axillary crease. Dilute epinephrine is injected along the planned incision to limit blood loss prior to prepping and draping (Fig. 45.5).
3. The skin is incised, and the subcutaneous tissue is developed using electrocautery. The deltopectoral interval is identified by finding the cephalic vein. We prefer to mobilize the vein medially, as this allows for easier retraction and protection proximally when working around the coracoid process.
4. Clavipectoral fascia and subdeltoid bursa are incised and removed to define the coracoid process, conjoint tendon, and pectoralis minor tendon.
5. The pectoralis minor, conjoined tendon (short head of biceps + coracobrachialis), and both the coracohumeral and coracoacromial ligaments are released from the coracoid process using bipolar electrocautery until the base of the coracoid is visualized. Care should be taken to avoid injury to the infraclavicular plexus and axillary artery that are coursing through the abundant fat just deep and medial to these tendinous structures (Fig. 45.6).
6. Remove the coracoid process at its base using a bone-biting rongeur (Fig. 45.7).

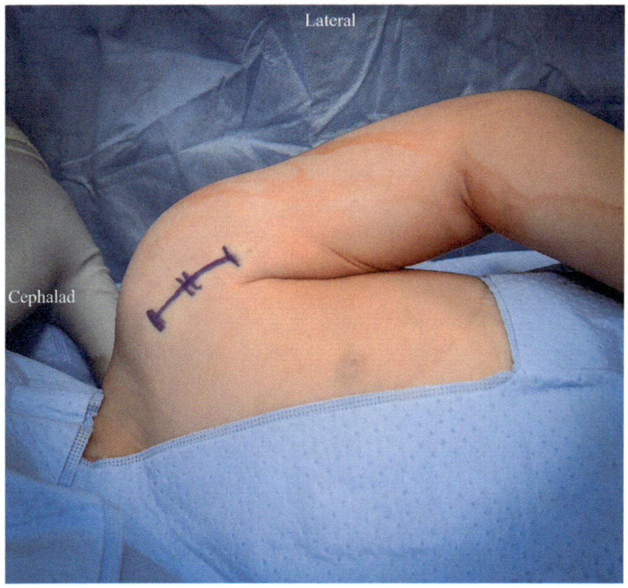

Fig. 45.5 The planned incision for anterior open shoulder release

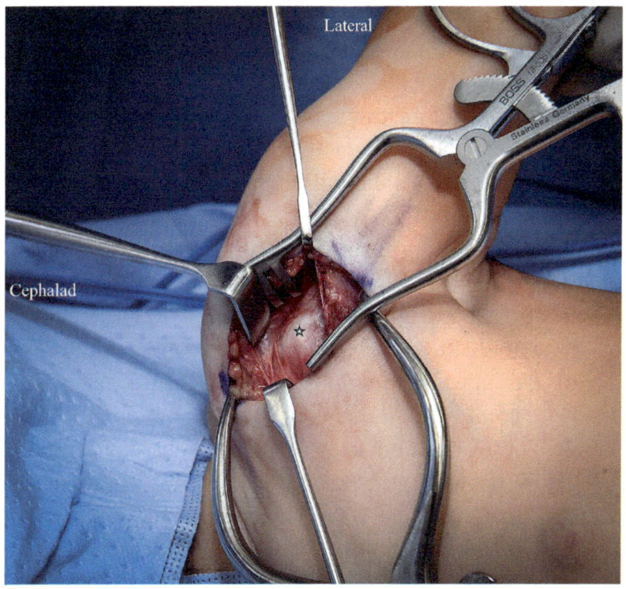

Fig. 45.6 The deltopectoral interval has been developed, and the coracoid (*star*) exposed with the origins of the pectoralis minor, coracobrachialis, and short head of the biceps brachii visible

7. With the coracoid removed, the subscapularis tendon is now better visualized. A peanut sponge can be used to bluntly dissect away remaining bursal tissue, better defining the upper rolled border of the subscapularis tendon. Placing the shoulder in external rotation facilitates identification of the taught subscapularis. Avoid medial dissection past the musculotendinous junction, as the axillary nerve travels over and superficial to the subscapularis muscle belly and is at risk of injury.

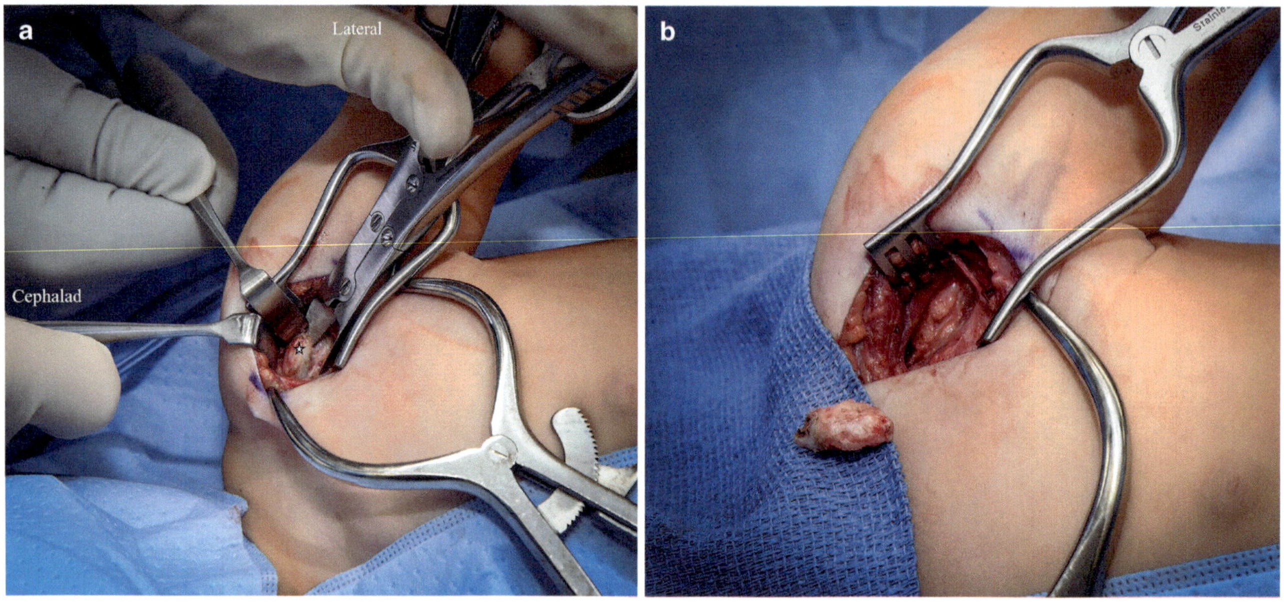

Fig. 45.7 The three muscular origins have been released from the coracoid with bipolar electrocautery. A bone-biting rongeur (**a**) is used to remove the coracoid process at its base (**b**)

8. Identify the rotator interval just cephalad to the rolled border, and then "pop" into the glenohumeral joint using a blunt instrument (e.g., freer elevator) while taking care not to injure the articular cartilage. A small effluent of joint fluid will confirm location within the joint.
9. Through the capsulotomy, use a right-angle hemostat to isolate the subscapularis tendon and anterior capsule from the underlying biceps tendon and labrum. Using bipolar electrocautery, an initial tenotomy is performed in the upper one-third of the subscapularis tendon (Fig. 45.8).
10. Do not release more than 50% of the subscapularis muscle, as complete or near-complete release of the muscle will lead to internal rotation weakness and loss of midline function. Additionally, the anterior-inferior labrum is in close proximity to the caudal portion of the subscapularis and joint capsule, and inadvertent injury will create anterior instability.
11. With the tendon released, the glenohumeral joint is inspected for the presence of the humeral head. The humeral head may appear absent upon first inspection due to its posteriorly subluxated position.
12. Moving posterior to the child, grab the affected arm around the elbow and brachium. This position creates a short lever arm through which an external rotation force can be applied, reducing the chance of creating an iatrogenic humerus fracture.
13. Slow but firm external rotation is applied while also providing an anterior translation force to the humeral head. This combined movement will reduce the humeral head back onto the glenoid. The humeral head should now be visualized in a reduced position when the shoulder is held in external rotation (Fig. 45.9).
14. If an internal rotation contracture remains, a small amount more of subscapularis muscle is released. Additionally, the pectoralis major should be inspected. If the pectoralis major is excessively tight in shoulder abduction and external rotation, the inferior tendinous portion should be fractionally lengthened.

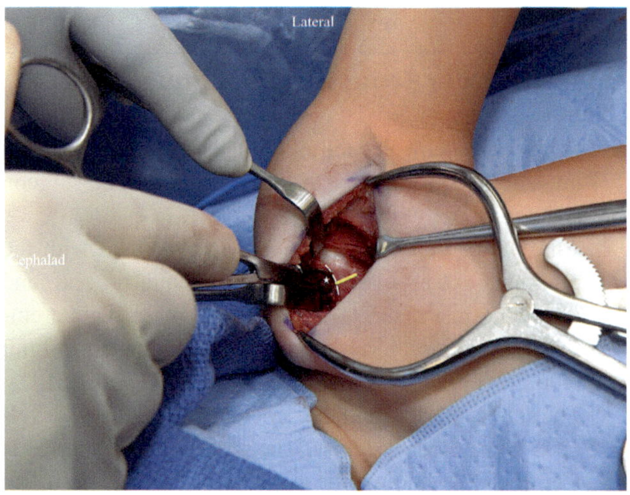

Fig. 45.8 With the coracoid removed, the upper rolled border of the subscapularis (*white hashed line*) is easily visible. The rotator interval (*star*) is just cephalad to the rolled border. A right-angle hemostat is placed through the interval and into the glenohumeral joint. The right angle is then opened, tensioning the subscapularis for the planned tenotomy (*yellow line*)

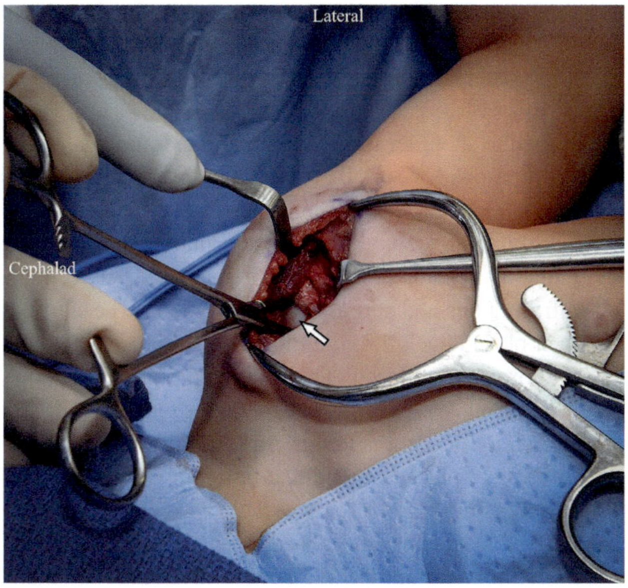

Fig. 45.9 The partial tenotomy is completed. With passive external rotation applied to the arm, the humeral head reduces and is easily visible through the capsulotomy (*arrow*)

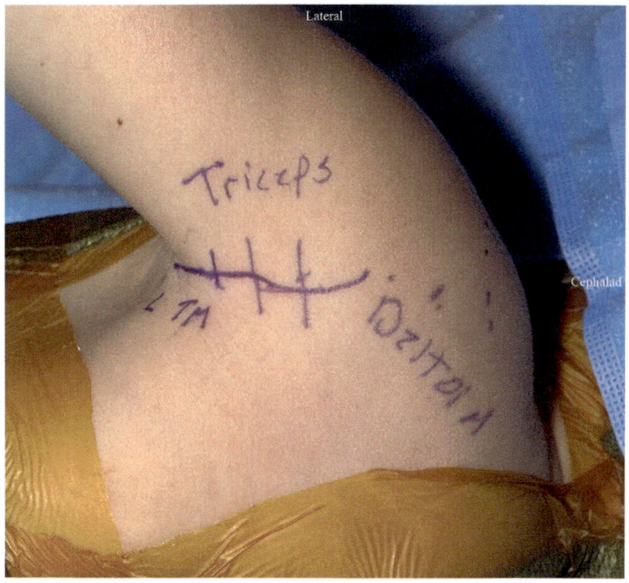

Fig. 45.10 The planned incision for posterior tendon transfer

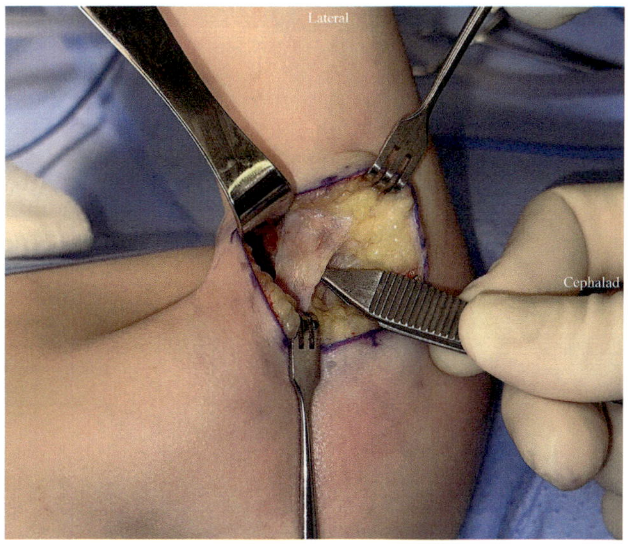

Fig. 45.11 The "confusing fascia" that overlays the true LD and TM tendons

Tendon Transfer Technique

1. The child remains in the lateral decubitus position.
2. A linear incision is planned starting 1 cm distal to the posterior-lateral corner of the acromion and extends to the posterior axillary crease. The incision is injected with 1:100,000 dilute epinephrine prior to prepping and draping (Fig. 45.10).
3. Skin is incised and subcutaneous tissue divided with electrocautery until the first layer of deep fascia is reached.
4. There is often a thick layer of "confusing fascia" superficial to the actual LD and TM tendons, so-called because one can easily mistake it for true tendon. It can be differentiated by its lack of muscular attachment. This must be isolated and divided to gain access to the true LD and TM tendons, which are often difficult to distinguish from one another and may appear as one combined tendon (Fig. 45.11).
5. A peanut sponge is used to bluntly dissect a plane along the tendon/s to their humeral insertion.
6. It is important to remember that the posterior humeral circumflex vessels and axillary nerve enter the quadrangular space just cephalad to the upper border of the teres major tendon. Similarly, at the level of the LD and TM humeral insertions, the radial nerve is just anterior and 1–2 cm medial as it travels proximal-to-distal and medial-to-lateral before entering the triangular interval just caudal to the teres major tendon (Fig. 45.12).
7. Define the cephalad and caudal borders of the LD and TM tendons. Use a right-angle hemostat to dissect anteriorly around the two tendons, allowing for passage of a penrose drain to encircle them.
8. Use the penrose to pull gentle traction and release the tendons with a cuff of periosteum using a protected tip bovie. The upper portion of the tendon may be released using scissors if the axillary nerve is too close to safely use electrocautery. Clamp the tendon/s to prevent their retraction into the wound (Fig. 45.13).
9. The interval between the posterior deltoid and triceps is developed, gaining entry into the subacromial space. A

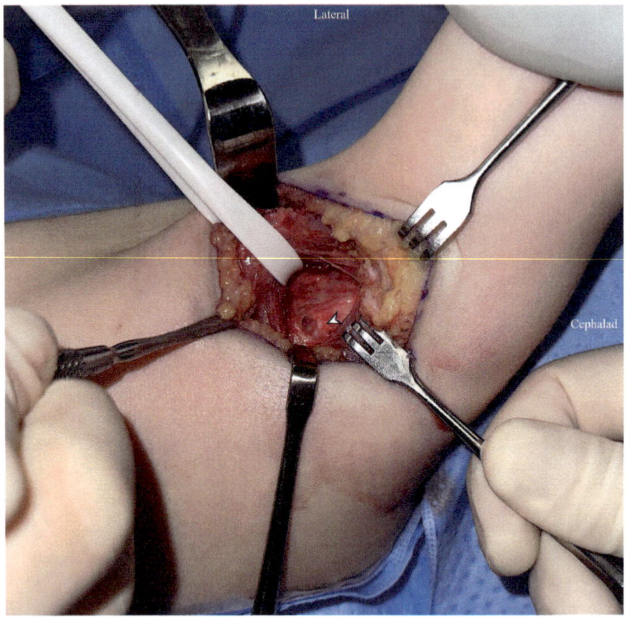

Fig. 45.12 The combined latissimus dorsi and teres major tendons are encircled with a penrose drain. The axillary nerve (*arrowhead*) is visible just anterior to the combined tendons

malleable or blunt Hohmann retractor can be placed through this interval and around the anterior humeral head, shoehorning the head in a posterior direction (Fig. 45.14).

10. Place the shoulder in 90° abduction and maximal external rotation. A #2 or #0 braided non-absorbable suture is placed first through the mid-portion of the tendon. A deep transosseous bite is then placed through the humeral head near the transitional area between the infraspinatus and supraspinatus insertions. The suture is then placed back through the tendon, where three locking throws are placed. This suture configuration allows for a strong grasping suture around the tendon while still allowing for knot sliding. An additional one or two sutures are placed in identical fashion to secure the tendon transfer (Fig. 45.15).
11. After the wounds are closed, a shoulder spica cast is placed to maintain the shoulder in external rotation and abduction.

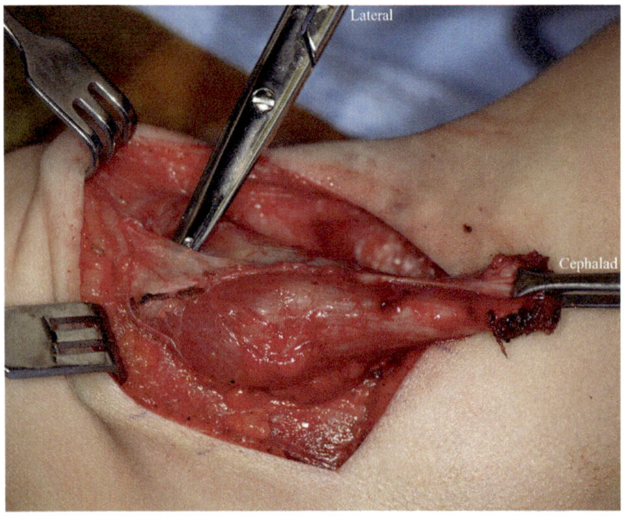

Fig. 45.13 The latissimus and teres major tendons are released from their humeral insertion. Light traction is applied, accentuating any areas of adhesion that may limit excursion if not released

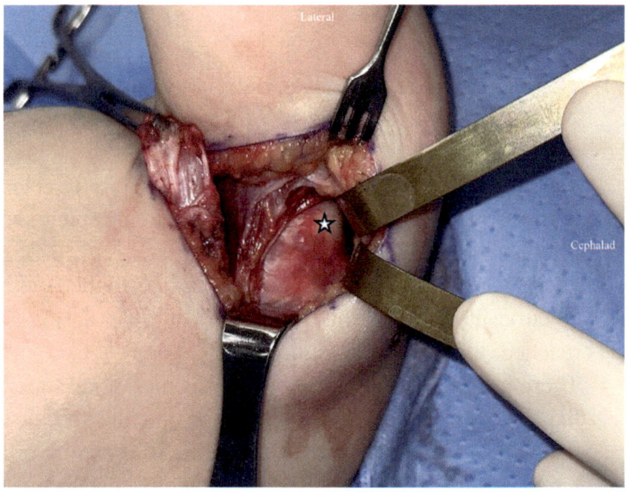

Fig. 45.14 The interval between the deltoid and triceps is developed to reach the subacromial space. A malleable retractor is used to shoehorn the humeral head (*star*) posteriorly

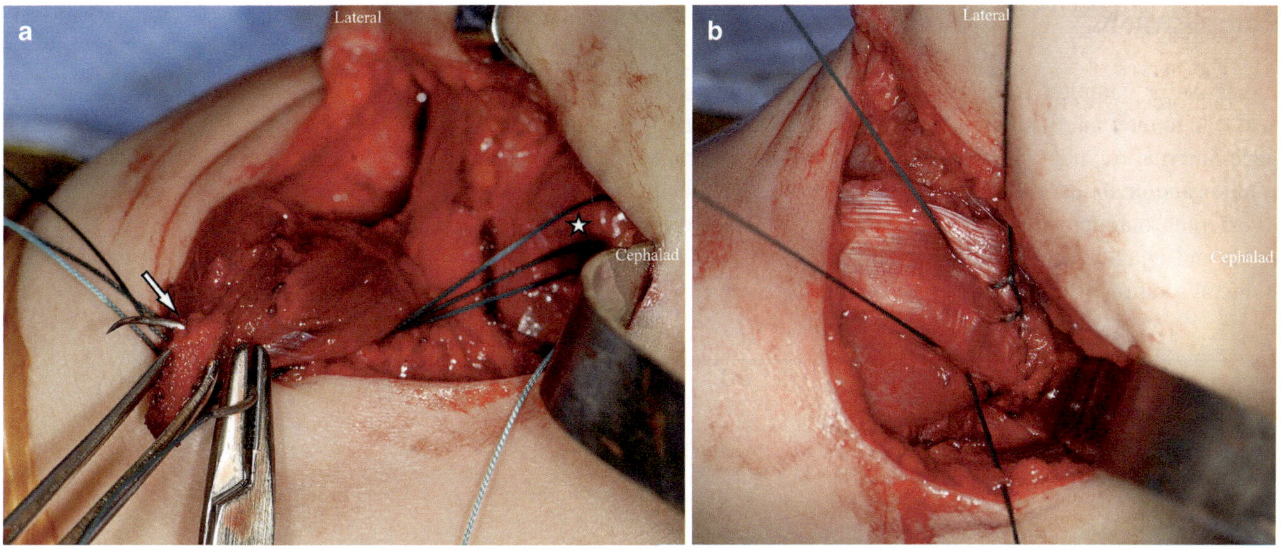

Fig. 45.15 (**a**) With the humeral head and rotator cuff exposed, a stich is first placed through the rotator cuff at the area of intended transfer (*star*). The suture is then thrown through the LD/TM tendon from deep to superficial (*arrow*), and then multiple running-locking sutures are placed from proximal to distal on the tendon. (**b**) Using a free-needle, the free end of the suture is placed through the tendon from deep-to-superficial in a single unlocked throw to allow for knot sliding. This suture configuration is repeated 1–2 more times to secure the transfer

Spica Cast

1. In children that are non-ambulatory, we prefer to use a soft casting material that allows for unravelling without a cast saw. A rigid fiberglass material is necessary for all ambulatory children.
2. A long arm cast is applied first with the elbow in 90° of flexion and neutral forearm rotation. Avoid the tendency to place the fiberglass too high on the brachium, as this will rub on the chest wall when the arm is placed into adduction.
3. A casting shirt is then applied to the child, and three towels are placed beneath the shirt to create additional space for the child's abdomen and thoracic expansion.
4. The child is then placed on a spica casting table. Only the head should be supported on the upper portion of the table, while the shoulders and chest are supported on the central removable beam.
5. If no tendon transfer was performed, we prefer to place the arm in mild adduction and external rotation. If a tendon transfer was performed, the shoulder must be positioned in abduction and external rotation to offload the transfer. An anterior translating force is also applied through the humerus to assist in maintaining glenohumeral reduction.
6. The distal extent of the cast should be a fingerbreadth proximal to the iliac crests. Cast padding is wrapped circumferentially around the abdomen, chest, around the affected shoulder, and down the arm. Wrapping around the affected shoulder will hold the spica cast in place.
7. Fiberglass is then wrapped in a similar fashion, with multiple rolls often being necessary.
8. With an initial layer of fiberglass applied, a wooden or fiberglass dowel is applied spanning from the abdomen to the anterior forearm and secured with more fiberglass wrapping.
9. The cast is allowed to harden, and the towels are removed. The child is sat up, and any fiberglass that could rub on the face or head is trimmed (Fig. 45.16).

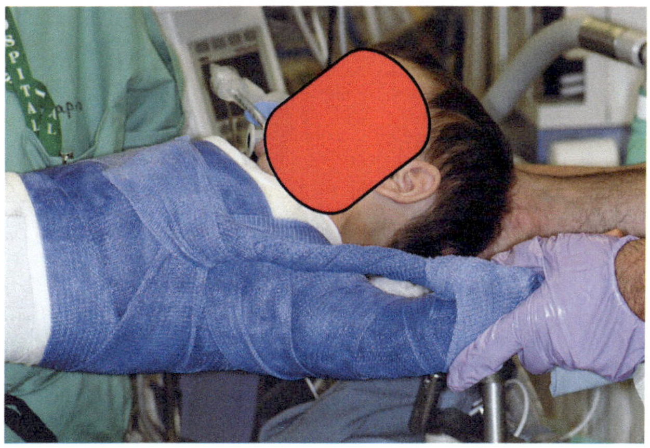

Fig. 45.16 A shoulder spica cast with bar support applied to maintain the arm in abduction and external rotation

Complications

Excessive or complete release of the subscapularis muscle will lead to internal rotation weakness. Preoperative or iatrogenic internal rotation weakness combined with an external rotation and/or abduction producing tendon transfer will lead to external rotation and abduction contracture. This is a difficult and equally debilitating problem that often requires humeral rotation osteotomy, or revision release, to remedy.

References

1. Donohue KW, Little KJ, Gaughan JP, Kozin SH, Norton BD, Zlotolow DA (2017) Comparison of ultrasound and MRI for the diagnosis of glenohumeral dysplasia in brachial plexus birth palsy. J Bone Joint Surg Am 99(2):123–132. https://doi.org/10.2106/JBJS.15.01116
2. Soldado F, Kozin SH (2005) The relationship between the coracoid and glenoid after brachial plexus birth palsy. J Pediatr Orthop 25(5):666–670. https://doi.org/10.1097/01.bpo.0000164873.41485.19
3. Abzug JM, Wyrick-Glover TO, Case AL, Zlotolow DA, Kozin SH (2019) Loss of midline function in brachial plexus birth palsy patients. J Pediatr Orthop 39(3):e232–e235. https://doi.org/10.1097/BPO.0000000000001251
4. Gu Y (1996) Functional motor innervation of brachial plexus roots. An intraoperative electrophysiological study. Chin Med J 109(10):749–751

Tendon Transfers for Lower Limb Nerve Injuries

46

Elise B. Raney, Eric J. Cotter, and Kathryn L. Williams

Indications

- Initial management of foot drop consists of ankle-foot orthoses (AFOs), lifestyle and activity modification, and physical therapy.
- Once patients have failed nonoperative management and/or nerve repair and have undergone thorough neurological evaluation and optimization, they are offered tendon transfers.
- Electrodiagnostic studies are helpful in determining the absence of recovery of the common peroneal nerve (CPN). A baseline study and at least one more to compare to the baseline should be utilized [1].
- Since recovery of nerve function can be seen up to 1 year following an insult to the CPN and/or nerve repair, it has been traditionally accepted to wait for at least 1 year after initial presentation before pursuing tendon transfers [2]. However, some groups prefer to do the tendon transfer at the same time as the nerve repair.

Contraindications

- Weak or absent posterior tibialis tendon strength (less than 4/5 muscle strength).
- Unstable, deformed, and/or severely arthritic tibiotalar joint, in which case a tibiotalar arthrodesis is preferred.
- Incomplete nerve injury with likelihood of recovery.
- Vascular insufficiency with high risk of poor wound healing.

Considerations

- Equinus contracture.
  - Nonoperative management includes Achilles stretching and botulinum toxin injections.
  - Operative management usually takes the form of tendo-Achilles lengthening (TAL).
    - Not always necessary, but typically required when foot drop occurs, as loss of active dorsiflexion eliminates the gastrocnemius–soleus' antagonist, leading to an Achilles contracture [3].
    - Preoperatively, if at least 10° of passive dorsiflexion is not obtainable, a tendo-Achilles lengthening is often performed [2].
- Flexible vs. fixed deformity.
  - Flexible deformity often corrects with tendon transfer alone.
  - Capsular release versus arthrodesis can be performed for fixed deformity.
- Toe contractures.
  - Claw toe deformities may become apparent once the ankle is dorsiflexed.
  - Flexor hallucis longus and flexor digitorum longus lengthening, or percutaneous tenotomies at the plantar toes, should be considered [3].

Supplementary Information The online version contains supplementary material available at https://doi.org/10.1007/978-3-031-73931-6_46.

E. B. Raney · E. J. Cotter
Department of Orthopedics and Rehabilitation, University of Wisconsin School of Medicine and Public Health, Madison, WI, USA
e-mail: cotter@ortho.wisc.edu

K. L. Williams (✉)
Foot and Ankle Division, Department of Orthopedics and Rehabilitation, University of Wisconsin School of Medicine and Public Health, Madison, WI, USA
e-mail: KWilliams@ortho.wisc.edu

A. S. Hanna (ed.), *Nerves: Anatomy, Exposures, and Techniques*, https://doi.org/10.1007/978-3-031-73931-6_46

Surgical Techniques

Posterior Tibialis Tendon (PTT) Transfer Through the Interosseous Membrane (IOM)

This is the preferred method, as the PTT is directly in-line from its muscle origin through the IOM to the lateral cuneiform. The lateral cuneiform is the preferred tendon anchor point, as it is slightly lateral to the midline of the foot, which promotes dorsiflexion and eversion, important in balancing the foot when a complete CPN palsy is present [4].

1. Position: The patient will be supine on a radiolucent operative table. It is helpful to have fluoroscopy available to identify bony landmarks.
2. A longitudinal medial midfoot incision over the navicular is performed to expose the main posterior tibial tendon insertion onto the navicular tuberosity (Fig. 46.1). The PTT is carefully elevated from the navicular tuberosity, along with the periosteum and distal accessory attachments, to maintain as much length as possible. Releases of the tendon proximally through the tarsal tunnel may be necessary. Once the tendon is completely released, the tendon should be debrided and tubularized so that it has a smooth tendon end to pass through the planned bone tunnel. A looped suture or suture placed in a Krakow fashion is placed in the distal tendon. The tendon is sized at this time in preparation for passage and fixation of the tendon within the lateral cuneiform.
3. A more proximal medial incision, cranial and posterior to the medial malleolus, is made just along the posteromedial aspect of the tibia. The flexor tendon sheath may need to be incised longitudinally to identify the posterior tibial tendon. The distal end of the PTT is then pulled into this more proximal medial incision.
4. A counter incision is then made at the distal third of the tibia, over its lateral border (Fig. 46.2). The soft tissues are dissected down to the level of the extensor muscle belly, which is retracted. The interosseous membrane is entered directly along the lateral and posterior borders of the tibia. A Kelly clamp is passed from the lateral to medial incision; the posterior neurovascular structures (tibial nerve and posterior tibial artery) being at risk, the clamp is passed directly on the posterior tibia.
5. The IOM opening is then widened by approximately 4 cm with the Kelly clamp in order to provide a safe passageway for the PTT by preventing adhesions and binding within the interosseous space. The suture on the end

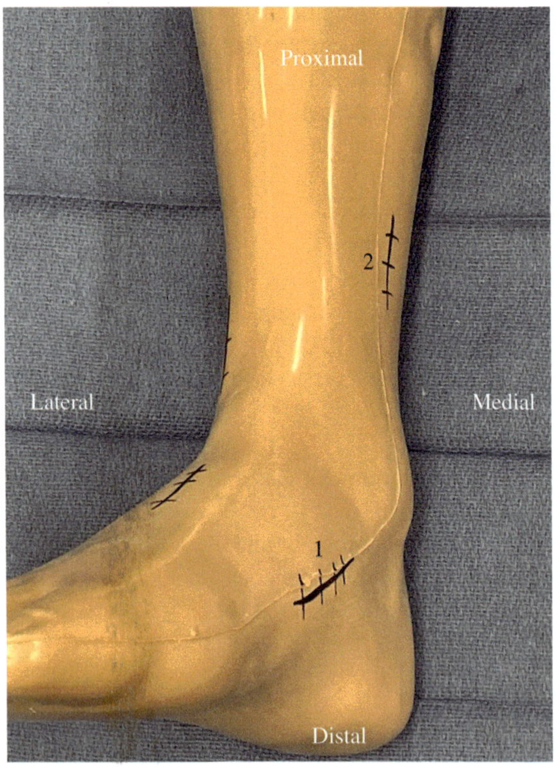

Fig. 46.1 A model demonstrating the surgical incisions. *1* is a 2–3 cm medial midfoot incision over the navicular, where the posterior tibialis tendon (PTT) inserts and is initially harvested. *2* is along the posteromedial aspect of the tibia, and the PTT is found here, and the tendon is pulled through this incision

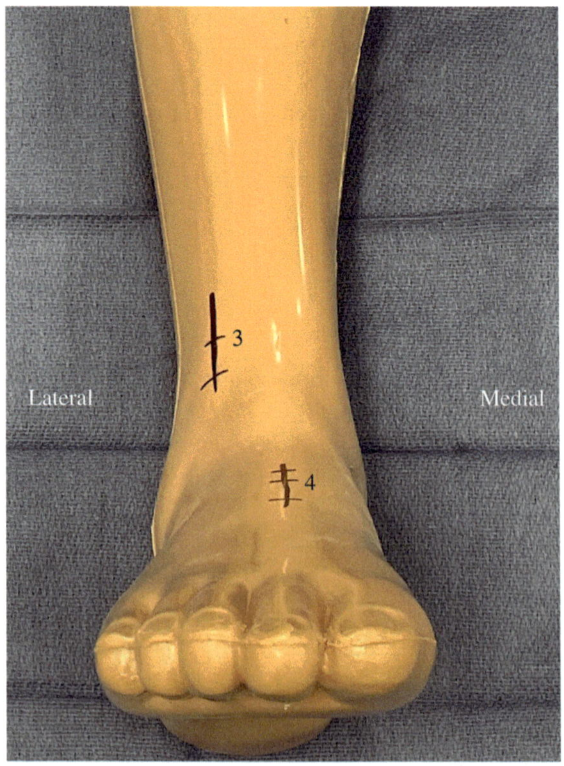

Fig. 46.2 A model demonstrating the surgical incisions. *3* is along the anterolateral aspect of the tibia. The PTT is pulled through the IOM and through this incision to bring it anteriorly. *4* overlies the lateral or middle cuneiform, where the PTT is finally inserted

of the tendon is grasped, and the tendon is transferred through the IOM into the anterolateral incision.

6. A dorsal incision is made directly over the lateral cuneiform, which can be identified with fluoroscopy (Fig. 46.3). The dissection is taken down to the level of the periosteum. A reaming guidewire is drilled in the center of the lateral cuneiform; the position can again be verified with fluoroscopy (Fig. 46.4). The guidewire is then drilled through the bone until it punctures the plantar aspect of the foot. A cannulated reamer is used to create a tunnel for the tendon fixation. The appropriately sized reamer is found from sizing the tendon; the bone tunnel diameter should be 0.5–1 mm larger than the size of the tendon. The tendon is then passed by placing the suture on the distal PTT through the eyelet of the guidewire, then pulling the guidewire through the lateral cuneiform and the plantar aspect of the foot. The ankle is then held in a neutral dorsiflexed position as the suture ends are pulled taut, and the interference screw is placed in the tunnel with the tendon (Fig. 46.5).
7. The suture ends are then cut close to the skin so that they retract under the plantar soft tissues. Wounds are closed per surgeon preference. A plaster splint is placed in the neutral dorsiflexed position.

Alternatively, the PTT can be transferred anterior to the tibia without going through the IOM. A disadvantage to this is that the PTT is not in direct line from its muscle origin to its anchor point in the foot, which will weaken its power [3].

An additional method of PTT transfer is the Bridle Procedure and consists of a posterior tibial tendon transfer through the IOM to the dorsum of the foot with a coaptation to the anterior tibialis tendon and a rerouted peroneus longus in front of the lateral malleolus [5].

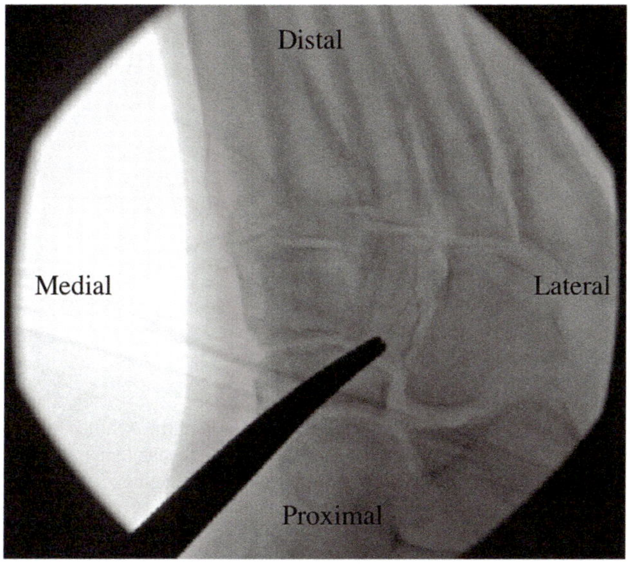

Fig. 46.3 Fluoroscopy showing intraoperative identification of the lateral cuneiform, the final site of insertion after tendon transfer

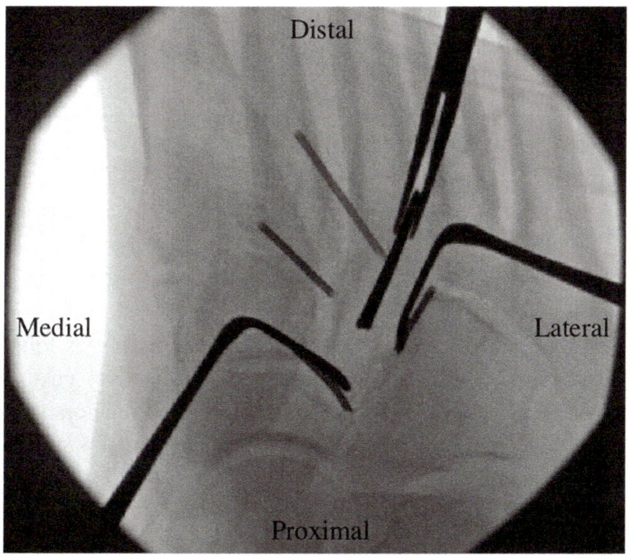

Fig. 46.4 Fluoroscopy demonstrating preparation of the lateral cuneiform. Needles are placed along the borders of the bone in order to enable centralizing of the guidewire used for reaming the tunnel for the tendon to be placed

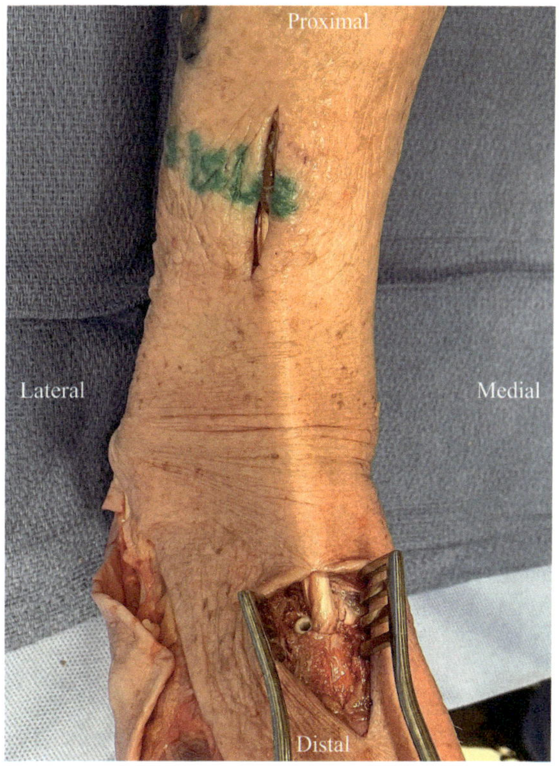

Fig. 46.5 Demonstration of the final construct after the PTT is brought through the IOM and fixated in the lateral or middle cuneiform with an interference screw

Tendo-Achilles Lengthening (TAL) for Equinus Contracture

This should be done before the PTT transfer, as persistent equinus contracture will make passage of the PTT into the cuneiform more difficult [3].

1. Position: Patient will be supine on a radiolucent operative table. The lower limb is elevated, and the foot is held in a dorsiflexed position by an assistant (Fig. 46.6).
2. An 11-blade scalpel is used to make a small stab incision in the central portion of the Achilles tendon approximately 2 cm above its insertion.
3. The blade is then turned 90° medially so as to cut the medial edge of the tendon.
4. Then, 2–3 cm proximal to the first incision, another stab incision is made with the knife turned laterally.
5. A third incision is made another 2–3 cm proximal along the tendon and again turned medially (Fig. 46.7a).
6. The foot/ankle is then dorsiflexed until the surgeon can feel the tendon has been lengthened and adequate passive dorsiflexion has been achieved (Fig. 46.7b).
7. Care should be taken to avoid complete disruption of the Achilles tendon by only transecting ~50% of the tendon at each cut so that it lengthens without complete rupture.

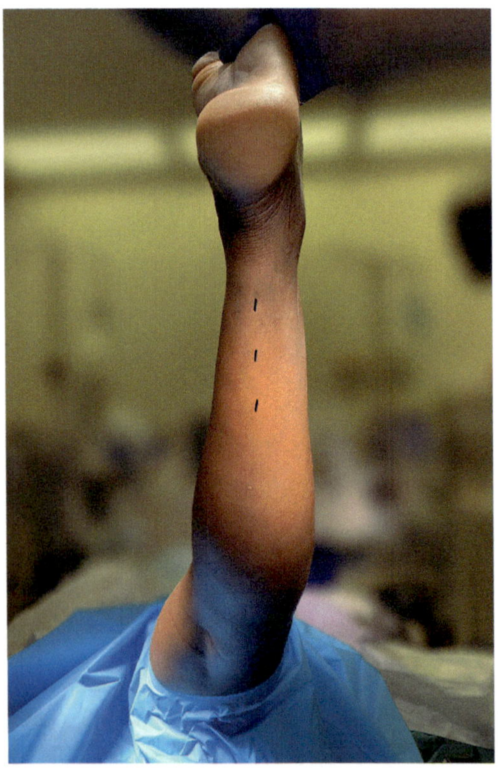

Fig. 46.6 Positioning and markings for skin incisions for a triple hemisection tendo-Achilles lengthening (TAL)

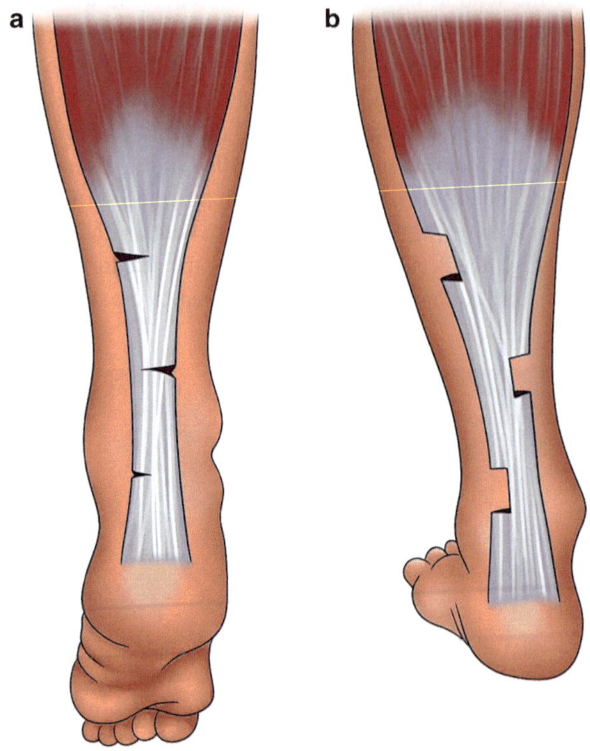

Fig. 46.7 Illustration demonstrating elongation of the Achilles following a triple hemisection TAL. (**a**) Demonstrates the stab incisions in the Achilles tendon. (**b**) After the actual lengthening with ankle dorsiflexion

However, it is the author's experience that, if it appears that a complete disruption has occurred, it is not necessary to "repair" the tendon as it will likely heal. Physical therapy aimed at Achilles rehabilitation should be considered in these cases, in conjunction with rehabilitation for the PTT transfer.

Postoperative Protocol

- 0–6 weeks post-op: Non-weight-bearing in a short-leg splint/cast.
- 6–12 weeks post-op: Weight-bearing as tolerated in a short-leg cast.
- 12 weeks to 6 months post-op: weight-bearing as tolerated in tall walking boot, then transitioned to custom AFO, and asked to use a night splint to maintain dorsiflexion. The patient will be braced for a minimum of 6 months after surgery.
- Physical therapy is usually recommended to facilitate recovery of active dorsiflexion and rehabilitation for Achilles lengthening, once range of motion and weight-bearing are allowed.

Outcomes

A handful of studies available demonstrate good to excellent results in small groups of patients:

- A 2017 study by Cho et al. compared 17 patients who underwent PTT transfer with matched controls and demonstrated significant improvement in 3 distinct functional outcome measures. This was despite achieving dorsiflexion strength that was only 33% normal and only 1 of 17 required an AFO postoperatively [6].
- Molund (2014) and Ho (2014) also demonstrated that despite postoperative strength measurements that were decreased compared to the contralateral limb, outcomes were good to excellent, with collectively 8 of 19 patients returning to a high activity level, including running [7, 8].
- To our knowledge, the longest follow-up study at a mean of 90 months by Yeap and colleagues showed that of 12 patients who underwent PTT transfer, 10 had good to excellent results and did not require an AFO postoperatively. Interestingly, 4 did develop an asymptomatic loss of the medial longitudinal arch [9].

Complications

- Infection: Can be superficial or deep, including osteomyelitis.
- Wound dehiscence: The wound must be healed before initiating active dorsiflexion.
- Failure of the tendon transfer anchor point.
  - Use of additional anchor points (other cuneiforms) or insertion into anterior tibialis tendon as a static transfer could be done if this occurs.
  - Additionally, tying over a button on the plantar foot is described but can have a high rate of plantar skin necrosis.
- Constriction and stenosis of the PTT within the narrow window in the IOM.
  - Transfer will act more like a static transfer, maintaining a more dorsiflexed position but will not allow for active dorsiflexion and plantarflexion.

References

1. Park JS, Casale MJ (2020) Posterior tibial tendon transfer for common peroneal nerve injury. Clin Sports Med 39(4):819–828. https://doi.org/10.1016/j.csm.2020.07.003
2. Wakefield CJ, Hamid KS, Lee S, Lin J, Holmes GB, Bohl DD (2021) Transfer of the posterior tibial tendon for chronic peroneal nerve palsy. JBJS Rev 9(7):1–10. https://doi.org/10.2106/JBJS.RVW.20.00208
3. Easley ME, Scott AT (2011) Tendon transfer for foot drop. In: Easley ME, Wiesel SW (eds) Operative techniques in foot and ankle surgery, 1st edn. Wolters Kluwer Health/Lippincott Williams & Wilkins, Philadelphia, PA, pp 1008–1024
4. Stevoska S, Pisecky L, Stadler C, Gahleitner M, Klasan A, Klotz MC (2023) Tendon transfer in foot drop: a systematic review. Arch Orthop Trauma Surg 143(2):773–784. https://doi.org/10.1007/s00402-021-04162-x. Epub 2021 Sep 15
5. Rodriguez RP (1992) The bridle procedure in the treatment of paralysis of the foot. Foot Ankle 13(2):63–69. https://doi.org/10.1177/107110079201300203
6. Cho BK, Park KJ, Choi SM et al (2017) Functional outcomes following anterior transfer of the tibialis posterior tendon for foot drop secondary to peroneal nerve palsy. Foot Ankle Int 38(6):627–633. https://doi.org/10.1177/1071100717695508. Epub 2017 Feb 1
7. Molund M, Engebretsen L, Hvaal K et al (2014) Posterior tibial tendon transfer improves function for foot drop after knee dislocation. Clin Orthop Relat Res 472(9):2637–2643. https://doi.org/10.1007/s11999-014-3533-x
8. Ho B, Khan Z, Switaj PJ et al (2014) Treatment of peroneal nerve injuries with simultaneous tendon transfer and nerve exploration. J Orthop Surg Res 9:67. https://doi.org/10.1186/s13018-014-0067-6
9. Yeap JS, Birch R, Singh D (2001) Long-term results of tibialis posterior tendon transfer for drop-foot. Int Orthop 25(2):114–118. https://doi.org/10.1007/s002640100229

47 Transposition of the Lateral Femoral Cutaneous Nerve After Ultrasound-Guided Wire Localization

Paul S. Page, Thomas M. Staniszewski, and Amgad S. Hanna

Indications

Meralgia paresthetica causes burning, tingling, numbness, allodynia, and/or hypesthesia in the anterolateral thigh. Diagnosis is most often made clinically. Nerve conduction studies are only helpful if the results are abnormal on the symptomatic side and normal on the contralateral side. Pain relief after lateral femoral cutaneous nerve (LFCN) injections aids in diagnosis. Surgery is indicated after failure of conservative therapy, including weight loss, injections, and avoidance of tight belts or pants. Simple decompression may preserve sensation but is associated with a 40–70% failure/recurrence rate. Neurectomy can be performed; this procedure results in numbness in the distribution of the nerve and potential risk for painful neuroma formation and deafferentation pain [1–3]. Here, we describe the transposition of the LFCN utilizing ultrasound-guide wire localization [4, 5]. The technique has been used by the senior author for over 10 years with ~90% success rate (Fig. 47.1). The anatomy of the nerve and its canal has already been detailed in Chap. 25.

Supplementary Information The online version contains supplementary material available at https://doi.org/10.1007/978-3-031-73931-6_47.

P. S. Page
Department of Neurological Surgery, University of Wisconsin School of Medicine and Public Health, Madison, WI, USA

Goodman Campbell Brain and Spine, Carmel, IN, USA

T. M. Staniszewski
Department of Neurological Surgery, University of Wisconsin School of Medicine and Public Health, Madison, WI, USA
e-mail: staniszewski@neurosurgery.wisc.edu

A. S. Hanna (✉)
Department of Neurosurgery, University of Wisconsin School of Medicine and Public Health, Madison, WI, USA

A. S. Hanna (ed.), *Nerves: Anatomy, Exposures, and Techniques*, https://doi.org/10.1007/978-3-031-73931-6_47

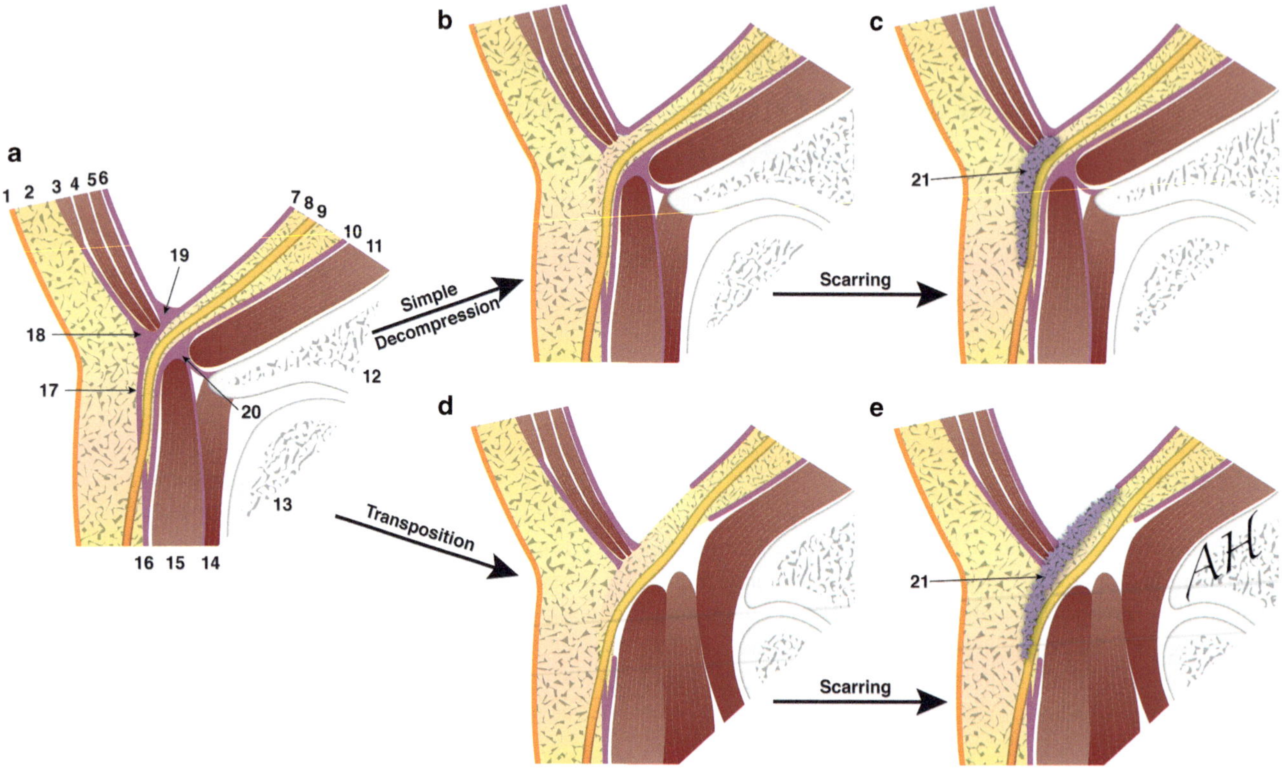

Fig. 47.1 Diagrammatic representation of the lateral femoral cutaneous nerve (LFCN) canal in an oblique sagittal view. *1* skin, *2* subcutaneous tissue, *3* external oblique, *4* internal oblique, *5* transversus abdominis, *6* transversalis fascia, *7* fascia iliaca superficial lamina, *8* retroperitoneal fat, *9* LFCN, *10* fascia iliaca deep lamina, *11* iliacus, *12* iliac bone, *13* femur, *14* rectus femoris, *15* Sartorius, *16* fascia lata, *17* LFCN canal, *18* inguinal ligament, *19* iliopubic tract, *20* thickening of the fascia deep to the LFCN. Copyright Amgad Hanna. Published with permission [10]. (**b**) After simple decompression, the deep fascia superficial to the nerve is released as well as the inguinal ligament. (**c**) When scar tissue (*21*) develops, the nerve is retethered into a position very similar to preoperative status in **a**. (**d**) With transposition, all components of the LFCN canal are opened: superficial and deep to the nerve, which is then mobilized medially for about 2 cm. After transposition, the nerve acquires a much straighter and relaxed course, has a softer muscular bed, and is further away from the ASIS, even after scarring (**e**). Copyright Wiley Periodicals. Published with permission [1]

Surgical Techniques

Ultrasound (US) has been used extensively to assist with nerve surgery [5–7]. Increased image resolution and diagnostic accuracy make it an indispensable tool for the nerve surgeon. The senior author has used US to localize nerves and small masses for over a decade.

Preoperative Wire Localization

1. The patient is scheduled for surgery the same day as placement of the wire localization. After routine preoperative marking, the patient is taken to an ultrasound suite, where ultrasound wire localization is completed with local anesthetic.
2. The LFCN is mapped below the inguinal ligament in its canal located superficial to the sartorius. In large patients, the nerve can be difficult to localize, and it may be helpful to find it more proximally at the level of the anterior superior iliac spine (ASIS) then follow it distally.
3. The US probe is placed in the transverse orientation of the nerve. A lateral to medial approach is taken to the nerve approximately 1 inch distal to the ASIS (Fig. 47.2a and b).
4. The wire is then placed deep to the nerve, once deployed the J-curve of the wire should hug the LFCN, which allows the nerve to be anchored and prevent migration.
5. Following wire placement, the ultrasound is used to measure the depth from the skin to the nerve (Fig. 47.2c). Additionally, the distance from the skin surface overlying the nerve to the skin entry site of the wire is measured. These two distances are reported to the surgeon to assist in incision planning. Sterile gauze and tape are applied to keep the area clean.

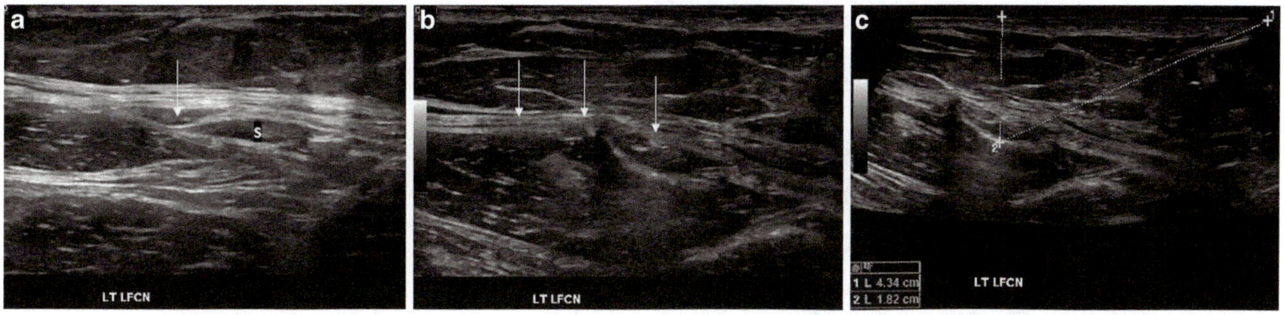

Fig. 47.2 The LFCN (*arrows*) is mapped using ultrasound guidance in a transverse (**a**) and longitudinal (**b**) fashion. Note the complete LFCN canal surrounding the nerve superficial to sartorius (*S*). (**c**) The depth of the wire tip from the skin surface and the distance from the wire entry point to the projected skin surface are measured and reported to the surgeon. These are used to mark the skin incision right on top of the nerve (wire tip)

Alternatives

- In recent years, we have started using smart clip application (Envisio navigation system; Elucent Medical). This can be applied a few days prior to surgery but is more expensive.
- If a good US machine is available in the operating room, with a good technician and an US reader (which could be a surgeon trained in US), localization can be done in the operating room rather than the radiology suite.
- Other surgeons have used methylene blue, but the problem is diffusion through the tissue, which reduces accuracy.

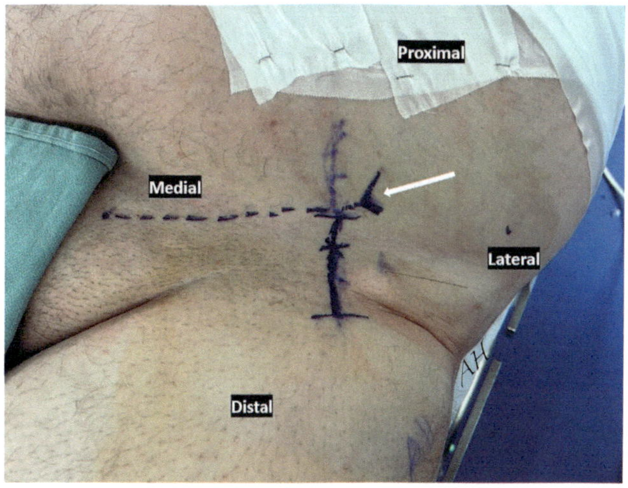

Fig. 47.3 Using the reported US measurements, a linear incision is planned along the course of the nerve. The inguinal ligament (*dashed line*) and ASIS (*arrow*) are identified and marked. Note the wire sticking out of the skin distal to ASIS

LFCN Transposition [8, 9]

1. The incision is marked based upon the provided ultrasound measurements (Fig. 47.3).
2. A linear incision is then made through the skin and superficial fascia obliquely in line with the nerve trajectory.
3. The wire is then palpable through the fat. Spreading with scissors allows the wire to come into visualization.
4. The wire is then visualized entering the deep fascia. Occasionally the other limb of the J wire can be seen or felt through the fascia (Fig. 47.4).
5. If the two limbs of the wire are seen, the incision can be made between these, if not the incision in the deep fascia should be made just medial to the wire entry in the deep fascia.
6. Once the nerve is identified, spreading along the nerve trajectory will identify the LFCN and its branches. All branches should be identified before pulling the wire out to avoid damaging the branches. The nerve should also be dissected proximally toward the inguinal ligament, this will allow more branches to be visualized and pro-

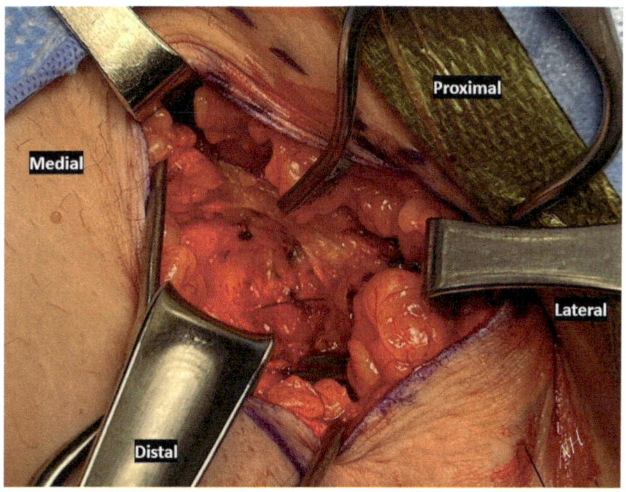

Fig. 47.4 After dissection through the superficial fascia, the wire is identified entering the deep fascia

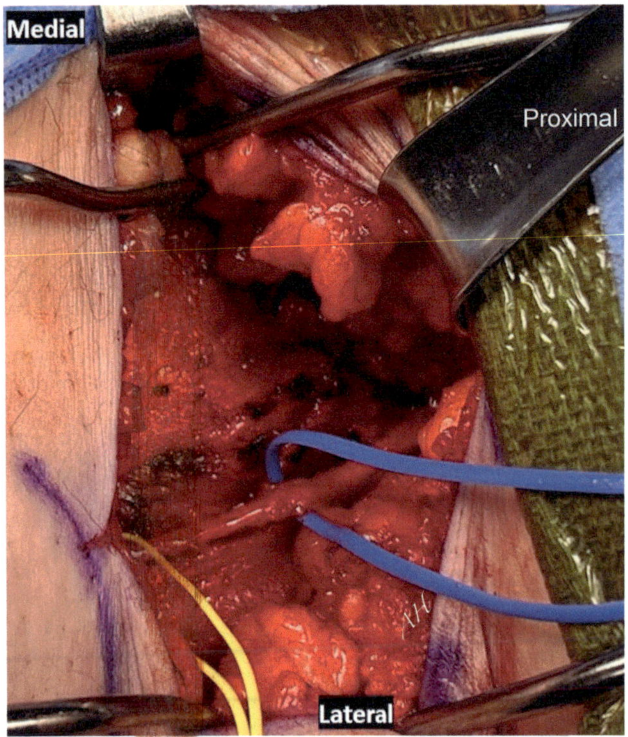

Fig. 47.5 The LFCN (*blue loop*) is identified as well as its branches

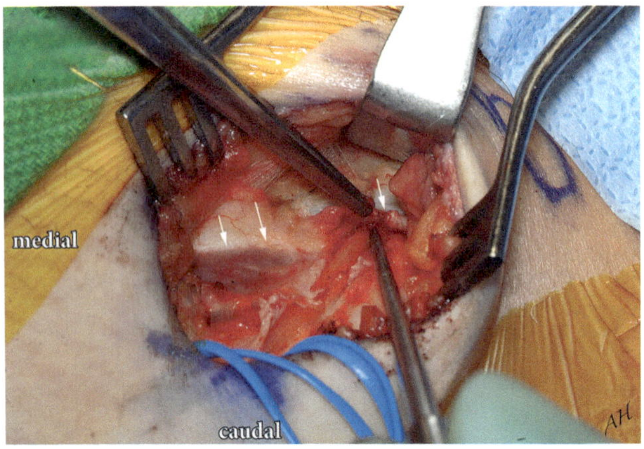

Fig. 47.6 Proximally, the nerve is observed under the inguinal ligament (*arrows*), tethering it against the ASIS. The inguinal ligament should be opened

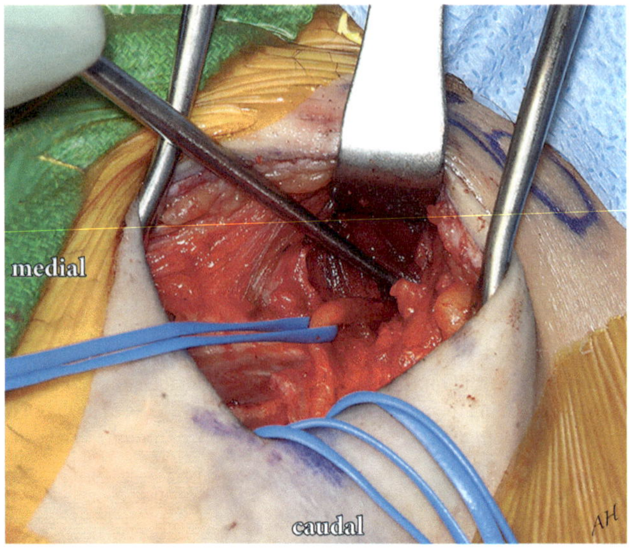

Fig. 47.7 The LFCN (*blue loop*) is completely released up to the retroperitoneal space. The deep fascia is opened superficial and deep to the nerve to ensure complete decompression

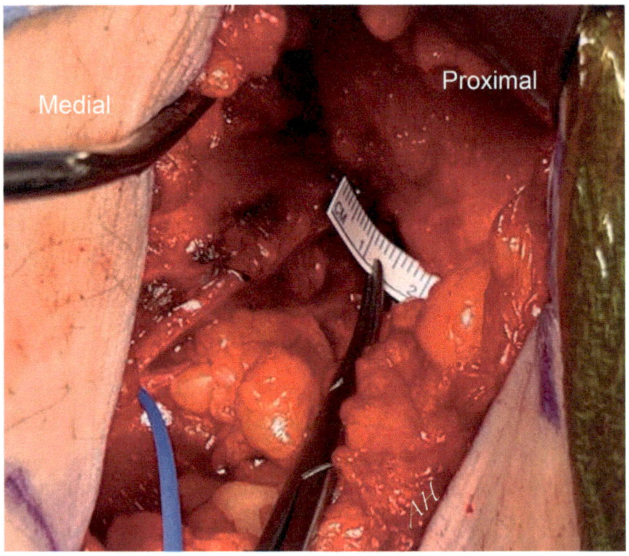

Fig. 47.8 The nerve is then transposed by approximately 2 cm medially away from the ASIS

tected. During this dissection the deep fascia deep to the nerve should be released (Fig. 47.5). The LFCN canal surrounds the nerve 360° (see also Chap. 25) and should be opened both superficial and deep to the nerve for full decompression and mobilization.

7. The dissection should be carried out distally and proximally. The latter involves releasing the inguinal ligament, being careful not to injure the ilioinguinal nerve or the vessels within the ligament (Fig. 47.6). It also involves cutting the duplicate fascia iliaca superficial and deep to the nerve (Fig. 47.7). Of note, despite opening the inguinal ligament, the authors have not observed any cases of hernia, likely because the opening is so lateral. There is a sagittal septum medial to sartorius that needs to be released as well prior to transposition.
8. Following releasing the nerve, it is then mobilized by approximately 2 cm medially away from the ASIS (Fig. 47.8). This should not be forced, but once enough release is done, rather let the nerve fall where it needs to go.

9. There are occasional cases where the nerve is too medial to transpose, in which case superficial and deep decompression by opening the fasciae superficial and deep to the nerve can be sufficient.
10. In most meralgia paresthetica patients, the LFCN is riding over the bone (ASIS). The deep decompression in that case involves cutting the fascia medial to ASIS (a slip from the inguinal ligament) in order to mobilize the nerve to the softer muscular bed deep to it.
11. A small drain is left in place and the wound is closed in 2 layers.

Complications

- Wound infection.
- Hematoma.
- Paresthesias.
- Failure to improve the symptoms. Look for other causes, like L3 radiculopathy. May attempt repeat injection of LFCN and consider nerve stimulation vs. neurectomy.

References

1. Hanna AS (2017) Lateral femoral cutaneous nerve transposition: renaissance of an old concept in the light of new anatomy. Clin Anat 30(3):409–412. https://doi.org/10.1002/ca.22849
2. Hanna A (2020) Letter to the editor. Meralgia paresthetica: what to do? J Neurosurg 132(6):2020–2021. https://doi.org/10.3171/2019.10.JNS192708
3. Hanna A, Hanna B (2018) Response to: anatomical considerations on transposition of the lateral femoral cutaneous nerve. Clin Anat 31(8):1222–1224. https://doi.org/10.1002/ca.23070. Epub 2018 Apr 30
4. Hanna A (2019) Transposition of the lateral femoral cutaneous nerve. J Neurosurg 130(2):496–501. https://doi.org/10.3171/2017.8.JNS171120. Epub 2018 April 13
5. Hanna AS, Ehlers ME, Lee KS (2017) Preoperative ultrasound-guided wire localization of the lateral femoral cutaneous nerve. Oper Neurosurg (Hagerstown) 13(3):402–408. https://doi.org/10.1093/ons/opw009
6. Frinkelstein ER, Buitrago J, Jose J, Levi AD, Xu KY, Burks SS (2023) Lower extremity peripheral nerve pathology: utility of preoperative ultrasound-guided needle localization before operative intervention. Skeletal Radiol 52(10):1997–2002. https://doi.org/10.1007/s00256-023-04347-y. Epub 2023 Apr 15
7. Haldeman CL, Baggott CD, Hanna AS (2015) Intraoperative ultrasound-assisted peripheral nerve surgery. Neurosurg Focus 39(3):E4. https://doi.org/10.3171/2015.6.FOCUS15232
8. Greeneway GP, Page PS, Ammanuel SG, Hanna AS (2023) Lateral femoral cutaneous nerve transposition. Neurosurg Focus Video 8(1):V8. https://doi.org/10.3171/2022.10.FOCVID2289. eCollection 2023 Jan
9. Staniszewski T, Buckley N, Hanna AS (2023. doi: 10.1227/ons.0000000000000903.Online ahead of print) Lateral femoral cutaneous nerve transposition with ultrasound-guided wire localization: 2-dimensional operative video. Oper Neurosurg (Hagerstown) 26:104
10. Hanna A (2017) The lateral femoral cutaneous nerve canal. J Neurosurg 126(3):972–978. https://doi.org/10.3171/2016.1.JNS152262. Epub 2016 Apr 22

48 Thoracic Outlet Syndrome

Kelsey M. Bowman and Amgad S. Hanna

Indications

Thoracic outlet syndrome (TOS) is a well-described constellation of symptoms resulting from compression of the brachial plexus and/or subclavian vessels in the anatomic region known as the thoracic outlet [1–3]. The thoracic outlet is the space between the supraclavicular fossa and the axilla and between the clavicle and first rib [3]. The clinical syndrome classically presents with pain, paresthesias, numbness, weakness, pallor, and/or cold sensation in the affected upper limb [1–3]. The compression causes symptoms involving multiple dermatomes and myotomes, differentiating it from cervical radiculopathy or peripheral neuropathy.

Clinically, patients present with numbness/tingling, weakness, and/or pain in the upper limb. The symptoms most commonly involve the distribution of the lower trunk of the brachial plexus. The symptoms are worst with the arms extended overhead. In extreme cases, a Gilliatt-Sumner (atrophic) hand may be seen. The patient may have a Tinel sign over the supraclavicular region or pectoralis minor. A positive Tinel sign at the elbow or wrist should prompt the clinician to consider alternative diagnoses of ulnar or median neuropathy, respectively. Additionally, there may be a positive scratch collapse test at the supraclavicular region or pectoralis minor as well [4]. Various provocative physical exam maneuvers have been described, including Roos (Fig. 48.1a and b), Adson's, and the costoclavicular test, in which the examiner assesses for radial pulse drop-off and reproduction of symptoms with particular arm maneuvers.

Diagnostic studies are aimed at identifying anatomic anomalies in the thoracic outlet region and/or provocation of symptoms with known maneuvers. Commonly used investigations include magnetic resonance neurography (MRN) of the brachial plexus (Fig. 48.1c and d), MR angiogram (MRA, Fig. 48.1e) of the chest with arms neutral and arms above the head, electrodiagnostic studies (rarely diagnostic but can help rule out other pathologies like ulnar neuropathy), cervical computed tomography (CT, Fig. 48.1f–h) (to evaluate for a cervical rib or elongated C7 transverse process and also rule out foraminal stenosis), and doppler ultrasonography with arms in various positions (to evaluate for positional vascular compression). Lastly, patients can be referred for steroid or botulinum toxin injection of the anterior scalene muscle. Symptomatic improvement with these injections helps the diagnosis and can give relief for a few months.

TOS is classically caused by compression of the brachial plexus (typically the lower trunk but any trunk can be involved), subclavian artery, and/or subclavian vein by the anterior and middle scalene muscles. The presence of an accessory scalene muscle (scalenus minimus, Fig. 48.1d and g), which is seen in 30–50% of patients with TOS [3], and other variations in scalene anatomy can contribute to the development of TOS. Bony anomalies, such as the presence of a cervical rib (Fig. 48.1h) or elongated C7 transverse process, are also implicated in some cases [1, 3], sometimes it's a membrane attached to these bony structures that compresses the neurovascular elements. Historically, TOS has been described as either "neurogenic"—caused by compression of the brachial plexus—or "vascular"—caused by compression of the subclavian artery and vein. However, given the close proximity of these structures within the thoracic outlet region, in our experience, most patients present with a combination of neurogenic and arterial, but could be predominantly vascular or neurogenic. Venous presentation can be different including arm swelling and deep venous thrombosis, since the vein travels separately anterior to anterior scalene, these may benefit from first rib resection. We have proposed the classification into venous thoracic outlet syndrome (VTOS) and non-venous thoracic outlet syndrome (NVTOS) [5].

Supplementary Information The online version contains supplementary material available at https://doi.org/10.1007/978-3-031-73931-6_48.

K. M. Bowman · A. S. Hanna (✉)
Department of Neurosurgery, University of Wisconsin School of Medicine and Public Health, Madison, WI, USA
e-mail: kbowman@uwhealth.org

A. S. Hanna (ed.), *Nerves: Anatomy, Exposures, and Techniques*, https://doi.org/10.1007/978-3-031-73931-6_48

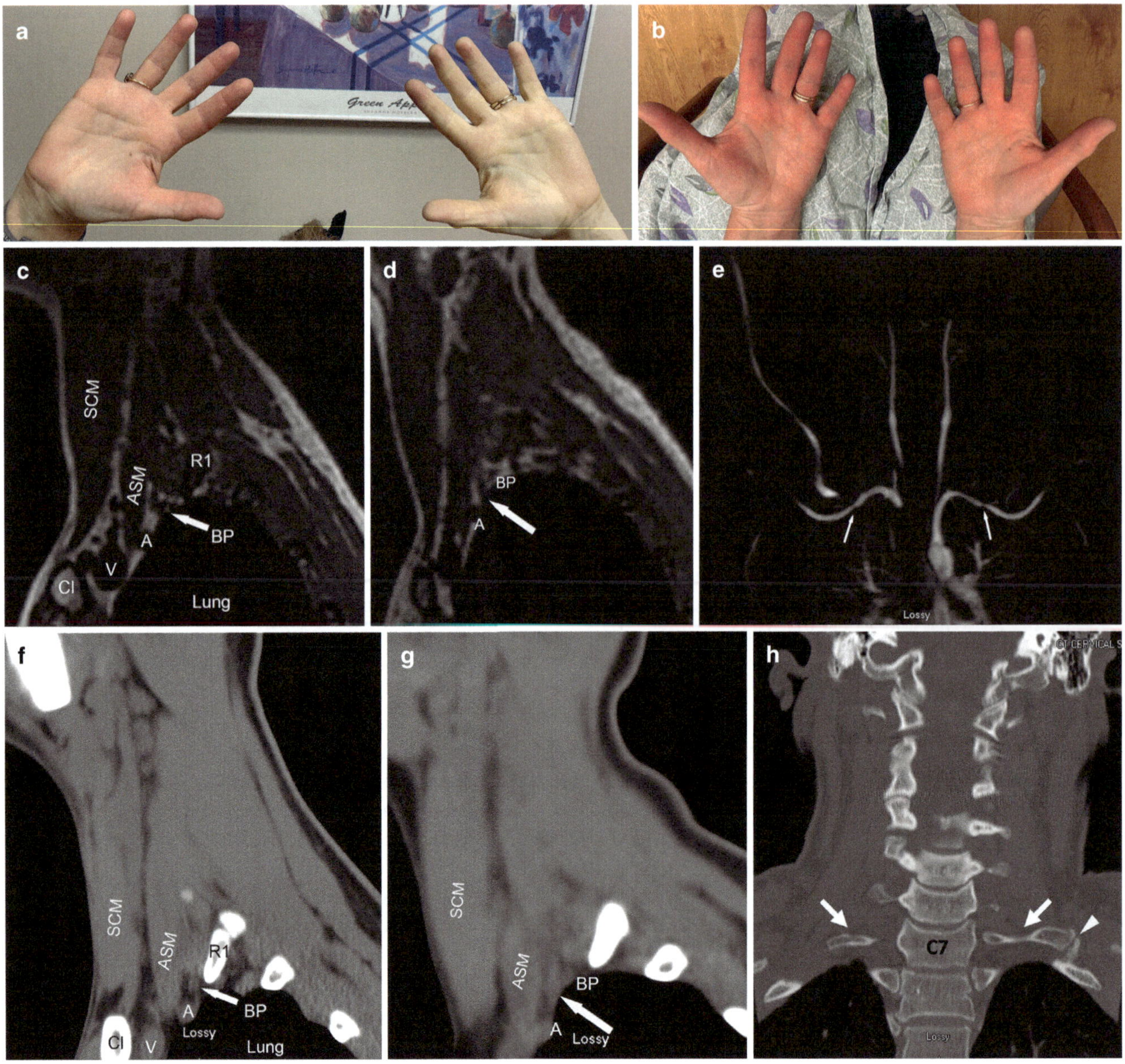

Fig. 48.1 Clinical and radiological findings in TOS from different patients. (**a**) Bilateral blanching of hands left > right while performing the Roos test. (**b**) The hand color returns to pink with the arms down. (**c**) Normal appearing sagittal MRI of the brachial plexus. (**d**) Scalenus minimus (*arrow*) is seen between the subclavian artery (*A*) and brachial plexus (*BP*). (**e**) MRA of the chest showing bilateral subclavian artery narrowing with the arms up (*arrows*). (**f**) Normal sagittal CT. (**g**) Sagittal CT showing scalenus minimus (*arrow*). (**h**) Coronal CT showing bilateral cervical ribs (*arrows*) in a patient with thoracic outlet syndrome; note the left cervical rib articulates with the first rib (*arrowhead*). *SCM* sternocleidomastoid, *ASM* anterior scalene muscle, *Cl* clavicle, *R1* first rib, *V* subclavian vein, *A* subclavian artery, *BP* brachial plexus

When patients meet the clinical and diagnostic criteria for thoracic outlet syndrome, a trial of conservative measures is attempted including physical therapy and scalene injections. If these fail, thoracic outlet decompression is offered. The most commonly performed surgery for thoracic outlet decompression at our institution is an anterior scalenectomy. Middle scalenectomy or cervical rib resection may be considered based on preoperative anatomic findings, but are not routinely performed. Refractory or recurrent cases may be treated with pectoralis minor release after this is tested with injections. We reserve first rib resection to recurrences or venous TOS. First rib resection for TOS has been associated with higher rates of complications, especially the transaxillary approach, it is not our preferred procedure for de novo TOS.

Surgical Technique

Anterior Scalenectomy

- **Positioning**
  The patient is positioned supine on the operating table. The head is turned to the contralateral side and slightly extended to best expose the supraclavicular region (Fig. 48.2), the back of the table is elevated to position the neck almost parallel to the floor. In this young population, a shoulder bump is rarely needed.
- **Incision**
  First, the external landmarks—midline, clavicle, mastoid process, posterior border of sternocleidomastoid (SCM), and external jugular vein—are marked. A horizontal curvilinear incision running within a skin crease 1 fingerbreadth above the clavicle is planned to expose the brachial plexus (Fig. 48.3).
- **Exposure**
  The skin incision is opened sharply, and the dissection is carried down through the subcutaneous tissues using Metzenbaum scissors until the platysma is encountered. The skin above the platysma is undermined in both directions (Fig. 48.4). The platysma is opened in the direction of its fibers and retracted with self-retaining retractors. The posterior border of SCM is then identified (Fig. 48.5). The external jugular vein is also identified and may be ligated with silk sutures and divided, if necessary. The dissection is continued along the posterior border of SCM. Next, the omohyoid is encountered (Fig. 48.6). Two sutures are placed into the muscle, which is then divided between the sutures. The suture strings are kept

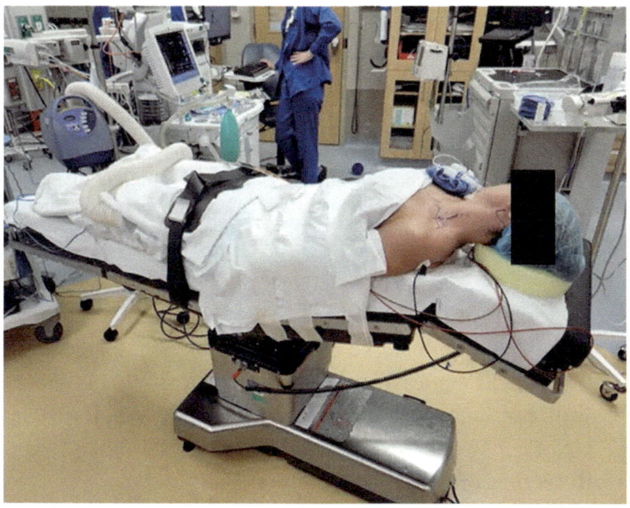

Fig. 48.2 The patient is positioned supine on the operating table, with the back up and head slightly extended and rotated to the contralateral side

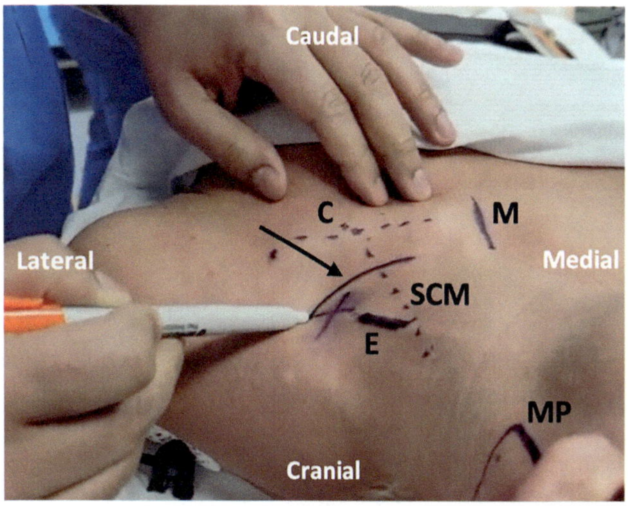

Fig. 48.3 The clavicle (*C*), midline (*M*), posterior border of sternocleidomastoid (*SCM*), mastoid process (*MP*), and external jugular vein (*E*) are marked. The curvilinear incision approximately 1 fingerbreadth above the clavicle is denoted with an arrow

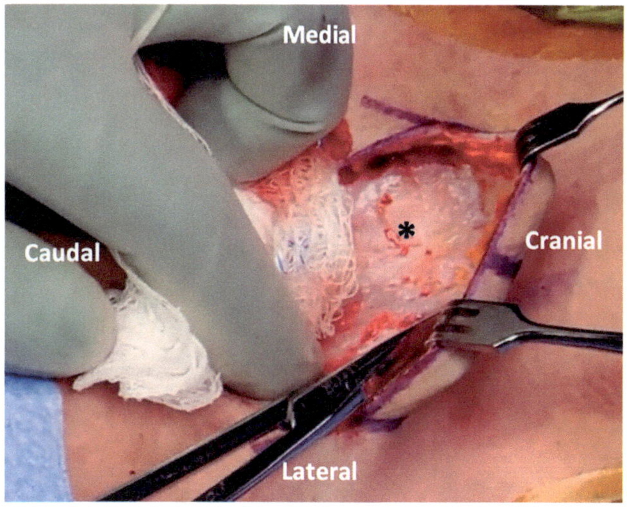

Fig. 48.4 The platysma is shown (*). The skin overlying the platysma is undermined in both a cranial and caudal direction

long and used for retraction of the muscle. These sutures will be tied together at the end of the case to reapproximate the two ends of the muscle. The fat pad is identified deep to the omohyoid and is retracted laterally. During dissection of the fat pad, the transverse cervical vessels are encountered; these should be ligated and divided.
- **Identification of the brachial plexus and subclavian vessels**
  Deep to the fat pad, the upper trunk of the brachial plexus is identified. The trifurcation of the upper (superior) trunk is seen, with the trunk dividing into the Suprascapular nerve, Posterior division, and Anterior

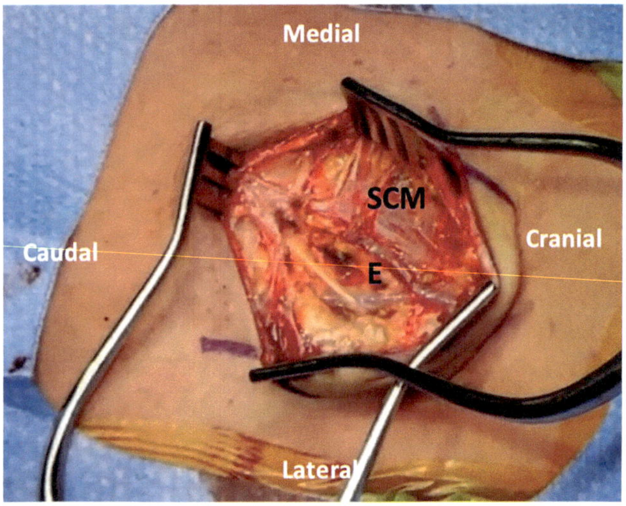

Fig. 48.5 After the platysma is opened along the length of its fibers, the posterior border of the sternocleidomastoid muscle (*SCM*) and external jugular vein (*E*) are identified. The external jugular vein can be ligated and divided as needed

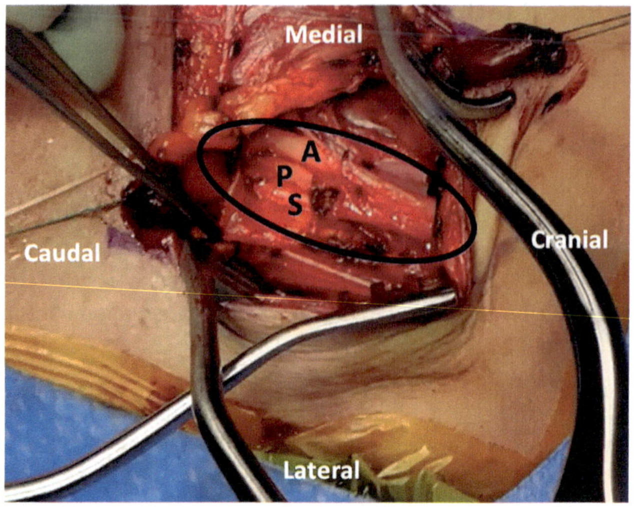

Fig. 48.7 After retraction of the fat pad and ligation of the transverse cervical vessels, the upper (superior) trunk of the brachial plexus is identified (*ellipse*). The upper trunk divides into three terminal branches: the suprascapular nerve (*S*), the posterior division (*P*), and the anterior division (*A*), hence the acronym *SPA*

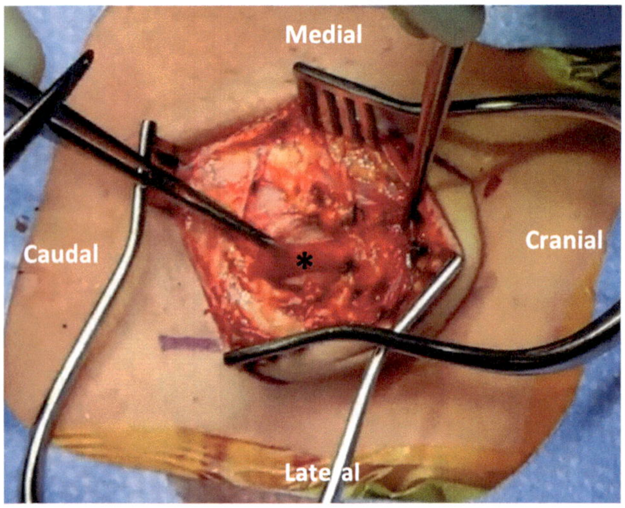

Fig. 48.6 The omohyoid is identified (*); sutures are tied around either end of the muscle; and the muscle is divided

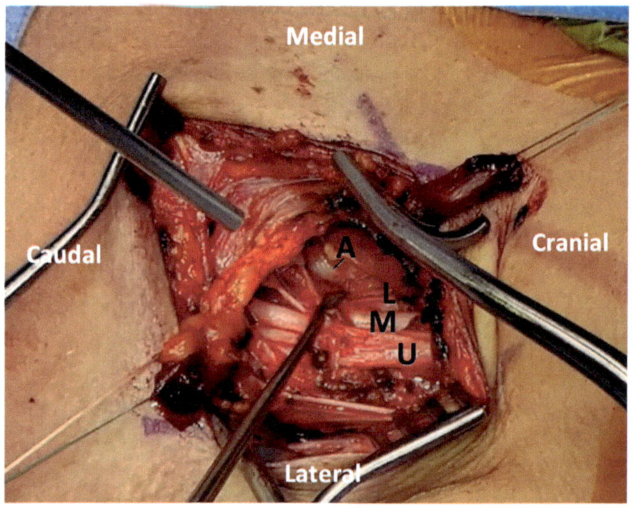

Fig. 48.8 The middle trunk of the brachial plexus (*M*) lies deep and caudal to the upper trunk (*U*). The lower (inferior) trunk (*L*) lies deep and caudal to that. The subclavian artery (*A*) can be identified running anterior to the lower trunk

division from cranial/posterior to caudal/anterior, respectively (Fig. 48.7). The order of these three branches can be best remembered using the acronym "SPA" [6]. The middle trunk lies deep/caudal to the upper trunk, and the lower (inferior) trunk lies deep/caudal to that (Fig. 48.8). The subclavian artery is anterior to the lower trunk and is typically palpated and/or seen before lower trunk.

- **Identification of the phrenic nerve**
  The anterior scalene muscle (ASM) is then identified near the medial aspect of the exposure. The phrenic nerve runs anterior to it in a cranial-lateral to caudal-medial direction. The phrenic nerve is identified and stimulated using a handheld, battery-operated, electrical stimulator. Chest wall rise and a change in end-tidal CO_2 waveform (see also Fig. 7.7b) are the expected responses.
- **Resection of the ASM**
  Once the exposure is complete, the resection of ASM is begun. Care is taken to remain underneath the fascia of the muscle to avoid phrenic nerve injury (Figs. 48.9 and 48.10). ASM is resected piecemeal using Metzenbaum

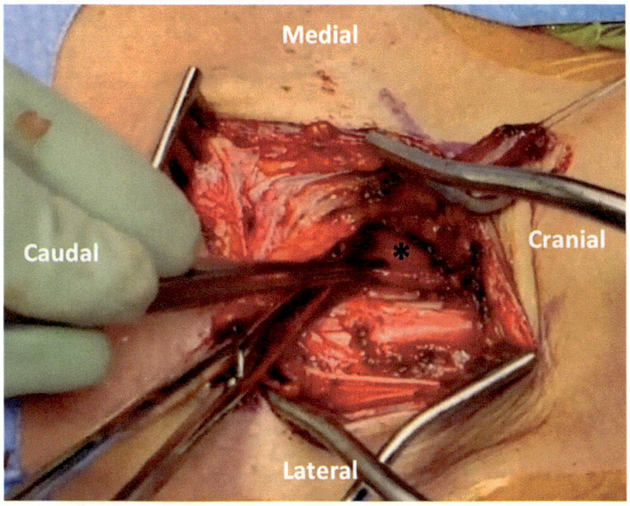

Fig. 48.9 The anterior scalene muscle (*) is cut and resected using Metzenbaum scissors. The phrenic nerve is not visualized here but is running from craniolateral to caudomedial, above the fascia that separates it from the anterior scalene muscle. Care should be taken to look for and protect accessory phrenic nerve(s) if present

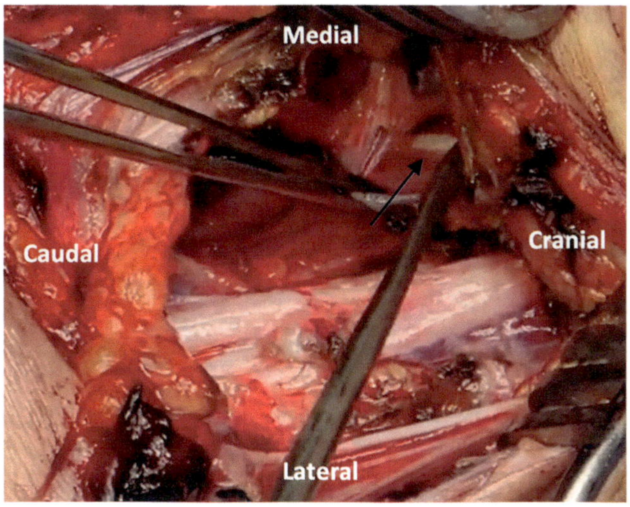

Fig. 48.10 The anterior scalene muscle has been completely removed. The fascia beneath the phrenic nerve is gently retracted to show the phrenic nerve (*arrow*)

scissors. Use of bipolar cautery is avoided to minimize the risk of thermal damage to the phrenic nerve and brachial plexus. Hemostatic packing and gentle irrigation can be used intermittently to control bleeding. If bipolar electrocautery is needed, it should be used judiciously and kept to a minimum to avoid injury to the phrenic nerve. The fascia deep to the anterior scalene is also divided and resected.

- **Additional decompression of the neurovascular bundle**

  After resection of ASM is complete, the trunks of the brachial plexus, as well as the subclavian artery, are inspected to identify any additional bands of constricting tissue (Fig. 48.11). Any such bands are divided. Additionally, any small vessels that appear to be causing compression of the plexus are also ligated and cut. The region is further inspected for any bony prominences behind the plexus, such as an elongated C7 transverse process or cervical rib that should be removed if identified using Kerrison rongeurs, with gentle retraction of middle and lower trunks. These bony components don't need to be completely resected but enough to decompress the neurovascular structures.
- **Closure**

  Once the brachial plexus and subclavian vessels have been fully decompressed, attention is turned to hemostasis, irrigation, and closure. A small drain to bulb suction is placed within the surgical bed. The ends of the omohyoid muscle are reapproximated using the two previously placed sutures. The fat pad is loosely approximated to the posterior border of SCM, and the platysma is closed with interrupted 3–0 Vicryl sutures. Inverted deep dermal sutures are placed in the subcutaneous tissue/dermis and the skin is closed with a running subcuticular 4–0 Monocryl stitch. Steri-strips are then placed over the incision.

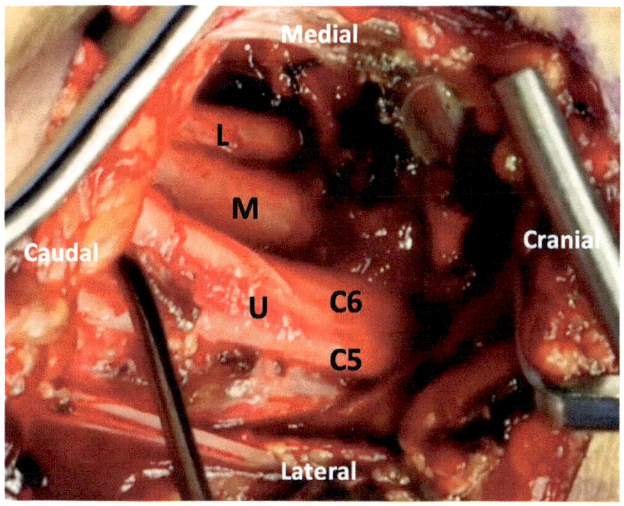

Fig. 48.11 Final view of the decompressed proximal brachial plexus. C5 and C6 nerves are seen joining to form the upper trunk (*U*). The decompressed middle (*M*) and lower (*L*) trunks are also seen

Pectoralis Minor (PM) Release

- **Positioning**
  The patient is positioned supine on the operating table, with the back of the table up and head slightly extended. The patient's head should be turned towards the contralateral side. If just pectoralis minor release is performed the arm should be abducted to open the infraclavicular space, if anterior scalenectomy is performed in the same session then the arm should be adducted so it doesn't get in the way.
- **Incision**
  For the infraclavicular approach to the brachial plexus, external landmarks are identified, including the clavicle and the deltopectoral groove. The deltopectoral groove is the palpable indentation between the deltoid and pectoralis major muscles. A linear incision is made along the deltopectoral groove (Fig. 48.12).
- **Exposure**
  The skin incision is opened sharply, and the dissection is carried down through the subcutaneous tissues using a combination of Metzenbaum scissors and electrocautery until the deltoid and pectoralis major are encountered. The deltoid is dissected from the pectoralis major muscle. The cephalic vein is identified in the groove between these two muscles (Fig. 48.13) and can be ligated and cut if needed. Next, the coracoid process is palpated. PM (medially, Fig. 48.14), the short head of the biceps brachii, and the coracobrachialis (laterally) attach to the coracoid process.
- **Release of PM**
  PM is identified as it inserts into the medial aspect of the coracoid process. The muscle is tagged with 2–0 Vicryl sutures, pulled anteriorly to protect the underlying neuro-

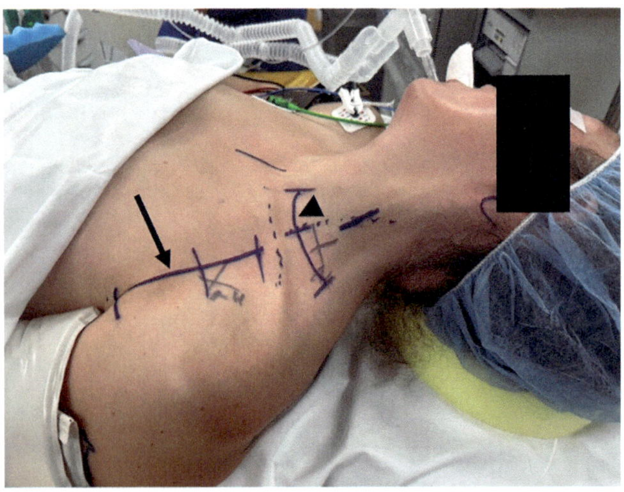

Fig. 48.12 The incision is planned along the deltopectoral groove (*arrow*). The incision for anterior scalenectomy is marked in this image as well (*arrowhead*)

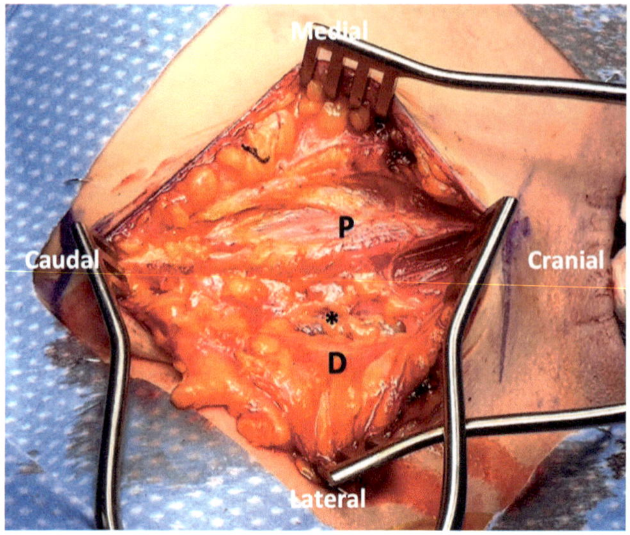

Fig. 48.13 The deltoid (*D*) and pectoralis major (*P*) are identified. The cephalic vein (*) can often be identified between these muscles

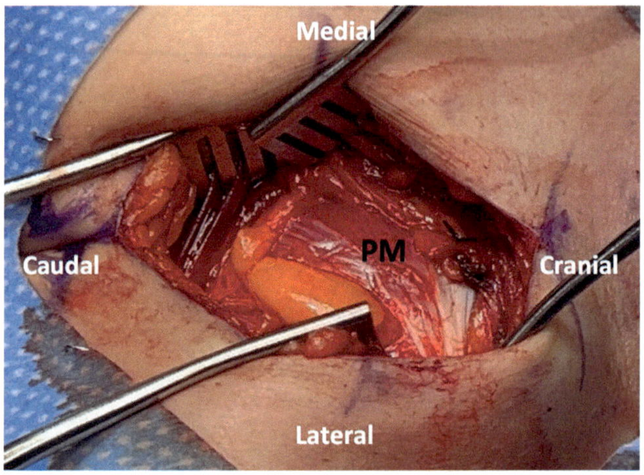

Fig. 48.14 After dissecting between the deltoid and pectoralis major, the pectoralis minor (*PM*) is identified, attaching to the medial aspect of the coracoid process

  vascular structures, and then transected (Fig. 48.15), alternatively a right-angled hemostat can be used to lift up the muscle belly before cutting it.
- **Identification of the brachial plexus**
  Once PM is released, a fat pad is identified underneath. The brachial plexus is identified within this fat pad. The infraclavicular approach to the brachial plexus exposes the cords and terminal branches of the plexus. The lateral cord can be identified after dissection through this fat pad. The lateral cord is formed from the combination of the anterior divisions of the upper and middle trunks. Terminal branches of the lateral cord include the musculocutaneous nerve and the lateral contribution to the median nerve (Fig. 48.16). Prior to the terminal branches,

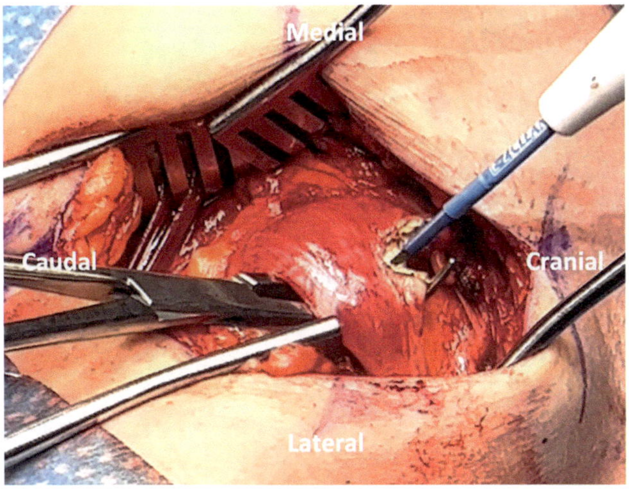

Fig. 48.15 The pectoralis minor muscle is lifted up with sutures or a right-angled hemostat, then divided with monopolar electrocautery

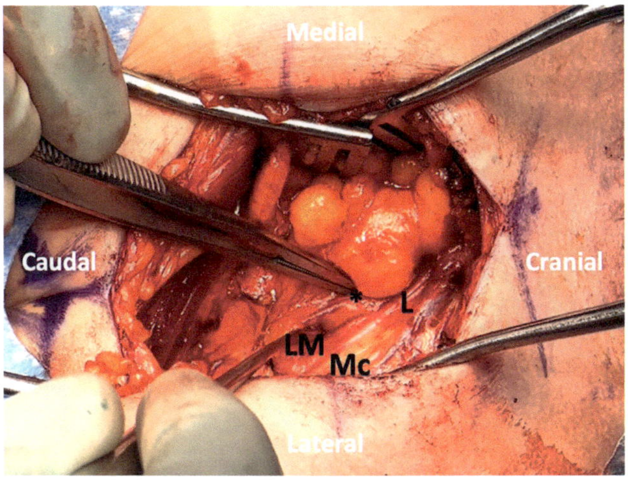

Fig. 48.16 The lateral cord is identified first (*L*), as it divides into its terminal branches, the musculocutaneous nerve (*Mc*) and the lateral contribution to the median nerve (*LM*). Axillary vessels also seen here (*). There is usually more than one lateral contribution to median nerve

it also gives off the lateral pectoral nerves. Posterolateral to the lateral cord, the posterior cord can be identified. The posterior cord is formed by the joining of the posterior divisions of the three trunks. Terminal branches of the posterior cord include the axially and radial nerves. The medial cord is formed from the continuation of the anterior division of the lower trunk and is found posteromedial to the axillary artery. The medial pectoral nerve, medial brachial cutaneous nerve, and medial antebrachial cutaneous nerve arise from the medial cord. It terminates as the ulnar nerve and the medial contribution to the median nerve. Of note, the terminal branches of the medial and lateral cords form an "M." Typically, the lateral

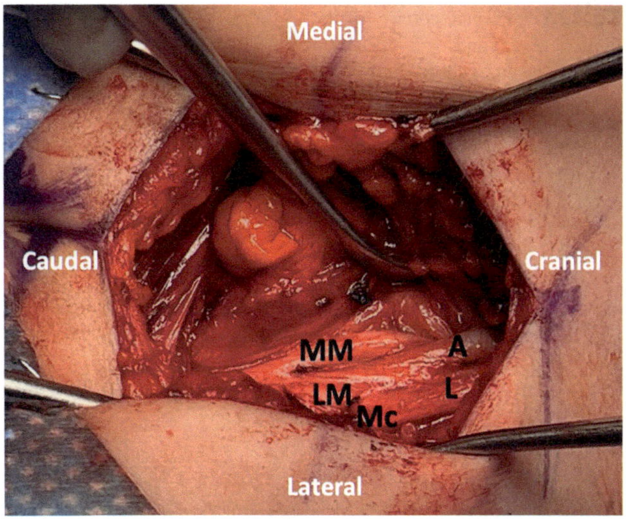

Fig. 48.17 Lastly, the terminal branches of the medial cord are exposed, including the medial contribution to the median nerve (*MM*). This can be followed proximally to identify the medial cord (not shown). The axillary artery (*A*) courses between the medial and lateral cords. Again shown are the musculocutaneous nerve (*Mc*), lateral contribution to the medial nerve (*LM*), and lateral cord (*L*)

cord is identified first; followed distally to the median nerve, the latter followed proximally and medially, leading to the medial contribution to the median nerve and then the medial cord (Fig. 48.17).

- **Additional decompression of the plexus**
  After PM is released, the cords and proximal terminal branches of the brachial plexus are inspected to identify any additional sites of compression. Any identified areas of compression are dissected and released. Additionally, any small vessels that appear to be causing compression of the plexus are also ligated and cut, special attention should be made to the medial contribution to the median nerve, more than often there is a vessel wrapping around it that should be released.
- **Closure**
  Once the brachial plexus has been fully decompressed, the wound is irrigated then closed in layers. Inverted deep dermal sutures are placed in the subcutaneous tissue/dermis, and the skin is closed with a running subcuticular 3–0 Monocryl stitch. Steri-strips are then placed over the incision. Usually, no drain is needed.

Complications

- Phrenic nerve injury—The phrenic nerve is susceptible to thermal injury or direct trauma. A postoperative chest X-ray can show an elevated hemidiaphragm (Fig. 48.18). This is usually well-tolerated but can rarely cause dyspnea, especially on exertion. Most of the time this resolves

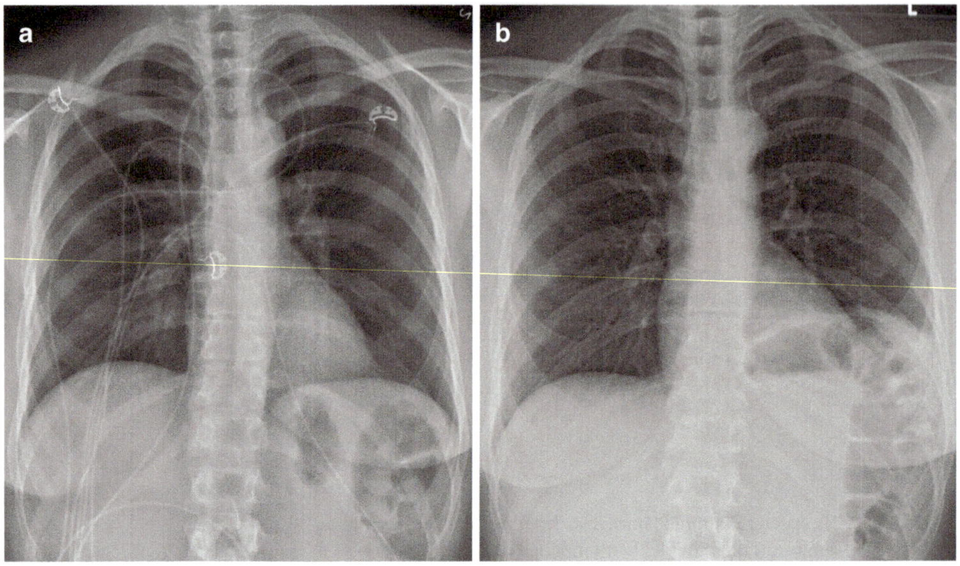

Fig. 48.18 Phrenic nerve injury. Pre- (**a**) and postoperative (**b**) chest X-ray showing left hemidiaphragm elevation after TOS decompression

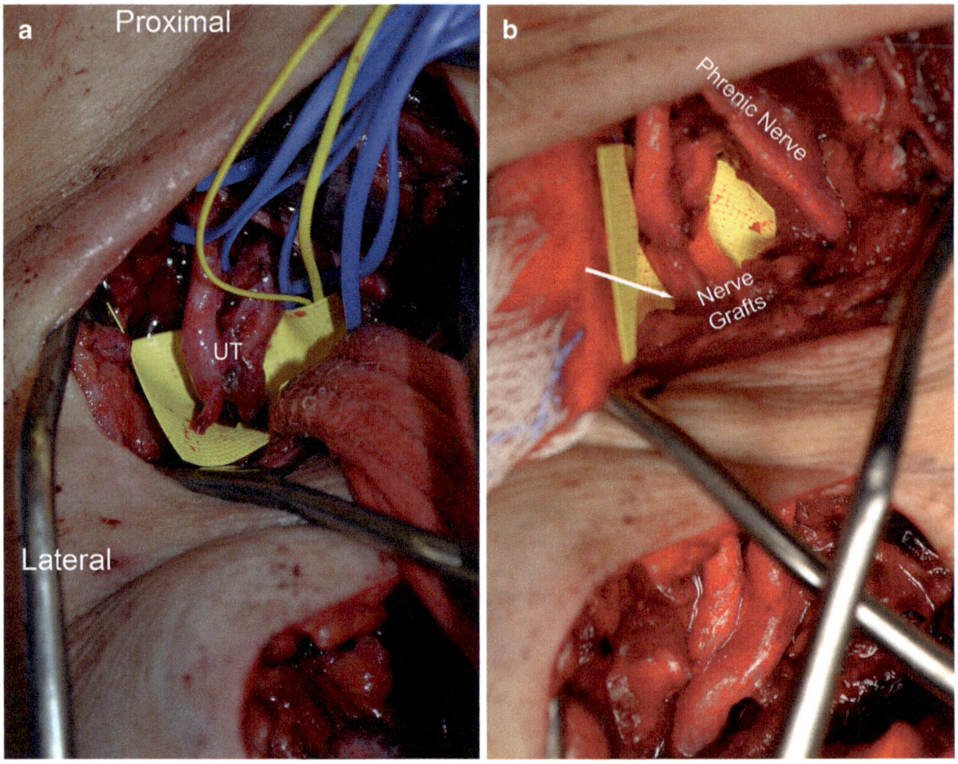

Fig. 48.19 Complete transection of the upper trunk (*UT*) of the brachial plexus during first rib resection via a supraclavicular approach before (**a**) and after (**b**) repair. The suprascapular nerve was directly repaired (*arrow*), while the posterior and anterior divisions required nerve grafts

spontaneously, even after a few months but may occasionally require diaphragmatic plication by thoracic surgery. We have not seen this complication since we have moved to the minimal bipolar technique. ASM is cut with scissors, bleeding points are packed with hemostatic agents, and if bipolar coagulation is needed, it should be kept to a minimum followed by copious irrigation to avoid thermal injury to the phrenic nerve.

- Pneumothorax on postoperative chest X-ray—Small pneumothorax could just be observed; large ones may require chest tube placement.
- Thoracic duct injury—The thoracic duct can be injured during dissection on the left side. An injury should be suspected if a milky fluid is seen within the wound, this can rarely occur on the right side. Injuries can be repaired directly with suturing, or fat patching, reinforced with

fibrin glue. A chyle leak from the wound postoperatively may require wound revision. If combined with pleural injury, it may lead to chylothorax.

- Bleeding due to vascular injury—including injury to the subclavian or axillary vessels, transverse cervical or suprascapular arteries, internal or external jugular veins.
- Iatrogenic brachial plexus injury—Temporary neurapraxia is not uncommon, especially if the middle and lower trunks are retracted for a long time to remove a cervical rib, or C7 transverse process. Retraction should be kept to a minimum. Nerve transection is seen with transaxillary, supraclavicular approach (Fig. 48.19), or infraclavicular approaches in a descending order. This occurs mostly during first rib resection, especially if no adequate brachial plexus exposure is done prior to the bony work. It is absolutely important to identify the brachial plexus and vessels prior to rib resection. Recent literature shows that anterior scalenectomy alone provides adequate decompression of TOS without the need for rib resection. The latter could be reserved for residual or recurrent symptoms.
- Wound infection—rare due to good vascularity of the skin in this area.

Common Abnormalities Encountered During Thoracic Outlet Surgery (Fig. 48.20)

- Hypertrophied ASM (Fig. 48.20b).
- Tight fascial band deep to ASM (Fig. 48.20c).
- Scalenus minimus, insinuates between subclavian artery and lower trunk (Fig. 48.20d).

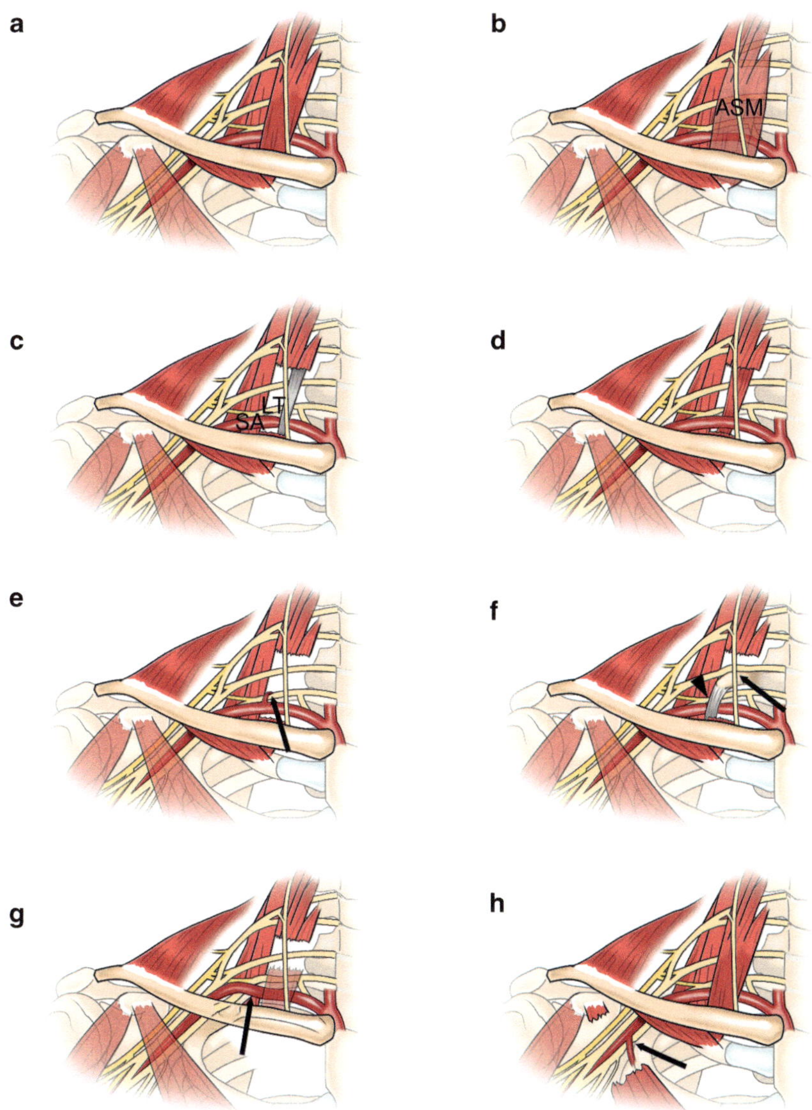

Fig. 48.20 Diagrammatic representation of the thoracic outlet and different pathologies encountered. (**a**) Normal thoracic outlet. (**b**) Hypertrophied anterior scalene (*ASM*). (**c**) Tight fascia deep to ASM compressing lower trunk (LT) and subclavian artery (*SA*) like a sling. (**d**) Scalenus minimus passes between SA and LT compressing it. (**e**) Abnormal vessel from SA wrapping around LT (*arrow*). (**f**) Cervical rib, or elongated transverse process of C7, with a band of tissue attached to it. The rib could compress the plexus from posterior (*arrow*), and the band could compress SA and LT anteriorly (*arrowhead*). (**g**) The first rib or a cervical rib may angle 90° to articulate with the next rib, raising the brachial plexus and SA and compressing them from below (*arrow*). (**h**) Abnormal vessel from the axillary artery wrapping around medial cord or medial contribution to median nerve (*arrow*). Copyright Amgad Hanna, published with permission

- Abnormal vessels (most often dorsal scapular) from subclavian vessels can wrap around lower or middle trunks (Fig. 48.20e).
- Cervical rib, or elongated transverse process of C7, usually associated with a membrane compressing subclavian artery and lower trunk (Fig. 48.20f).
- Abnormal first rib angling down and articulating with second rib, lifting and compressing subclavian artery and lower trunk (Fig. 48.20g).
- Abnormal vessels from axillary artery wrapping around medial cord or medial contribution to median nerve, deep to pectoralis minor (Fig. 48.20h) [7].
- Supraclavius could be encountered during the approach, but its causative implication is questionable [8].
- Narrow costoclavicular space has also been reported.

References

1. Li N, Dierks G, Vervaeke HE, Jumonville A, Kaye AD, Myrcik D et al (2021) Thoracic outlet syndrome: a narrative review. J Clin Med 10(5):962. https://doi.org/10.3390/jcm10050962
2. Klaassen Z, Sorenson E, Tubbs RS, Arya R, Meloy P, Shah R, Shirk S, Loukas M (2014) Thoracic outlet syndrome: a neurological and vascular disorder. Clin Anat 27(5):724–732. https://doi.org/10.1002/ca.22271. Epub 2013 May 29
3. Kuhn JE, Lebus VGF, Bible JE (2015) Thoracic outlet syndrome. J Am Acad Orthop Surg 23(4):222–232. https://doi.org/10.5435/JAAOS-D-13-00215
4. Cheng CJ, Mackinnon-Patterson B, Beck JL, Mackinnon SE (2008) Scratch collapse test for evaluation of carpal and cubital tunnel syndrome. J Hand Surg Am 33(9):1518–1524. https://doi.org/10.1016/j.jhsa.2008.05.022
5. Maghrabi H, Ansari D, Eslami A, Hanna AS (2025) Rib-sparing anterior scalenectomy versus first rib resection for the treatment of thoracic outlet syndrome: a retrospective cohort study of morbidity and outcomes. Oper Neurosurg
6. Hanna A (2016) The SPA arrangement of the branches of the upper trunk of the brachial plexus: a correction of a longstanding misconception and a new diagram of the brachial plexus. J Neurosurg 125:350–354. https://doi.org/10.3171/2015.5.JNS15367. Epub 2015 Nov 27
7. Hanna A, Bodden LO, Siebiger GRL (2018) Neurogenic thoracic outlet syndrome caused by vascular compression of the brachial plexus: a report of two cases. J Brachial Plex Peripher Nerve Inj 13(1):e1–e3. https://doi.org/10.1055/s-0037-1607977. eCollection
8. Greeneway GP, Page PS, Navarro MA, Hanna AS (2022) Supraclavius muscle observed during anterior scalenectomy for thoracic outlet syndrome: a report of two cases and review of the literature. Surg Neurol Int 13:600. https://doi.org/10.25259/SNI_806_2022. eCollection 2022

49 Entrapments of the Pudendal Nerve, Nerve to the Obturator Internus, and Ganglion Impar

Aaron G. Filler

Introduction

Pain, numbness, and motor dysfunction in the pelvic and genital area can arise from a variety of reasons; however, it is important to appreciate that treatable nerve impingement syndromes do play a considerable role. It is important to differentiate between various causes of non-discogenic back pain (Fig. 49.1). Nerve structures that can be involved pose significant technical challenges to treatment and require advanced skills for nerve identification and management of these disorders.

Recognition and treatment of pudendal nerve entrapment syndrome has an extended history [1, 2], and the first large-scale study was published in 1998 [3]. There are now numerous general publications covering various aspects of diagnosis and treatment [4–8]. However, the success rate in treatment of pudendal neuralgia had not been satisfactory [9–11] until diagnostics and surgical approaches were substantially reconsidered and new approaches applied to both diagnostics and nerve decompression methodology [12, 13]. One problem in the past was a lack of appreciation that there are several subtypes with different anatomic bases and presentations [8, 14–17]. Further, the surgical anatomy of the pudendal nerve itself is subject to significant individual variation [18].

Targeted pudendal nerve injections with the use of electrodiagnostic technique [19], C-arm fluoroscopy [20, 21], and computerized tomography (CT) scanning have been described [22–24]. Diagnosis has also relied on pudendal nerve latency testing [25, 26], but diagnostic imaging really played very little role in the past. A 2008 large-scale study on treatment of this condition using magnetic resonance neurography (MRN) (Figs. 49.2, 49.3, and 49.4) [13, 27–29], open magnetic resonance imaging (MRI)-guided injections [30, 31], and newer minimal access surgical techniques provided significant clarification [12].

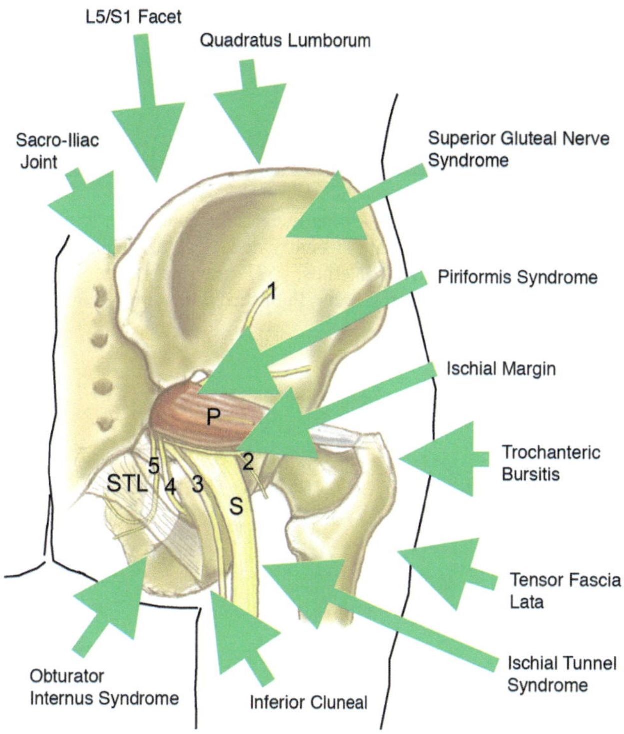

Fig. 49.1 Different causes of non-discogenic "back pain." *1* superior gluteal nerve, *2* inferior gluteal nerve, *3* posterior cutaneous nerve of the thigh, *4* nerve to obturator internus, *5* pudendal nerve, *P* piriformis, *S* sciatic nerve, *STL* sacrotuberous ligament. Copyright Journal of Neurosurgery. Published with permission. Adapted from Filler 2009 [14]

Pudendal nerve entrapment can be categorized into four major categories on the basis of the location of the entrapment [8, 14]; they are as follows:

Type I: exclusively at the level of the piriformis muscle in the sciatic notch only.
Type II: at the level of the ischial spine and sacrotuberous ligament.

A. G. Filler (✉)
Institute for Nerve Medicine, Santa Monica, CA, USA
e-mail: afiller@nervemed.com

A. S. Hanna (ed.), *Nerves: Anatomy, Exposures, and Techniques*, https://doi.org/10.1007/978-3-031-73931-6_49

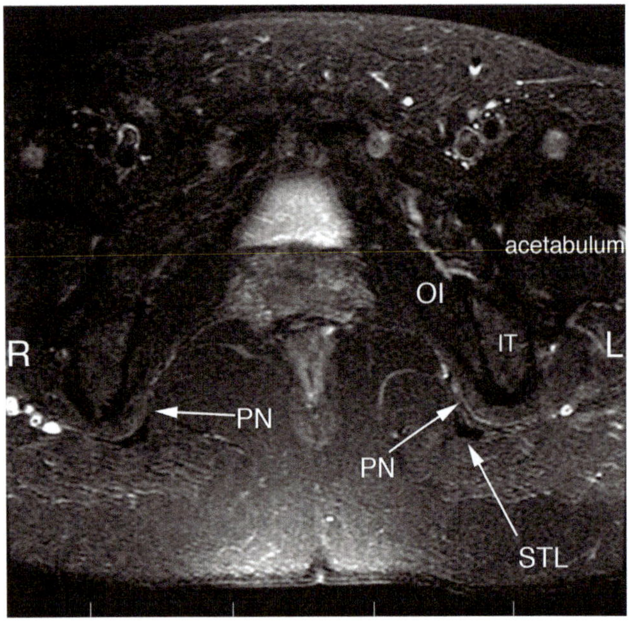

Fig. 49.2 MR neurogram showing increased signal of the left pudendal nerve (*PN*) just proximal to its entry into Alcock's canal. *IT* ischial tuberosity, *OI* obturator internus, *STL* sacrotuberous ligament. Copyright Journal of Neurosurgery. Published with permission [14]

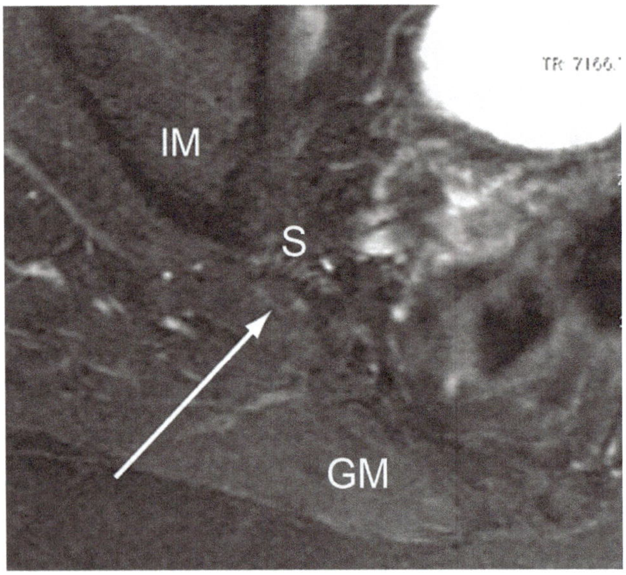

Fig. 49.3 Axial MRI shows increased T2 signal of the sciatic nerve (*S*) as it passes between the piriformis tendon (*arrow*) and the ischial margin (*IM*). *GM* gluteus maximus. Copyright Elsevier. Published with permission [8]

Type III: in Alcock's canal on the medial surface of the obturator internus.
Type IV: at distal branches.

In addition, some patients present with prominent autonomic symptoms such as burning with light contact in the skin as well as complex sexual dysfunctions such as persistent genital arousal or urinary function abnormalities. In these patients, involvement of the ganglion impar (inferior hypogastric ganglion) on the deep surface of the sacrococcygeal joint is likely.

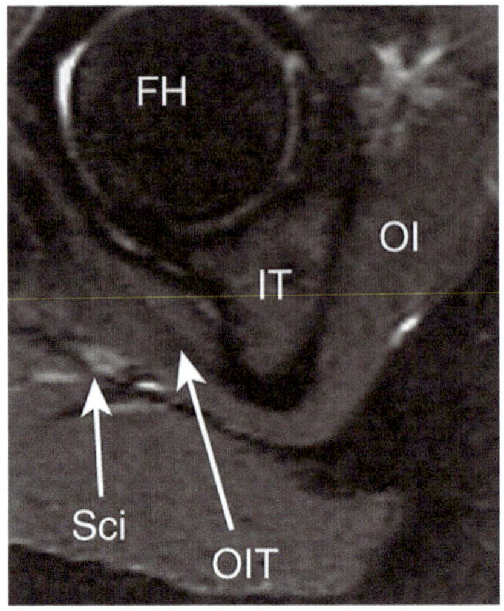

Fig. 49.4 Axial MRI showing the sciatic nerve (*Sci*) relationship to the obturator internus tendon (*OIT*). *FH* femoral head, *OI* obturator internus, *IT* ischial tuberosity. Copyright Elsevier. Published with permission [8]

Presentation

The symptoms of pudendal nerve entrapment involve pain, dysfunction, and numbness in all or part of the distribution of the nerve. This distribution encompasses the saddle area between the legs, including the genitalia, rectum, and terminal urinary tract, as well as pelvic floor musculature. In addition, sexual dysfunction and sphincter dysfunction are often seen. Sexual dysfunctions included female continuous arousal as well as lack of sensation, male impotence, and dyspareunia. Aggravation by sitting is common when the obturator internus or piriformis muscles are involved, but there is not always a positional trigger. Many cases are unilateral, even though some patients have difficulty identifying the laterality of pain in midline urogenital structures; bilateral pudendal entrapment does occur, however, in more than 25% of cases. In a previous study, patients' age ranged from 8 to 82 years, and there was no significant sex preponderance [12].

Physical Examination

The most common physical finding in pudendal syndromes is sensitivity to palpation at the obturator internus muscle elicited by manual compression on the deep medial aspect of the ischial tuberosity. Reproduction of symptoms with straight leg raising is rare. Adduction of the thigh and passive internal or external rotation of the hip may reproduce pain in the supine position. Resisted abduction or adduction of the thigh in the seated position also elicited symptoms in some individuals [14].

Many patients with ganglion impar involvement have significant tenderness with movement of the coccyx. This symptom is distinct from coccygeus muscle pain lateral to the coccyx, which arises from irritated pudendal branches.

Management with Open MRI-Guided Injections

Depending on the location of the entrapment, injection targets include the piriformis muscle, the obturator internus muscle, and the pudendal nerve at the following points: at the ischial margin or ischial spine, at the sacrotuberous ligament, or at small branch takeoffs from Alcock's canal, including the rectal branch in the ischiorectal fossa, at the urogenital diaphragm, and at the "crows foot" distal branching area at the outlet of Alcock's canal.

In patients obtaining no alteration of symptoms from dense proximal pudendal nerve block, open MRI can be used to guide injection via a lateral sub-coccygeal approach to block the impar ganglion to rule out autonomically driven, non-pudendal saddle area pain syndromes. This approach is similar to paramedian approaches [32] rather than transcoccygeal approaches [33, 34].

Impar ganglion blocks have been considered treacherous in the past because of the proximity and variability in position of the bowel wall immediately adjacent to the ganglion. The open MRI approach from lateral to the ganglion is safe and reliable for this type of block and has the benefit of providing excellent visualization of the adjacent bowel wall. This lateral approach may also be performed under fluoroscopic and ultrasonographic guidance, although the non-MRI techniques are associated with somewhat greater risks because the closely apposed and constantly moving nearby bowel structures may be perforated by the needle if these structures cannot be adequately visualized.

In cases which present a significant autonomic profile of symptoms (bilaterality, urinary/sexual dysfunction, burning sensation in the skin, sensitivity to the light touch of clothing) but in which a block of the impar ganglion does not interrupt the symptoms, another location to assess is the more distal inferior hypogastric plexus ("DIHP"). A common point of entrapment/irritation for this plexus is just medial and distal to the ischial spine. For this reason, if an impar ganglion block does not provide a suppressive effect on the autonomic symptoms, then an injection directed to a point distal and medial to the tip of the ischial spine may be warranted. Importantly, elements of the DIHP include some nerve elements that pass from the superior hypogastric ganglion (which is located anterior to the L5/S1 interspace). This explains the presence of distal pelvic/genital autonomic symptoms despite a dense block of the impar ganglion.

As many spine surgeons are aware, damage to the superior hypogastric plexus can occur during an anterior L5/S1 fusion or artificial disk replacement resulting in sexual dysfunction. Similarly, this provides a route for distal genital autonomic symptoms to persist immediately following a dense impar ganglion block. Injection of hyaluronidase (such as Hylenex®) deep and distal to the ischial spine can relieve symptoms arising in the inferior hypogastric plexus.

Surgical Management of Pudendal Nerve Entrapment

The need to include the following components of the operation for pudendal nerve entrapment varies according to the etiologic subtype: piriformis muscle resection, partial section of the sacrotuberous ligament, neuroplasty (and/or partial neurolysis) of the nerve to the obturator internus in the retro-sciatic space along with dilation of Alcock's canal in the obturator internus/Alcock's canal. Intra-operative EMG monitoring of muscles innervated by the pudendal nerve, sciatic nerve, nerve to the obturator internus, and inferior gluteal and superior gluteal nerves is essential for nerve identification.

Procedures can be performed using minimal access approaches on an outpatient or overnight stay basis [35]. The surgical approach for patients with piriformis muscle involvement is described below (see also Chap. 26) [30].

Step-By-Step Surgical Methodology for Pudendal Nerve Decompression

Placement of the Incision

An incision useful for most cases is carried out in the prone position. The first step is to position the incision relative to a pre-incision X-ray after the patient has been positioned prone on bolsters under general anesthesia. As with any prone case, care is taken to cushion and protect skin over prominent bones, such as at the anterior superior iliac spine and at the chin. A pair of thick bolsters (about 8 in. in diameter) running from shoulder to hips and careful attention to avoiding pressure on the ASIS, forehead, and chin is helpful.

Palpation is used to locate approximately the location of the superior tip of the greater trochanter. The skin is then marked with a small scratch, and two 18-gauge needles are placed on the skin surface so that they are cross each other at a 90° angle directly over the small skin scratch. A posterior to anterior (PA) X-ray is then obtained with care to assure the X-ray source is directly over the crossed needles in order to minimize any parallax.

These steps allow confident, correct, and precise location of the landmark at the tip of the greater trochanter. For a piriformis surgery (in patients who have only an entrapment at the greater sciatic notch involving the piriformis muscle), a three-centimeter incision is then made commencing at the scratch point over the tip of the greater trochanter and proceeding medially and superiorly at a 45° angle.

For most pudendal cases, however, the focus will be in the lesser sciatic notch and the retro-sciatic space. For this typical type of pudendal surgery, the landmark of the tip of the greater trochanter will be a bit too superior and lateral to be optimal. Therefore, once the landmark X-ray is obtained, the surgeon should mark a point on the skin that is two centimeters inferior and medial to the tip of the greater trochanter mark. This more inferior and medial starting point is then marked with a skin scratch and an incision line—about 3 cm in length—and proceeding medially and superiorly at a 45° angle is marked out.

Placement of EMG Electrodes for Intraoperative Monitoring

Prior to surgery, it is absolutely mandatory that a number of electrode pairs are placed by an experienced electrodiagnostic technologist to ensure reliable identification and the ability to distinguish among the various nerves in the area. The electrodes should be placed as follows: (a) Superior gluteal nerve/gluteus medius: four centimeters below the iliac crest and superior to the center of the sciatic notch. (b) Tensor fasciae latae (TFL, just inferior to the greater trochanter) for the TFL branch of the superior gluteal nerve. (c) Inferior gluteal nerve/gluteus maximus—this pair can be inserted at the lateral margin of the gluteal crease. (d) Obturator internus, this identification is critical, so we use two electrode pairs: one pair is placed above the gluteal crease about three centimeters lateral to midline (medial portion of obturator internus), and a second pair is placed just above the gluteal crease about six centimeters lateral to midline (lateral portion of the obturator internus). For the pudendal nerve, perianal electrodes are placed. To monitor the sciatic nerve, electrode pairs should be placed for biceps femoris short head, semimembranosus, semitendinosus, gastrocnemius, tibialis anterior, medial foot, and lateral foot. Additionally, a more anteriorly placed thigh electrode pair for the vastus lateralis (femoral nerve) is useful. Sterile electrode tips with a Tegaderm should be used with alcohol prep in advance at each site. The wires should be carefully gathered and placed where they will not be damaged or displaced by any table-fixed retractor clamps.

Initial Approach to the Gluteal Fascia

The previously placed skin scratches are used to draw the incision plan with crossed marks to optimize skin-edge alignment during closure. After prep and drape with iodine (alcohol preps can seep under the tegaderms and short out the electrodes), an Ioban drape is applied, and the skin is injected with 0.75% marcaine without epinephrine. A three-to-five-centimeter incision is then made with a number 15 blade, skin-edge hemostasis is obtained, and then a Bovie coagulator in cautery mode is used to progress through the adipose tissues below the skin surface. The electricity causes some muscle reaction just as the gluteal fascia is reached, and the Bovie coagulator is then set aside, not to be used again until just before final skin closure.

Adipose tissues are cleared from the gluteal fascia along a path about 1 cm in width to facilitate later closure of the fascia. The gluteal fascia is then punctured, and the tip of a tonsil clamp (with a gently curving tip that is blunt and not sharp) is passed through the puncture to elevate a strip of the fascia from the underlying muscle. A Malis bipolar coagulator is then used to pre-hemostase the fascia along a line, and then the linear three-to-five-centimeter incision is made in the gluteal fascia using Metzenbaum (Metz) scissors. Subsequent robust closure of this fascia is the key to rapid and comfortable post-operative recovery with early and full mobilization.

Non-destructive Advance Through the Gluteal Musculature

Progress is then made gradually through the gluteal muscles using a gloved finger, the tonsil clamp to spread tissues, the Malis bipolar, and the Metz scissors. Do not cut through the gluteal muscles with a Bovie. Doing so can result in a wholly unnecessary permanent gait impairment. Patiently working through natural planes in the gluteal muscles will eventually bring the surgeon to the pre-piriformis fascia. This avoids any significant harm to the gluteus maximus and assures a rapid, smooth post-operative recovery (the patient should be up and comfortably walking at least by the morning after surgery).

Visualization and Exposure of the Pre-Piriformis Fascia (Surgeon's View)

Arrival at the pre-piriformis fascia is detected by the observation of a layer of yellow adipose tissue beneath a hard, clear membrane. At this point, the approach must pause while self-retaining retractors are put in place. Depending on the individual patient, this tissue level will be between five and eight centimeters below the skin surface. It is imperative to have fixed control of the muscle opening to allow for delicate exploration and manipulation of the nerves below. A Shadowline retractor system with four blades (as for an anterior cervical discectomy) usually works well at this stage, but a table-fixed retractor is usually necessary to properly reach the pudendal nerve for safe and extensive decompression. An example is the TeDan retractor, which essentially holds the retractor at the necessary angles as the surgery progresses and allows for correction of the tendency of the retractor blades to toe-in at depth, with rigid, adjustable attachment to a rail of the operating room table.

Making and Retracting a Flap of the Pre-Piriformis Fascia

Once the retractors are in place, the optimal next step is to carefully elevate a flap based on the pre-piriformis fascia. The location of nerve elements varies considerably with patient anatomy. Critical motor nerve elements may be immediately in contact with the pre-piriformis fascia, or they may be deep to it by two to three centimeters. Only the nerve stimulator probe (Medtronic Prass Xomed Flush-tip or similar probe) can safely identify them, and it must be deployed along the surface of the pre-piriformis fascia to check for any nerve elements immediately below the fascia that are not visible due to being embedded in the pre-piriformis fat pad. This fascia is a very thin but substantial, nearly transparent layer.

After the initial exploration of the fascia surface with the stimulator probe—the fascia is punctured with the tip of the tonsil clamp, beginning on the superior and lateral corners of the intended flap, and the tonsil is used to advance below the fascia, progressing medially towards the superior and medial corners of the flap. Once any nerve element is cleared from adherence to the deep surface of the flap in this fashion, the Malis bipolar is used to coagulate the superior side of the flap, and it is cut with Metz scissors. This process is then repeated, progressing from the supero-medial corner to the infero-medial corner of the flap. Then the third and final step is to repeat this progressing from the infero-medial corner to reach the infero-lateral corner. Once these incisions in the pre-piriformis fascia are completed, the flap itself is elevated carefully from underlying tissues, repetitively assuring that no nerve element is adherent to the deep surface of the flap as it is elevated. Once it is elevated, the lateral retractor blade is repositioned to retract the flap, and the medial retractor blade is repositioned to retract the cut medial edge of the fascia. The superior and inferior blades are similarly repositioned to help retract the superior and inferior margins of the fascia.

Initial Identification of Nerve Elements in the Pre-Piriformis Fat Pad

At this point, another survey of the exposed pre-piriformis fat pad is carried out by very slowly and gently advancing the stimulator probe (set to one milliamp) along a series of linear courses, advancing it slowly into the fat pad. In this fashion, it should be possible to identify the sciatic nerve without risk of injury to it, and then the superior gluteal nerve near the superior margin of the flap (it is superior to the piriformis muscle), and the inferior gluteal nerve (which is generally just inferior to the sciatic nerve). Once the sciatic nerve is located by the probe, gradual progress is made through the fat pad to bring the postero-superior surface of the sciatic nerve into view. Once an initial very small view of the sciatic nerve is appreciated visually (with Loupe magnification and a headlight)—the superior and posterior surfaces can be carefully and gently brought completely into view by gently dissecting the deep and inferior surface of the pre-piriformis fat pad from the sciatic nerve postero-superior surface. If there are also superior gluteal nerve symptoms to be treated (gluteus medius pain up to the iliac crest or TFL pain descending from the greater trochanter), then the superior gluteal nerve is then more fully identified (initially locating it with the stimulator probe) and at least its inferior surface brought into view.

Piriformis Muscle Resection When Indicated

If there is piriformis muscle pain, then a piriformis muscle resection is carried out by first assuring there is no split nerve/split muscle configuration (no portion of the sciatic nerve passing through the piriformis muscle). This step involves injecting the muscle with marcaine, encircling it with a 0-Silk tie (Fig. 49.5a), and then carefully and slowly progressing to cut through the muscle by small serial steps of coagulation with the Malis and cuts with the Metz along the proximal portion of the muscle while keeping the sciatic nerve and superior gluteal nerve in view [30]. A second progressive incision with recurrent hemostasis by the Malis then severs the tendon of attachment to the greater trochanter. If there is a split/muscle, split/nerve configuration—then the deeper muscle segment (which effectively passes intra-neural through the sciatic nerve in some cases) is first very carefully resected, carefully avoiding any traction, excess pressure, or heat application to any component of the sciatic nerve. Variably, the remaining segment of the piriformis muscle superior to the split nerve components may also need to be resected. Nota bene that there are several sub-variants as to whether, from inferior to superior, it is nerve, muscle, nerve, muscle or muscle, nerve, muscle, nerve progressing from inferior to superior in this field of view.

Mapping of Nerve Elements in the Retro-Sciatic Space (Surgeon's View)

Once the sciatic nerve postero-superior surface is in view (Fig. 49.5b) (and any piriformis resection and/or neuroplasty of the superior gluteal nerve is completed), the surgeon then proceeds to carry out an initial mapping of the nerve elements immediately inferior to the sciatic nerve. These nerve elements are typically just inferior to the sciatic nerve and may be either or both posterior and/or anterior to the posterior aspect of the sciatic nerve course.

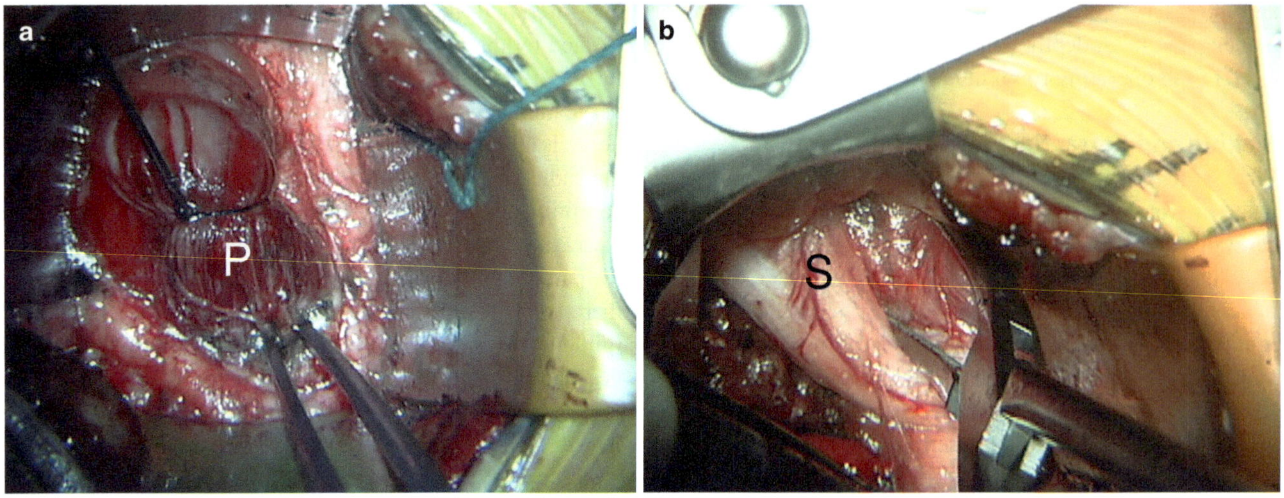

Fig. 49.5 Piriformis resection. (**a**) A ligature is placed around the muscle to protect the sciatic nerve before bipolar coagulation and cutting of the piriformis (*P*). (**b**) Surgical release of the sciatic nerve (*S*) Copyright Journal of Neurosurgery. Published with permission. Adapted from Filler 2005 [30]

Separation of the Inferior Gluteal Nerve, Nerve to the Obturator Internus from Vessels

Often, the other elements are in direct contact with the sciatic nerve. However, there may be a number of complex venous and arterial structures intertwined with the inferior gluteal nerve and the nerve to the obturator internus here as well. It is critically important to proceed gradually and carefully with this step, as extensive bleeding arising from the midst of the inferior gluteal, sciatic, and obturator internus nerves can obscure the field. When bleeding occurs, there is no place here for blind coagulation; everything is extremely eloquent. Use cottonoids, gel foam, and gentle pressure to patiently bring any bleeding vessel under control. Generally, this step of identification of the inferior gluteal nerve and the nerve to the obturator internus can be carried out with no bleeding at all.

Any nerve elements adherent to a vessel should be carefully separated from the vessel. In some cases, a varicose and dilated vein will have a nerve element stretched and flattened over the surface of the vein, and it is imperative to gradually coagulate the vein and to separate the nerves from the vein surface. Some patients have pain linked to dilation of veins with activity: as blood flow causes vein dilatation, nerves get stretched, causing pain, so that separation of these nerve elements from the vessels is helpful to assure a good result from the surgery.

Neuro-Diagnostic Stimulation for Full Identification of Each Nerve Element

The stimulator is used repeatedly during these steps to identify the branches of the inferior gluteal nerve and the nerve to the obturator internus based on stimulation. Ideally the medial and lateral obturator internus transcutaneous muscle electrodes fire together with stimulation of the nerve to the obturator internus. If there is also gluteus medius firing, then that branch of the nerve to the obturator internus cannot be subject to partial neurolysis without affecting the gluteus medius function. Similarly, if stimulation of any neural element that appears to be associated with the obturator internus or the gluteus medius leads to a response in the anal sphincter—then that nerve element is assumed to be involved with the pudendal nerve and also cannot be subject to any partial neurolysis. There may be more than one branch or major component of these nerves in the retro-sciatic space.

Identification and Initial Assessment of the Pudendal Nerve in the Retro-Sciatic Space

Once there is substantial mobilization of the inferior gluteal nerve and the nerve to the obturator internus as well as mobilization, separation, and sometimes coagulation of associated veins and arteries (which are similar to just larger than the caliber of the nerves)—attention is turned to the pudendal nerve itself. The pudendal nerve is generally unitary but may be found in two or three separate branches in some cases. It is identified substantially by response to stimulation-causing activity of the anal sphincter, and the electrodiagnostic technologist must constantly call out the identity of the reacting muscle or the expected nerve identified as the exploration for the pudendal nerve is carried out.

Neuroplasty of the Pre-Spinous Portion of the Pudendal Nerve in the Retro-Sciatic Space

The pudendal nerve generally has a segment that runs parallel to the inferior gluteal and obturator internus nerves but is inferior to, and often posterior to, the nerve to the obturator internus. There is considerable variation. In many patients, a proximal portion of the pudendal nerve is adherent to the deep surface of the sacrotuberous ligament. It is recommended that a neuroplasty include mobilizing the pudendal nerve from the sacrotuberous ligament completely. That ligament can form a roof over the area of dissection (from the point of view of the surgeon using this approach), and it is often necessary to carefully and progressively incise the superior margin of the sacrotuberous ligament in this area to better expose the pudendal nerve. Ideally, the pudendal nerve is mobilized in a gradual, progressive fashion, from the sciatic notch towards the ischial spine. It may also be adjacent to the sciatic nerve at its more proximal portions near the greater sciatic notch.

Mobilization and Decompression of the Pudendal Nerve at the Level of the Ischial Spine and Sacrospinous Ligament

Attention is then turned to the ischial spine, the sacrospinous ligament, and the lesser sciatic notch. Careful and gentle dissection with the tonsil clamp will identify an opening just posterior to the sacrospinous ligament through which the ischiorectal fossa can be accessed and through which the pudendal nerve travels. For orientation, the surgeon should keep in mind that the sacrotuberous ligament is closest to the surgeon (posteriorly placed), then the pudendal nerve passes, and then the sacrospinous ligament is anterior to the nerve (deepest from the surgeon's view). The pudendal nerve then turns so that it becomes anterior and the sacrospinous ligament becomes posterior as the nerve traverses the lesser sciatic notch and enters the ischiorectal fossa. The traverse of the pudendal nerve towards the lesser sciatic notch and its entry into the ischiorectal fossa is a common area of entrapment. Ideally, any vessels crossing and restricting the pudendal nerve and any fibrous adhesions along this portion of the pudendal nerve course should be carefully and completely released so that the pudendal nerve has full mobility, commencing at its exit from the greater sciatic and then reaching the lesser sciatic notch. In many patients, the entire symptomatic entrapment is in this "pre-sacrospinous" portion of the nerve.

Neuroplasty of the Pudendal Nerve in the Ischiorectal Fossa Distal to the Ischial Spine

Once the pudendal nerve is fully mobilized along its course from the greater sciatic notch to the lesser sciatic notch, it is necessary to commence exploration and evaluation of the portion of the pudendal nerve that crosses the sacrospinous ligament to reach the ischiorectal fossa, where it will enter a fascia along the medial surface of the obturator internus muscle, which becomes Alcock's canal more distally. From this angle of approach, the surgeons "view" into the lesser sciatic notch is essentially along the "barrel" of the Alcock's canal—this is essentially a "magic angle" approach so that the canal can be gently dilated from this point of view—using the tips of the tonsil clamp—to a depth of two to three centimeters, thus carefully mobilizing some of the obturator internus muscle fascia that surrounds the pudendal nerve in the ischiorectal fossa.

Resection of Any Involved Margin of the Ischial Spine or Sacrospinous Ligament

In many patients with pudendal nerve entrapment, the impingement includes the point of traverse posterior to the sacrospinous ligament and anterior to the sacrotuberous ligament by which the nerve travels from the retro-sciatic space and into the ischiorectal fossa. If an impingement at the margin of the sacrospinous ligament is observed/appreciated, then the (anteriorly placed) inferior margin of the ligament can be notched as follows: the pudendal nerve is carefully moved and then held out of its normal position, and a No. 11 scalpel blade, scissors, or a Kerrison punch is used to notch the inferior aspect of the ligament. Some urological surgeons have advocated cutting the sacrospinous ligament or partially resecting the tip of the ischial spine—however, this may result in some sense of pelvic instability in some patients. It is usually sufficient to notch the ligament and/or the ischial spine to mobilize the pudendal nerve for patients with this location of entrapment.

"Magic-Angle" Approach for Decompression within the Proximal Alcock's Canal

This medial transgluteal approach also offers an excellent "magic angle" access along Alcock's canal in that the line of approach is parallel to the canal. The surgeon accomplishes a view of the course of the pudendal nerve as it progresses in its fascial sheath on the deep surface of the obturator internus muscle. However, this view is "end on" and "along the 'barrel' of the fascial sheath/nerve" from proximal to distal. This angle makes it possible to noninvasively access the canal to progressively dilate it. Reliance on careful, repeated electrodiagnostic guidance is helpful. The surgeon is therefore able to reach through the lesser sciatic notch and mobilize several centimeters of the post-spinous pudendal nerve course with progressive, careful openings of a long tonsil clamp.

Modified and More Inferior Approach

In patients with distal branch entrapments (e.g., isolated penile numbness), the incision is centered between the ischial spine and the ischial tuberosity; this approach takes the surgeon directly to the sacrotuberous ligament. Once the ligament is exposed, the pudendal nerve can be accessed distally along the course of Alcock's canal as well as along its proximal approach to the lesser sciatic notch. In patients with a dense adhesion of the pudendal nerve to the deep surface of the sacrotuberous ligament, it is possible to carry out a partial or complete section of the ligament to access the nerve, as some have advocated [11], but most entrapments can be released without sectioning of this major structural ligament. Hruby and colleagues [16] have also described direct anterior approaches for decompression of small distal sensory branches of the pudendal nerve.

Hemostasis and Placement of Anti-Adhesion Agents/Materials

Once the neuroplasty is complete, hemostasis is assured, and the area is irrigated extensively with gentamicin irrigation at body temperature (avoid bacitracin irrigation as it may inflame the nerves in patients with a TNF [tumor necrosis factor] autoimmune neuritis). Next, numerous small pieces (0.5–1 cm cut squares) of Seprafilm® are placed in plentiful amount and in many layers around all dissected nerve and muscle surfaces that are deep to the pre-piriformis fascia. The retractors are then removed, and hemostasis is again assured. The gluteal fascia is closed with interrupted sutures of 0-Vicryl.

Decompression of the Inferior Hypogastric (Impar) Ganglion for Treatment of Urogenital Pain and Dysfunction

Irritative and compressive syndromes affecting the inferior hypogastric (impar) ganglion are important considerations for a neurosurgeon. In a patient presenting with saddle area numbness as well as bowel/bladder retention or incontinence—immediate attention is drawn to the possibility of cauda equina syndrome. This is reasonable because early surgical intervention can avoid making a temporary situation into a serious permanent disability. However, if the lumbar imaging demonstrates no physical basis for any possibility of a cauda equina, the surgeon should do a physical examination of the sacrococcygeal joint (pain or aggravation of symptoms with pressure on the coccyx) and consider an MR neurography of the sacrococcygeal area.

Injection of the impar ganglion can be carried out by a lateral approach, which will allow for testing for relief of autonomic pain in the perineum and genitalia (Fig. 49.6) [12, 14, 36]. Use of steroids or hyaluronidase may help improve symptoms. Botulinum toxin injection has also been advocated for prolonged ganglion treatment [37–39]. Diagnostics and treatments directed at the impar ganglion should be considered when treatment directed at the pudendal nerve [14, 40] fails to affect the principal pain symptoms.

Filler [41] described a trans-coccygeal approach which allows for decompression and mobilization of the impar ganglion without acquiring the potential risks and complications of a coccygectomy. This was reported to be effective for treatment of a variety of impar ganglion symptoms, including incontinence, retention, sexual dysfunction, burning pain, and urethral symptoms [14].

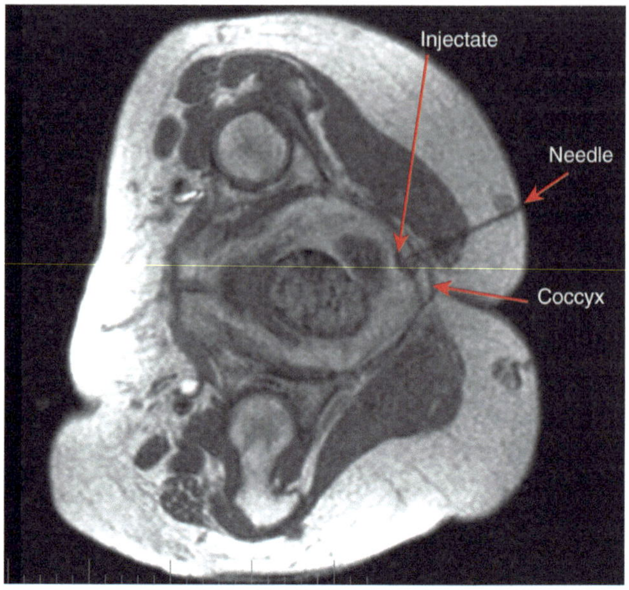

Fig. 49.6 Ganglion impar injection, open MRI-guided. Copyright Elsevier. Published with permission [36]

Surgical Method for Decompression of Ganglion Impar

- In detail, for impar ganglion syndromes with coccygeal pain or coccygeal fracture that cannot be expected to improve with treatment of the pudendal entrapment alone, good relief can be obtained with a modified partial coccygectomy. This procedure differs from older coccygectomy methods in that it preserves all of the attachments of the pelvic floor to the tip of the coccyx and does not call for any substantial mobilization or removal of most of the coccyx.
- A small midline incision—approximately 2 centimeters in length—is made that is centered over the mobile point of the coccyx relative to the stable inferior margin of the sacrum. This point can alternately be verified and identified radiologically, but a PA and lateral X-ray will most likely be required. The approach to the periosteum can be made with a Bovie coagulator, but the periosteum itself should be coagulated with a Malis and incised with a #15 or #11 scalpel blade.
- The periosteum of the coccyx is formally opened over the first coccygeal segment with a midline incision from the inferior margin of the last sacral segment to the superior margin of the second coccygeal segment. Sutures are passed through each of the left and the right incision margins so that the cut margins of the incised periosteum can be retracted to expose the central portion of the first coccygeal segment.
- Next, using a Midas Rex with a standard drill bit such as an MR8 3 mm bit or similar drill, a subtotal removal, pri-

marily of the first coccygeal segment only, is achieved. This can be completed with a one- or two-millimeter Kerrison punch, relying also on exploration with a small Karlin FA (forward angled) or BA (back angle) or Epstein curette. This is performed along with the removal of any anterior osteophytes at the sacrococcygeal joint and at the superior margin of the second coccygeal segment. Next, a 4–0 FA (forward-angled) cervical curette or similar instrument is used to mobilize the impar ganglion on the deep surface of the sacrococcygeal joint area.

- Following this, hemostasis is accomplished with bone wax and thrombin-soaked Gelfoam. Marcaine without epinephrine is then applied. It is then imperative to suture closed the periosteal incision and to fully and individually close all associated fascial layers with a full abundance of sutures. The skin is closed with both a subcutaneous interrupted layer of 3–0 Vicryl and a subcuticular continuous layer of 4–0 Vicryl. Nylon skin sutures placed as a series of horizontal mattress knots further assure the integrity of the closure at this low midline location. A layer of cyanoacrylate closure covered by steri-strips in multiple layers additionally secured with adhesive fluid such as Mastisol®. A small square sterile gauze is placed, covered with a small Tegaderm, and the edges of the Tegaderm are further secured with two-inch paper tape carefully trimmed to exclude the ano-rectal area.
- The integrity of the closure is especially critical. This is because the incision is invariably near the rectum and highly susceptible to inadvertent postoperative contamination by the patient. In addition, the natural anatomy of the buttock tends to pull the skin edges apart when a patient sits. It is not clear that a horizontal incision faces any less stress, but a careful closure as described will generally be completely effective.

Summary

Although many nerve specialists did not receive training in pudendal nerve surgery, this type of treatment is best carried out by a nerve specialist. The detailed approach provided in this chapter should be sufficient to allow surgeons to add this class of treatment to their repertoire. Patients with these conditions are often suffering severely, and outcomes are generally quite satisfactory. The techniques involved are consistent with somatic and autonomic nerve treatments elsewhere in the body and should become accessible once the particulars of the anatomy in the retro-sciatic space and the relevant adjacent anatomical area are understood and appreciated.

References

1. Darget R (1955) Treatment of pelvic pain by the enervation by gluteal route of the pudendal nerve. J Urol Medicale Chir 61(1–2):98–101. Le traitement des algies pelviennes par l'enervation par voie fessiere du nerf honteux
2. Turner ML, Marinoff SC (1991) Pudendal neuralgia. Am J Obstet Gynecol 165(4 Pt 2):1233–1236. https://doi.org/10.1016/s0002-9378(12)90733-4
3. Robert R, Prat-Pradal D, Labat JJ, Bensignor M, Raoul S, Rebai R et al (1998) Anatomic basis of chronic perineal pain: role of the pudendal nerve. Surg Radiol Anat 20(2):93–98. https://doi.org/10.1007/BF01628908
4. Antolak SJ Jr, Hough DM, Pawlina W, Spinner RJ (2002) Anatomical basis of chronic pelvic pain syndrome: the ischial spine and pudendal nerve entrapment. Med Hypotheses 59(3):349–353. https://doi.org/10.1016/s0306-9877(02)00218-9
5. Ramsden CE, McDaniel MC, Harmon RL, Renney KM, Faure A (2003) Pudendal nerve entrapment as source of intractable perineal pain. Am J Phys Med Rehabil 82(6):479–484
6. Benson JT, Griffis K (2005) Pudendal neuralgia, a severe pain syndrome. Am J Obstet Gynecol 192(5):1663–1668. https://doi.org/10.1016/j.ajog.2005.01.051
7. Popeney C, Ansell V, Renney K (2007) Pudendal entrapment as an etiology of chronic perineal pain: diagnosis and treatment. Neurourol Urodyn 26(6):820–827
8. Filler AG, Gilmer HS (2022) Chapter 278. Piriformis syndrome, obturator internus syndrome, pudendal nerve entrapment and other pelvic entrapments. In: Winn HR (ed) Youmans & Winn neurological surgery, 8th edn. Elsevier, Philadelphia, PA, pp 2151–2160
9. Mauillon J, Thoumas D, Leroi AM, Freger P, Michot F, Denis P (1999) Results of pudendal nerve neurolysis-transposition in twelve patients suffering from pudendal neuralgia. Dis Colon Rectum 42(2):186–192. https://doi.org/10.1007/BF02237125
10. Beco J, Climov D, Bex M (2004) Pudendal nerve decompression in perineology: a case series. BMC Surg 4:15. https://doi.org/10.1186/1471-2482-4-15
11. Robert R, Labat JJ, Bensignor M, Glemain P, Deschamps C, Raoul S et al (2005) Decompression and transposition of the pudendal nerve in pudendal neuralgia: a randomized controlled trial and long-term evaluation. Eur Urol 47(3):403–408. https://doi.org/10.1016/j.eururo.2004.09.003
12. Filler AG (2008) Diagnosis and management of pudendal nerve entrapment syndromes: impact of MR Neurography and open MR-guided injections. Neurosurg Q 18(1):1–6
13. Filler AG (2022) Chapter 275. Imaging for peripheral nerve disorders. In: Winn HR (ed) Youmans & Winn neurological surgery, 8th edn. Elsevier, Philadelphia, PA, pp 2114–2127
14. Filler AG (2009) Diagnosis and treatment of pudendal nerve entrapment syndrome subtypes: imaging, injections, and minimal access surgery. Neurosurg Focus 26(2):E9. https://doi.org/10.3171/FOC.2009.26.2.E9
15. Shafik A (1994) Pudendal canal decompression in the treatment of erectile dysfunction. Arch Androl 32(2):141–149. https://doi.org/10.3109/01485019508987835
16. Hruby S, Ebmer J, Dellon AL, Aszmann OC (2005) Anatomy of pudendal nerve at urogenital diaphragm--new critical site for nerve entrapment. Urology 66(5):949–952. https://doi.org/10.1016/j.urology.2005.05.032
17. Loukas M, Louis RG Jr, Hallner B, Gupta AA, White D (2006) Anatomical and surgical considerations of the sacrotuberous ligament and its relevance in pudendal nerve entrapment syndrome. Surg Radiol Anat 28(2):163–169. https://doi.org/10.1007/s00276-006-0082-3. Epub 2006 Feb 7

18. Mahakkanukrauh P, Surin P, Vaidhayakarn P (2005) Anatomical study of the pudendal nerve adjacent to the sacrospinous ligament. Clin Anat 18(3):200–205. https://doi.org/10.1002/ca.20084
19. Naja MZ, Al-Tannir MA, Maaliki H, El-Rajab M, Ziade MF, Zeidan A (2006) Nerve-stimulator-guided repeated pudendal nerve block for treatment of pudendal neuralgia. Eur J Anaesthesiol 23(5):442–444. https://doi.org/10.1017/S026502150623028X
20. Abdi S, Shenouda P, Patel N, Saini B, Bharat Y, Calvillo O (2004) A novel technique for pudendal nerve block. Pain Physician 7(3):319–322
21. Choi SS, Lee PB, Kim YC, Kim HJ, Lee SC (2006) C-arm-guided pudendal nerve block: a new technique. Int J Clin Pract 60(5):553–556. https://doi.org/10.1111/j.1742-1241.2006.00836.x
22. Thoumas D, Leroi AM, Mauillon J, Muller JM, Benozio M, Denis P et al (1999) Pudendal neuralgia: CT-guided pudendal nerve block technique. Abdom Imaging 24(3):309–312. https://doi.org/10.1007/s002619900503
23. Calvillo O, Skaribas IM, Rockett C (2000) Computed tomography-guided pudendal nerve block. A new diagnostic approach to long-term anoperineal pain: a report of two cases. Reg Anesth Pain Med 25(4):420–423. https://doi.org/10.1053/rapm.2000.7620
24. Hough DM, Wittenberg KH, Pawlina W, Maus TP, King BF, Vrtiska TJ et al (2003) Chronic perineal pain caused by pudendal nerve entrapment: anatomy and CT-guided perineural injection technique. AJR Am J Roentgenol 181(2):561–567. https://doi.org/10.2214/ajr.181.2.1810561
25. Amarenco G, Kerdraon J (1999) Pudendal nerve terminal sensitive latency: technique and normal values. J Urol 161(1):103–106
26. Robert R, Labat JJ, Riant T, Khalfallah M, Hamel O (2007) Neurosurgical treatment of perineal neuralgias. Adv Tech Stand Neurosurg 32:41–59. https://doi.org/10.1007/978-3-211-47423-5_3
27. Filler AG, Kliot M, Howe FA, Hayes CE, Saunders DE, Goodkin R et al (1996) Application of magnetic resonance neurography in the evaluation of patients with peripheral nerve pathology. J Neurosurg 85(2):299–309. https://doi.org/10.3171/jns.1996.85.2.0299
28. Filler AG, Maravilla KR, Tsuruda JS (2004) MR neurography and muscle MR imaging for image diagnosis of disorders affecting the peripheral nerves and musculature. Neurol Clin 22(3):643–682., vi-vii. https://doi.org/10.1016/j.ncl.2004.03.005
29. Filler AG, Howe FA, Hayes CE, Kliot M, Winn HR, Bell BA et al (1993) Magnetic resonance neurography. Lancet 341(8846):659–661. https://doi.org/10.1016/0140-6736(93)90422-d
30. Filler AG, Haynes J, Jordan SE, Prager J, Villablanca JP, Farahani K et al (2005) Sciatica of nondisc origin and piriformis syndrome: diagnosis by magnetic resonance neurography and interventional magnetic resonance imaging with outcome study of resulting treatment. J Neurosurg Spine 2(2):99–115. https://doi.org/10.3171/spi.2005.2.2.0099
31. Filler AG (2008) Piriformis and related entrapment syndromes: diagnosis & management. Neurosurgical Clinics of North America 19:609–622, vii. https://doi.org/10.1016/j.nec.2008.07.029
32. McAllister RK, Carpentier BW, Malkuch G (2004) Sacral postherpetic neuralgia and successful treatment using a paramedial approach to the ganglion impar. Anesthesiology 101(6):1472–1474. https://doi.org/10.1097/00000542-200412000-00032
33. Munir MA, Zhang J, Ahmad M (2004) A modified needle-inside-needle technique for the ganglion impar block. Can J Anaesth Nov 51(9):915–917. https://doi.org/10.1007/BF03018890
34. Toshniwal GR, Dureja GP, Prashanth SM (2007) Transsacrococcygeal approach to ganglion impar block for management of chronic perineal pain: a prospective observational study. Pain Physician 10(5):661–666
35. Rey D, Oderda M (2015) The first case of robotic pudendal nerve decompression in pudendal nerve entrapment syndrome. J Laparoendosc Adv Surg Tech A Apr 25(4):319–322. https://doi.org/10.1089/lap.2014.0013
36. Filler AG (2022) Peripheral nerve treatments for central and autonomic disorders. In: Winn HR (ed) Youmans & Winn neurological surgery, 8th edn. Elsevier, Philadelphia, PA, pp 2236–2241. (chapter 289)
37. Naumann M, So Y, Argoff CE, Childers MK, Dykstra DD, Gronseth GS et al (2008) Assessment: botulinum neurotoxin in the treatment of autonomic disorders and pain (an evidence-based review): report of the Therapeutics and Technology Assessment Subcommittee of the American Academy of Neurology. Neurology 70(19):1707–1714. https://doi.org/10.1212/01.wnl.0000311390.87642.d8
38. Jabbari B (2008) Botulinum neurotoxins in the treatment of refractory pain. Nat Clin Pract Neurol 4(12):676–685. https://doi.org/10.1038/ncpneuro0948
39. Lim SJ, Park HJ, Lee SH, Moon DE (2010) Ganglion impar block with botulinum toxin type a for chronic perineal pain—A case report. Korean J Pain 23(1):65–69. https://doi.org/10.3344/kjp.2010.23.1.65
40. Dellon AL, Coady D, Harris D (2015) Pelvic pain of pudendal nerve origin: surgical outcomes and learning curve lessons. J Reconstr Microsurg 31(4):283–290. https://doi.org/10.1055/s-0034-1396896
41. Filler AG (2019) Chapter 11. Piriformis syndrome and other nerve entrapments of the posterior pelvis. In: Wilson TJ, Yang LJ-S (eds) Peripheral nerve surgery (neurosurgery by example). Oxford University Press, New York, NY, pp 99–106

Abdominal Cutaneous Nerve Entrapment Syndrome (ACNES)

50

Armin Edalatpour, Allison J. Seitz, Brian H. Gander, and Jacqueline S. Israel

Surgical Anatomy

The rectus abdominis muscle (RA) is innervated by eight separate nerves arising from the 5th to 12th thoracic spinal levels. These somatic nerves each have a dorsal branch innervating the back musculature, a lateral branch, and a ventral branch that supply the abdominal wall (Fig. 50.1).

Abdominal wall skin receives innervation from the cutaneous branches of the six lowest intercostal nerves and sub-

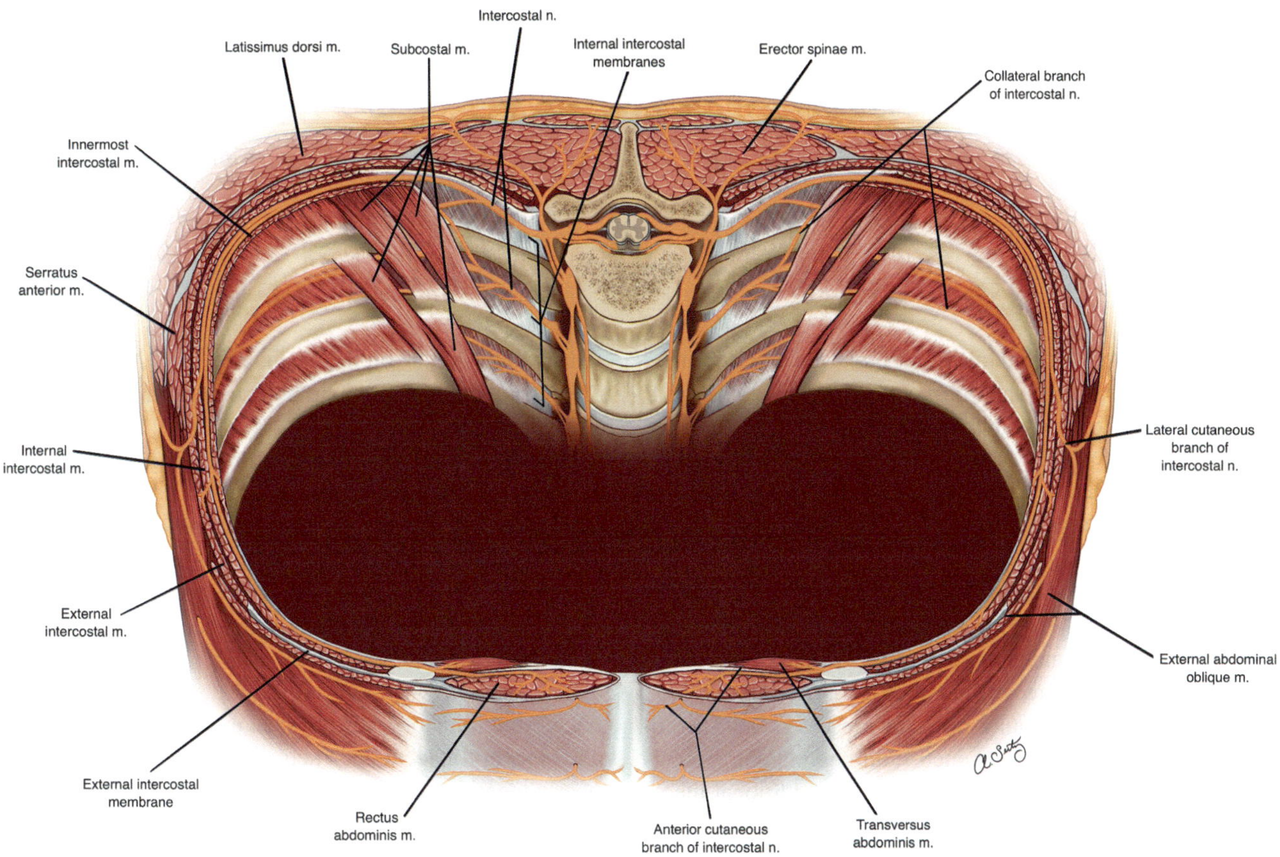

Fig. 50.1 Axial cut of the abdominal wall. The anterior cutaneous branch of the intercostal nerve traverses the rectus abdominis muscle and the anterior rectus sheath

Supplementary Information The online version contains supplementary material available at https://doi.org/10.1007/978-3-031-73931-6_50.

A. Edalatpour · A. J. Seitz · B. H. Gander · J. S. Israel (✉)
Division of Plastic and Reconstructive Surgery, Department of Surgery, University of Wisconsin Hospitals and Clinics, Madison, WI, USA
e-mail: edalatpour@surgery.wisc.edu; ASeitz2@uwhealth.org; gander@surgery.wisc.edu; israel@surgery.wisc.edu

A. S. Hanna (ed.), *Nerves: Anatomy, Exposures, and Techniques*, https://doi.org/10.1007/978-3-031-73931-6_50

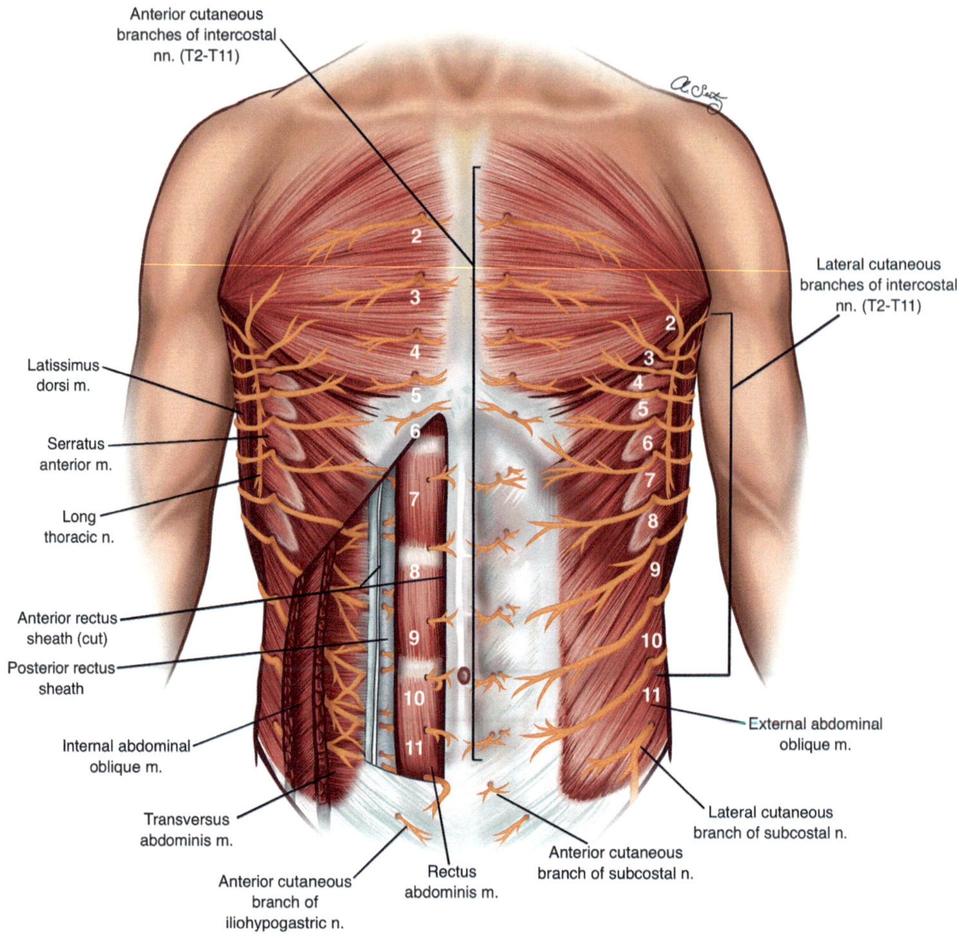

Fig. 50.2 Anatomy of the anterior abdominal wall demonstrating the thoraco-abdominal intercostal nerves. Note the lateral and anterior cutaneous branches relative to the abdominal wall muscles

costal nerve (7th to 12th thoracic nerves). The anterior ones traverse the RA and the anterior rectus fascia (Fig. 50.2) and are subject to entrapment in this location.

Pathophysiology

While there is limited data regarding exact pathophysiology, the symptoms experienced in ACNES are felt to be attributable to entrapment and compression of the anterior cutaneous branch of the intercostal nerve as it traverses the RA or its fascia [1]. A debilitating cycle of muscle spasm, nerve kinking, swelling, and worsened compression/entrapment can result in chronic, debilitating pain [1]. Additional theorized causes of ACNES include focal neuroma formation related to laparoscopic port sites or penetrating trauma, stretch due to pregnancy, and infections including herpes zoster [1, 2].

Diagnostic Approach

The Carnett test is a previously validated examination maneuver that can be used to assess abdominal wall pain [3]:

- Lay patient supine on the exam table.
- Identify the point of maximal tenderness and apply firm, constant pressure.
- Ask patient to cross arms and raise their head, shoulder, and chest off the table to contract the abdominal muscle (may also raise both legs off the exam table as alternative). Resultant reproduced and/or worsening pain is considered a positive test, suggesting an abdominal wall etiology. A negative test may indicate intra-abdominal pathology [3].

A thorough history and physical examination, combined with injection of local anesthetic and ultrasonography, can properly identify ACNES. Injection of local anesthetic at the trigger point (e.g., 3–5 cc of 1% lidocaine) can have two main benefits. First, pain relief after injection can rule out other causes, including visceral sources of pain. Second, up to 20% of patients may experience long-term pain relief from local injection [1]. Ultrasonography can detect a mass, abscess, hematoma, tissue edema, hernia, or other etiologies at the trigger point [4]. Lastly, if the cause of abdominal pain is unclear or an intra-abdominal etiology is expected, an abdominal computerized tomography (CT) scan should be considered.

Nonoperative Treatment

Oral nonsteroidal anti-inflammatory drugs, muscle relaxants, and antispasmodics can be helpful in some patients [4]. Trigger point injection with local anesthesia (lidocaine or bupivacaine), corticosteroids, and/or onabotulinumtoxinA (Botox) can be both diagnostic and therapeutic in certain patient populations [1, 4]. While there is very little data available regarding various treatment options, providers should consider additional modalities, including activity modification, alternative nonrestrictive clothing, occupational or physical therapy, and/or vibration/desensitization.

Surgical Technique

For patients who have exhausted nonoperative treatment, surgical intervention can be beneficial. The terminal branches of the affected intercostal nerves can be decompressed and/or removed at the level of the anterior rectus sheath.

1. A transverse incision is designed, directly over the trigger point at the lateral anterior abdominal wall. The incision is made through the skin, subcutaneous tissue, and Scarpa's fascia.
2. The anterior rectus abdominis fascia (anterior rectus sheath) and the neurovascular bundle(s) are identified (Fig. 50.3).

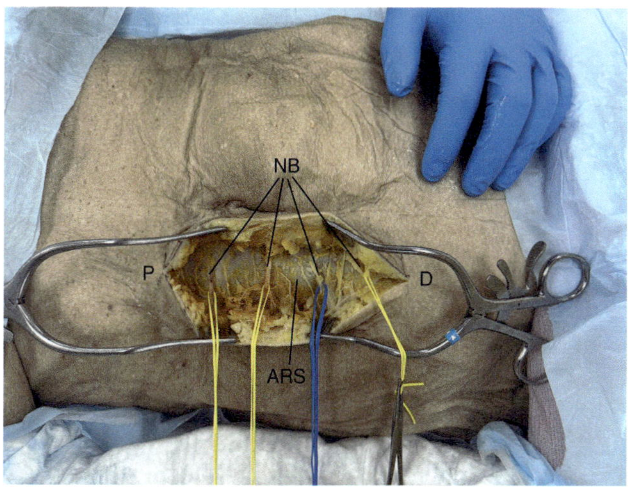

Fig. 50.3 A large longitudinal incision demonstrates the anatomy of multiple intercostal nerves. When performing surgical release, a smaller, transverse incision can be used. The dissection is performed through skin, subcutaneous tissue, and Scarpa's fascia down to the anterior rectus sheath (*ARS*). The neurovascular bundles (*NB*) are then dissected and released circumferentially at the fascial foramen. A segment of nerve can be excised (neurectomy) and the adjacent vessels cauterized. *P* proximal, *D* distal

3. The oval-shaped neurovascular opening at the level of the anterior rectus abdominis fascia is identified and enlarged.
4. The neurovascular bundle is released/decompressed circumferentially at its fascial foramen.
5. Neurectomy can be performed, excising a segment of nerve. The adjacent vessels may be cauterized using bipolar cautery.
6. Following neurectomy and cauterization of the vessels, the neurovascular bundle is allowed to retract through the RA.
7. The above steps can be repeated for the nerves above and/or below the trigger point.

Complications/Sequelae

1. Persistent, worsened, and/or recurrent symptoms.
2. Wound dehiscence/delayed wound healing and/or infection.
3. Seroma.
4. Hematoma.
5. Paresthesia of overlying skin.
6. Neuroma formation at the site of nerve ligation/cauterization.

References

1. Scheltinga MR, Roumen RM (2018) Anterior cutaneous nerve entrapment syndrome (ACNES). Hernia 22(3):507–516. Epub 2017 Dec 21. https://doi.org/10.1007/s10029-017-1710-z
2. Boelens OB, Scheltinga MR, Houterman S, Roumen RM (2011) Management of anterior cutaneous nerve entrapment syndrome in a cohort of 139 patients. Ann Surg 254(6):1054–1058. https://doi.org/10.1097/SLA.0b013e31822d78b8
3. Carnett J (1926) Intercostal neuralgia as a cause of abdominal pain and tenderness. Surg Gynecol Obstet 42:625–632
4. Shian B, Larson ST (2018) Abdominal wall pain: clinical evaluation, differential diagnosis, and treatment. Am Fam Physician 98:429–436

Nerve Decompressions for Migraine

51

Pradeep K. Attaluri, Shady Elmaraghi, Robert E. George, Ellen C. Shaffrey, and Ahmed M. Afifi

Indications

Patients with chronic migraines and refractory headaches require a multidisciplinary team to elucidate a proper diagnosis and formulate a comprehensive treatment plan. Accurate diagnosis of migraine headaches relies on patient history and physical examination. In many cases, the patients can point to and describe the originating location of their symptoms at one of the sensory nerves in the head and neck, which is the first step in determining if they are indeed a candidate for nerve decompression. A physical examination can support the diagnosis if triggering their headache pattern results from pressure at the known anatomical nerve sites. Patients can have various trigger sites, including occipital, frontal, and temporal areas.

Conservative therapies must be exhausted before becoming a surgical candidate. Conservative treatments for acute symptom management include over-the-counter analgesics, prescription triptans, ergots, and calcitonin gene-related peptide (CGRP) antagonists [1, 2]. Preventative therapies include serotonin and norepinephrine reuptake inhibitors (SNRIs), tricyclic antidepressants (TCAs), and anticonvulsant medications [2]. Radiofrequency ablation is another technique pain management specialists use to help alleviate migraine attacks. By the time they are referred to a surgeon for management, the use of a local anesthetic can aid in the diagnosis during an active migraine attack, as patients should feel relief within 5–10 min. The use of botulinum toxin can also assist in diagnosing muscular trigger sites. However, the effects of botulinum toxin can take up to 1 week to be perceived, and negative responses must be interpreted with caution [2]. Hand-held doppler can identify vascular triggers that can be contributing to migraine pathology.

Supplementary Information The online version contains supplementary material available at https://doi.org/10.1007/978-3-031-73931-6_51.

P. K. Attaluri · E. C. Shaffrey
Division of Plastic Surgery, Department of Surgery, University of Wisconsin-Madison, Madison, WI, USA
e-mail: pattaluri@uwhealth.org; shaffrey@wisc.edu

S. Elmaraghi
Department of Plastic Surgery, Vanderbilt Health, Nashville, TN, USA
e-mail: shady.elmaraghi@outlook.com

R. E. George · A. M. Afifi (✉)
Division of Plastic and Reconstructive Surgery, Department of Surgery, University of Wisconsin-Madison, Madison, WI, USA
e-mail: rgeorge@uwhealth.org; afifi@surgery.wisc.edu

Surgical Anatomy

The greater occipital nerve (GON) requires adequate nerve decompression at multiple locations (Fig. 51.1). At its most proximal location, point 1 is on average 77 mm inferior to occipital protuberance (OP) and 20 mm lateral to the midline, where the GON is being compressed by the musculofascial tissue surrounding the obliquus capitis inferior muscle [1]. Points 2 and 3 represent the entry and exit of the nerve into the semispinalis capitis. These are 59 mm inferior and midline, and 30 mm inferior and 17 mm lateral to the OP, respectively [1]. Points 4 and 5 are the entry and exit from the trapezius, and the nerve is located 24 mm inferior to the OP and 21 mm lateral to the midline and 4 mm inferior to the OP and 37 mm lateral to the midline, respectively [1]. Point 6 is the potential compression of the GON by the occipital artery along its course [1]. Clinically, many surgeons recognize the nerve crossing over the nuchal ridge as an important compression point, as it coincides with points 5 and 6. There is usually a lymph node at this location, and a tight fascial sheath covers the nerve.

The lesser occipital nerve (LON) location is not as anatomically consistent but is generally found at the lateral border of the sternocleidomastoid (SCM) muscle, a few centimeters below the skull base. As it travels cephalad, it becomes more superficial and courses anteriorly. There is significant variation in the anatomy of this nerve, and it can be quite challenging to find [4].

A. S. Hanna (ed.), *Nerves: Anatomy, Exposures, and Techniques*, https://doi.org/10.1007/978-3-031-73931-6_51

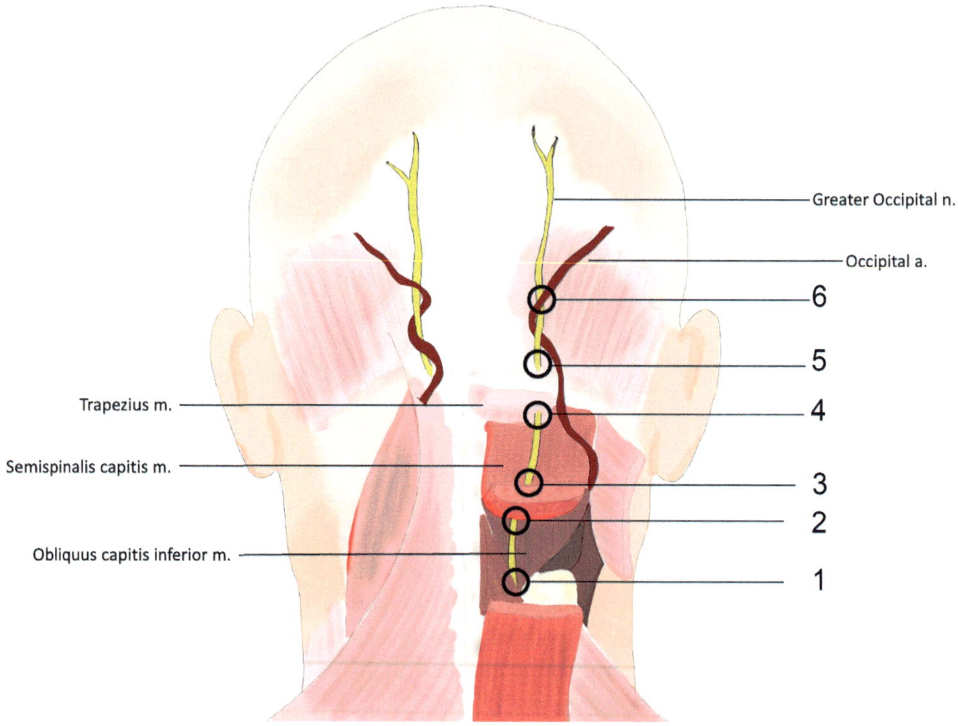

Fig. 51.1 Six anatomical compression points of the greater occipital nerve for occipital migraines. (1) Obliquus capitis inferior, (2 and 3) entry and exit semispinalis capitis, (4 and 5) entry and exit trapezius, and (6) crossing of the occipital artery

The third occipital nerve (TON) branches from the posterior division of the third cervical nerve. It can be found approximately 3 mm lateral to the occipital protuberance. Moreover, it pierces the trapezius and ultimately courses to the skin in the medial occipital area. Similar to the lesser occipital nerve, there are anatomical variations [4].

The supraorbital nerve (SON) has multiple points of compression, including a narrow bony supraorbital foramen, a tight supraorbital notch, fascial bands, an adjacent supraorbital artery, or the corrugator muscles.

The supratrochlear nerve (STN) has three well-known compression points: the nerve entrance into the brow through the frontal notch or foramen, the entrance of the nerve through the corrugator supercilii, and the exit of the nerve from the corrugator.

The auriculotemporal nerve (ATN) is a branch of the third division of the trigeminal nerve (V3) that has the potential to be compressed within the soft tissue of the temple by the superficial temporal artery.

The zygomaticotemporal nerve (ZTN), a terminal branch of the trigeminal nerve's second division (V2), has multiple possible compression points as it traverses through deep and superficial structures. Bony compression points include the zygomatic bone foramen, which is 17 mm lateral and 6 mm cephalad to the lateral orbital commissure. The muscular compression points include various locations within the temporalis muscle due to branching of the ZTN. The fascial compression point consists of the deep temporal fascia. Lastly, the vascular compression point includes the superficial temporal artery.

Surgical Technique

GON and LON Decompression

At our institution, we use a single modified transverse incision to capture both the GON and LON and utilize the addition of fat flaps to decompress the nerves further.

1. The patient is placed in a prone position with the arms tucked at the side and adequate padding to prevent pressure injuries.
2. The incision is placed 2.5 cm caudal to the external occipital protuberance and extends to the posterior edge of the SCM to capture the LON (Fig. 51.2). In bilateral cases, the incision will span the length of the distance between the posterior edges of the bilateral SCM.
3. Using a 15-blade, make the skin incision and elevate skin flaps in a cephalad and caudad direction in a plane just deep to the hair follicles. The depth is important to leave the fat intact over the trapezius fascia (Fig. 51.3).
4. This deep fat will be raised as a medially based vascularized flap off the trapezius fascia in a lateral to medial direction, stopping 1 cm lateral to the midline (Fig. 51.4). The flap usually measures 4 cm in length and 2 cm in

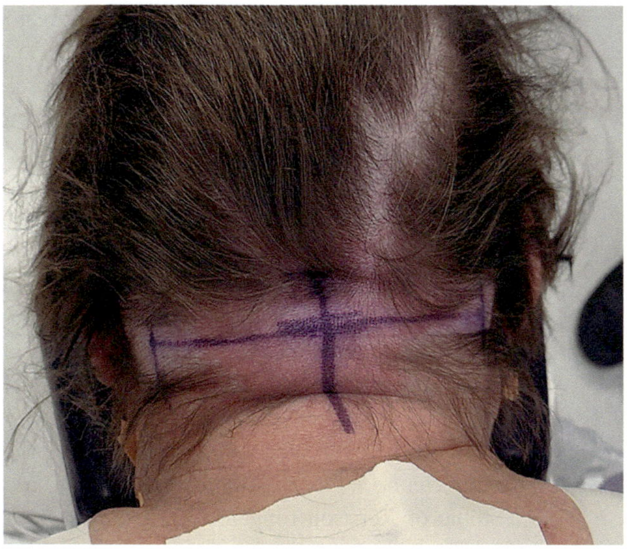

Fig. 51.2 Incision placement 2.5 cm caudal to the external occipital protuberance

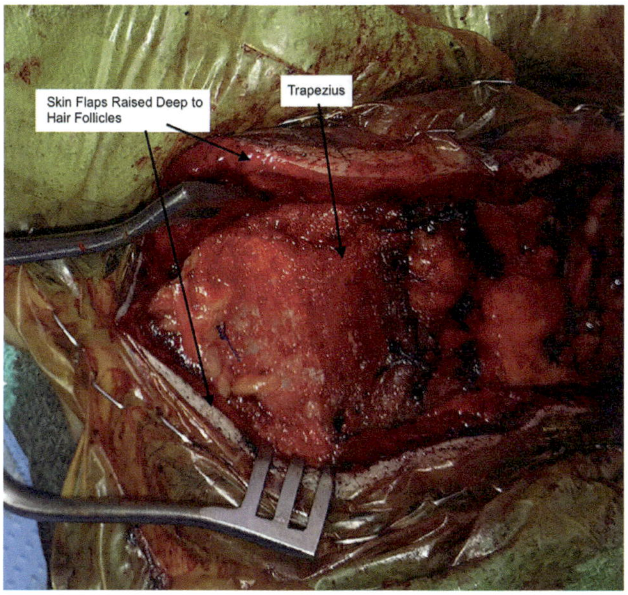

Fig. 51.3 Elevate skin flaps in a plane just deep to the hair follicles in order to leave the fat intact over the trapezius fascia

width. Leave the fat flap attached to the deeper tissues over the nuchal ligament.

5. Then, divide the trapezius fascia and muscle with a vertical incision just lateral to the base of the flap. At this point, the GON should be identified. If the third occipital nerve is present, this can either be transected or decompressed.
6. The GON is then followed proximally through the trapezius (obliquely oriented fibers) to the semispinalis muscle (vertically oriented fibers).

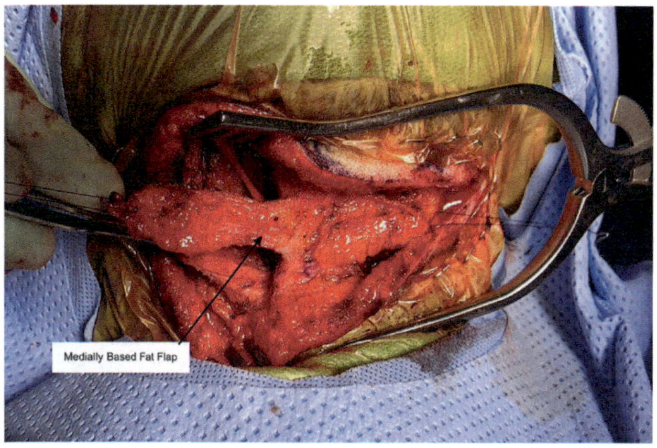

Fig. 51.4 Deep fat will be raised as a medially based vascularized flap off the trapezius fascia in a lateral to medial direction, stopping 1 cm lateral to the midline

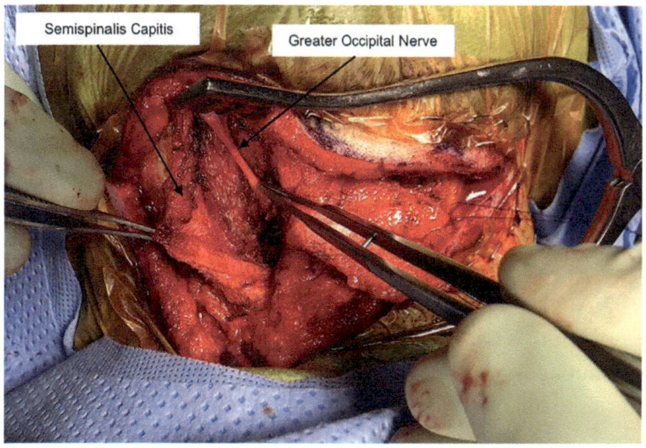

Fig. 51.5 A rectangular cuff of semispinalis capitis muscle between the median raphe and nerve can be removed along with a separate small segment lateral to the nerve

   (a) A rectangular cuff of semispinalis muscle between the median raphe and nerve can be removed along with a separate small segment lateral to the nerve (Fig. 51.5).

7. Fascial bands and the obliquus capitis at the base of the nerve are then decompressed.
8. Then, a small cuff of trapezial fascia and muscle is removed and incised at the entrance to the trapezial tunnel. At this point, the nerve is followed distally as it moves into a subcutaneous position (Fig. 51.6).
9. If the occipital artery or veins are compressing the nerve, cauterization or ligation of the vessels is performed.
10. The LON is identified at the posterior border of the SCM, roughly 2.5 cm caudal to the nuchal ridge and just deep to the deep fascia of the muscle.
11. At this point, decompression or neurectomy can be performed on the LON.

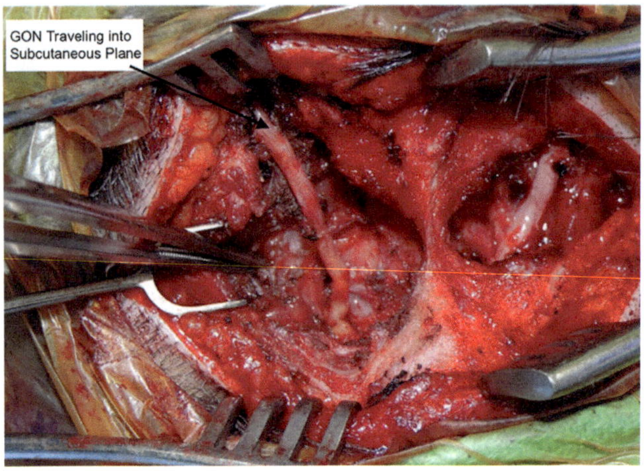

Fig. 51.6 A small cuff of trapezial fascia and muscle is removed and incised at the entrance to the trapezial tunnel. At this point, the nerve is followed distally as it moves into a subcutaneous position

12. The fat flaps that were preserved at the beginning of the case are now used to wrap the GON. The flap is passed deep, then lateral, and finally superficial to the nerve, making sure to use the distal edge of the flap to cover the nerve as it crosses the nuchal ridge.
    (a) There are modifications that can be made to the fat flaps that can be used to cover the nerve at various compression points.
13. After meticulous hemostasis is obtained, placement of a drain is decided upon. Close the wound with 3–0 monocryl in the deep dermal layer and a 4–0 monocryl for subcuticular closure.

It should be noted that the GON surgery can also be done through a vertical midline incision. The steps of nerve decompression are very similar, except that the fat flap would be based on the skin and is oriented vertically.

SON and STN Decompression

Regarding frontal trigger sites, a standard upper eyelid blepharoplasty incision is the most common approach.

1. The patient is placed in a supine position with the arms tucked at the side and adequate padding to prevent pressure or nerve-related injuries.
2. An upper eyelid blepharoplasty incision is designed and made using a 15 blade. Next, using a Colorado tip bovie, the exposure is deepened to a sub-orbicularis plane.
3. Dissection is carried out in a cephalad direction in the plane just below the orbicularis muscle (superficial to the orbital septum) towards the orbital rim. The orbicularis retaining ligament is released, exposing the corrugator and depressor muscles.
4. At this point, we prefer to remove the corrugator muscle and fill the void at the conclusion of the case using abdominal fat.
5. We should identify the SON and STN at this level and follow the nerves proximally and distally.
    (a) If the supraorbital or supratrochlear arteries are found to be compressing the nerves, these vessels can be ligated or coagulated using cautery.
    (b) If a supraorbital notch or frontal notch with fascial bands is identified, these bands can be released sharply to decompress the nerves.
    (c) If a supraorbital or frontal foramen are found, these foramina can be safely decompressed using a 2 mm osteotome or Kerrison rongeur to remove the compressive bony structure.
6. It is crucial to ensure meticulous hemostasis, and closure can be obtained using a single layer 5–0 fast absorbing gut suture to close the upper blepharoplasty incision.

ATN and ZTN Decompression

1. The patient is placed in a supine position with the arms tucked at the side and adequate padding to prevent pressure or nerve-related injuries.
2. When decompressing the auriculotemporal nerve:
    (a) Make a small 1.5 cm incision in the pre-auricular area around the point of maximum pain. Using tenotomy scissors, perform a blunt dissection through the subcutaneous tissues and identify the point of intersection for the superficial temporal artery and the auriculotemporal nerve. This artery and nerve complex can be ligated proximally and distally to the area of the nerve-artery intersection.
3. When decompressing the zygomaticotemporal nerve:
    (a) Start by making a 3 cm incision that is 8–10 mm behind the temporal hairline.
    (b) Using blunt dissection, continue the dissection deep to the deep temporal fascia.
    (c) Open the inferior temporal septum to expose the inferior temporal compartment that contains the ZTN, sentinel vessels, and temporal branch of the facial nerve.
        (i) If the patient described pre-operative pulsating pain, the sentinel vein can be ligated.
    (d) Widen the exit of the ZTN through the temporal muscle and fascia, ensuring full release of any constricting bands.

Complications

Larger caliber nerves such as the GON, STN, and SON will primarily undergo decompression as there is higher morbidity associated with neurectomy. Smaller nerves such as the LON, ATN, and ZTN can safely be divided with minimal morbidity. During the pre-operative visit, there must be a thorough discussion with the patient about strategies for decompression vs. neurectomy and subsequent plans for the transected nerve endings to prevent neuroma formation [3]. Other complications include, but are not limited to, bleeding, hematoma, seroma, infection, dehiscence, and neuroma formation.

References

1. Afifi AM, Carbullido MK, Israel JS, Sanchez RJ, Albano NJ (2019) Alternative approach for occipital headache surgery: the use of a transverse incision and "W" flaps. Plast Reconstr Surg Glob Open 7(4):e2176. https://doi.org/10.1097/GOX.0000000000002176. eCollection 2019 Apr
2. Hatef DA, Gutowski KA, Culbertson GR, Zielinski M, Manahan MA (2020) A comprehensive review of surgical treatment of migraine surgery safety and efficacy. Plast Reconstr Surg 146(2):187e–195e. https://doi.org/10.1097/PRS.0000000000007020
3. Afifi AM, Peled ZM, Janis JE (2020) Surgical management of chronic headaches and migraines. Springer, Switzerland
4. Lee M, Lineberry K, Reed D, Guyuron B (2013) The role of the third occipital nerve in surgical treatment of occipital migraine headaches. J Plast Reconstr Aesthet Surg 66(10):1335–1339. https://doi.org/10.1016/j.bjps.2013.05.023. Epub 2013 Jun 2

Nerve Tumors: Benign, Rare, and Malignant

52

Nora F. Dengler, Maria T. Pedro, Allison M. Grayev, and Amgad S. Hanna

Types

Most nerve tumors are benign. Most of them originate from the nerve sheath, such as schwannomas and neurofibromas. They either occur sporadically or as part of neurofibromatosis (NF) 1 or 2, or schwannomatosis, sometimes called NF3 (Table 52.1) [1]. More rare benign nerve tumors include perineuriomas, lipomas, aggressive fibrosis (desmoid tumors), paragangliomas, and hemangiomas. Malignant peripheral nerve sheath tumors (MPNST) are rare but more common in NF1, especially in patients with high tumor loads and plexiform neurofibromas. Intermediate stages such as ANNUBPS are sometimes difficult to diagnose and may need a surgical strategy that differs from that in MPNST [2]. Metastatic tumors include metastatic breast cancer to the brachial plexus, perineural spread of prostate cancer, and lymphoma. The recognition of a nerve tumor and knowledge of different tumor types are relevant to prevent misdiagnosis and mistreatment.

Supplementary Information The online version contains supplementary material available at https://doi.org/10.1007/978-3-031-73931-6_52.

N. F. Dengler
Fakultät für Gesundheitswissenschaften Brandenburg, Medizinische Hochschule Brandenburg Theodor Fontane, Bad Saarow Klinik für Neurochirurgie, HELIOS Klinik Bad Saarow Charité – Universitaetsmedizin, Berlin, Germany
e-mail: nora.dengler@charite.de

M. T. Pedro
Sektion Periphere Nerven, Klinik für Neurochirurgie, Universitaetsklinik Ulm am Bezirkskrankenhaus, Günzburg, Germany
e-mail: maria-teresa.pedro@uni-ulm.de

A. M. Grayev
Department of Radiology, University of Wisconsin School of Medicine and Public Health, Madison, WI, USA
e-mail: grayev@wisc.edu

A. S. Hanna (✉)
Department of Neurosurgery, University of Wisconsin School of Medicine and Public Health, Madison, WI, USA

A. S. Hanna (ed.), *Nerves: Anatomy, Exposures, and Techniques*, https://doi.org/10.1007/978-3-031-73931-6_52

Table 52.1 Neurogenetic syndromes associated with nerve tumors

Syndrome, incidence, genetics	Criteria
Neurofibromatosis type 1 (*von Recklinghausen*) 1:3000 NF1 gene (chromosome 17)	Two or more out of the following: • ≥6 café au lait patches of the skin • ≥2 neurofibroma or one plexiform neurofibroma • Axillary or inguinal freckling • ≥2 iris hamartoma (Lisch nodules) • Optic nerve glioma • Bony dysplasia or pseudarthrosis • First-degree relative with NF1 [3, 4]
Neurofibromatosis type 2 (*NF2-associated schwannomatosis*) 1:25,000 NF2 gene (chromosome 22)	One out of the following: • Bilateral vestibular schwannomas • Identical NF2 gene pathogenic variant in two anatomically different NF2-related tumors (schwannoma, meningioma, and/or ependymoma) (Mosaic NF2 <50% allele variants in a blood sample) or Presence of two major or one major and two minor criteria *Major criteria* • Unilateral vestibular schwannoma • First-grade relative with NF2-associated schwannomatosis • ≥2 meningioma • NF2 pathogenic variant in non-affected tissue (e.g., blood) *Minor criteria* • Ependymoma, one meningioma, or non-vestibular schwannoma • Juvenile subcapsular or cortical cataract, or retinal hamartoma [5]
Schwannomatosis 1:69,000 Pathogenic variants of SMARCB1 or LZTR1 gene	One out of the following: • >1 schwannoma or hybrid tumor and a SMARCB1 (or LZTR1) pathogenic variant in non-affected tissue (e.g., blood) • Presence of the same SMARCB1 or LZTR1 pathogenic variant in two schwannomas or hybrid tumors [5]

Imaging

MRI (≥3T) and high-resolution nerve ultrasound (HNUS) can be used as both allow for anatomic localization of nerve tumors and may suggest a tumor type [6]. For deep-seated tumors, for example, in the retroperitoneum, MRI is advantageous, but in superficial locations, HNUS has the advantage of easy and fast availability. The differentiation between benign nerve tumors, ANNUBP, and MPNST by imaging alone is challenging. Morphological criteria that are indicative of malignancy include invasiveness, ill-defined margins, tumor heterogeneity, and large tumor size. MRI ADC (apparent diffusion coefficient) and F18-FDG-PET may help to quantitatively assess tumor metabolism to guide in differentiating tumor entities, especially in patients with NF1 [7]. MR tractography can be used to define normal tracts from tumor.

Treatment Strategy

1. Surgery for benign tumors should aim at preserving function. Whenever possible, the parent nerve should be preserved, and only the fascicle(s) harboring the tumor are sacrificed (described below). Small cutaneous nerves can be sacrificed, especially with neurofibromas.
2. In neurofibromatosis or schwannomatosis, only symptomatic or fast-growing tumors need resection.
3. Dumbbell tumors may require a combined intradural/extradural procedure. The need for spine stabilization depends on the extent of bony resection and the level of the spine.
4. Surgery for MPNST should aim at preserving life. Function can be sacrificed to obtain an oncological resection with negative margins. It requires a team approach with an oncologic surgeon, medical oncologist, radiation oncologist, and a rehabilitation team.
5. Recently, MEK inhibitors (selumetinib) showed reduction in size of inoperable plexiform neurofibromas.

Technique of Removal of a Benign Nerve Sheath Tumor [1]

1. Expose the nerve harboring the tumor based on clinical (Fig. 52.1) and imaging (Fig. 52.2) localization. Intraoperative ultrasound can be used to assist in localizing small and deep tumors. Individual nerve exposures are discussed in Parts III and IV of this book.
2. Once the nerve and the tumor are exposed (Fig. 52.3), the tumor surface is mapped with a **nerve stimulator** to identify a safe entry zone free of fascicles.
3. The nerve sheath is opened using tenotomy or microscissors.

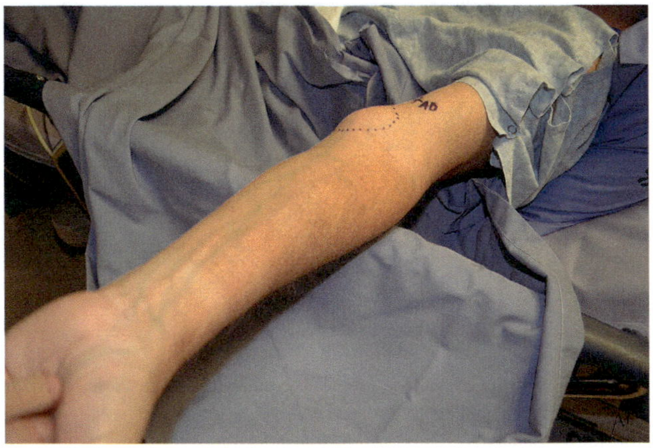

Fig. 52.1 This patient presented with a tender mass (*dotted circle*) in the left arm

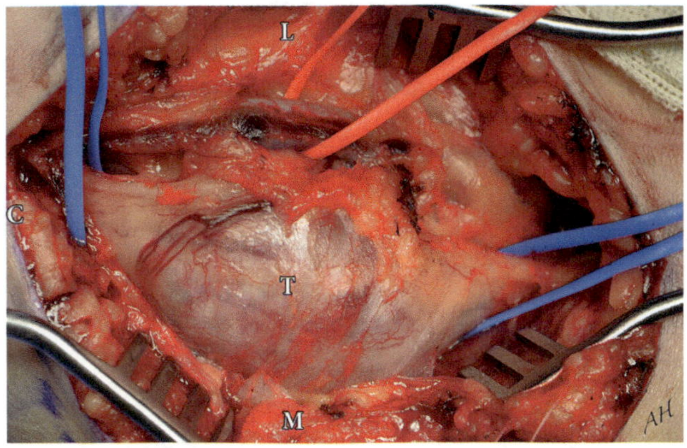

Fig. 52.3 Operative view of the tumor (*T*) within the median nerve (*blue loops*). The brachial vessels are in the *red loop*. *M* medial, *L* lateral, *C* cranial. Using a nerve stimulator, the tumor is mapped for a safe entry zone

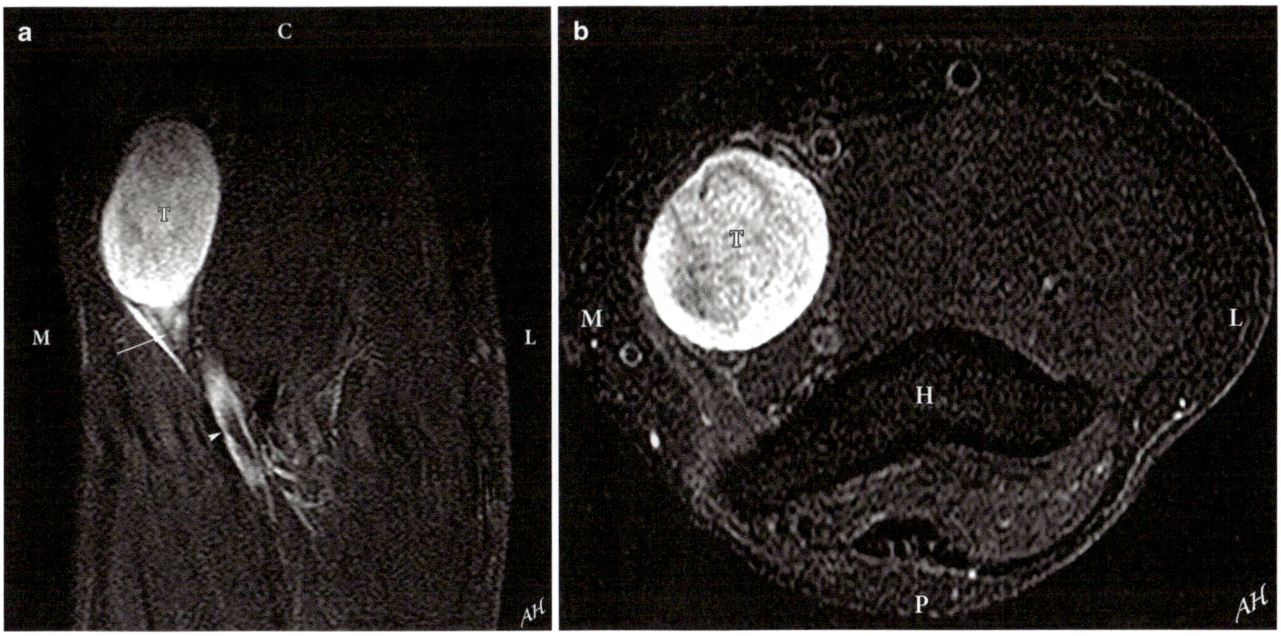

Fig. 52.2 Coronal (**a**) and axial (**b**) T2-weighted STIR MRI of the left arm showing a tumor (*T*) along the median nerve (*arrow*). Note brachial vessels (*arrowhead*). *M* medial, *L* lateral, *C* cranial, *P* posterior, *H* humerus

4. Identify the plane between the pseudocapsule and the tumor capsule. This is a safe plane that allows dissection of the tumor with preservation of most bystander fascicles within and outside the pseudocapsule (Fig. 52.4). A spatula or Roton 8 is used for this dissection.
5. At the 2 poles of the tumor, one or more fascicles are seen entering and exiting the tumor (Fig. 52.5). Stimulation is used to confirm these are non-motor fascicles. They can then be coagulated with bipolar coagulation, cut, and the tumor is then removed (Fig. 52.6). Small tumor fascicles with minor motor response on stimulation can still be resected as long as redundant response is obtained from the remaining fascicles left untouched.
6. **Biopsy is not indicated** in straight-forward benign nerve sheath tumors and can in fact be detrimental. Levi et al. reported more neurological deficits after biopsy for benign nerve sheath tumors. Dissection can also be difficult with additional scar tissue [8].
7. **Piecemeal resection** is sometimes needed in large tumors of important mixed nerves. This prevents too much retraction or traction on the normal fascicles. **Ultrasonic aspirator** can help debulk the tumor before dissecting the periphery.
8. **Microscope magnification** is sometimes helpful if the dissection is tedious.

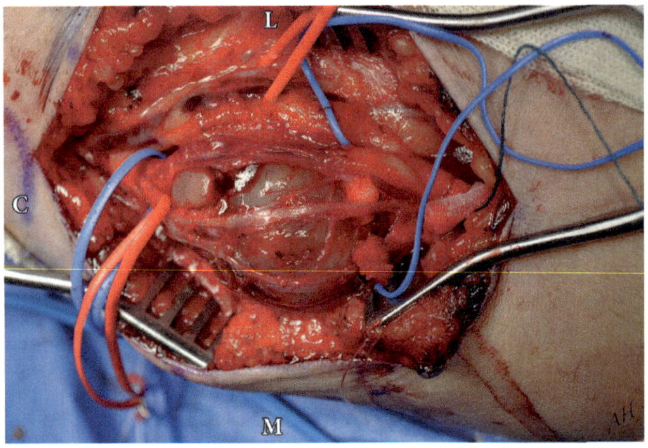

Fig. 52.4 Dissection around the tumor capsule allows preservation of all normal-functioning fascicles

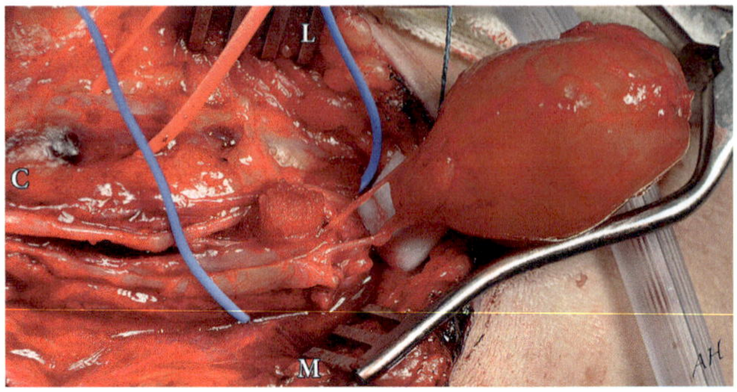

Fig. 52.5 Further dissection reveals the pathological fascicles entering the tumor. These can be coagulated and cut. Stimulation usually reveals non-motor fascicles

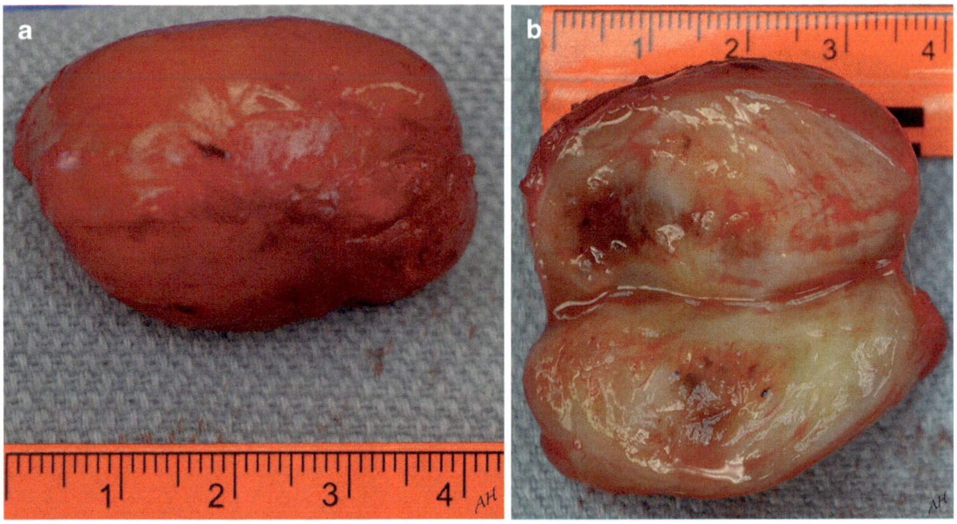

Fig. 52.6 Gross appearance (**a**), and cut surface (**b**) of the tumor, note the brownish yellow appearance, pathology revealed a schwannoma. Neurofibromas appear grayish white on cut surface

Peculiarities in Rare and Malignant Tumors

Certain clinical or morphological criteria are indicative of more rare or malignant tumors of nerves, that may lead to a change in surgical strategy.

Perineurioma (Fig. 52.7)

Deficit of motor function in younger patients and long-distance enlargement or distension of a nerve on MRI or HNUS are usually indicative of perineurioma. A biopsy under neuromonitoring may help differentiate a perineurioma from chronic inflammatory demyelinating polyneuropathy (CIDP). Epineurectomy or secondary reconstructive strategies for motor function (e.g., nerve transfers vs. tendon transfers) are indicated in some cases [2]. Wilson et al. argued that the MRI criteria are so compelling that biopsy is not indicated [9]. Resection and grafting is sometimes indicated in very short segment disease, and partial involvement of one or a few nerve fascicles.

Lipoma (Fig. 52.8)

Clinical signs are similar to those of compressive neuropathy (pain, loss of sensory and/or motor function) in extraneural and intraneural lipomas. On MRI, they are circumscribed fatty masses. In contrast, nerve lipomatosis presents on MRI with massive diffuse fatty nerve enlargement and is sometimes accompanied by excessive growth in the nerve territory (*Macrodystrophia* lipomatosa). In the case of symptomatic lipomatous nerve lesions or documented size progression, exploration should be performed with the aim of histopathological confirmation and decompression of the nerve. In focal tumors, a complete resection under intraoperative neuromonitoring (IONM) may be possible, but this is not achievable in nerve lipomatosis [2].

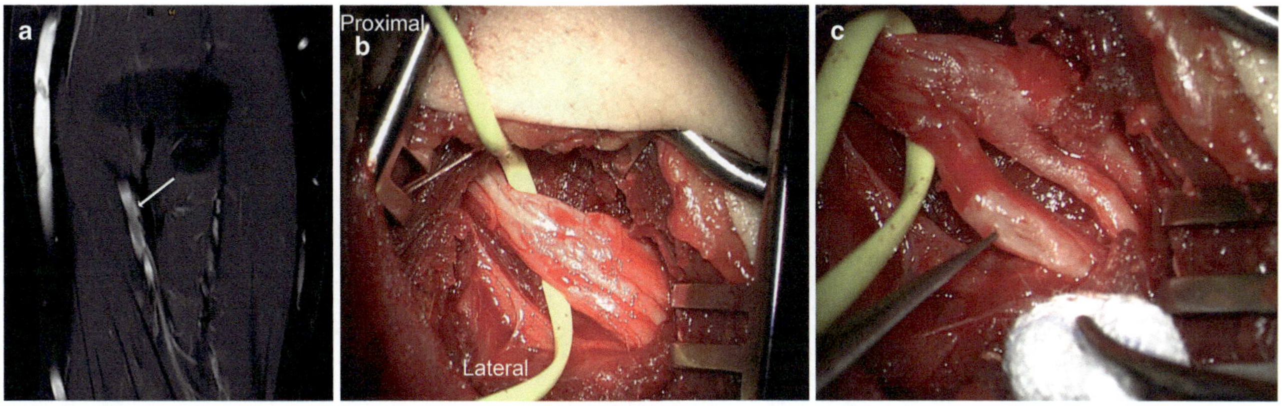

Fig. 52.7 (**a**) T2-weighted MRI showing increased signal of the radial nerve (*arrow*). (**b**) Right distal radial nerve exposure (*yellow loop*) showing enlargement of the nerve. (**c**) Interfascicular dissection for fascicular biopsy. This revealed perineurioma of the ramus profundus nervi radialis (*surgical forceps pointing to a supinator branch of the deep radial nerve*)

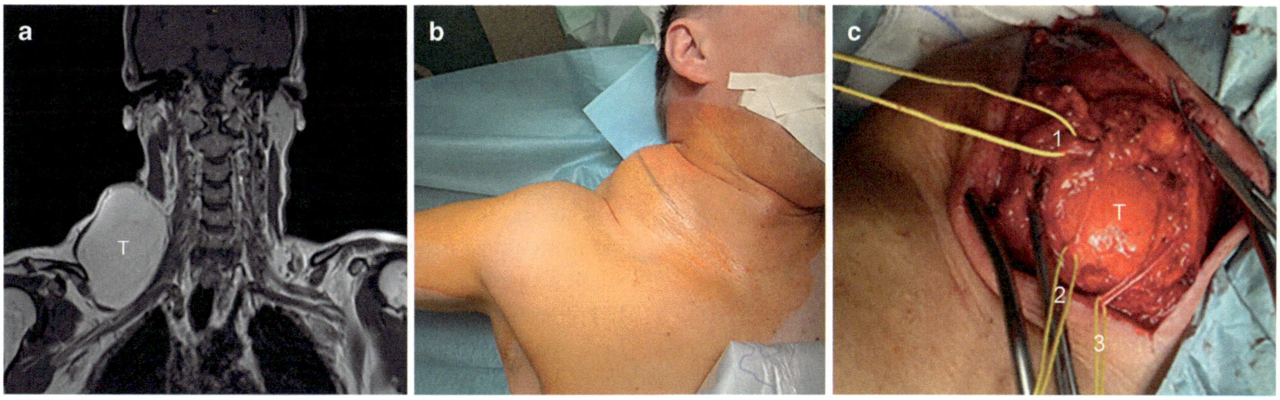

Fig. 52.8 (**a**) T1-weighted MRI showing right-sided tumor (*T*), mostly supraclavicular with an infraclavicular component, and similar signal intensity to subcutaneous fat. (**b**) Intraoperative photograph with the patient positioned supine and the head turned to the left. (**c**) Following exposure, the tumor (*T*) is exposed and appears to be associated with C6/upper trunk. *1* C5, *2* and *3* cervical plexus. Pathology revealed a lipoma

Desmoid Tumor (Aggressive Fibromatosis) (Fig. 52.9)

Aggressive fibromatosis (also called desmoid tumors) are benign connective tissue proliferations with aggressive growth and recurrence. It can also be localized intraneurally and then usually presents as sensory and motor function loss and/or pain. In some cases, a tumor-like lesion is palpable. It often affects women of childbearing age, growth induction due to pregnancy has been reported, and they could develop after the diagnosis of a neuromuscular choristoma. On MRI, an infiltratively growing lesion appears, which often does not enhance with contrast but could heterogeneously enhance. In contrast to other nerve tumors, no central necrosis formation has been reported. Surgical therapy aims for histopathologic confirmation, and often only partial resection is possible to preserve neural function. Other or additional therapeutic options are postoperative radiotherapy (risk of late radiation consequences), chemotherapy (e.g., tyrosine kinase inhibitors), and/or anti-estrogenic therapy [2]. Malignant transformation of desmoid tumors may occur in rare cases, and an association with familial adenomatous polyposis was shown. Recent studies support the view that malignant transformation stems from the mutated desmoid tumor cells in some cases, but in others, sarcoma transformation after local radiation of a desmoid tumor has been reported [10].

Hemangioma

Hemangioma usually present due to sensory and motor function loss of the affected nerve and pain. The ulnar and median nerve are most frequently affected. The MRI shows a hyper-

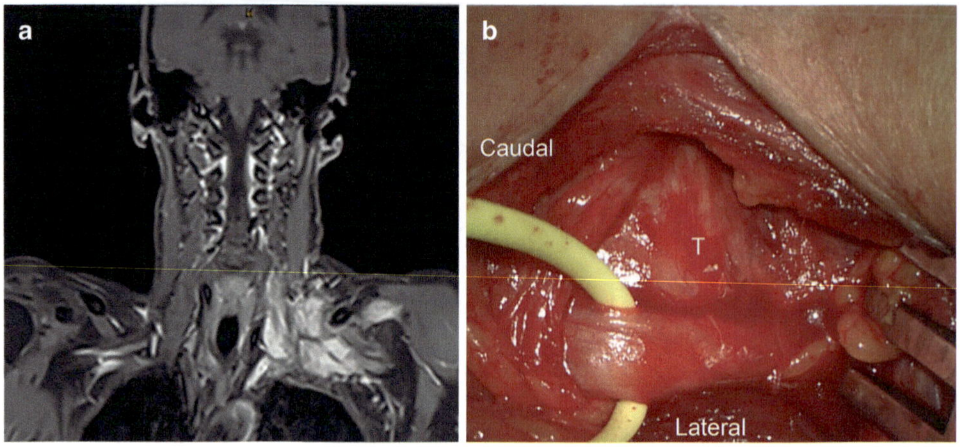

Fig. 52.9 (**a**) T1-weighted MRI with contrast shows heterogeneously-enhancing tumor of the left brachial plexus. (**b**) Intraoperative view shows that the tumor (*T*) is involving the C5 spinal nerve (*yellow loop*). Pathology revealed a desmoid tumor

intense signal with clear contrast uptake in association to a nerve. The exact location in relation to the nerve and fascicles determines the risk of surgical resection [2]:

- Type 1: Intraneural extrafascicular, low risk.
- Type 2: Intraneural intrafascicular, high risk.
- Type 3: Extraneural and intraneural, surgical risk depends on the location of the intraneural section as well as the complexity of blood flow.

Paraganglioma

Paragangliomas are most often located in the head and neck region and then present with loss of cranial nerve function and/or a palpable mass. The MRI shows contrast uptake and good vascularization. In the HNUS, calcified phleboliths and a pendulum flow of the blood within the vessels during tumor compression can be identified. Before surgical resection, an embolization and/or a multidisciplinary approach are helpful. In some cases, in order to preserve function, residual tumor may be left, in which case, radiation and/or nerve reconstruction may be necessary [2].

Ganglion Cysts (Fig. 52.10)

Ganglion cysts present with pain to touch, swelling, and a loss of sensory and/or motor function. The MRI shows a circumscribed cystic lesion in association with a nerve. Some classic MRI signs such as the "tail" or signet ring sign have been described. In HNUS, a hypoechoic, septated, cystic formation with nerve fascicles displaced to the periphery can be detected. Surgical treatment includes the opening of the cyst with decompression of the nerve (in intraneural cysts, IONM is recommended) and disconnecting the articular branch to prevent recurrence. Partial resection of the superior tibio-fibular joint can be performed to prevent recurrence, in cases involving the peroneal nerve [2].

Endometriosis of Nerves

In some cases, endometriosis can cause neuropathy of a pelvic nerve, most often detected in the sciatic nerve. Imaging studies support the hypothesis of perineural spread. Other hypotheses include retrograde menstruation, lymphogenous or hematogenous spread, and coelomic or Mullerian duct metaplasia [11]. The pathogenesis is important to choose treatment options as some endometric lesions require estrogen for growth and some being progesterone resistant. Treatment options include symptomatic for pain relief, medical therapy (contraception), and/or surgery (resection of endometriosis), open vs endoscopic.

ANUBP

ANUBP usually occur in patients with neurofibromatosis type 1. They are atypical neurofibromas that do not fulfill the criteria for MPNST (rare individual cases have been detected in patients without NF1). Their clinical appearance lies within the spectrum between neurofibroma and MPNST. On MRI, the presentation may be heterogenous. On F18-FDG, cases of lower and higher SUV values have been described. The concept of surgical treatment may be challenging due to the difficulty in making a reliable preoperative diagnosis, and possible tumor heterogeneity. A complete resection with the aim of preserving nerve function under neuromonitoring is advised [2].

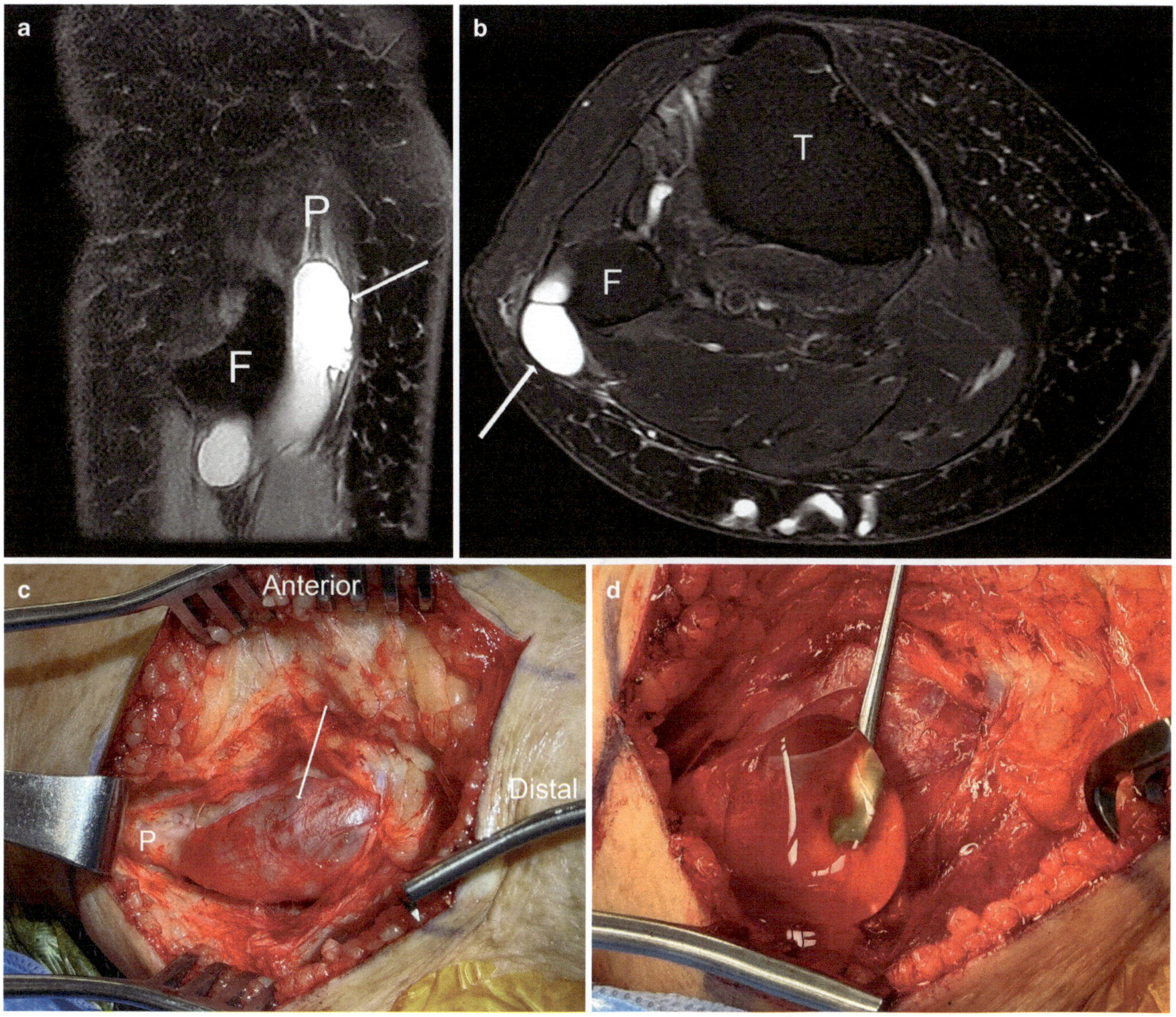

Fig. 52.10 Intraneural ganglion cyst (*arrow*). (**a**) Sagittal proton density and (**b**) axial T2 MRI showing intraneural ganglion cyst of the right peroneal nerve (*P*). *T* tibia, *F* fibula. (**c** and **d**) Surgical views before and during draining of the cyst, respectively. Note the synovial fluid coming out in (**d**)

MPNST (Figs. 52.11 and 52.12)

MPNST usually presents with a painful, palpable, and only slightly displaceable swelling. Motor deficits and a rapid increase in tumor size are indicative of MPNST. Infiltrative growth, blurred borders, heterogeneous enhancement with contrast, and surrounding edema may be seen on MRI. The locally infiltrative growth can also be detected on HNUS [6]. The F18-FDG PET or MRI (ADC) is helpful to differentiate the different tumor entities, especially in NF1 patients [7]. An SUVmax >6 is suggestive of malignancy. An interdisciplinary evaluation, surgery—preferably resection with negative margins whenever possible, radiotherapy and chemotherapy, as well as functional reconstruction may be necessary [2].

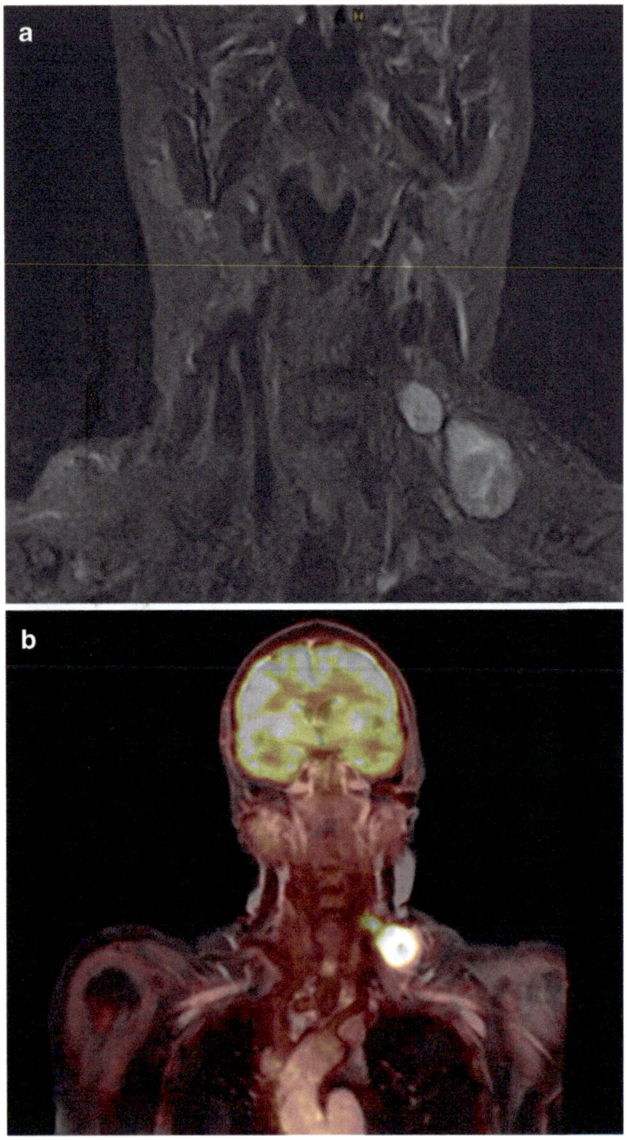

Fig. 52.11 (**a**) T1-weighted MRI with contrast shows a contrast-enhancing left brachial plexus tumor. (**b**) F18-FDG-PET with high tracer uptake of the tumor. Pathology revealed MPNST

Fig. 52.12 (**a**) NF1 patient (same as in Fig. 52.11) positioned for surgery for a left-sided tumor of the brachial plexus that has been previously explored. (**b**) Intraoperative view with the tumor (*T*) exposed. Pathology revealed MPNST

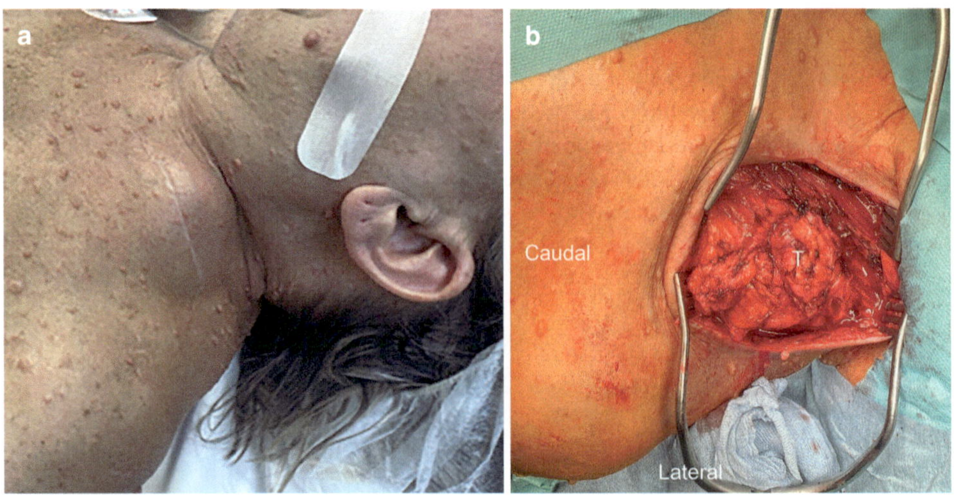

Metastatic Tumors

Solid tumors, leukemia, and lymphoma (Fig. 52.13) can infiltrate nerves and nerve plexuses, causing severe neurological deficits and pain. Differentiation between neoplastic plexopathies and radiation plexopathy, especially in breast cancer (Fig. 52.14) and Pancoast tumors (Fig. 52.15), invading the brachial plexus, can be challenging. Presence of Myokymia on electrodiagnostic studies is suggestive of radiation plexopathy. Recent studies provide evidence that the infiltration of the lumbosacral plexus in prostate cancer (Fig. 52.16), via perineural spread, may be underestimated. High-resolution MRI and PET imaging may be helpful for the diagnosis [13, 14].

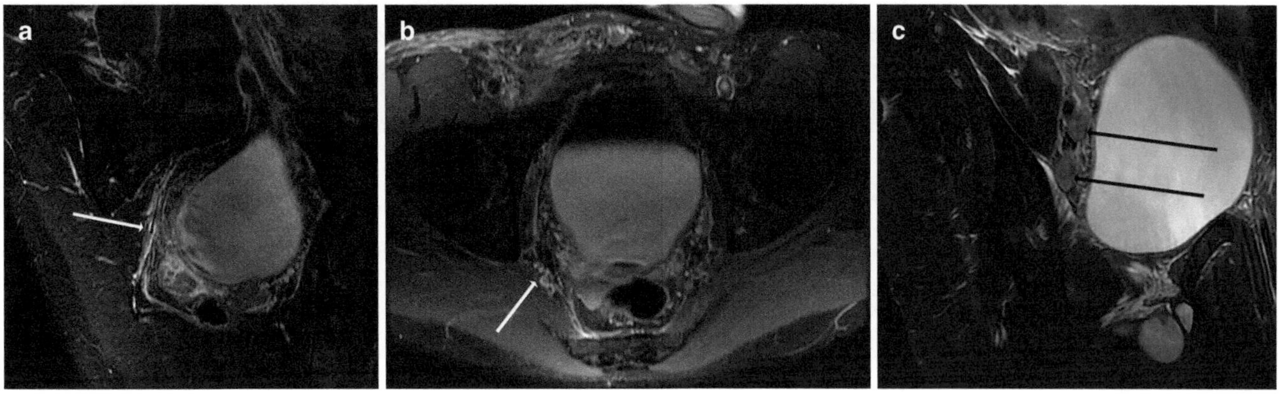

Fig. 52.13 35-year-old male with anaplastic large cell lymphoma. (**a** and **b**) Coronal and axial T1 IDEAL (Iterative Decomposition of water and fat using Echo Asymmetry and Least squares estimation) [12] MRI with contrast showing enhancement of the right sciatic nerve (*white arrow*). (**c**) Coronal T2 showing pelvic lymph nodes (*black arrows*)

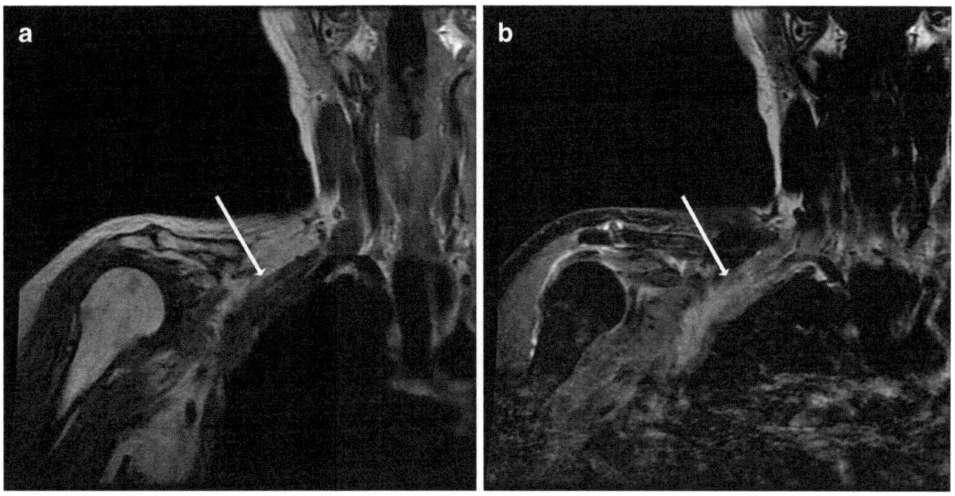

Fig. 52.14 63-year-old female with breast cancer recurrence with involvement of the right infraclavicular brachial plexus. T1 coronal MRI pre- (**a**) and post- (**b**) contrast showing enhancing tumor involving the right brachial plexus (*arrow*)

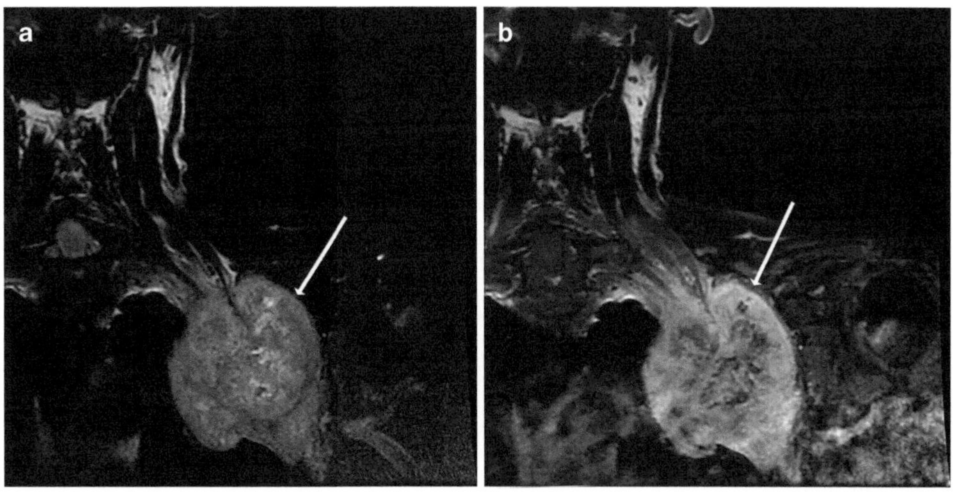

Fig. 52.15 72-year-old male with left lung apex tumor infiltrating the brachial plexus. Coronal T2 MRI (**a**) and T1 post-contrast (**b**) showing heterogeneously enhancing tumor involving the lung apex and the left brachial plexus (*arrow*), with central necrosis. The tumor was a metastatic sarcomatoid carcinoma

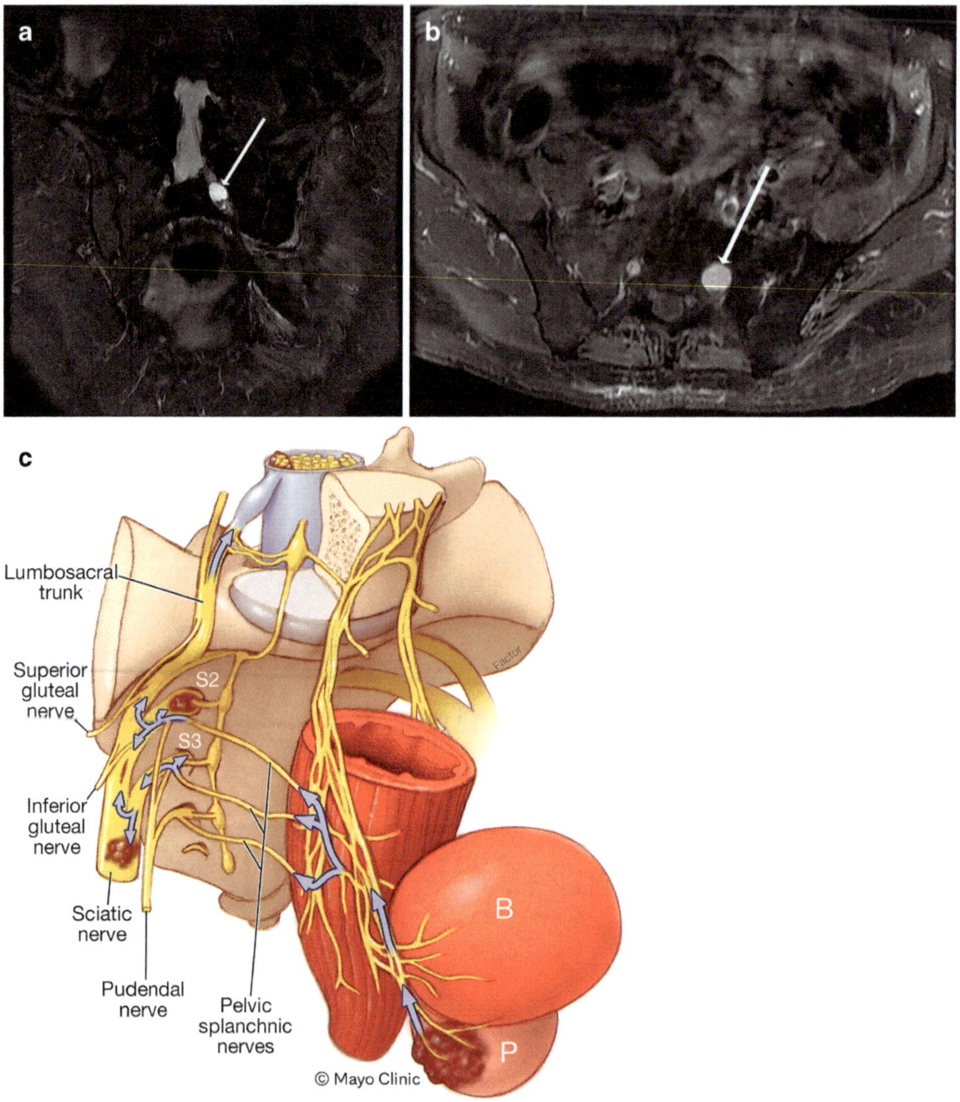

Fig. 52.16 79-year-old male with recurrent prostate cancer. (**a**) T2 coronal MRI showing increased signal of the left S1 nerve. (**b**) Axial T1 with contrast showing enhancement of the left S1 nerve. (**c**) Diagram depicting the mechanism of perineural spread of prostate cancer. *B* bladder, *P* prostate. (Used with permission of Mayo Foundation for Medical Education and Research. All rights reserved [14])

References

1. Kim DH, Murovic JA, Tiel RL, Moes G, Kline DG (2005) A series of 397 peripheral nerve sheath tumors: 30-year experience at Louisiana State University Health Sciences Center. J Neurosurg 102(2):246–255. https://doi.org/10.3171/jns.2005.102.2.0246
2. Dengler NF, Pedro MT, Kolbenschlag J (2024) Treatment interdisciplinarity of tumorous and tumor-like lesions of peripheral nerves. HaMiPla
3. Ferner RE, Huson SM, Thomas N, Moss C, Willshaw H, Evans DG, Upadhyaya M et al (2007) Guidelines for the diagnosis and management of individuals with neurofibromatosis 1. J Med Genet 44(2):81–88. https://doi.org/10.1136/jmg.2006.045906. Epub 2006 Nov 14
4. Farschtschi S, Mautner VF, McLean ACL, Schulz A, Friedrich RE, Rosahl SK (2020) The neurofibromatoses. Dtsch Arztebl Int 117(20):354–360
5. Plotkin SR, Messiaen L, Legius E, Pancza P, Avery RA, Blakeley JO, Babovic-Vuksanovic D, Ferner R, Fisher MJ, Friedman JM, Giovannini M, Gutmann DH, Hanemann CO, Kalamarides M, Kehrer-Sawatzki H, Korf BR, Mautner VF, MacCollin M, Papi L, Rauen KA, Riccardi V, Schorry E, Smith MJ, Stemmer-Rachamimov A, Stevenson DA, Ullrich NJ, Viskochil D, Wimmer K, Yohay K, International Consensus Group on Neurofibromatosis Diagnostic Criteria (I-NF-DC), Huson SM, Wolkenstein P, Evans DG (2022) Updated diagnostic criteria and nomenclature for neurofibromatosis type 2 and schwannomatosis: an international consensus recommendation. Genet Med 24(9):1967–1977. https://doi.org/10.1016/j.gim.2022.05.007
6. Lefebvre G, Le Corroller T (2023) Ultrasound and MR imaging of peripheral nerve tumors: the state of the art. Skeletal Radiol 52(3):405–419. https://doi.org/10.1007/s00256-022-04087-5
7. Ahlawat S, Blakeley JO, Rodriguez FJ, Fayad LM (2019) Imaging biomarkers for malignant peripheral nerve sheath tumors in neu-

rofibromatosis type 1. Neurology 93(11):e1076–e1084. https://doi.org/10.1212/WNL.0000000000008092
8. Perez-Roman RJ, Burks SS, Debs L, Cajigas I, Levi AD (2020) The risk of peripheral nerve tumor biopsy in suspected benign etiologies. Neurosurgery 86(3):E326–E332. https://doi.org/10.1093/neuros/nyz549
9. Wilson TJ, Howe BM, Stewart SA, Spinner RJ, Amrami KK (2018) Clinicoradiological features of intraneural perineuriomas obviate the need for tissue diagnosis. J Neurosurg 129(4):1034–1040. https://doi.org/10.3171/2017.5.JNS17905. Epub 2017 Dec 1
10. Verschoor AJ, Cleton-Jansen AM, Wijers-Koster P, Coffin CM, Lazar AJ, Nout RA, Rubin BP et al (2015) Radiation-induced sarcomas occurring in desmoid-type fibromatosis are not always derived from the primary tumor. Am J Surg Pathol 39(12):1701–1707. https://doi.org/10.1097/PAS.0000000000000510
11. Siquara De Sousa AC, Capek S, Amrami KK, Spinner RJ (2015) Neural involvement in endometriosis: review of anatomic distribution and mechanisms. Clin Anat 28(8):1029–1038. https://doi.org/10.1002/ca.22617. Epub 2015 Sep 9
12. Grayev A, Reeder S, Hanna A (2016) Use of chemical shift encoded magnetic resonance imaging (CSE-MRI) for high resolution fat-suppressed imaging of the brachial and lumbosacral plexuses. Eur J Radiol 85(6):1199–1207. https://doi.org/10.1016/j.ejrad.2016.04.002
13. Gwathmey KG (2018) Plexus and peripheral nerve metastasis. Handb Clin Neurol 149:257–279. https://doi.org/10.1016/B978-0-12-811161-1.00017-7
14. Hébert-Blouin MN, Amrami KK, Myers RP, Hanna AS, Spinner RJ (2010) Adenocarcinoma of the prostate involving the lumbosacral plexus: MRI evidence to support direct perineural spread. Acta Neurochir 152(9):1567–1576. https://doi.org/10.1007/s00701-010-0682-x. Epub 2010 May 15

Surgical Approaches to Retroperitoneal Tumors

53

Thomas Kretschmer and Christian Heinen

General [1–3]

Preoperative diagnosis and grade are frequently unclear (especially benign vs. malignant). Nevertheless, surgical strategy and goal are influenced by entity (benign vs. malignant, function sparing vs. palliative/life prolonging). The tumor is located within or near the lumbosacral plexus or its branches. The dissection is challenging due to depth and risk for functional damage: voiding, sphincters, vascular/genitourinary injury, or gluteal/lower extremity muscular and sensory deficits.

Indication

- Newly discovered mass of unclear entity or under suspicion of malignancy
- Related symptoms or deficits (pain, functional)
- Risk of malignant transformation in NF I patients
- Size, large masses

Tumor Types in the Retroperitoneum [4]

- Primary lesions: Mesenchymal tumors (including sarcoma and neurogenic tumor) account for approximately half of all. Liposarcomas and leiomyosarcomas represent approximately 80% of all adult retroperitoneal sarcomas. Parasympathetic tumors, extragonadal germ cell tumor, lymphoid tumors, cystic vestigial tumors, desmoid, solitary fibrous tumors, PEComas (Perivascular epithelioid cell neoplasms), deep angiomyxomas (infra-peritoneal), lymphangioma, and rarely hemangioma.
- Secondary lesions: metastatic carcinoma, adenopathy, lymphoma.
- Classification: fatty tumors, smooth muscle tumors, fibroblastic and myofibroblastic tumors, striated muscle tumors, vascular tumors, nerve tumors, extraskeletal osseous and cartilaginous tumors, uncertain tumor differentiation, unclassified/undifferentiated sarcomas (rare in retroperitoneum).

Tumor Frequency [2]

Nerve tumor of retroperitoneal space is rare: Benign schwannoma 0.7–2.7%, retroperitoneal sarcoma 0.51/100,000 persons per year. Malignant retroperitoneal tumors have poor survival rates and are prone to severe deficits after surgery. Reported are a 22% complication rate with substantial blood loss, urinary retention, reoperation due to surgery related complications in 14%, and a 4% mortality rate in 500 retroperitoneal soft tissue sarcomas. One-third of all retroperitoneal tumors are reported as sarcomas; among these, 3% were listed as MPNST. A 32.8-month survival rate in 35 patients with limb preservation and limb amputation hemipelvectomy is reported in malignancy.

Approach Selection [2]

Dictated by tumor location in three anatomical planes on imaging as well as prior surgery. Authors' classification for anterior abdominal approach choice: relation of tumor growth to virtual anatomical lines (Fig. 53.1) on a coronal/axial and sagittal magnetic resonance imaging (MRI): sacral promontory, medial and lateral psoas borders, and inguinal ligament.

T. Kretschmer
Department of Neurosurgery and Neurorestoration, Federal State Hospital Klinikum, Klagenfurt, Austria
e-mail: Thomas.kretschmer@kabeg.at

C. Heinen (✉)
Department Neuro-, Spine- and Nerve Surgery, Christliches Krankenhaus, Quakenbrück, Germany
e-mail: C.heinen@ckq-gmbh.de; christian.heinen@uol.de

A. S. Hanna (ed.), *Nerves: Anatomy, Exposures, and Techniques*, https://doi.org/10.1007/978-3-031-73931-6_53

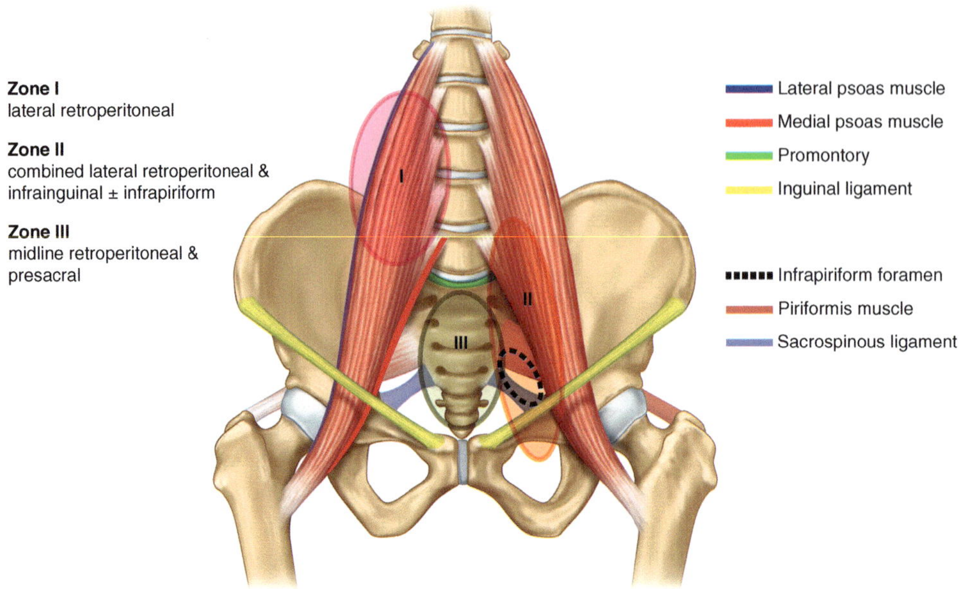

Fig. 53.1 Anterior landmarks that help to choose for anterior abdominal approaches to retroperitoneal tumor: *blue* lateral psoas border, *red* medial psoas border, *green* sacral promontory, *yellow* inguinal ligament. **Zones** define areas above (**I**) and below promontory (**II** and **III**) that are ± apt for certain approaches and combinations thereof. If tumor extends into spinal canal, neuroforamen, through infrapiriform foramen, or infrainguinal to medial thigh, approach combinations are helpful. Examples for anterior combinations are lateral retroperitoneal and infrainguinal approach; for anterior and dorsal approaches, midline retroperitoneal and dorsal trans-spinal. (Artwork by Thomas Kretschmer©, adapted and reprinted with permission from "Neurosurgery" [2])

If above promontory in coronal and sagittal views, lateral retroperitoneal flank incision is preferred (**Zone I**, Fig. 53.1). If below promontory (deep in pelvis), choice between lateral retroperitoneal and transperitoneal depends on relation of mass to medial and lateral psoas border (since this also defines proximity to iliac artery and other structures at risk). If below and above promontory but mainly lateral (**Zone II**), still lateral retroperitoneal is preferred because of ease and reduced morbidity of approach. If tumor mass is below promontory and completely central (**Zone III**), transperitoneal is preferred. If the tumor is large and extends into other compartments, approaches can be combined without the need for extensive transperitoneal exposure. Examples: a) Tumor follows femoral/obturator nerve route-combination with infrainguinal approach (separate incision, connection of ports via retractors or endoscope); b) tumor follows sciatic nerve route-combination with subgluteal/transgluteal approach [5]. We might combine two to three approaches. It might be necessary to combine an anterior with a posterior approach. In such a case, patient positioning needs to be carefully considered; it is often possible to circumvent the need for repositioning and redraping.

The more medial the tumor is situated in relation to the psoas muscle, the closer it is to the iliac vessels. This increases the necessity for room and good vascular control and swings the pendulum towards midline transperitoneal. Dependent on overall risk estimation, and if in doubt, midline large transperitoneal is chosen as it can deliver a maximum of dissection room.

Many approaches have been described to tackle retroperitoneal tumors, among them transperitoneal, retroperitoneal, dorsal, and trans-sacral variations. However, there are only a few reports on approaches and combinations. Our systematic approach attempts to define tumor extension on imaging with relation to pertinent landmarks first and then choosing from the below-listed approach modules accordingly (Figs. 53.1, 53.2, 53.3, and 53.4). Our choice is influenced by anatomical landmarks, expected pathology, surgical risk and previous surgery, extent of resection, general condition of the patient, and the patient's wishes (e.g., radicality vs. function sparing in the case of expected malignancy).

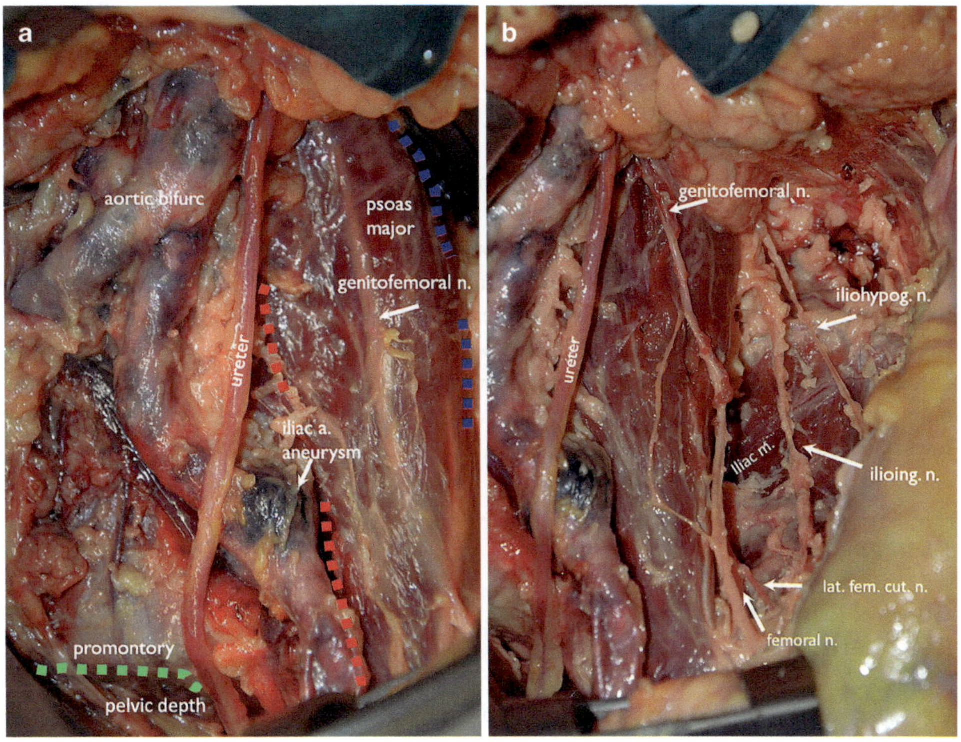

Fig. 53.2 Left retroperitoneal space. (**a**) Mid to lateral retroperitoneal space, mainly above sacral promontory with major landmarks: promontory (*green*), psoas medial (*red*) and lateral (*blue*) borders, and guiding structures genitofemoral nerve, ureter, aortic bifurcation, and iliac artery. (**b**) Further lateral retroperitoneal space with psoas, ilioinguinal and iliohypogastric nerves, and iliacus muscle. Lateral femoral cutaneous nerve coming off from only marginally visible femoral nerve lateral to lower psoas

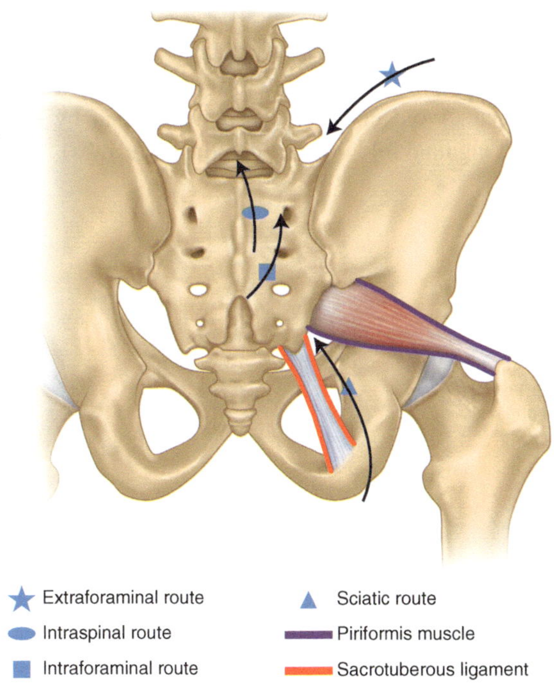

Fig. 53.3 Coronal dorsal view of tumor growth routes. Each route (*arrows*) stands for a separate approach module that can be combined with an anterior approach, if tumor extension necessitates. (Artwork by Thomas Kretschmer©, adapted and reprinted with permission from "Neurosurgery" [2])

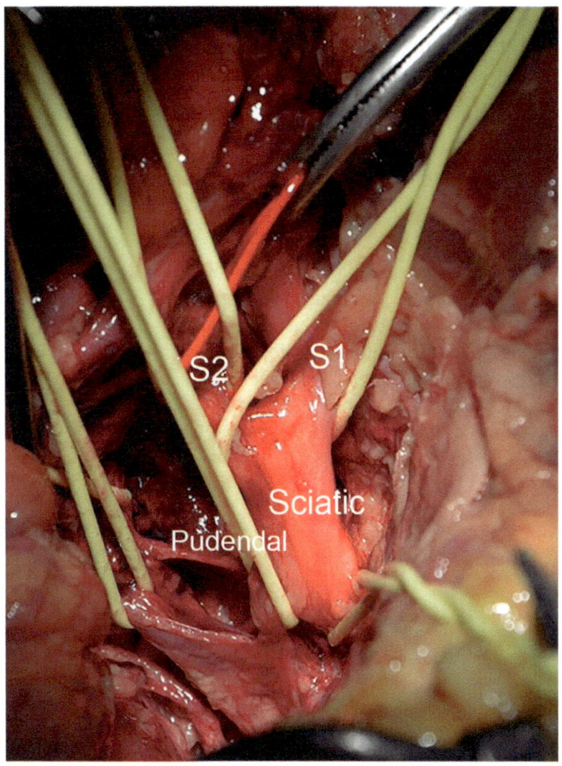

Fig. 53.4 Left sacral plexus (partial), deep view into retroperitoneal pelvis, below promontory, with S1 and S2 roots forming sciatic nerve and branching to pudendal nerve

Anatomy

Lateral abdominal wall consists of external oblique running obliquely from superolateral to inferomedial towards rectus sheath, internal oblique immediately beneath from inferolateral to superomedial, and transversus running horizontally directly beneath it.

Anterior abdominal wall with rectus abdominis has continuous rectus sheaths meeting in the midline at linea alba: in the upper 2/3 of abdomen strong fibrous anterior and posterior rectus sheaths, in the lower 1/3 only strong anterior sheath with fibrofatty layer called transversalis fascia between peritoneum and rectus. The arcuate line marks the lower border of the posterior rectus sheath.

Approaches

General Principles to Abdominal Retroperitoneal Exposures

Choice strongly affects how straight forward or difficult the operation will be. One factor is how well an incision can adapt to more extensive dissection. More length can help and should be appropriate besides versatile fixed retractor systems with different choices of blade lengths and widths.

Incisions should be in layers, avoiding visceral injury and enabling pristine anatomical closure later. There is no special dietary preparation needed; enemas defeat the purpose and just negatively influence the fluid balance. After previous laparotomies, small bowel adhesions should be envisioned and incisions planned accordingly, most likely avoiding the previous incision.

Closure should be meticulous to prevent incisional hernia, wound dehiscence, or visceral injury. Sutures through fascia, if possible, layered closure (vs. mass closure); small bites with short travel; visualization of needle; starting from each end of a fascial closure and meeting in the middle increases closure safety (especially for long midline transperitoneal incisions; in addition to interrupted retention sutures every 3–5 cm). Depending on exposure size and hemostasis, placement of drains should be considered (retroperitoneal, intrapelvic, below abdominal wall). A normal diet is started on the first postoperative day.

Authors prefer their own approaches; however, in selected cases like previous intraperitoneal surgery and repeat transperitoneal exposure, we work in interdisciplinary teams.

Lateral Abdominal to Flank Incision (Figs. 53.5, 53.6, 53.7, and 53.8) [2]

Opening space between pelvis and rib cage by flexing the table, use of kidney bump, or inflatable roll (Fig. 53.8).

1. Flank incision with tailored length; palpate anterior superior iliac spine and twelfth rib and place incision in-between. Avoid entering the inguinal canal by staying above inguinal fold (at least two fingerbreadths).

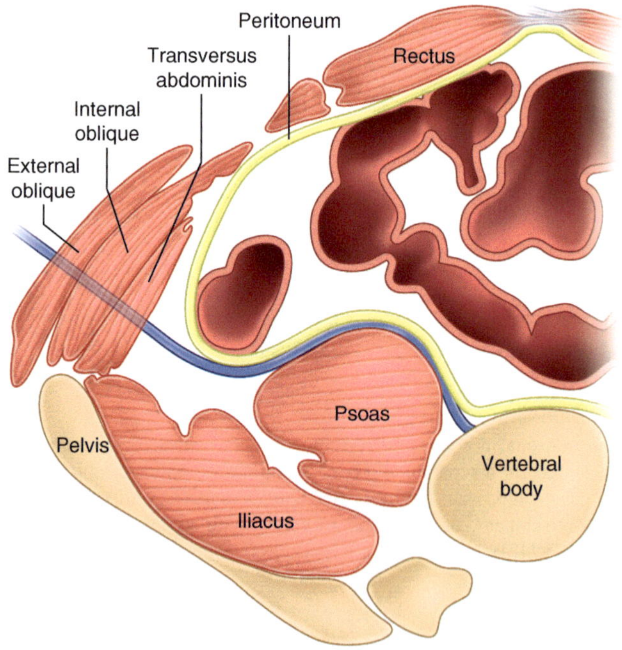

Fig. 53.5 Lateral retroperitoneal dissection pathway. The *blue line* represents the approach through the muscular layers of the abdominal wall (external oblique, internal oblique, and transversus abdominis) at a flank level above the anterior superior iliac spine. (Copyright (Artwork by) Thomas Kretschmer©, published with permission)

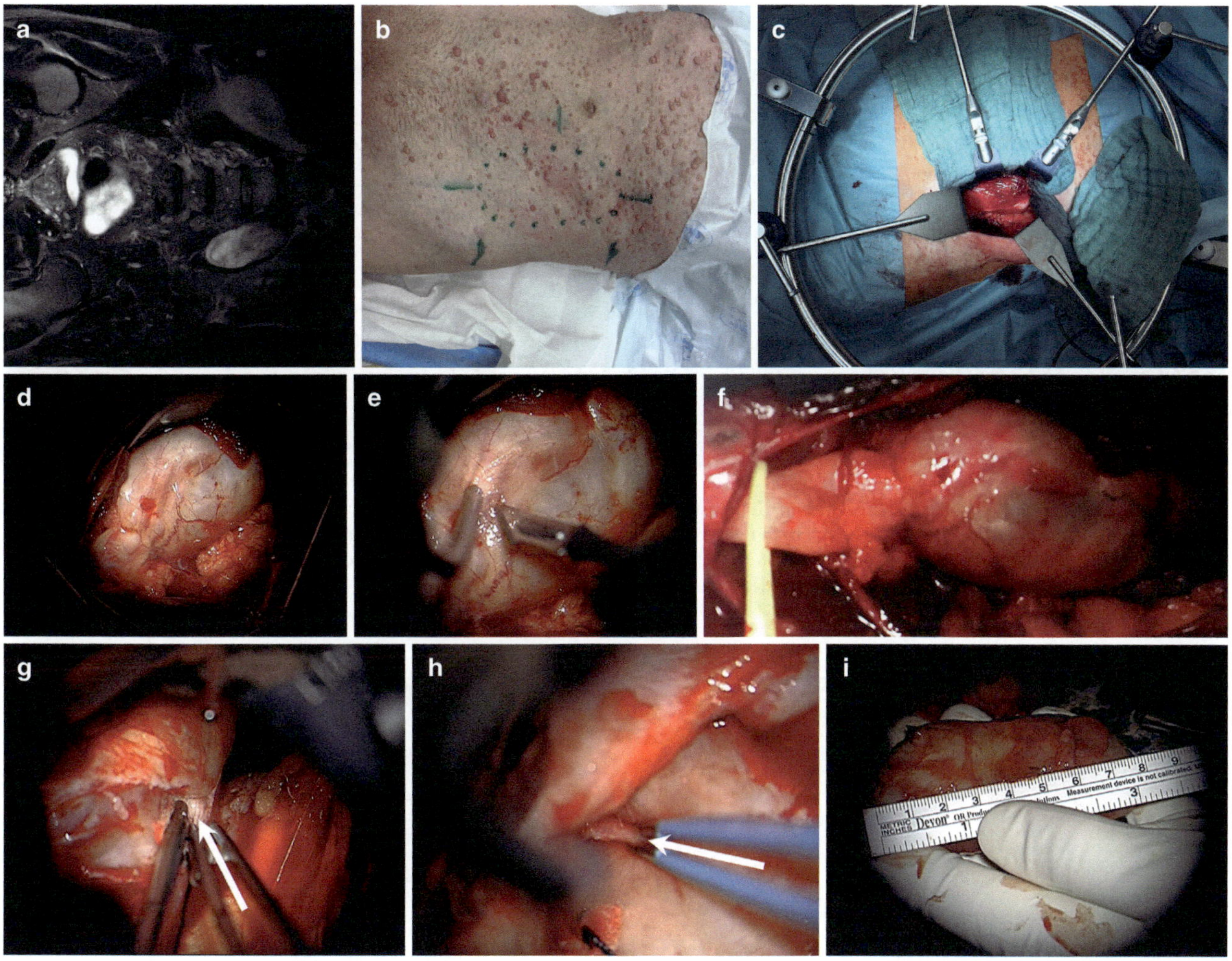

Fig. 53.6 Left lateral retroperitoneal approach covering Zone I > II for benign Peripheral Nerve Sheath Tumor (PNST) in NF1 patient. (**a**) Tumor bulk on coronal MRI; caudal end of tumor is reaching further than depicted (beginning of promontory level). (**b**) Patient placed supine head on the right image side. Tumor outline as per ultrasound. (**c**) Incision centered over tumor for microsurgical work on caudal or cranial end retraction can be adjusted accordingly with ring retractor system. (**d**) Central tumor portion in direct view. (**e**) Incision at tumor equator in fascicle-free area. (**f**) Developed caudal tumor pole with adjusted retraction. *Yellow loop* femoral nerve distal to tumor. (**g**) Caudal tumor outleading fascicle (*arrow*). (**h**) Cranial tumor inleading fascicle of tumor origin (*arrow*) (**i**) Delivered tumor with length about 9 cm

2. Layers:
   (a) Skin-subcutaneous fat, including Scarpa's fascia.
   (b) External oblique muscle/aponeurosis with sharp division to avoid injury to ilioinguinal or iliohypogastric nerves from pulling.
   (c) Internal oblique muscle, divide blunt or with diathermy, repositioning of retractors for clear sight might be necessary, ilioinguinal and iliohypogastric nerves covered by fibrous tissue might become visible.
   (d) Transversus abdominis muscle.
3. Opening the three muscle layers by combination of incision and retraction respecting the fiber direction, sustain clean edges to enable meticulous closure in layers on the way out (prevention of hernia). After division of the muscle layers, the blunt dissection goes through the extraperitoneal fat until the peritoneum is reached and retracted medially, then follow a path aiming towards vertebrae dissecting along the iliacus and psoas on the lateral side (Fig. 53.5). Psoas muscle and genitofemoral nerve running anterior to it are major landmarks (Figs. 53.2 and 53.9).

   Avoid injury to ilioinguinal or iliohypogastric nerves (Fig. 53.9a).

   Careful retraction, hemostasis, attention to detail allow for recognition of each layer.
4. Placement of self-held retractors with abdominal cloth to shelter bowel surface; during dissection repositioning and

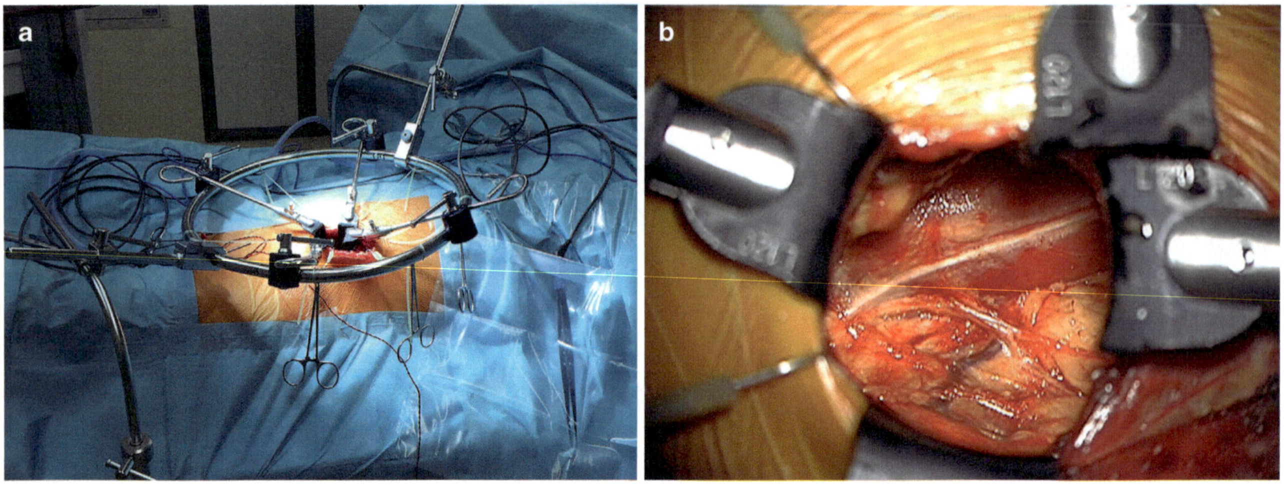

Fig. 53.7 Left lateral retroperitoneal approach Zone II, adjustable for Zones I and III. Patient placed supine head on the right image side. (**a**) Ring retractor system, fixed to the operating table, with polyaxial possibility for adjustment of changeable retractor blades of different lengths. (**b**) A look into the created retroperitoneal cavity after medial mobilization and retraction of fat and peritoneal sac; direct view onto the white genitofemoral nerve coursing anteriorly on the psoas muscle

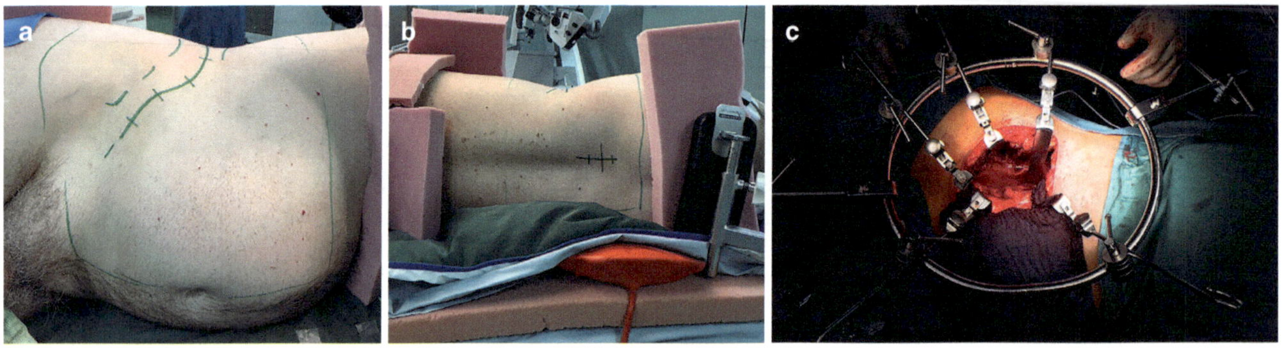

Fig. 53.8 Combined lateral retroperitoneal and trans-spinal approach for tumor extending into spinal canal. (**a**) Lateral decubitus position with markings of incision on flank/abdomen (only ventral portion used), *interrupted, below incision mark* iliac crest, *mark above incision* rib margin. (**b**) Dorsal approach with skin incision marked (*vertical line*), inflatable bag (orange), to open angle between pelvis and rib cage at flank. (**c**) Retroperitoneal view on psoas in exposure center, Zone II

exchange of retractor blades (longer vs. shorter) might be necessary.

5. Identification of bladder and ureter, ±uterus and adnexa, iliac vessels, tumor region; in lateral approach, psoas muscle and genitofemoral nerve on top is the important landmark structure to locate femoral nerve, iliac vessels, and ureter.

   Avoid superior hypogastric plexus (presacral nerve): situated anterior to vertebral body L5 and sacral promontory ± above and anterior of bifurcation of abdominal aorta, forms left and right hypogastric nerve; lesions affect continence (urinary and fecal) and normal sexual function including erection and ejaculation (improper closing of the bladder neck with resulting retrograde ejaculation).

   Avoid inferior hypogastric plexus (pelvic plexus or pelvic ganglion): it gives rise to prostatic plexus/uterovaginal plexus, which is paired left and right and located on either side of rectum/sides of rectum and vagina; lesions may cause urinary dysfunction/incontinence and impair micturition and sexual function.
6. Tumor resection: developing tumor circumference, pertinent anatomy, in and outleading plexal elements and lumbosacral plexus by use of dissection and intraoperative stimulation.

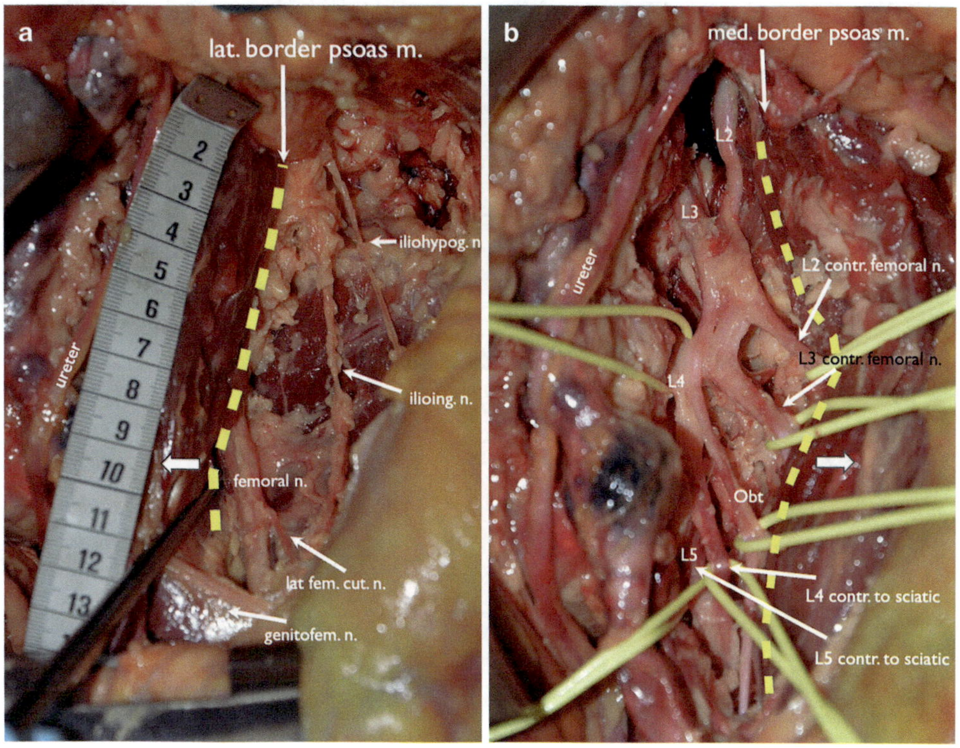

Fig. 53.9 Nerve anatomy around the left psoas muscle and lumbar plexus. (**a**) Psoas shifted medially allows to visualize the underlying femoral nerve and branching of lateral femoral cutaneous nerve. (**b**) Psoas shifted laterally opens lumbar plexus contributions to femoral (*L2, L3, contr.*) and sciatic nerve (*L4, L5, contr.*), and branching of obturator nerve (*Obt*) from L4

Transperitoneal Midline Vertical (Figs. 53.10 and 53.11) [2]

1. Vertical inferior midline and periumbilical incision for larger exposure.
2. Opening along linea alba, avoiding transmuscular if possible

   Details: skin incision knife, subcutaneous fat "cut" diathermy-pulling on both sides of wound edges for easier fat separation, controlled division of linea alba fascia-finger dissection between preperitoneal space and fascia
3. Opening of peritoneum and bowel mobilization to the side

   Details: division of peritoneum (glistening white structure) with diathermy, grasp peritoneum and pull upwards, an option to use two fingers underneath to shelter the intestines. For maximum exposure in the pelvis, the division of linea alba can extend to pubic symphysis.
4. Placement of self-retaining table-mount retractors with abdominal cloth to protect bowel.
5. Identification of bladder and ureter, ±uterus and adnexa, iliac vessels, tumor region. The sacral promontory and iliac vessels are the landmarks to define the other structures.
6. Developing plane of tumor capsule, in- and outleading fascicles, and adjacent lumbosacral plexus by use of dissection and intraoperative nerve stimulation.

Infrainguinal

See Chaps. 24 and 30.

Posterior Approaches (Figs. 53.3 and 53.8b) [2]

- Transgluteal (see Chap. 26)
- Subgluteal [5]
- Trans-sacral
- Translaminar (Fig. 53.8b)
- Transforaminal

Combined Approaches [2]

Any of the above abdominal approaches can be combined with a dorsal or more distal one (Fig. 53.12, approach algorithm). In such a case, there are usually two to three access ports that are used to enlarge the overall exposure. Positioning and draping are then accordingly adapted. If, for example, a retroperitoneal approach is combined with posterior translaminar access, a lateral decubitus position provides access for both, obviating the need for repositioning and redraping (Fig. 53.10).

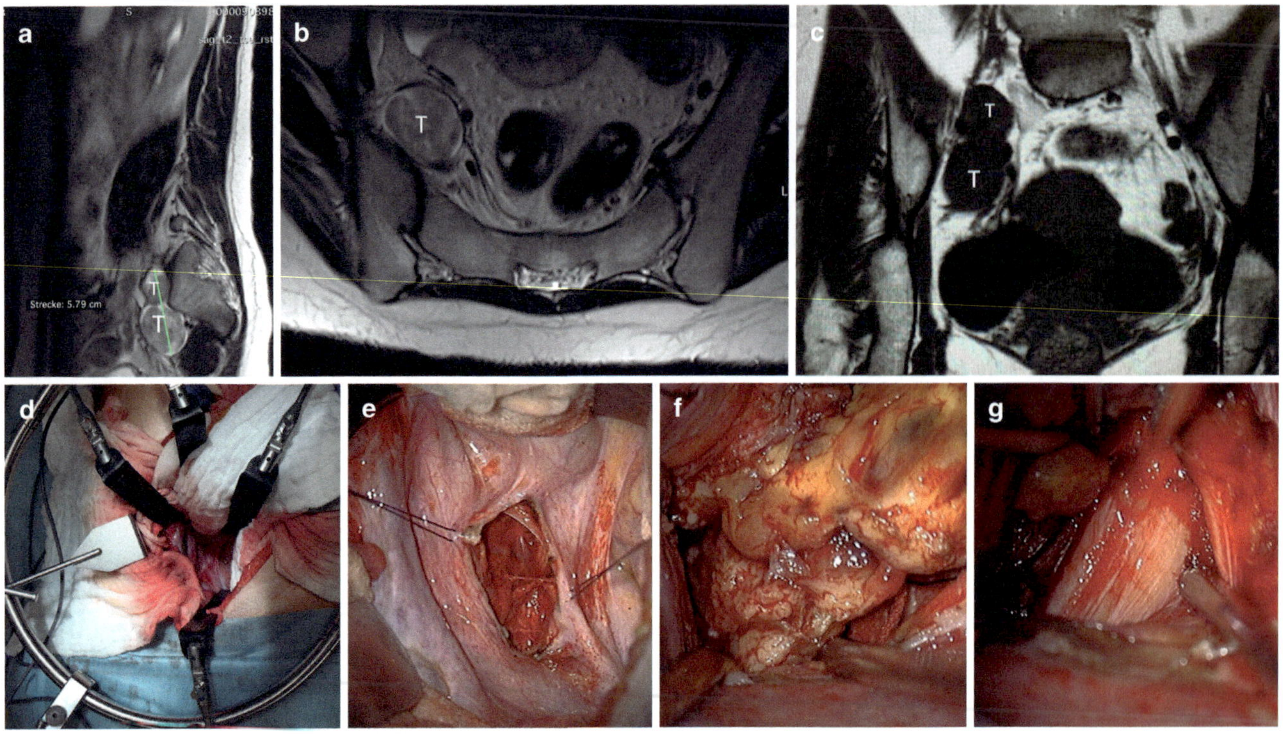

Fig. 53.10 Midline transperitoneal approach, retroperitoneal Zone III. Chosen for right L5/S1 PNST with intact motor function due to previous retroperitoneal surgery. Midline chosen for larger exposure, and vascular control in anticipation of adhesions and potential scars. Surgeon positioned on left patient side, with view and dissection trajectory from midline to lateral for vascular control during nerve dissection. (**a**–**c**) MRI showing right, bilobular PNST tumor (*T*) above and below promontory (**a** sagittal view), crossing medial psoas border line towards middle (**b** axial view), above inguinal canal and infrapiriform foramen (**c** coronal). (**d**) Vertical incision, midline transperitoneal approach, after having mobilized the viscera (behind white cloth held back by lower retractor). (**e**) View after opening peritoneal sheath. (**f**) Some of the PNST developed. (**g**) Looking from intraperitoneal onto sciatic nerve in the retroperitoneal space, caudal to tumor mass to have nerve control and be able to follow nerve up proximal towards tumor

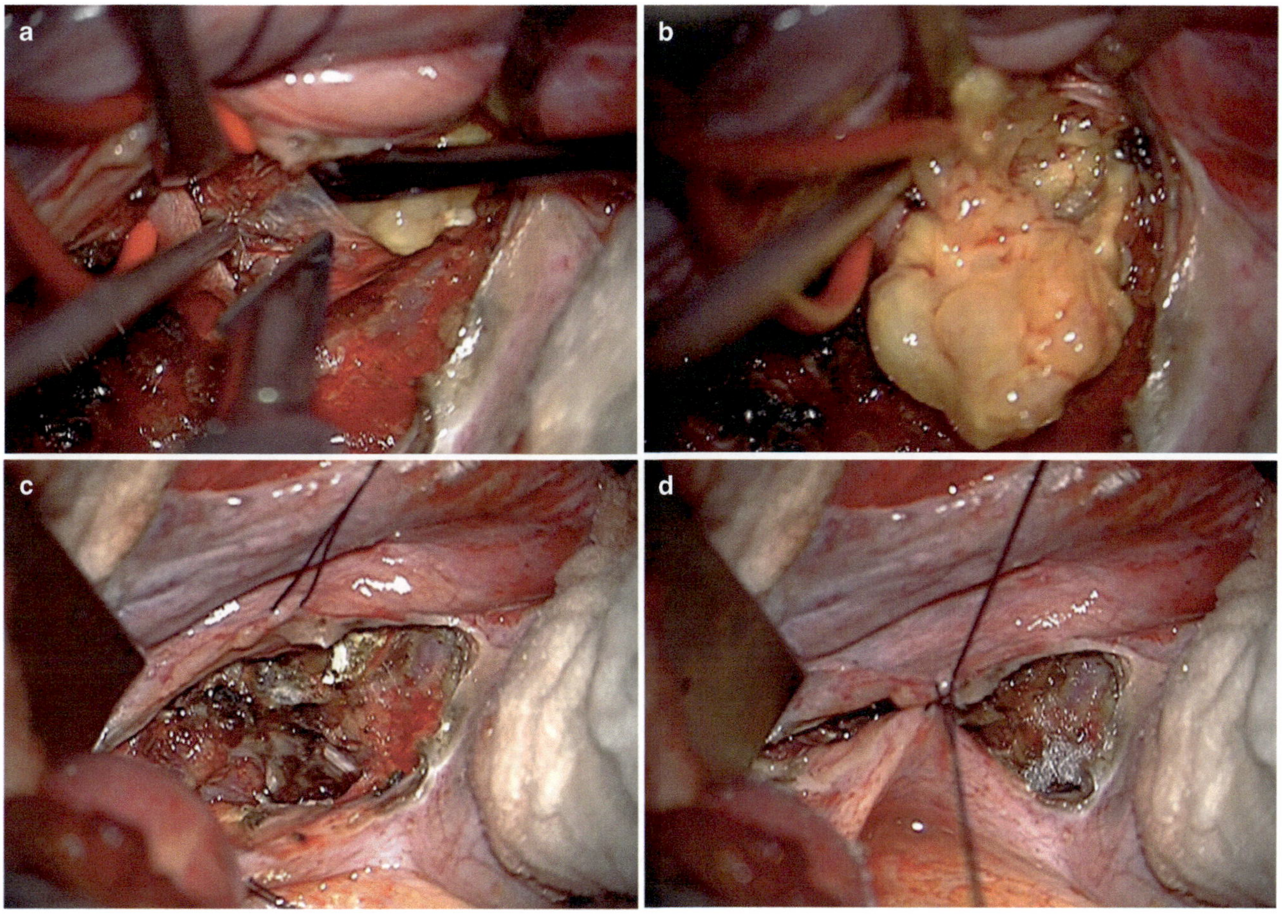

Fig. 53.11 Deep into midline transperitoneal approach from Fig. 53.10. (**a**) Detailing vascular control after using a vascular mini-Doppler for detection (*red vessel loop*) and sharp dissection. (**b**) Final proximal piecemeal tumor resection. (**c**) View after resection. (**d**) Closure of peritoneal sheath

Landmarks to Guide Anterior Approach Choice (Figs. 53.1, 53.2, and 53.12)

- Promontory
- Sacrum/ilium
- Lumbosacral spine/neuroforamina
- Psoas muscle
- Piriformis muscle
- Inguinal ligament/canalis obturatorius
- Aortic bifurcation, iliac artery
- Genitourinary tract and hypogastric plexus
- Bladder, rectum, bowels, uterus, and adnexa

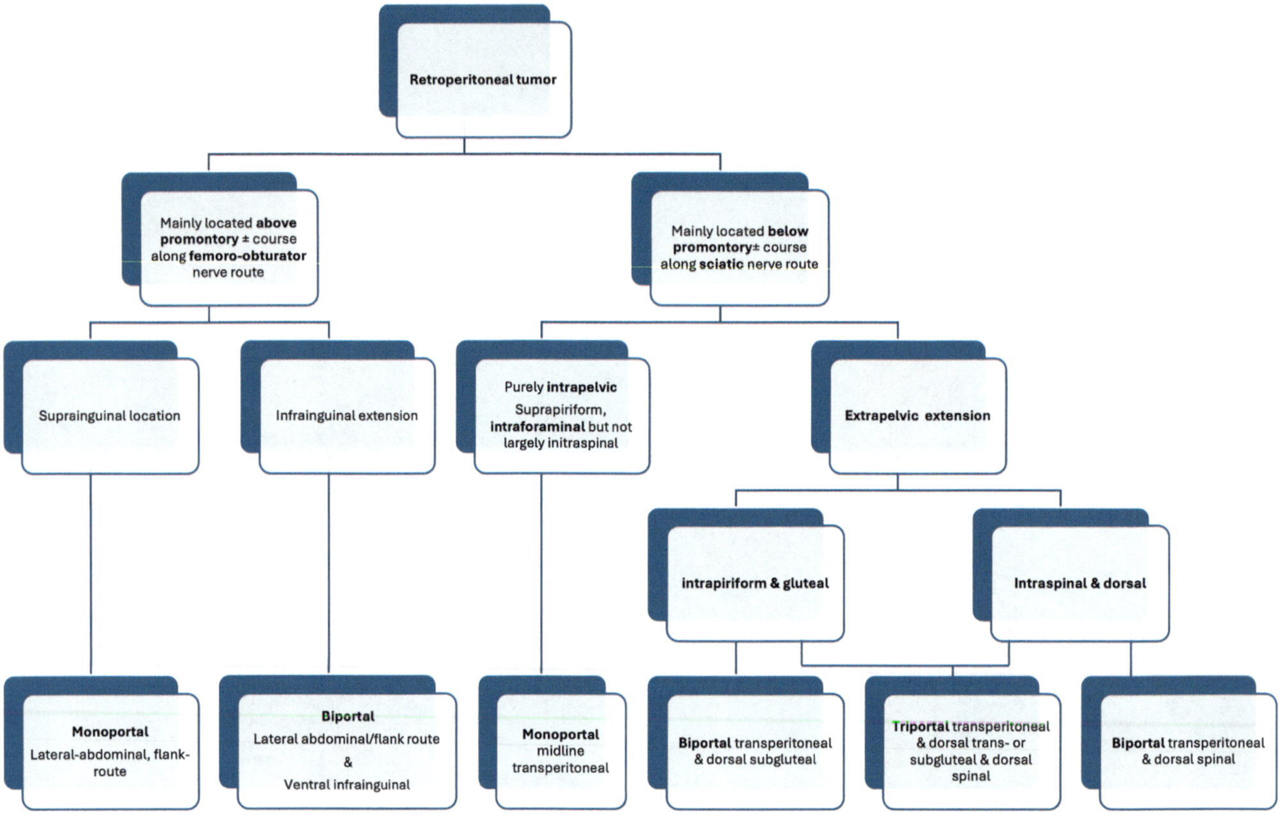

Fig. 53.12 Approach choice and combinations depending on tumor location, above or below promontory, and extension into other "compartments": along femoral/obturator or sciatic route to inguinal, infrapiriform, or intraspinal

Nerve Anatomy and Variation

Regular, guiding nerve anatomy is depicted on Fig. 53.2 (relation to retroperitoneal space landmark structures), Fig. 53.4 (deeper, in retroperitoneal pelvis), Fig. 53.9 (lumbar plexus), Fig. 53.13, and Fig. 53.14 (sacral plexus and magnification).

Lumbosacral Plexus anatomy, however, is not always as distinct as it seems. On the brachial plexus for comparison, more detailed anatomical work on variations is available. Numerous variants of "textbook anatomy" exist, and only a part of them is described. Some variants that we encountered and found relevant are (Figs. 53.15, 53.16, and 53.17):

- Split lumbar plexus with complete separation of L 1/2/3 to femoral/obturator nerve (no L4 contribution to femoral nerve; textbook L2–4), and L4/5/S1/2/3 to sciatic nerve (Fig. 53.14).
- Lateral femoral cutaneous nerve origin is variable. It can come directly off the femoral nerve (Figs. 53.2b, 53.15r, and 53.16l) or originate from L1/2 (Fig. 53.15l).
- Fiber exchange between the femoral and obturator nerves is possible.

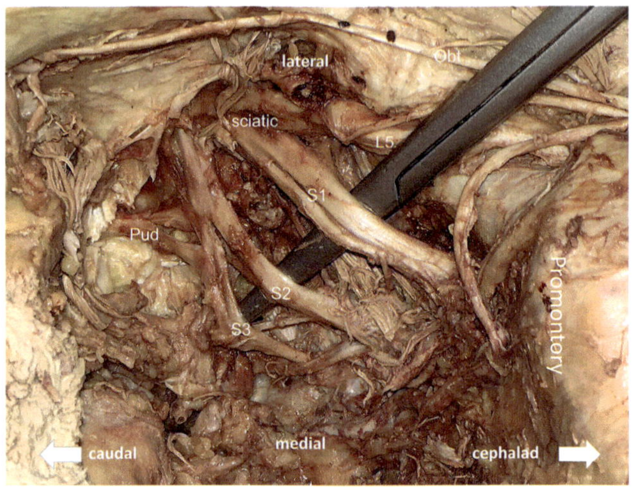

Fig. 53.13 Right sacral plexus overview

- Sciatic nerve with L3 contribution is possible (textbook L4/5/S1–3 contribute to sciatic).
- Sciatic nerve formation is variable and can be different on the left and right of the same individual (e.g., long or short course of S1–3 from neuroforamen until contribution to sciatic) (Fig. 53.17).

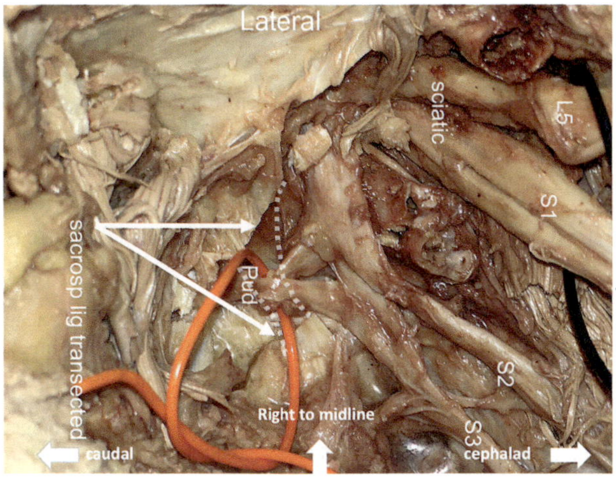

Fig. 53.14 Magnified view of right sacral plexus (enlarged from Fig. 53.13), pointing out the transected sacrospinous ligament edges. The sacrospinous ligament (*dotted lines*) roofs ventral to pudendal nerve (*Pud, orange loop)*

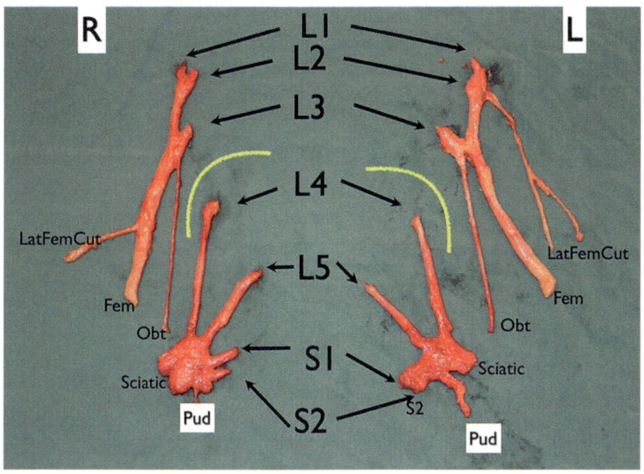

Fig. 53.15 Lumbosacral plexus, anatomical variations. Complete separation of L1–L3 to femoral/obturator nerve from L4, L5, sacral to sciatic nerve (*yellow line*). Branching of lateral femoral cutaneous nerve from femoral nerve on right, from L1/2 on left

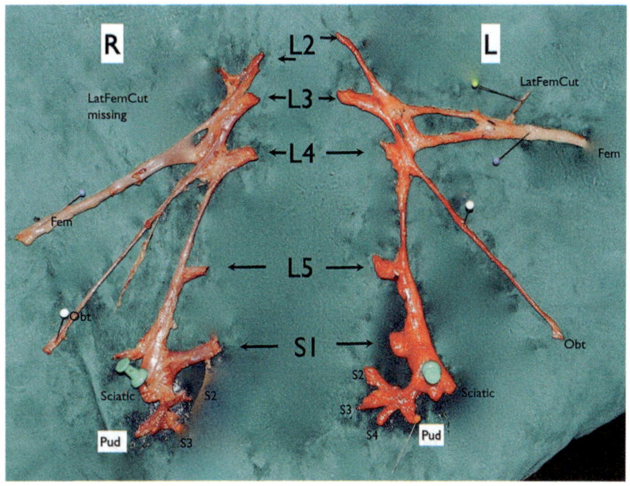

Fig. 53.16 Lumbosacral plexus anatomy. Lateral femoral cutaneous nerve directly coming off femoral nerve on left with visible connection to L2 and L3

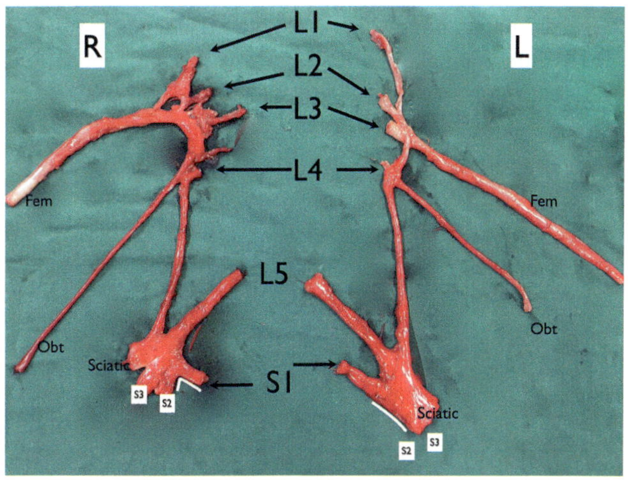

Fig. 53.17 Lumbosacral plexus anatomy. Above L5 is a more symmetrical pattern; distal to L5 is not as symmetrical. *White line* S2 and 3 inflows into sciatic

Risk and Stress Reduction

- Self-retaining retractor systems enabling strong pull with long blades that can be moved and fixed polyaxially, resting of hands
- Long (micro-) instruments
- Appropriate light in the depth
- High-resolution ultrasound and mini doppler for tumor and vessel detection
- Bladder and sphincter monitoring

Avoiding and Managing Complications

- Intraoperative nerve stimulation, running EMG of key muscles, including sphincters (if potentially affected), optional functional bladder, anal sphincter monitoring [6, 7]
- Interdisciplinary setup if not familiar with abdominal approaches
- Vascular surgeon in standby
- Vascular tray at hand for potential 3–10 mm caliber vessels (comparable to carotid at neck) repair, sutures 4-0 to 7-0, atraumatic larger size clamps with long handle, long forceps, long needle holder

References

1. Benato A, D'Alessandris QG, Murazio M, Pacelli F, Mattogno PP, Fernández E et al (2023) Integrated neurosurgical management of retroperitoneal benign nerve sheath tumors. Cancers 15(12):3138. https://doi.org/10.3390/cancers15123138
2. Heinen C, Schmidt T, Kretschmer T (2020) Decision making in retroperitoneal nerve sheath and nerve-associated tumors: a modular approach. Neurosurgery 87(3):E359–E369. https://doi.org/10.1093/neuros/nyaa020
3. Rasulić L, Grujić J, Lepić M, Savić A, Samardžić M (2020) Commentary: decision making in retroperitoneal nerve sheath and nerve-associated tumors: a modular approach. Neurosurgery 87(3):E370–E372. https://doi.org/10.1093/neuros/nyaa067
4. Improta L, Tzanis D, Bouhadiba T, Abdelhafidh K, Bonvalot S (2020) Overview of primary adult retroperitoneal tumours. Eur J Surg Oncol 46(9):1573–1579. https://doi.org/10.1016/j.ejso.2020.04.054
5. Heinen CPG, Schmidt T, Kretschmer T (2015) Endoscopically assisted piriformis-to-knee surgery of sciatic, peroneal, and tibial nerves: technical note. Neurosurgery 11(Suppl 2):37–42; discussion 42. https://doi.org/10.1227/NEU.0000000000000621
6. Guedes-Correa JF, Torrao Junior F, De Souza Moreira CA, Pirez Amorim RM (2018) The importance of intraoperative neurophysiological monitoring for resection of lumbosacral plexus tumors, vol 28. Neurol Psychiatry Brain Res, pp 7–12. https://doi.org/10.1016/j.npbr.2018.01.050
7. Kneist W, Ghadimi M, Runkel N, Moesta T, Coerper S, Benecke C et al (2023) Pelvic intraoperative neuromonitoring prevents dysfunction in patients with rectal cancer: results from a multicenter, randomized, controlled clinical trial of a NEUROmonitoring System (NEUROS). Ann Surg 277(4):e737–e744. https://doi.org/10.1097/sla.0000000000005676

Laparoscopic Approach to the Lumbosacral Plexus and Pelvic Autonomic Nerves

54

Nucelio Lemos, Gustavo L. Fernandes, and Augusta Morgado-Ribeiro

Introduction

The improvement in the quality of laparoscopy imaging and advances in anatomical studies allowed for the development of a new clinical subspecialty named Neuropelveology. Among other applications, Neuropelveologists utilize the laparoscopic approach to treat nerve entrapments on the intrapelvic portions of the lumbosacral plexus [1].

The clinical workup for the diagnosis of intrapelvic nerve entrapments is essentially based on the anamnesis, focused on determining if the patient's complaint correlates with dermatomes and myotomes of the intrapelvic bundles of the lumbosacral plexus [2].

The main symptoms suggestive of intrapelvic nerve entrapments are:

- Pain in the dermatomes of the nerves of the lumbosacral plexus,
- Vaginal/rectal foreign body sensation,
- Refractory urinary urgency associated with single-sided pain on the dermatomes of the nerves of the lumbosacral plexus,
- Refractory dyschezia (difficulty/pain with defecation) or proctalgia (rectal/anal pain), and/or
- Vesical/rectal tenesmus.

Whenever one or more of these symptoms are present, a careful assessment of the lumbosacral plexus must be performed, and the patient must only be taken to surgery after the exact site of entrapment (topographic diagnosis) has been defined [3]. The topography of the entrapment must also be confirmed with a low-volume diagnostic block. While pain distribution is key for topographical diagnosis, its characteristics, eliciting, and ameliorating factors will provide hints to the etiology of the entrapment. The main causes of intrapelvic nerve entrapments are aberrant bundles of the piriformis muscle originating medial to the sacral foramina, neurovascular conflict, fibrosis, tumors, and endometriosis. Urodynamic study is used to help differentiate between proximal and distal entrapments of the S3/S4 nerves. Magnetic Resonance Neurography (MRN) is of little use for diagnosing intrapelvic nerve entrapments, although high definition abdominopelvic (visceral) MR protocols can provide some insight on the etiology of the entrapment. Some promising initial results have been obtained with pelvic MR tractography.

Anatomical Nerve Groups

Anatomically, we divide the intrapelvic portions of the lumbosacral into three groups:

- *Proximal*: the nerve bundles proximal to the crossing of the internal iliac veins, namely the proximal portions of the sacral nerves, the pelvic splanchnic nerves, the inferior hypogastric plexus, the hypogastric nerves, and the superior hypogastric plexus.
- *Distal*: those fibers distal to the crossing of the internal iliac vein, namely the obturator, superior and inferior gluteal, sciatic and pudendal nerves, the distal portions of the sacral nerve roots and the nerve to the levator ani muscle, and the lumbosacral trunk.

Supplementary Information The online version contains supplementary material available at https://doi.org/10.1007/978-3-031-73931-6_54.

N. Lemos (✉)
Temerty Faculty of Medicine, University of Toronto, Toronto, ON, Canada
e-mail: nucelio.lemos@utoronto.ca

G. L. Fernandes
Department of Gynecologic Oncology at Santa Casa, São Paulo, Brazil
e-mail: gustavo.fernandes@increasing.com.br

A. Morgado-Ribeiro
Neuropelveology at UNIFESP, São Paulo, Brazil
e-mail: augusta.morgado@increasing.com.br

A. S. Hanna (ed.), *Nerves: Anatomy, Exposures, and Techniques*, https://doi.org/10.1007/978-3-031-73931-6_54

– *Lateral*: the genitofemoral nerve and the nerves lateral to the psoas muscle, namely the femoral, lateral femoral cutaneous, ilioinguinal, and iliohypogastric nerves.

In the following paragraphs, we describe the steps for the laparoscopic access to such portions of the plexus.

General Principles of Laparoscopic Surgery

Laparoscopic access to the pelvic cavity is achieved by insufflating the abdomen with CO_2 at a pressure of 15 mmHg. A 10 mm camera port is placed in the umbilicus, and 3–4 ancillary 5 mm ports are placed in the lower abdomen. After a general survey of the abdominal cavity and lysis of adhesions is performed, the retroperitoneal spaces are developed as described in the sections below.

Proximal Approach

Indications [3, 4]

- Explore and approach entrapments of the proximal portions of the sacral nerves.
- Treatment of deep infiltrating parametrial endometriosis.
- Nerve-sparing techniques of the pararectal space.

Step-by-Step Dissection

1. Incise of the parietal peritoneum at the midline, just over the sacral promontory.
2. Develop the retrorectal space and identify the presacral fascia and the hypogastric nerve (Fig. 54.1).
3. Open the presacral fascia lateral to the hypogastric nerve to develop the presacral space (Fig. 54.2).
4. Expand the dissection of the presacral space laterally towards the hypogastric fascia (lateral limit of presacral space).
5. Open the hypogastric fascia, revealing the piriformis underneath.
6. Identify the sacral nerves coursing in an antero-distal direction over the ventral surface of the piriformis (Fig. 54.3). Of note, about 30% of the population have a variant piriformis muscle bundle originating medial to the sacral foramina, causing the sacral nerves to have an intramuscular course.
7. Identification of the different sacral nerves can be confirmed by intraoperative stimulation with intraoperative neuromonitoring or observation of the motor response:
   (a) S2—outward rotation of the leg, plantar flexion of the foot and lateral toes, and clamp-like squeeze of the anal sphincter from anterior to posterior

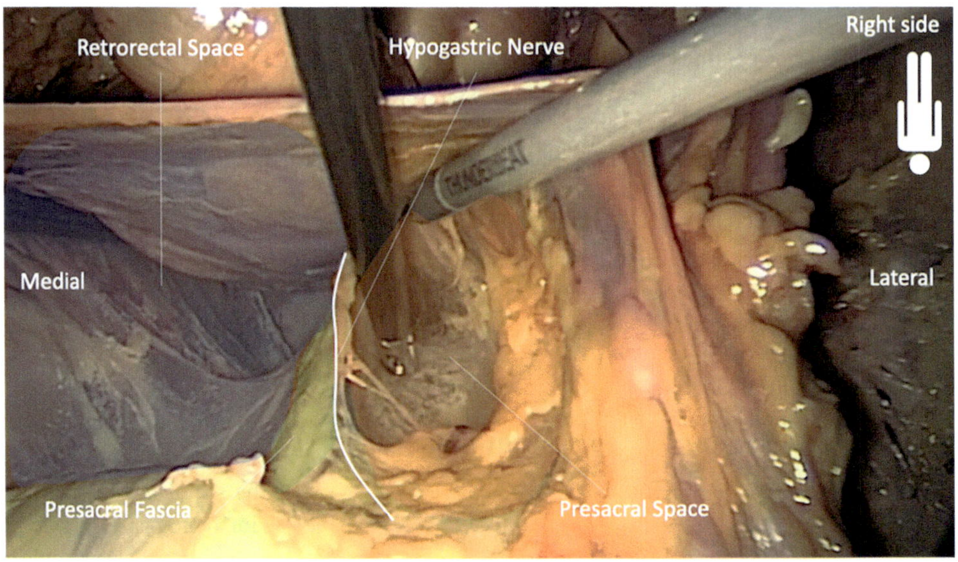

Fig. 54.1 Retrorectal space medially (left). Opened presacral fascia and hypogastric nerve showing the developed the presacral space laterally (right)

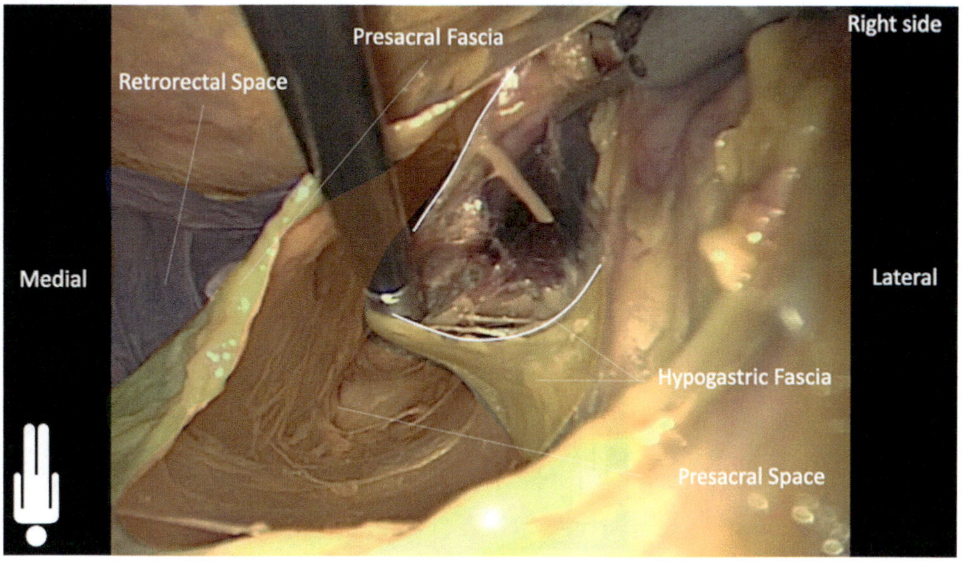

Fig. 54.2 Presacral fascia limiting the retrorectal space posteriorly (left) and the developed presacral space anteriorly (right), limited by the opened hypogastric fascia

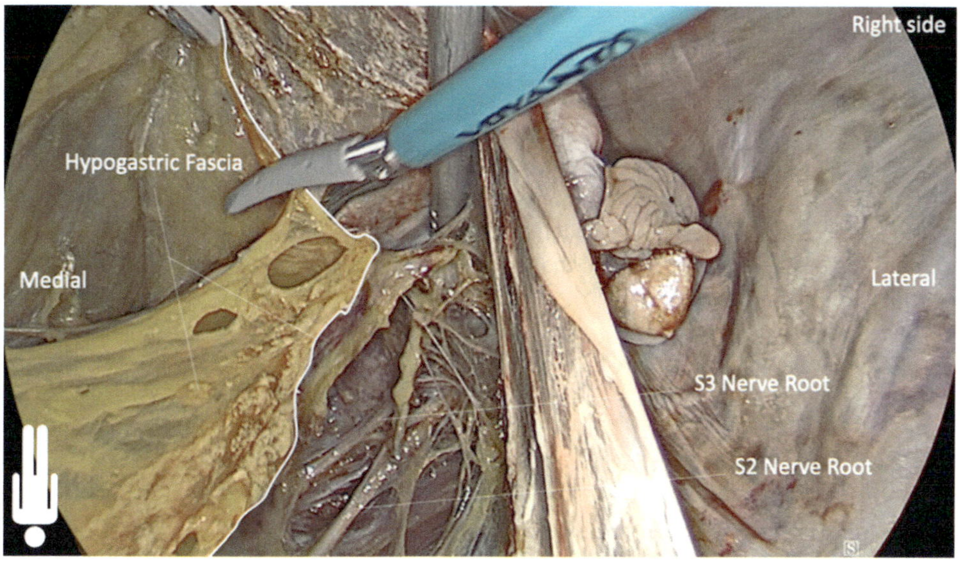

Fig. 54.3 Opened hypogastric fascia medially (left), revealing the sacral roots underneath (right)

(b) S3—deepening and deepening of the buttock groove and marked flexion of the large toe and less important flexion of other toes
(c) S4—anal sphincter contraction

8. Following the sacral nerves ventrally will expose the pelvic splanchnic nerves sprouting out just before the crossing under the internal iliac vein (Fig. 54.4).

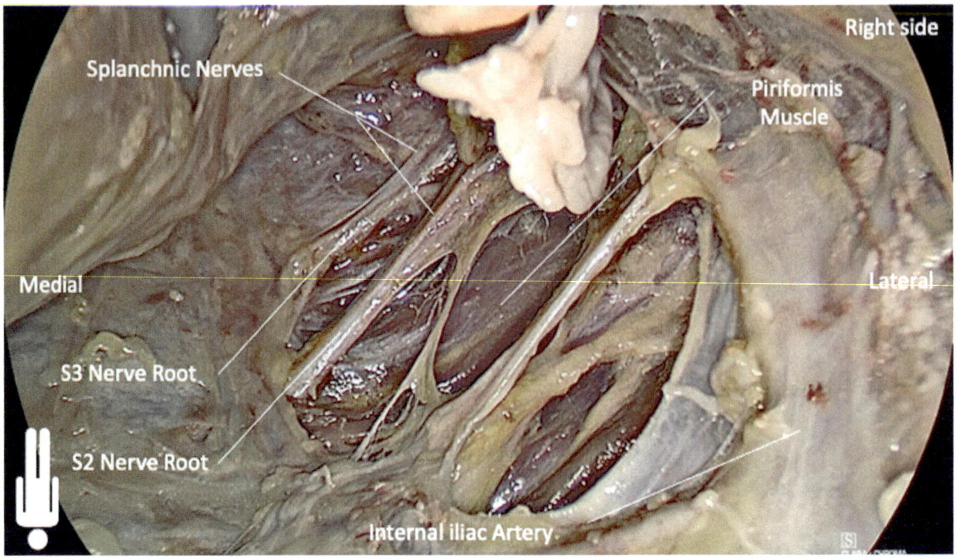

Fig. 54.4 Sacral nerves coursing in an antero-distal direction over the ventral surface of the piriformis muscle, pelvic splanchnic nerves sprouting out its ventral surface just before the crossing under the internal iliac vein

Distal Approach

Indications

- Treatment of deep infiltrating parametrial endometriosis.
- Laparoscopic release of the obturator, superior and inferior gluteal, sciatic and pudendal nerves, the distal portions of the sacral nerves and the nerve to the levator ani, and the lumbosacral trunk [5].
- Laparoscopic implantation of neuromodulators for rehabilitation of spinal cord-injured patients.

Step-by-Step Dissection

1. Peritoneal incision between the external iliac vessels and the psoas muscle to develop the obturator space and the iliolumbar fossa (Fig. 54.5).
2. Find the abdominal origin of the obturator nerve under the medial aspect of the psoas muscle.
3. Identify the lumbosacral trunk above the sacroiliac joint.
4. Extend the dissection distally into the obturator and the retropubic spaces.
5. Following the lumbosacral trunk, progressively dissect the sciatic perineurial fat and expose the superior gluteal and sciatic nerves (Fig. 54.6).
6. Carry forward with the dissection and medial retraction of the internal iliac vessels to expose the distal S3/S4 nerves between the inferior gluteal and pudendal vessels.
7. Identify the sacrospinous ligament and proximal pudendal nerve.
8. To expose the interligament and intracanal portions of the pudendal nerve, transect the sacrospinous ligament, retract the iliococcygeus, and carefully open the pudendal (Alcock's) canal (Figs. 54.7 and 54.8).

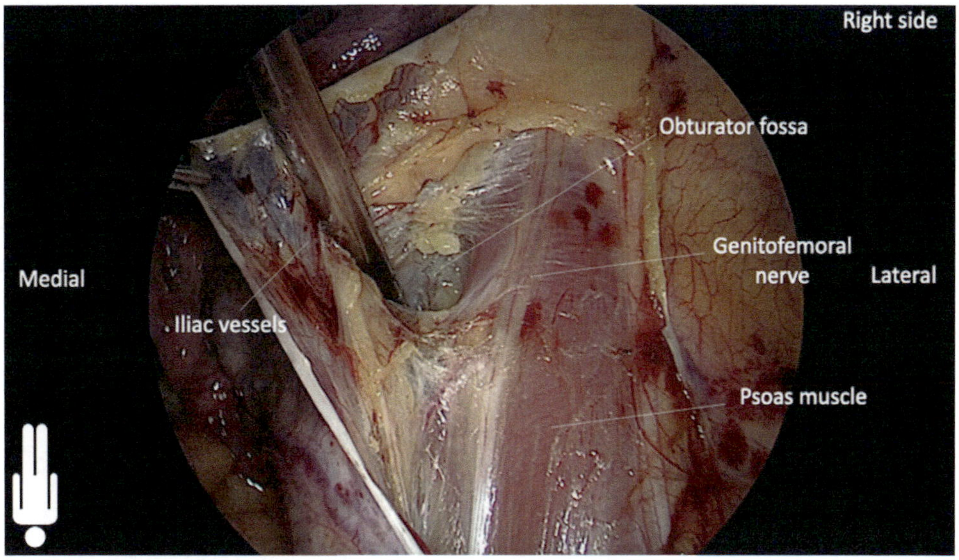

Fig. 54.5 Peritoneal incision between the external iliac vessels and the psoas muscle to develop the obturator space and the iliolumbar fossa

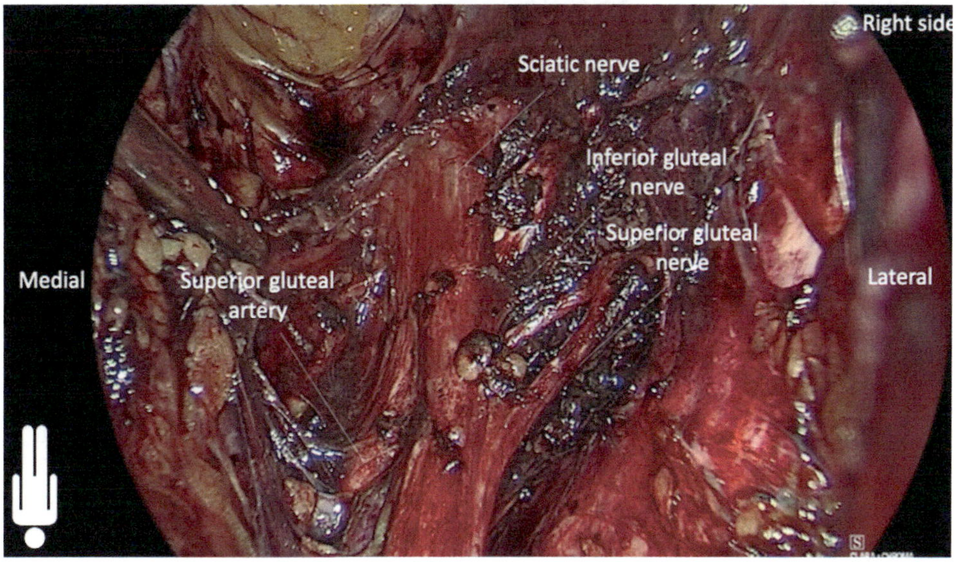

Fig. 54.6 Exposure of sciatic nerve and gluteal nerves and vessels

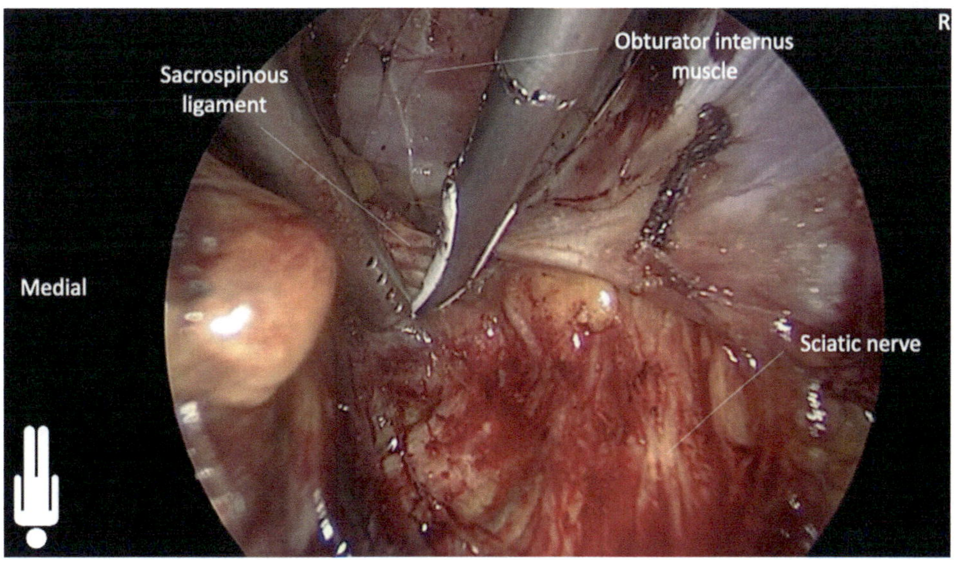

Fig. 54.7 Section of the sacrospinous ligament

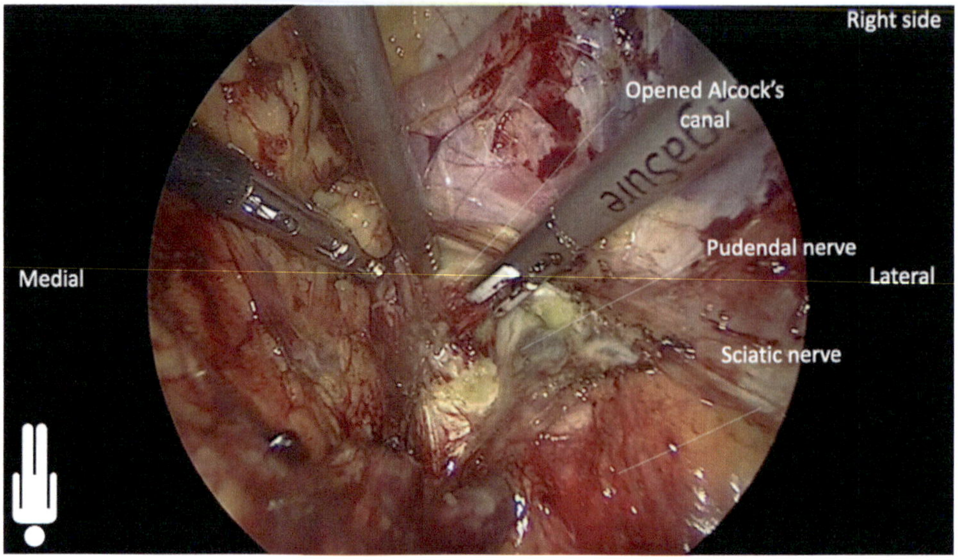

Fig. 54.8 Opening of the Alcock's canal and exposure of the pudendal nerve

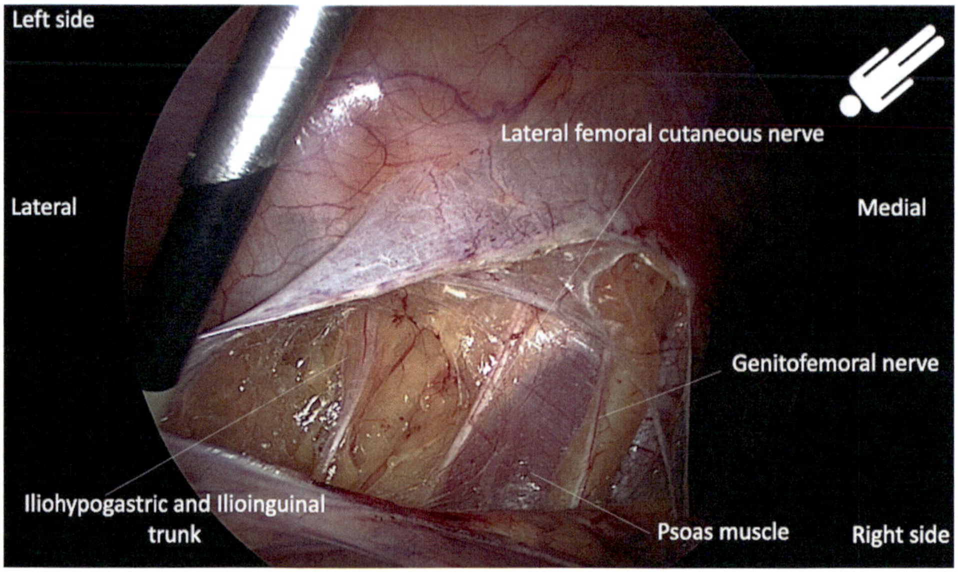

Fig. 54.9 Exposure of genitofemoral, lateral femoral cutaneous, ilioinguinal, and iliohypogastric nerves

Lateral Approach

Indications

- Laparoscopic neurolysis of the genitofemoral nerve and the nerves lateral to the psoas muscle, namely the femoral, lateral femoral cutaneous, ilioinguinal, and iliohypogastric nerves.
- Perform neurectomies as indicated for pain.
- Laparoscopic implantation of neuromodulators for rehabilitation of spinal cord-injured patients.

Step-by-Step Dissection

1. Incise the peritoneum over the psoas muscle to identify the genitofemoral nerve.
2. Develop the parieto-psoic space and identify the fascia transversalis and the lateral femoral cutaneous nerve running in parallel to the psoas muscle.
3. Extend the dissection proximally and identify the ilioinguinal and iliohypogastric nerves (Fig. 54.9).
4. Pierce the fascia transversalis between the lateral femoral cutaneous nerve and the psoas muscle and identify the femoral nerve.

Complications

In our series, overall complication rate was 16.7%. These included:

- pudendal nerve transection/tear,
- genitofemoral traction neuropathy,
- incisional hernia, and
- adhesion of the distal portion of the transected piriformis muscle to the deep gluteal portion of the sciatic nerve requiring a transgluteal endoscopic procedure.

References

1. Possover R, Chiantera. (2004) The "Laparoscopic Neuro-Navigation"—LANN: from a functional cartography of the pelvic autonomous neurosystem to a new field of laparoscopic surgery. Minim Invasive Ther Allied Technol 13(5):362–367. https://doi.org/10.1080/13645700410005392
2. Lemos N, D'Amico N, Marques R, Kamergorodsky G, Schor E, Girão MJ (2016) Recognition and treatment of endometriosis involving the sacral nerve roots. Int Urogynecol J 27(1):147–150. https://doi.org/10.1007/s00192-015-2703-z. Epub 2015 Apr 25
3. Lemos N, Souza C, Marques RM, Kamergorodsky G, Schor E, Girão MJ (2015) Laparoscopic anatomy of the autonomic nerves of the pelvis and the concept of nerve-sparing surgery by direct visualization of autonomic nerve bundles. Fertil steril 104(5):e11–e12. https://doi.org/10.1016/j.fertnstert.2015.07.1138. Epub 2015 Aug 8
4. Possover M, Chiantera V, Baekelandt J (2007) Anatomy of the sacral roots and the pelvic splanchnic nerves in women using the LANN technique. Surg Laparosc Endosc Percutan Tech 17(6):508–510. https://doi.org/10.1097/SLE.0b013e31812f81e4
5. Lemos N, Sermer C, Fernandes G, Morgado-Ribeiro A, Rossos A, Zhao ZY et al (2021) Laparoscopic approach to refractory extraspinal sciatica and pudendal pain caused by intrapelvic nerve entrapment. Sci Rep 11(1):10820. https://doi.org/10.1038/s41598-021-90319-y

Intraneural Ganglion Cysts

55

Amgad S. Hanna

Mechanism of Formation

Intraneural ganglion cysts typically arise from a degenerated joint. Synovial fluid builds under pressure and exits the joint through an articular branch of a nerve (Fig. 55.1). This can spread retrograde to involve the parent nerve. The classic example is the common peroneal nerve and the superior tibiofibular joint (Fig. 55.2).

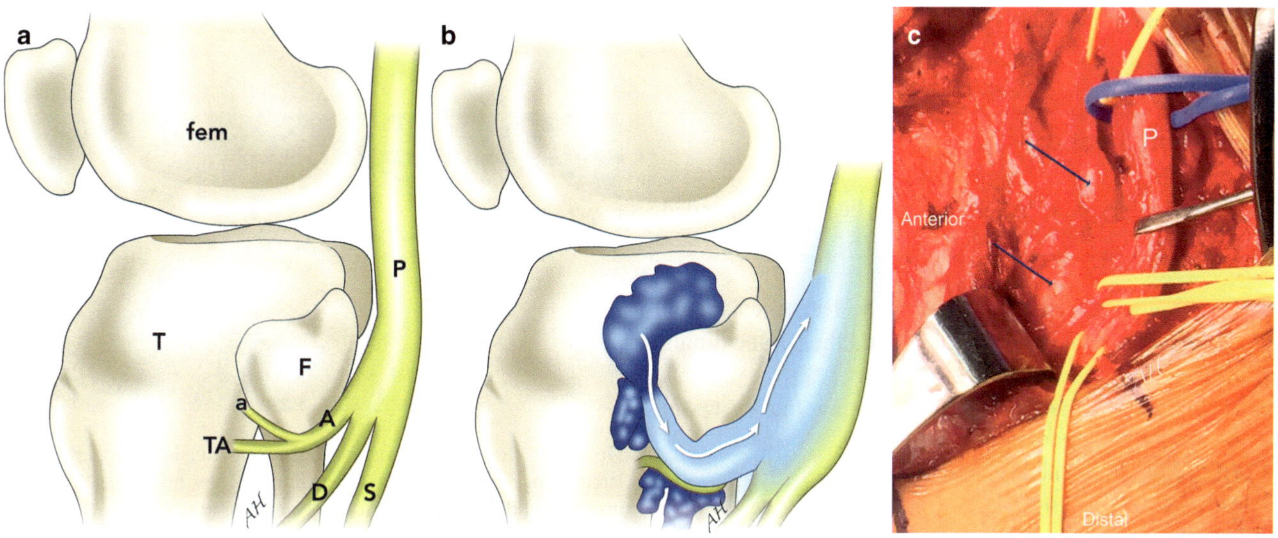

Fig. 55.1 (**a**) Normal branching of the peroneal nerve (*P*). *S* superficial peroneal, *D* deep peroneal, *A* articular trunk, *TA* tibialis anterior branch, *a* articular branch proper. *T* tibia, *F* fibula, *fem* femur. (**b**) Intraneural ganglion cyst formation. Arthritis of the superior tibiofibular joint causes synovial fluid buildup under pressure and retrograde filling of the nerve (*arrows*). *Light blue* intraneural ganglion cyst, *dark blue* extraneural cysts. Copyright Amgad Hanna. Published with permission. (**c**) Ganglion cysts (*arrows*) associated with left peroneal nerve (*P*)

Supplementary Information The online version contains supplementary material available at https://doi.org/10.1007/978-3-031-73931-6_55.

A. S. Hanna (✉)
Department of Neurosurgery, University of Wisconsin School of Medicine and Public Health, Madison, WI, USA

A. S. Hanna (ed.), *Nerves: Anatomy, Exposures, and Techniques*, https://doi.org/10.1007/978-3-031-73931-6_55

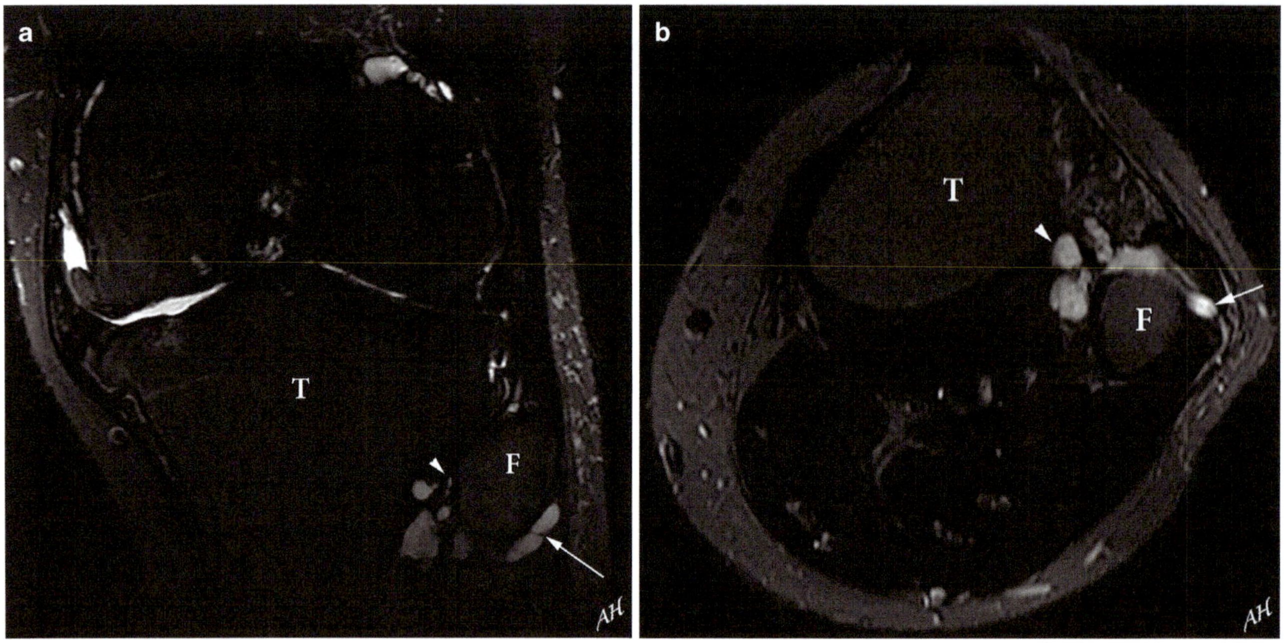

Fig. 55.2 Coronal (**a**) and axial (**b**) T2-weighted fat-saturated MRI of the left knee showing ganglion cyst along the left peroneal nerve (*arrow*) and in the superior tibiofibular joint (STFJ) (*arrowhead*). *T* tibia, *F* fibula

Treatment Strategy

To prevent recurrence, the following has been recommended: **4Ds**

1. **D**ecompress the nerve by releasing the deep fascia around the nerve as well as the fascia around the peroneal muscles overlying the nerve.
2. **D**rain the intraneural cyst by opening the cyst wall through its thinnest part.
3. **D**isconnect the articular branch.
4. **D**rill the related joint, possibly.

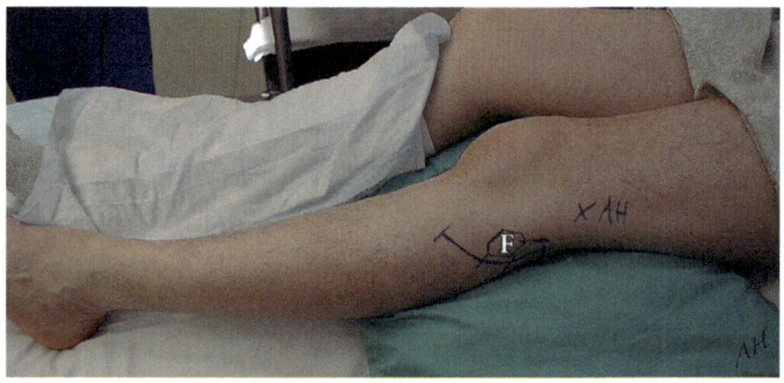

Fig. 55.3 The patient is positioned supine with a bump under the ipsilateral hip. *F* marks the surface anatomy of the fibular head with the insertion of the biceps femoris tendon cranial to it

Surgical Technique for Peroneal Intraneural Ganglion Cyst [1]

1. The patient is positioned supine with a bump to allow access to the anterior and the lateral aspects of the knee joint (Fig. 55.3).
2. The common peroneal nerve and its branches are exposed (Chap. 28) (Fig. 55.4). The incision is extended more anteriorly to access the superior tibio-fibular joint (STFJ). Care should be taken when using the scalpel or the Bovie cautery since the nerve can be ballooned and very superficial.
3. The nerve is thicker than usual, and the wall can be very thin from cystic dilatation.

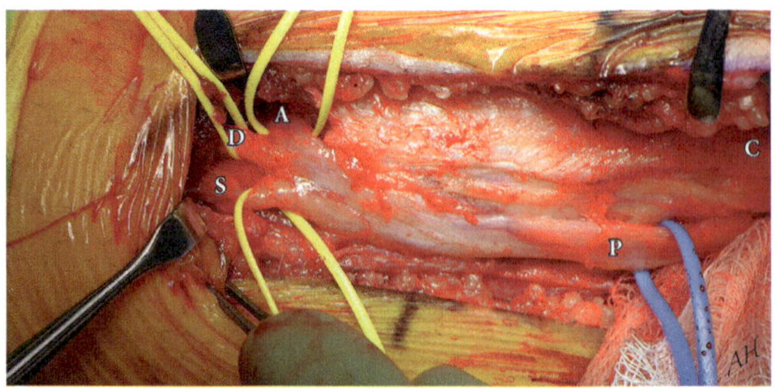

Fig. 55.4 The common peroneal (fibular) nerve (*P*) is exposed with its terminal branches: superficial (*S*), deep (*D*), and articular (*A*) trunk. Note the dilated articular branch and the adjacent peroneal nerve. *C* cranial. The nerve sheath should be opened to drain the cyst

4. The intraneural cyst can be decompressed using an 11-blade; a slit is made along the nerve axis, and the synovial fluid is expressed out. This allows further dissection without nerve damage.
5. The nerve is followed distally until its trifurcation (superficial peroneal, deep peroneal, and articular trunk). The articular trunk gives off a tibialis anterior motor branch before becoming pure sensory. The articular branch is then followed till the STFJ.
6. The STFJ can be resected or fused. Resection is achieved by removal of the articular surface of the fibular head (Fig. 55.5). Some bone growth substitute (e.g., demineralized bone matrix) can be placed in the resected joint space to enhance fusion. Some surgeons skip this step and are content with resection of the articular branch.
7. The articular branch proper is then resected (Fig. 55.6).

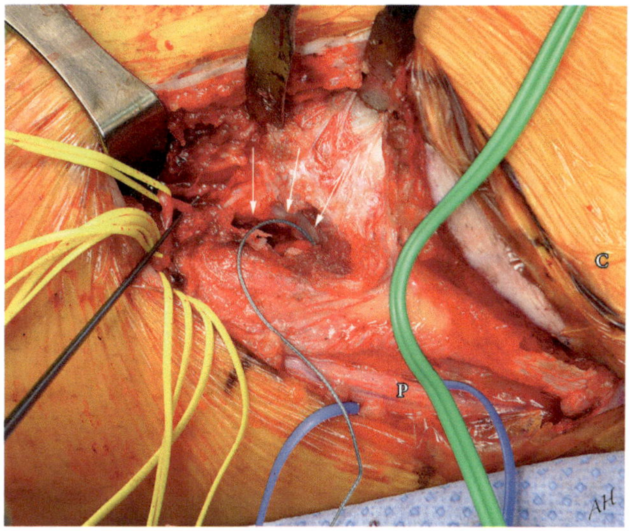

Fig. 55.6 The branch entering the STFJ from the articular branch is identified (*nerve hook*) and resected. Note that the STFJ has been resected (*arrows*), wax was used to stop bleeding from the bony surface. *P* common peroneal nerve, *C* cranial

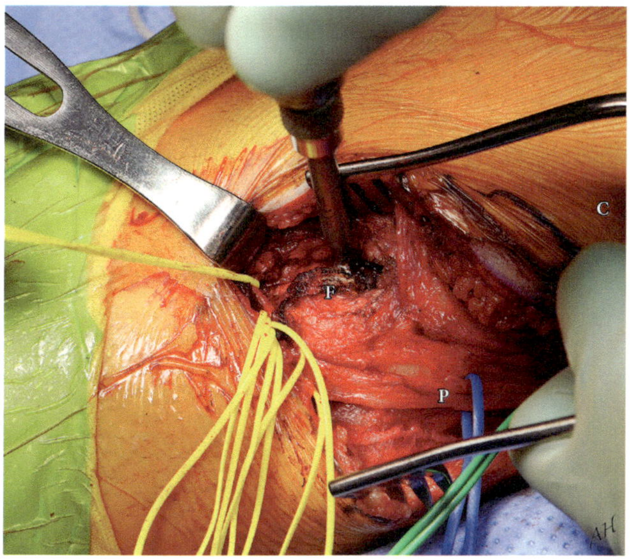

Fig. 55.5 The STFJ is resected using a drill. *F* fibular head, *P* common peroneal nerve, *C* cranial

Reference

1. Spinner RJ, Desy NM, Rock MG, Amrami KK (2007) Peroneal intraneural ganglia. Part I. Techniques for successful diagnosis and treatment. Neurosurg Focus 22(6):E16

56 Flaccid Facial Paralysis

Adolfo Zamora-Madrazo and Shai M. Rozen

Guiding Principles

"Time is muscle" in the setting of complete facial paralysis. In patients with acute (<72 h) and subacute (72 h to 12–18 months) facial paralysis, the main goal is to salvage the patient's own mimetic muscles. This may be accomplished through primary neurorrhaphy (e.g., sharp lacerating trauma), nerve grafting when a nerve gap precluding tension-free coaptations exists, and/or nerve transfers. Interposition nerve grafting is performed in patients in which (1) both the proximal and distal facial nerve stumps can be visualized, (2) nerve continuity to the brain proximally and mimetic muscles distally remains, and (3) tension-free coaptation is not possible, thus excluding primary neurorrhaphy. When the proximal facial nerve stump is not visualized (e.g., intratemporal facial nerve injury), a local nerve transfer is performed often in combination with a cross-facial nerve graft (CFNG) from the healthy side with the purpose of increasing synchroneity and possibly spontaneity. In patients presenting with long-standing facial paralysis (i.e., 18–24 months), salvage of mimetic muscle is less likely, and introduction of a new neuromuscular unit via a free muscle transplant or local muscle transfer is indicated [1].

Supplementary Information The online version contains supplementary material available at https://doi.org/10.1007/978-3-031-73931-6_56.

A. Zamora-Madrazo
Department of General Surgery, Hospital General de México
Dr. Eduardo Liceaga, Ciudad de méxico, Mexico

S. M. Rozen (✉)
Department of Plastic and Reconstructive Surgery, University of Texas Southwestern Medical Center, Dallas, TX, USA
e-mail: Shai.Rozen@UTSouthwestern.edu

Intersegmental Facial Nerve Graft

Indication

Patients with acute or subacute facial paralysis with identified proximal and distal facial nerve stumps (e.g., sharp laceration), where tension-free primary coaptation is not feasible, thus disqualifying primary neurorrhaphy [1].

Surgical Technique

1. In trauma cases, whether a preauricular incision is made or whether the wound is directly explored depends on the clinical scenario and the experience and preference of the surgeon. In other settings, a preauricular incision is advised.
2. Perform a preauricular incision with a 15-blade and achieve hemostasis with bipolar electrocautery. Clean bloodless surgical planes are important for the identification of nerve branches and to avoid unnecessary trauma.
3. The first 0.5 cm of the dissection is performed in a subcutaneous plane, and the remainder of the dissection is performed in the superficial musculoaponeurotic system (SMAS) plane, just superficial to the parotid-masseteric fascia. It is important to leave the sub-SMAS fat attached to the SMAS so the facial nerve branches are more readily identified deep to the parotid-masseteric fascia before innervating the mimetic muscles of the midface on their deep surface (Fig. 56.1).
4. Parotid dissection can be done either in a retrograde or anterograde approach, with reference to the anterior border of the parotid gland. In proximal facial nerve injuries, retrograde dissection is preferred, whereas anterograde dissection is more likely to benefit in a scenario of distal injury of the facial nerve branches.
5. After parotid dissection, confirm availability of both proximal and distal facial nerve stumps, and reconsider if

A. S. Hanna (ed.), *Nerves: Anatomy, Exposures, and Techniques*, https://doi.org/10.1007/978-3-031-73931-6_56

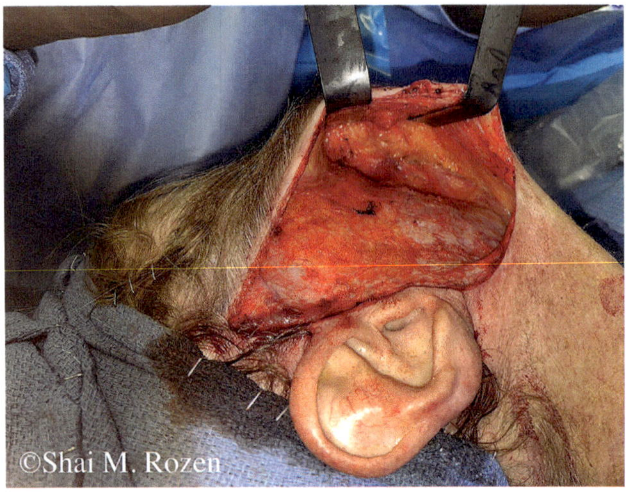

Fig. 56.1 Preauricular incision and sub-SMAS dissection. It is important to leave the sub-SMAS fat attached to the SMAS. SMAS superficial musculoaponeurotic system. (Used with permission of Shai M. Rozen, MD for Medical Education and Research. All rights reserved)

the gap excludes primary neurorrhaphy after sufficient mobilization of both stumps.
6. Any of the following is a good potential nerve graft donor: the sural nerve is identified 2 cm posterior to the lateral malleolus, the great auricular nerve at the mid-third of the sternocleidomastoid 3 cm inferior to the earlobe, the lateral antebrachial cutaneous nerve (LABC) near the cephalic vein in the proximal aspect of the lateral forearm, or the anterior division of the medial antebrachial cutaneous nerve (MABC) anterior to the basilic vein.
7. Donor nerve can be readily harvested under loupe magnification (3.5×–4.5×) with fine tenotomy scissors.
8. Using a microscope, the stumps of the injured nerve should be freshened in a guillotine fashion with a new 15-blade on top of a tongue depressor, and then meticulous tension-free epineural coaptation with a 10-0 to 11-0 nylon suture is performed.

Complications

1. Failure to restore motion of paralyzed neuromuscular units
2. Sensory deficit from nerve graft donor site
3. Neuroma of donor site

Masseter Nerve Transfer

Indication

A donor nerve is a branch or a section of a nerve in the region of the injured facial nerve which may be directly coapted to the distal injured nerve but does not have the function of the original injured nerve, in this case, the facial nerve. Options include the masseter nerve (V2 cranial nerve [CN] branch), the hemi-hypoglossal nerve (XII CN), and the spinal accessory nerve (XI CN). In fact, the first nerve transfer reported was in 1903 by Sir Charles Alfred Ballance on an 11-year-old boy with facial nerve palsy after surgery for otitis media. He performed an end-to-side facial to spinal accessory nerve transfer in 1895 in St Thomas Hospital, London. The main indication is in patients with acute or subacute facial paralysis with an unavailable proximal facial nerve stump (e.g., intracranial or intratemporal nerve injury). A nerve transfer may be done as part of a "babysitter procedure" in which the local nerve transfer provides sufficient axonal load to salvage the neuromuscular unit until a cross-facial nerve graft has achieved complete axonal growth to potentially provide additional synchroneity and possible spontaneity (i.e., an emotional smile) [2, 3].

Surgical Technique

1. Perform a preauricular incision with a 15-blade and achieve hemostasis with bipolar electrocautery.
2. The first 0.5 cm of the dissection is performed in a subcutaneous plane, and the remainder of the dissection is performed in the SMAS plane, just superficial to the parotid-masseteric fascia. It is important to leave the sub-SMAS fat attached to the SMAS so the facial nerve branches are more readily identified deep to the parotid-masseteric fascia before innervating the mimetic muscles of the midface on their deep surface.
3. Dissection of the masseter nerve begins safely when considering four constant anatomical landmarks: the zygomatic arch, mandibular condyle, mandibular notch, and coronoid process [2] (Fig. 56.2).
4. Dissection proceeds through the parotid while preserving all paralyzed facial nerve branches since these will be coapted to the donor masseter nerve. Dissection then proceeds deep into the superficial and middle portions of the masseter muscle until the anterior (often called oblique) branch of the masseter nerve is identified. It is cut as distally as possible to allow easy coaptation on the surface of the parotid.
5. Once the recipient facial nerve is chosen (this may be a specific branch or a more proximal trunk), it is cut proximally and coapted to the masseter donor nerve under a microscope with a 9-0 nylon suture.

Complications (Rare)

1. Failure to restore motion of paralyzed neuromuscular units due to technical failure, lack of axonal growth

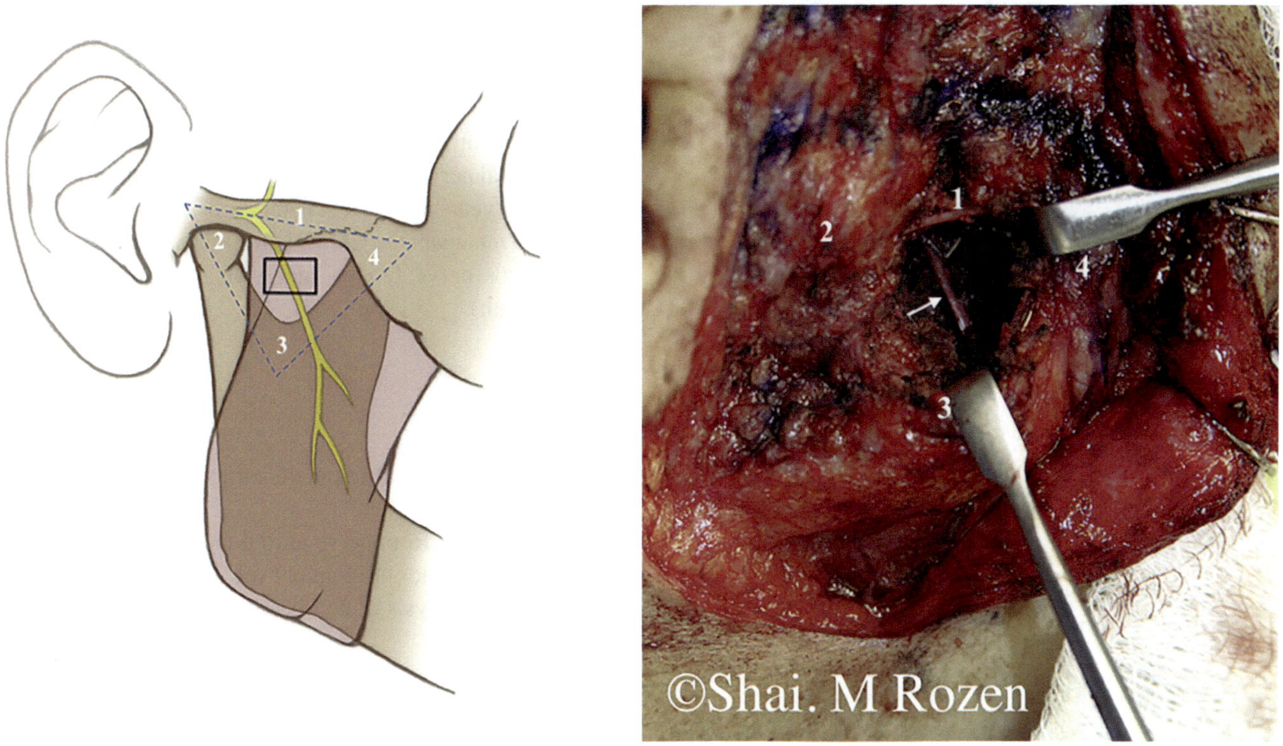

Fig. 56.2 Masseter nerve dissection. Four constant anatomical landmarks for identifying the masseter nerve (*arrow*): zygomatic arch (*1*), mandibular condyle (*2*), mandibular notch (*3*), and coronoid process (*4*). (Used with permission of Shai M. Rozen, MD for Medical Education and Research. All rights reserved [2])

through the coaptation (i.e., neurotoxic agents given with chemotherapy), or failure of the surgeon to identify discontinuity of the facial nerve into the mimetic muscles.
2. Parotid leak.

Cross-Facial Nerve Graft (CFNG)

Indication

A CFNG can be used in several settings. It may be used as part of a babysitter procedure with a nerve transfer in patients with acute or subacute facial paralysis and an unavailable proximal facial nerve stump. In cases with long-standing facial paralysis, a CFNG can also be used to innervate a muscle transplant (i.e., gracilis) in the paralyzed hemiface, coaptating it to a healthy donor facial nerve branch in the non-paralyzed hemiface [5].

Sural Nerve Harvesting

1. Identify the sural nerve midway between the lateral malleolus and the Achilles tendon and harvest via several skip incisions in an ascending fashion (Fig. 56.3) if both lateral and medial sural nerve contributions are needed. Otherwise, the nerve may be harvested via 1 or 2 incisions with a nerve stripper or endoscopically.
2. Harvesting both the tibial and peroneal contributions to the sural nerve provides additional graft material and may be used as two grafts after internal separation within the sural nerve is performed.

Facial Dissection and Nerve Grafting

1. On the non-paralyzed hemiface, perform a preauricular incision with a 15-blade and achieve hemostasis with bipolar electrocautery. Clean, bloodless surgical planes are important for the identification of nerve branches and to avoid unnecessary trauma.
2. The first 0.5 cm of the dissection is performed in a subcutaneous plane, and the following dissection is performed in the SMAS plane, just superficial to the parotid-masseteric fascia. It is important to leave the sub-SMAS fat attached to the SMAS so the facial nerve branches are more readily identified deep to the parotid-masseteric fascia before innervating the mimetic muscles of the midface on their deep surface.
3. Once the anterior border of the parotid gland is reached (unto the mobile SMAS), the individual facial nerve

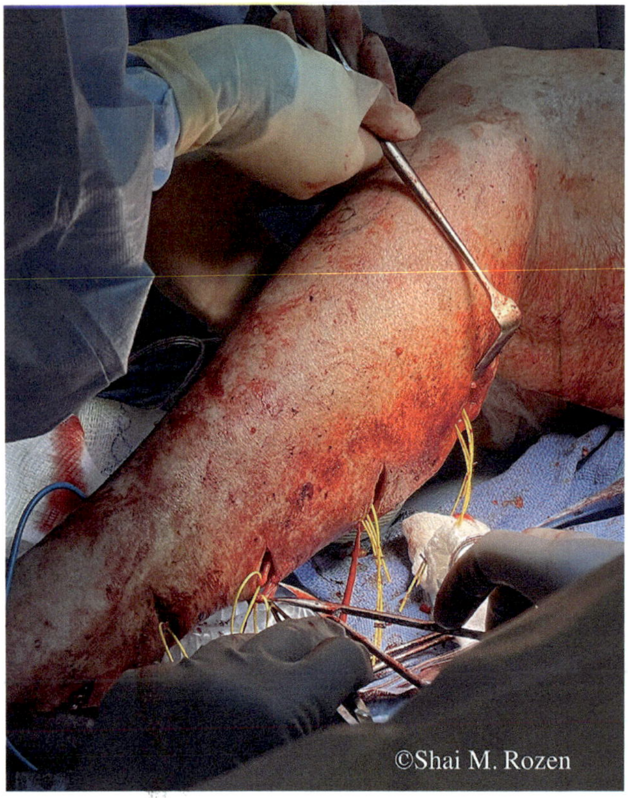

Fig. 56.3 Sural nerve harvest. Skip incisions in an ascending fashion. (Used with permission of Shai M. Rozen, MD for Medical Education and Research. All rights reserved)

branches can be identified, and the facial nerve is stimulated and mapped.

4. Choosing a correct donor branch necessitates two conditions: (1) The branch needs to perform the correct function. (2) Redundancy in function is needed so sacrifice of the branch will not cause paralysis of the normal side.
5. Once the donor branches are identified, dissection converts into the subcutaneous plane, dissecting towards the modiolus and the upper lip.
6. On the paralyzed hemiface, the preauricular incision and initial dissection are performed in a similar sub-SMAS fashion beyond the mobile SMAS.
7. Subcutaneous dissection is performed toward the upper lip, and small incisions are made either on the upper gingival buccal sulcus above the first or second molars or in the nares.
8. Passing the CFNG from one hemiface to the other can be done using one of several techniques. The sural nerve may be attached to a 6 Fr red rubber feeding tube, which has been passed between the previously performed hemiface incisions, then pulled, or the nerve may simply be pulled with a long and thin tendon passer.
9. On the non-paralyzed hemiface, after meticulous freshening of the CFNG end with a fresh blade, perform a meticulous tension-free epineural coaptation of the CFNG to the selected healthy facial nerve branch(es) with 10-0 to 11-0 nylon sutures in an end-to-end fashion.
10. The surgeon may choose to coapt the CFNG to the recipient facial nerve branch(es) on the paralyzed hemiface or do so a year later as a separate procedure. In a muscle transplant, coapt the CFNG to the muscle nerve (e.g., the obturator nerve branch innervating a gracilis muscle transplant).

Complications

1. Failure to restore motion of paralyzed neuromuscular units
2. Sensory deficit from nerve graft donor site
3. Neuroma of donor or recipient site
4. Iatrogenic paralysis of non-paralyzed healthy hemiface

Two-Stage Partial Gracilis Muscle Transplant

Indication

Muscle transplants and local muscle transfers are indicated in patients without viable neuromuscular units due to long-standing facial paralysis (i.e., >12–18 months) or significant soft tissue injury of the mimetic muscles (i.e., trauma or tumor extirpation).

Surgical Technique

One-stage muscle transplants can be performed by innervating the muscle with an ipsilateral non-facial nerve (V, XI, XII CN). However, the only nerve that can display emotion with spontaneity is the contralateral facial nerve. Although in some cases a muscle transplant can be performed in one stage coapting it to the contralateral facial nerve, the most common procedure is a two-stage procedure in which a CFNG is attached to a healthy non-paralyzed facial nerve branch and banked for 6–12 months on the contralateral palsied side, at which time a new muscle transplant is introduced and coapted to the previously placed CNFG or dually innervated with the CFNG and another ipsilateral non facial nerve [4, 6].

1. The face is prepared concomitantly with the muscle dissection. You must have the recipient vessels (facial artery and vein in most cases) and insertion sutures at the lip and nose prepared prior to muscle transplantation to minimize ischemia time (Fig. 56.4).

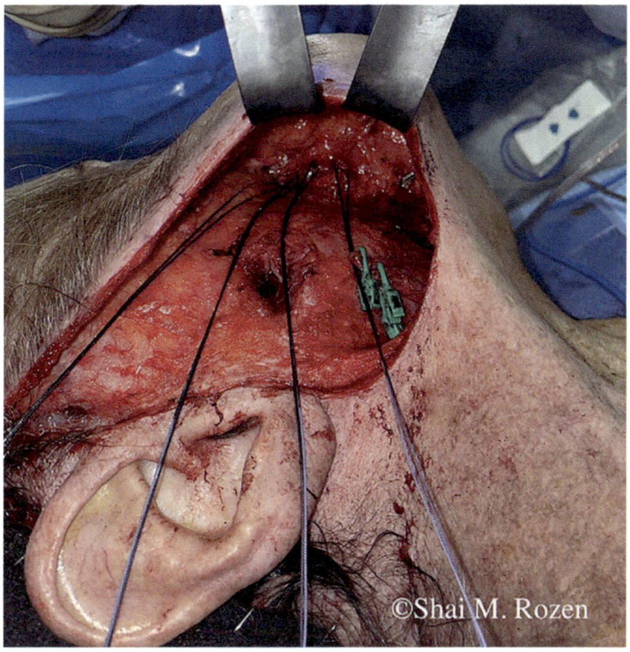

Fig. 56.4 Sutures anchored to the lip and the nose prior to muscle transplantation. Green clips placed on facial artery and vein in preparation of vascular anastomoses. (Used with permission of Shai M. Rozen, MD for Medical Education and Research. All rights reserved)

2. Measure the length of muscle needed from the modiolus to the temporalis fascia above the zygomatic arch and add 2 additional cm. The additional cm on each end of the muscle is used for baseball stitches to help avoid ripping of the sutures through the muscle during inset.
3. Palpate the posterior border of the adductor longus while the knee is flexed in 90° and in abduction. Mark a line 2.5 cm posteriorly.
4. After the skin incision is performed and the saphenous vein is preserved, the gracilis muscle and the adductor longus muscle are identified. The gracilis muscle is freed along its anterior and posterior borders while carefully identifying the major pedicle anteriorly.
5. Identify and dissect cranially and anteriorly the anterior branch of the obturator nerve (Fig. 56.5).
6. Dissect the neurovascular pedicle to the medial circumflex source vessel while ligating any branches into the adductor longus.
7. The gracilis muscle is split lengthwise around 35–50% of its width, sequentially cutting the caudal segment followed by the cranial segment of the gracilis flap.
8. Each muscle ending is sutured with 0-0 Vicryl in a baseball stitch fashion to decrease muscle slip once the muscle is transplanted in the face.
9. Make sure the recipient nerve and facial vessels are prepared in the face prior to transferring the muscle.
10. The obturator nerve and the vascular pedicle are cut and the muscle is transferred to the face.

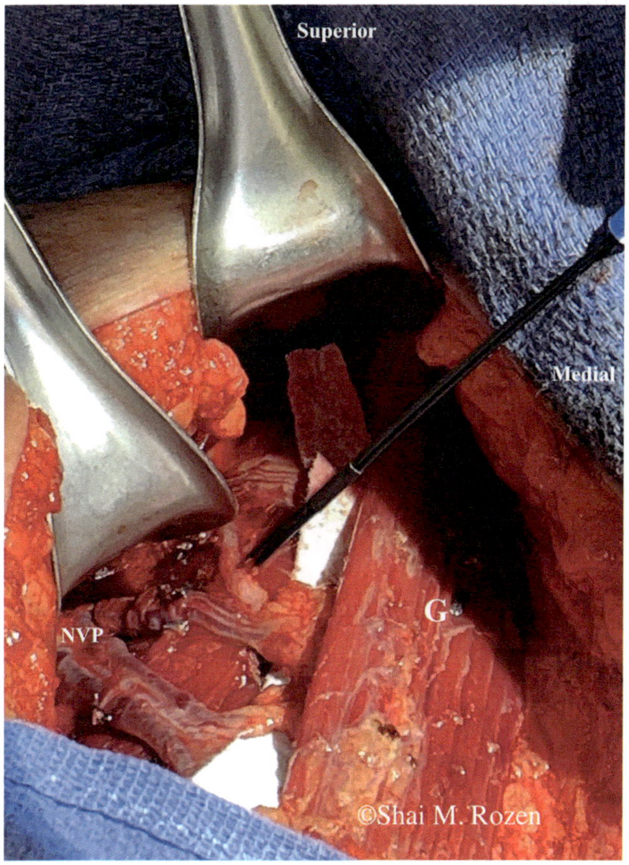

Fig. 56.5 Gracilis (G) and neurovascular pedicle (NVP). A neurostimulator is pointing at the obturator nerve. (Used with permission of Shai M. Rozen, MD for Medical Education and Research. All rights reserved)

11. Using a previously placed 1-0 Vicryl suture into the upper lip and nasal base, the muscle is parachuted into the face and secured into the modiolus, mid-upper lip, anterior upper lip close to the philtrum, and nasal root. Then suture the superior edge of the muscle, the new muscle origin, to the temporalis fascia (Fig. 56.6).
12. Under magnification, perform venous and arterial anastomoses, as well as tension-free coaptation with 10-0 nylon suture of the obturator nerve stump to CFNG and/or the masseter nerve.

Complications

1. Failure to restore motion
2. Vascular compromise of the muscle transfer
3. Increased bulkiness of the face
4. Misplaced muscle transfer and incorrect vector leading to asymmetry

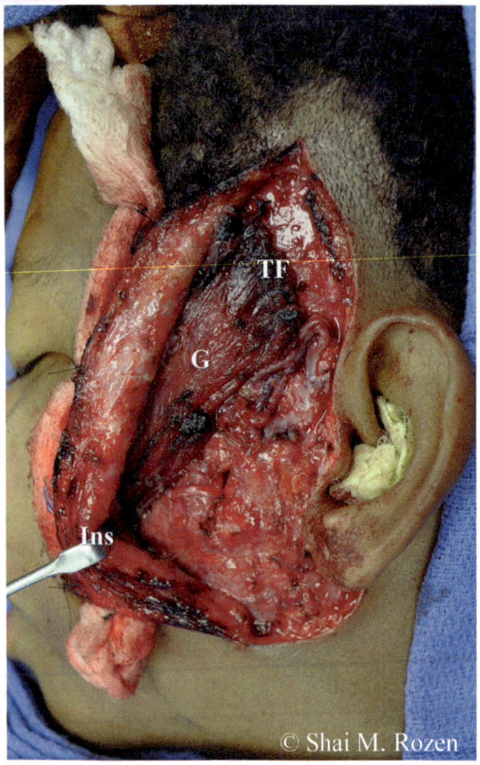

Fig. 56.6 Gracilis (*G*) muscle transplant in place. The temporalis facia (*TF*) becomes the new muscle origin. Likewise, the modiolus, mid-upper lip, anterior upper lip, and the nasal root become the new insertion point (*Ins*). (Used with permission of Shai M. Rozen, MD for Medical Education and Research. All rights reserved)

References

1. Brown S, Isaacson B, Kutz W, Barnett S, Rozen SM (2019) Facial nerve trauma: clinical evaluation and management strategies. Plast Reconstr Surg 143(5):1498–1512. https://doi.org/10.1097/prs.0000000000005572
2. Cheng A, Audolfsson T, Rodriguez-Lorenzo A, Wong C, Rozen S (2013) A reliable anatomic approach for identification of the masseteric nerve. J Plast Reconstr Aesthet Surg 66(10):1438–1440. https://doi.org/10.1016/j.bjps.2013.04.009
3. Krag AE, Rozen SM (2021) Nerve transfers to the facial nerve. In: Tzou C-HJ, Rodríguez-Lorenzo A (eds) Facial palsy: techniques for reanimation of the paralyzed face. Springer International Publishing, Cham, pp 79–88. https://doi.org/10.1007/978-3-030-50784-8_8
4. Rozen S, Saba SC (2017) Free muscle transfer for long-standing facial palsy. In: Anh Tran T, Panthaki ZJ, Hoballah JJ, Thaller SR (eds) Operative dictations in plastic and reconstructive surgery. Springer International Publishing, Cham, pp 337–340. https://doi.org/10.1007/978-3-319-40631-2_80
5. Rozen SM (2017) Facial reanimation: basic surgical tools and creation of an effective toolbox for treating patients with facial paralysis: part B. Nerve transfer combined with cross-facial nerve grafting in the acute facial palsy patient. Plast Reconstr Surg 139(3):725–727. https://doi.org/10.1097/prs.0000000000003128
6. Rozen SM (2017) Facial reanimation: basic surgical tools and creation of an effective toolbox for treating patients with facial paralysis. Part a: functional muscle transfers in the long-term facial palsy patient. Plast Reconstr Surg 139(2):469–471. https://doi.org/10.1097/prs.0000000000003025

Facial Synkinesis

57

Y. Edward Wen and Shai M. Rozen

Indications

Synkinesis is a condition of concomitant involuntary mimetic muscle movement, hypertonicity, and possibly hypotonicity in separate facial zones as a result of facial nerve damage and aberrant reinnervation. The etiology of synkinesis may vary greatly, but the clinical presentation is similar, albeit with different degrees of severity. Conventional naming lists the area of voluntary movements before the region of involuntary movement. Voluntary smiling with involuntary eye closure (i.e., oral-ocular synkinesis) and voluntary eye closure with involuntary perioral contraction (i.e., oculo-oral synkinesis) are the most prevalent synkinetic facial motions.

Though there is a plethora of synkinesis grading systems, uniformity and consensus are lacking. Most clinicians utilize some form of subjective grading system, such as the Ross et al. classification system [1].

1. None: no synkinesis or mass movement
2. Mild: slight synkinesis
3. Moderate: obvious but not disfiguring synkinesis
4. Severe: disfiguring synkinesis/gross mass movement of several muscles

Indications for treatment may range from facial deformity during animation and, in severe cases, during repose, pain due to constant facial and neck muscle spasm, blepharospasm, speech impediment, and oral incompetence during eating.

Generally, three questions should be considered: should hypertonic muscles be weakened, should hypotonic muscles be strengthened, and should muscle and/or nerve (groups) be removed in order to rebuild with a subsequent muscle transfer?

Treatment strategies usually combine chemo-denervation (e.g., botulinum toxin injections), physical therapy, and surgery. These should be tailored to each patient based on their chief complaints, severity of synkinesis, and specific goals, which may vary. Therefore, a thorough history and physical examination are pertinent. Frequently, a graded intervention approach with most patients is helpful but may not fit all individuals, as some patients will ask for more involved approaches upfront. A comprehensive discussion about treatment strategies should include not only chemo-denervation and physical therapy, which have an essential role but limited lasting effect in some patients, but also all surgical options, including myectomies, neurectomies, and muscle transplants. These are important to mention early on since some conservative surgical approaches may not provide the desired result for a specific individual and should be perceived by the patient as a staged approach rather than a failed approach.

The following text will discuss the different surgical techniques currently used in the treatment of synkinesis.

Depressor Anguli Oris (DAO) Myectomy [2, 3]

Anatomy and Considerations

1. The DAO receives innervation from both lower buccal and marginal mandibular facial nerve branches, whereas the depressor labii inferioris muscle is predominantly innervated by marginal mandibular facial nerve branches (Figs. 57.1 and 57.2). This may partially explain why DAO hypertonicity and depressor labii inferioris weakness are frequently and concomitantly reported in synkinetic patients.

Supplementary Information The online version contains supplementary material available at https://doi.org/10.1007/978-3-031-73931-6_57.

Y. E. Wen · S. M. Rozen (✉)
Department of Plastic and Reconstructive Surgery, University of Texas Southwestern Medical Center, Dallas, TX, USA
e-mail: yuanedward.wen@utsouthwestern.edu; Shai.Rozen@UTSouthwestern.edu

A. S. Hanna (ed.), *Nerves: Anatomy, Exposures, and Techniques*, https://doi.org/10.1007/978-3-031-73931-6_57

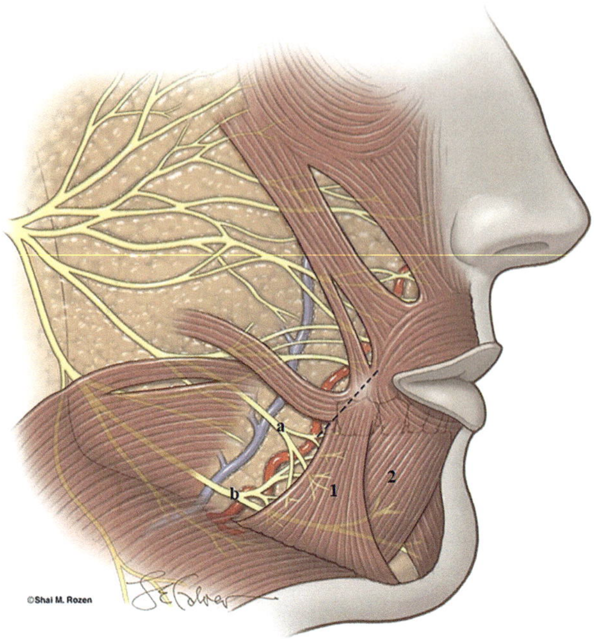

Fig. 57.1 The depressor anguli oris muscle (DAO) (1) receives innervation from both lower buccal (a) and marginal mandibular (b) facial nerve branches, whereas the depressor labii inferioris muscle (2) is only innervated by marginal mandibular facial nerve branches. From their mandibular origin to insertion into the modiolus, the DAO fibers consistently passed anterior to the first mandibular molar. As indicated by the dotted line, the intraoral mucosal incision for DAO myectomy should begin 1 cm inferolateral to the modiolus and extend toward the sulcus anterior to the first mandibular molar. (Used with permission of Shai M. Rozen, MD for Medical Education and Research. All rights reserved [3])

2. Transcutaneous lidocaine injection in the spastic DAO muscle that is palpated during a strong open mouth smile (string sign) can be conducted in the clinic to predict myectomy results (Fig. 57.3) [2].
3. Increased modiolus resting position, closed-mouth smile modiolus angle and excursion, open-mouth smile modiolus angle, excursion, dental show, and decreased lower lip height deviation may be seen after DAO myectomies (Fig. 57.3).
4. An intraoral approach is utilized to avoid a visible scar (Figs. 57.4 and 57.5).

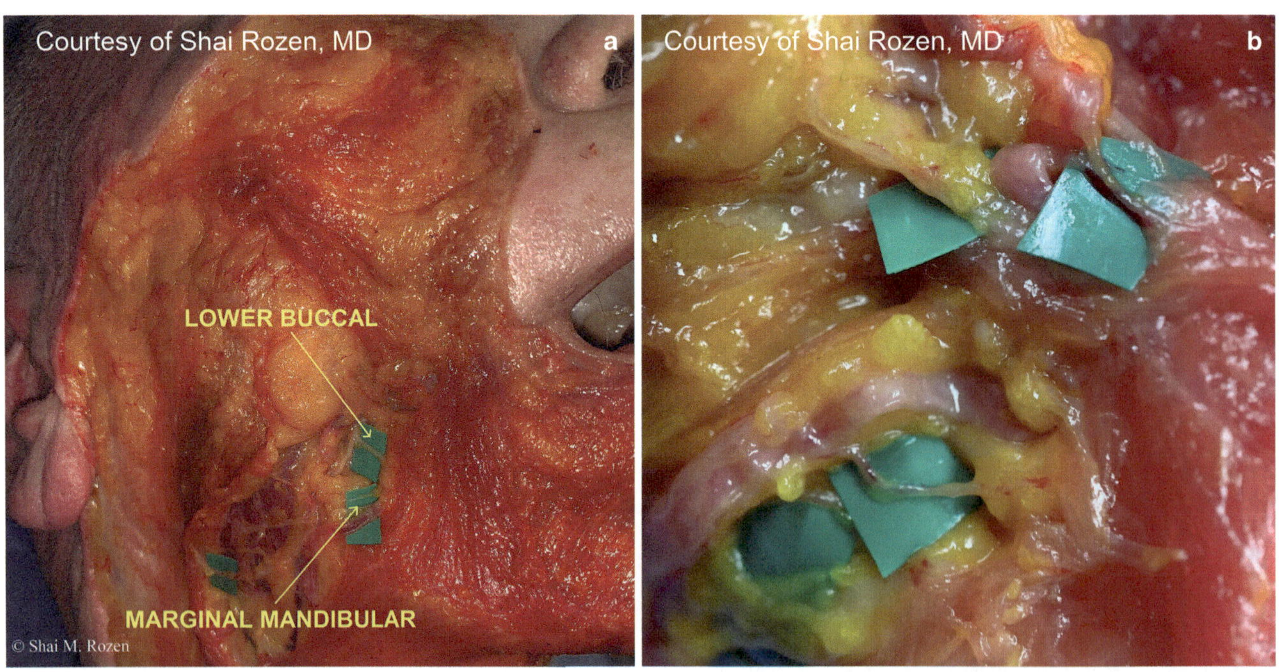

Fig. 57.2 (**a**) A cadaver hemi-face is shown with the sub-superficial muscular aponeurotic system (SMAS) dissected, followed by the perioral muscle complex dissection, and finally with the neurovascular supply to the DAO and depressor labii inferioris muscles exposed. Arrows indicate the lower buccal and marginal mandibular branches of the facial nerve that supply the DAO. (**b**) Magnification of A, showing the DAO's neurovascular supply. (Used with permission of Shai M. Rozen, MD for Medical Education and Research. All rights reserved [3])

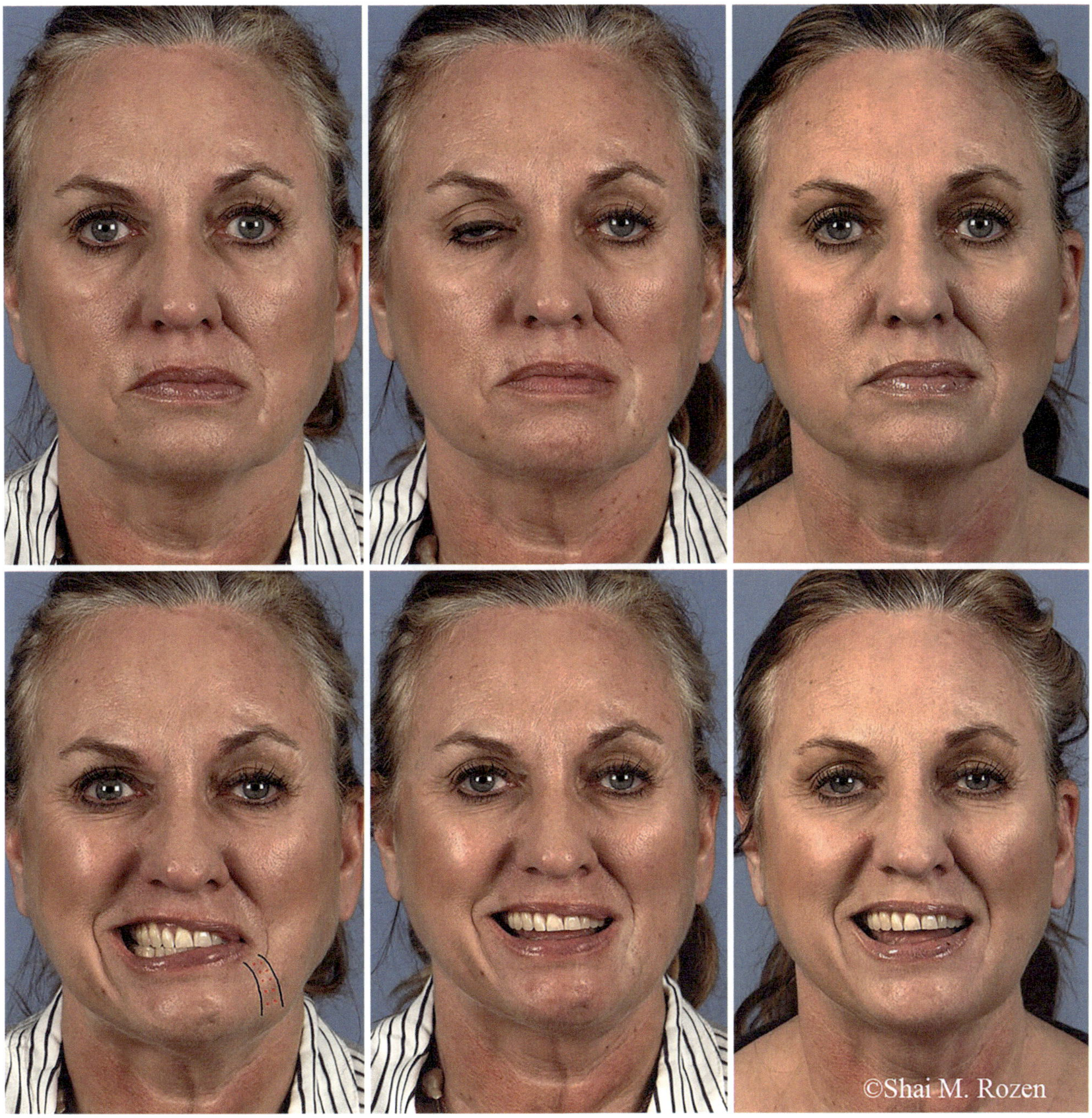

Fig. 57.3 A 55-year-old woman with Bell's palsy and left-sided incomplete facial paralysis and synkinesis (patient 1). (Used with permission of Shai M. Rozen, MD for Medical Education and Research. All rights reserved [3])
(Above, left) She is shown in repose upon initial presentation
(Above, center) Next, she is shown in repose 15 min after left DAO lidocaine block. Take note of the small injection sites on the skin
(Above, right) Finally, she was photographed in repose 77 days after left DAO myectomy
(Below, left) Prior to intervention, there was initial hypertonicity of the DAO and weakness of the depressor labii inferioris muscle on the left side when smiling. The strong downward pull of the modiolus due to the hypertonic DAO, as well as the elevation of the left lower lip due to depressor labii inferioris weakness, can be seen. During a full-effort smile, the black lines denote the palpable tense DAO (i.e., the string sign). The injection site along the tense depressor anguli oris is indicated by the red dots
(Below, center) 15 min after lidocaine block of the hypertonic DAO on the left side, the smile angle and maxillary teeth exposure showed improvement. Take note of the small injection sites on the skin
(Below, right) The improvements in smile angle and maxillary teeth exposure replicated 77 days after left DAO myectomy

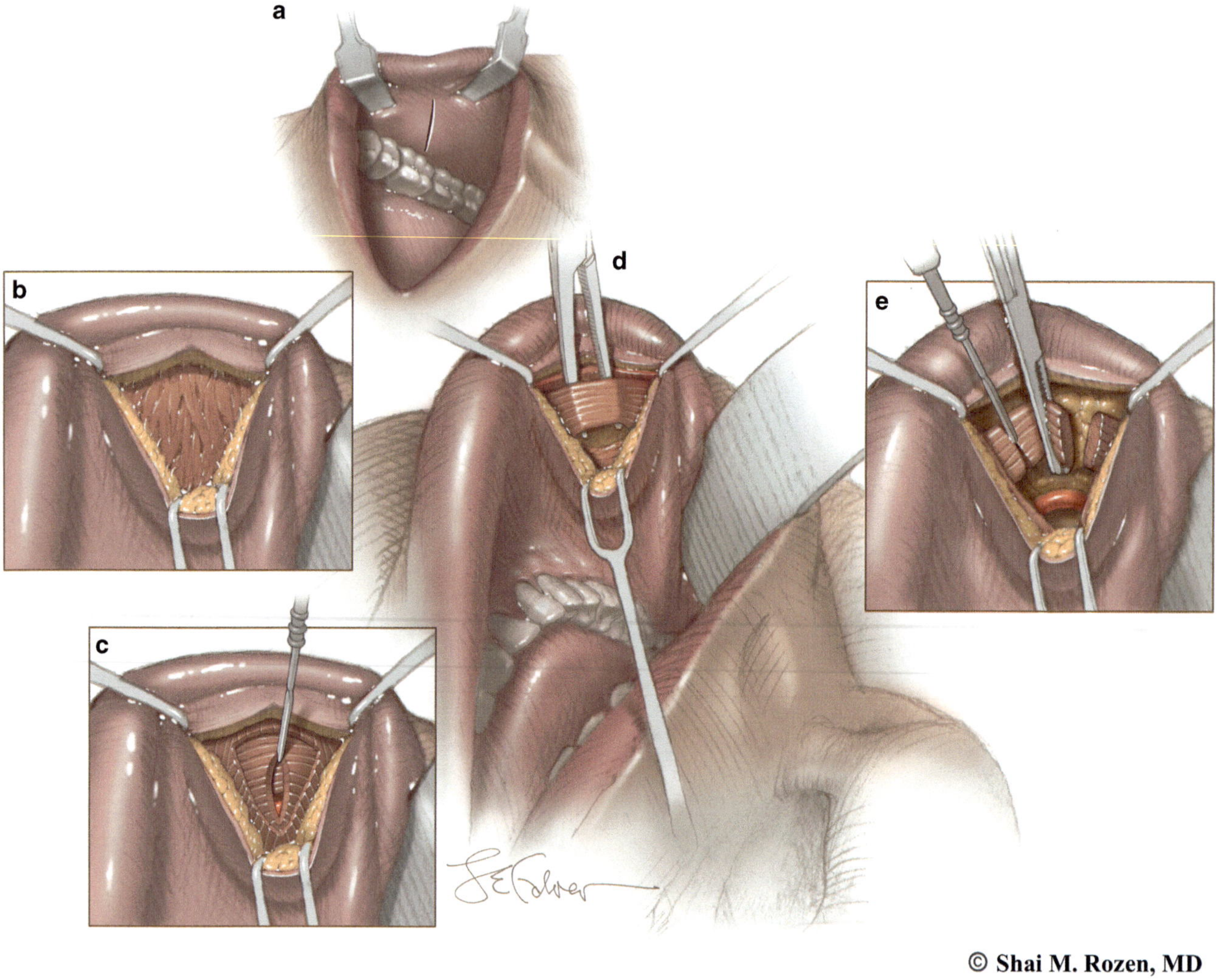

Fig. 57.4 (**a**) The planned intraoral approach to the DAO for myectomy is depicted in this illustration. A line anterior to the first mandibular molar is planned 0.5–1.0 cm inferolateral to the modiolus. (**b**) After a full-thickness incision is made through the mucosa, the buccinator muscle fibers should be immediately visible (**c**) and with the orbicularis oris coming into view next anteriorly. (**d**) Following transection of the buccinator and orbicularis muscle fibers, the DAO is seen anteriorly. (**e**) A 1.0–1.5 cm segment of the cranial DAO is carefully resected, avoiding injury to the facial artery laterally. (Used with permission of Shai M. Rozen, MD for Medical Education and Research. All rights reserved)

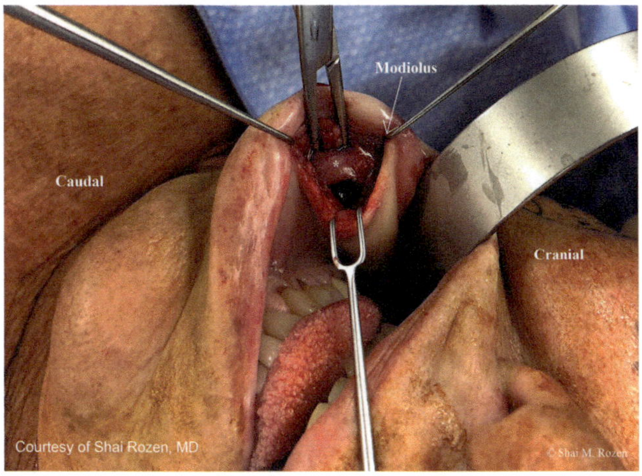

Fig. 57.5 A female patient with right facial synkinesis and DAO hypertonicity is shown with her DAO dissected and exposed (*) before myectomy. The fibers of the anterior buccinator and orbicularis muscles have been transected previously. A 1.0–1.5 cm segment of the DAO is excised caudally from the "tubularized" insertion point cranially near the modiolus. The next layer encountered is the subcutaneous fat layer, which verifies that the DAO has been completely myectomized. (Used with permission of Shai M. Rozen, MD for Medical Education and Research. All rights reserved [3])

Technique

1. Surgery may be performed under local or general analgesia.
2. Ten minutes prior to incision, inject with 8–10 mL of 1:1000 epinephrine along the muscle border with 1% lidocaine intraorally.
3. Protect the eyes with lubrication.
4. Prep with Betadine or another antiseptic, then drape in a sterile fashion.
5. A 4 cm incision is made 0.5–1.0 cm inferolateral to the modiolus and prolonged along a line anterior to the first mandibular molar, as depicted by the dashed black line in Fig. 57.1 with the incision shown in Fig. 57.4a.
6. After a full-thickness incision is made through the mucosa, the buccinator muscle fibers should be immediately visible, with the orbicularis oris muscle fibers following anteriorly (Figs. 57.4b and c).
7. After transecting the anterior buccinator and orbicularis muscle fibers, the DAO should be identifiable underneath or anteriorly, towards its insertion in the modiolus (Fig. 57.4d).
8. Through an areolar plane between the orbicularis oris and the DAO muscles, dissection proceeds circumferentially from cranial to caudal; it is of note that the superior DAO fibers are more tubularly arranged and therefore easier to isolate (Fig. 57.5).
9. A 1.0–1.5 cm segment of the cranial DAO is resected with care taken to avoid the facial artery lateral to the DAO's lateral border (Fig. 57.4e).
10. When all muscle fibers of the DAO are resected, a subcutaneous fat layer should be seen, verifying complete DAO resection.
11. Closure is performed in layers from deep to superficial with 3-0 Vicryl sutures at the muscle layer, followed by 4-0 chromic catgut interrupted and/or continuous sutures.

Potential Complications (Infrequent)

1. Paresthesia (temporary)
2. Infection/abscess
3. Hemorrhage/hematoma

DAO to Depressor Labii Inferioris (DLI) Muscle Transfer [4] (a Variation on DAO Myectomy)

Anatomy and Considerations

1. The main neurovascular perforators enter laterally, in the inferior two-thirds of the DLI, from the facial artery and marginal mandibular branches. The medial DAO overlaps with the deeper DLI fibers by about 70% [3].
2. At the juncture of the upper and middle thirds of the DAO, another neurovascular pedicle with facial artery and lower facial nerve buccal branches penetrates the muscle [3].
3. Because the major source of motor innervation (the marginal mandibular nerve) is likely diminished in synkinesis, it is critical to protect the lower buccal branches (i.e., the cranial neurovascular bundle).
4. Compared to DAO myectomy, DAO to DLI transfer produced similar results in terms of increased smile excursion but has yet to demonstrate effective lower lip depression [4].
5. The goal of this technique is to transfer the hypertonic DAO muscle into the DLI muscle insertion, simultaneously eliminating unwarranted DAO hyperactivity and enhancing lower lip depression via augmentation of the weak DLI muscle insertion [4].

Technique

1–8. As above under DAO myectomy.

9. The dissection is carried as far cranially as feasible towards the modiolus, taking care to retain the aforementioned

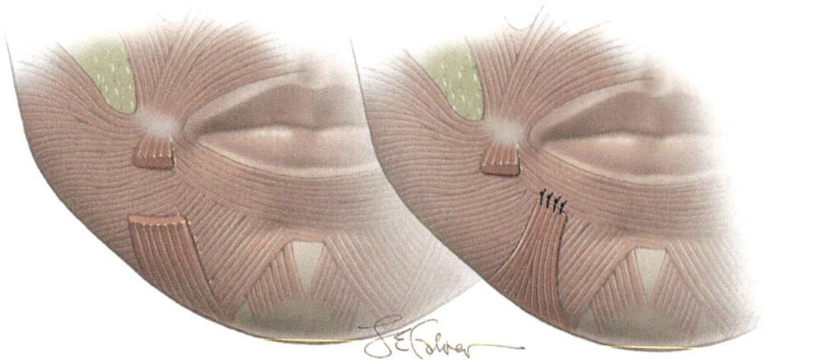

Fig. 57.6 The myectomy of the DAO (left) and its transfer to the insertion of the depressor labii inferioris (right) are depicted in this illustration. (Used with permission of Shai M. Rozen, MD for Medical Education and Research. All rights reserved [4])

second neurovascular pedicle that inserts into the cranial third of the DAO and to avoid the facial artery lateral to the DAO's lateral border.

10. The cranial third of the DAO is then excised to free the muscle, while the approximately caudal two-thirds of the muscle is still attached to its lower perforators from the facial vessels.
11. Next, the inferior portion of the DAO is transferred superomedially to where the DLI inserts into the orbicularis oris and oversewn with 1–2 layers of running sutures using 3-0 Vicryl. (Fig. 57.6).
12. When satisfied with the positioning of the transfer, irrigate, maintain hemostasis, and begin closure as above.

Complications

1. Paresthesia (temporary)
2. Infection/abscess
3. Hemorrhage/hematoma

Neurectomy (of Synkinetic Branches of the Facial Nerve) [5]

Anatomy and Considerations

1. The thought behind selective neurectomies is to excise aberrant facial nerve branches, which may contribute to synkinesis.
2. A quality nerve stimulator that can create reliable tetany is of great importance for accurate facial nerve mapping.
3. This technique is complementary to myectomies, but its long-term results still need to be thoroughly evaluated in high-quality studies as some degree of recurrence is occasionally observed.

Technique

1. Sequential compressive devices (SCDs) are applied to the lower limbs.
2. Protect eyes with lubrication.
3. Examine and protect all pressure points.
4. Short-acting or no paralytics should be used to allow for intraoperative stimulation.
5. The face is prepped with Betadine and draped in a sterile fashion.
6. Insert foley if surgery is planned for longer than 4 h (only if performed concomitantly with other procedures).
7. Preauricular rhytidectomy incision extending superiorly to the temporal region, then extending inferiorly with a retro-ramus approach.
8. Elevate the skin flap to about 0.5 cm and then raise a composite skin-superficial muscular aponeurotic system (SMAS) flap dissecting in the sub-SMAS plane.
9. The sub-SMAS is lifted anteriorly to the mobile SMAS anterior to the parotid gland.
10. The cervical, marginal mandibular, buccal, and zygomatic nerve branches of the facial nerve are mapped with a nerve stimulator as they leave the parotid gland, deep to the parotid-masseteric fascia.
11. Identify synkinetic movements such as oculo-oral synkinesis or oral-ocular synkinesis (i.e., stimulation of cervical and lower buccal branches causing unwarranted periorbital and frontalis contractions).
12. Verify existing innervation redundancies prior to any neurectomy.
13. Neurectomize the synkinetic branches (Fig. 57.7).
14. Return SMAS to the original position.
15. Begin layered closure with 4-0 Monocryl and 5-0 nylon.

Complications (Very Rare)

1. Paresthesia
2. Parotid leak
3. Infection/abscess
4. Hemorrhage/hematoma

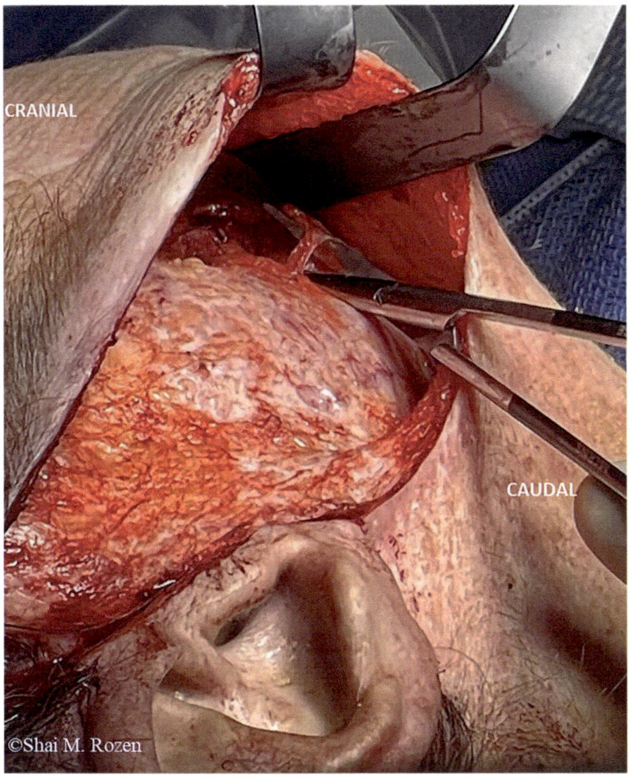

Fig. 57.7 In the sub-SMAS plane, a synkinetic buccal branch is identified, activated with the neurostimulator, and then neurectomized after innervation redundancy is confirmed. (Used with permission of Shai M. Rozen, MD for Medical Education and Research. All rights reserved)

Cross-Facial Nerve Graft (CFNG), Myectomy, and/or Neurectomy Followed by Free Functional Muscle Transfers (FFMTs) [6]

Anatomy and Considerations

For the most severe cases of synkinesis, a combination of extensive myectomy, neurectomy, and CFNG are used in the first stage, and then after at least 6–9 months, a FFMT (e.g., gracilis) for facial reanimation is used in the second stage.

Technique and Complications

1. Myectomy: Refer to the aforementioned myectomy technique in this chapter.
2. Neurectomy: Refer to the aforementioned neurectomy technique in this chapter.
3. CFNG: Refer to the section in the flaccid facial paralysis Chap. 56.
4. FFMT: Refer to the section in the flaccid facial paralysis Chap. 56.

References

1. Ross BG, Fradet G, Nedzelski JM (1996) Development of a sensitive clinical facial grading system. Otolaryngol Head Neck Surg 114(3):380–386. https://doi.org/10.1016/s0194-5998(96)70206-1
2. Krag AE, Glick S, Hembd A, Rozen SM (2021) The effect of depressor anguli oris muscle block on facial symmetry in synkinetic facial paralysis patients and its role in preoperative assessment. Plast Reconstr Surg 147(3):455–465. https://doi.org/10.1097/prs.0000000000007674
3. Krag AE, Dumestre D, Hembd A, Glick S, Mohanty AJ, Rozen SM (2021) Topographic and neural anatomy of the depressor anguli oris muscle and implications for treatment of synkinetic facial paralysis. Plast Reconstr Surg 147(2):268e–278e. https://doi.org/10.1097/prs.0000000000007593
4. Halani SH, Sanchez CV, Hembd AS, Mohanty AJ, Reisch J, Rozen SM (2022) Depressor anguli oris myectomy versus transfer to depressor labii inferioris for facial symmetry in synkinetic facial paralysis. J Reconstr Microsurg 38(4):328–334. https://doi.org/10.1055/s-0041-1732350
5. Azizzadeh B, Irvine LE, Diels J, Slattery WH, Massry GG, Larian B et al (2019) Modified selective neurectomy for the treatment of post-facial paralysis synkinesis. Plast Reconstr Surg 143(5):1483–1496. https://doi.org/10.1097/prs.0000000000005590
6. Chuang DC, Chang TN, Lu JC (2015) Postparalysis facial synkinesis: clinical classification and surgical strategies. Plast Reconstr Surg Glob Open 3(3):e320. https://doi.org/10.1097/gox.0000000000000283

58 Corneal Neurotization

Simeon C. Daeschler, Asim Ali, and Gregory H. Borschel

Indications

The main indication for corneal neurotization is neurotrophic keratopathy in the anesthetic eye, either acquired or congenital. Whereas conventional ophthalmic management aims at preventing disease progression and mitigating symptoms of neurotrophic keratopathy [1], corneal neurotization offers a potentially definitive treatment option by rerouting sensory nerve fibers and thereby restoring corneal innervation [2, 3]. It also enhances the potential for corneal transplantation success.

Patient selection criteria include (1) impaired or absent corneal innervation, (2) the presence of neurotrophic keratopathy, (3) unlikely spontaneous corneal reinnervation based on the cause of corneal denervation (e.g., congenital trigeminal hypoplasia) and/or a prolonged period of time has passed since the causal event (at least 1 year), (4) availability of an appropriate sensory donor nerve (contra- or ipsilateral), and (5) the absence of active eye infection (viral, bacterial, or mycotic).

Contraindications for corneal neurotization are uncontrolled local infections, active corneal epithelial ulcerations (Mackie stage 2 or 3) and below normal levels of sensation in the skin area supplied by the donor nerve.

Supplementary Information The online version contains supplementary material available at https://doi.org/10.1007/978-3-031-73931-6_58.

S. C. Daeschler
Department of Hand, Plastic and Reconstructive Surgery, Burn Center, BG-Trauma Center, University of Heidelberg, Ludwigshafen/Rhine, Germany

A. Ali
Department of Ophthalmology and Vision Sciences, University of Toronto and The Hospital for Sick Children, Toronto, ON, Canada
e-mail: asim.ali@sickkids.ca

G. H. Borschel (✉)
Division of Plastic Surgery, Riley Hospital for Children, Indianapolis, IN, USA
e-mail: gborsche@iu.edu

Surgical Technique

The patient is under general anesthesia and placed in a supine position. The endotracheal tube is directed caudally to give access to the eye and forehead. The face and one leg (nerve graft harvesting site) are prepped and draped. The affected eye(s) is prepared with povidone-iodine ophthalmic solution (never chlorhexidine!) and the contralateral normal eye receives a temporary, protective tarsorrhaphy.

1. The sural nerve is approached 2 cm posterior and 2 cm proximal to the lateral malleolus through a 1–2 cm horizontal skin incision. The nerve is mobilized with scissors, transected as far distally as possible, and the distal end of the proximal segment is passed through the orifice of the nerve stripper device. The nerve stripper is then advanced with gentle rotation in cranial direction as far as the nerve graft length is required while avoiding traction to the graft. The nerve is transected proximally through a second skin incision, and the graft is harvested (Fig. 58.1). The proximal end of the graft is labeled and placed in moist sterile gauze until further use. Skin incisions are closed.
2. This step can be performed by a second team simultaneously with the nerve graft harvest. The contra- or ipsilat-

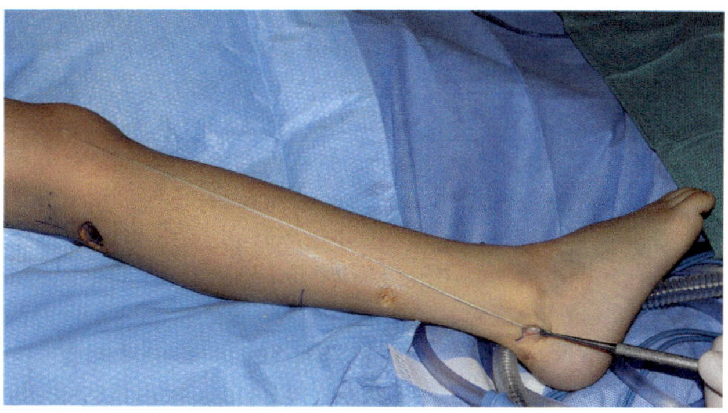

Fig. 58.1 Harvested sural nerve through three small incisions using a nerve stripper device

A. S. Hanna (ed.), *Nerves: Anatomy, Exposures, and Techniques*, https://doi.org/10.1007/978-3-031-73931-6_58

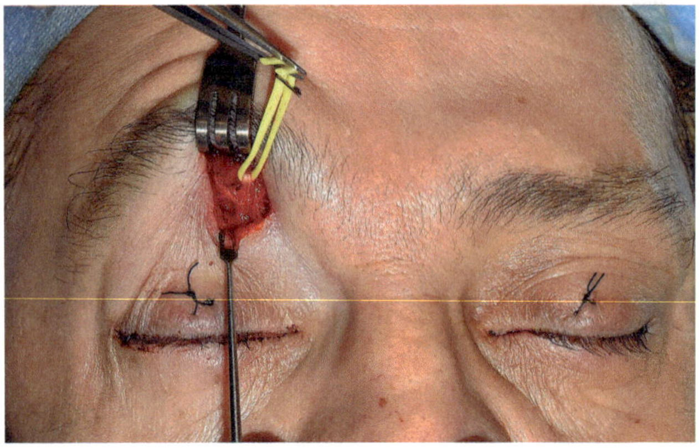

Fig. 58.2 The supraorbital nerve (*yellow loop*) has been identified on the healthy side as a suitable axon donor based on its larger caliber, offering a reasonable size match to the harvested sural nerve graft

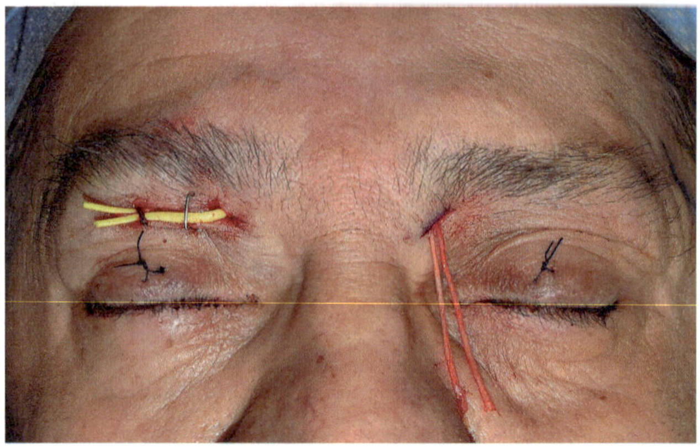

Fig. 58.3 Two sural nerve graft cables are subcutaneously tunneled across the nasal rim towards the affected eye

eral supraorbital and supratrochlear [4] nerves are approached via a 2 cm transverse sub-brow incision starting 1.5 cm lateral to the facial midline and extending to the mid-pupillary line (Fig. 58.2). The supraorbital nerve may be expected 2 cm lateral to the facial midline, whereas the supratrochlear nerve usually runs 0.2–1.0 cm medial to the supraorbital nerve (1.0–1.8 cm lateral to facial midline). The corrugator supercilii muscle is then exposed and carefully dissected with scissors to locate and expose both nerves. The larger nerve is chosen as axon donor. If both are small in caliber, both are used as donor nerves.

3. The diameter of the nerve graft ideally matches the donor nerve. When the nerve graft is thin, two parallel nerve graft cables can be used. The length of each cable is defined by placing the graft on the patient's face: one end of the graft is touching the donor nerve and the graft is placed horizontally above the nasal rim up to the mid-pupillary line of the affected eye, angling 90° in a caudal direction and coursing up to the nasal alar base (Fig. 58.3). As a rule of thumb, this distance provides sufficient length for tensionless nerve grafting and permits unrestricted globe excursion. For ipsilateral corneal neurotization, the ipsilateral nasal ala can be used as a landmark.
4. A reversed nerve graft orientation is used. A 1 cm transverse skin incision is made at the cranio-medial orbital rim right below and parallel to the brow of the affected eye. A subcutaneous tunnel is established over the cranial nasal bridge to the donor nerve incision using blunt dissection. The nerve graft is grasped at the proximal end (previously marked) and subcutaneously tunneled from the donor site towards the affected eye (Fig. 58.3). The donor nerve skin incision is temporarily closed with sterile strips to prevent desiccation of the donor nerve and the nerve graft.

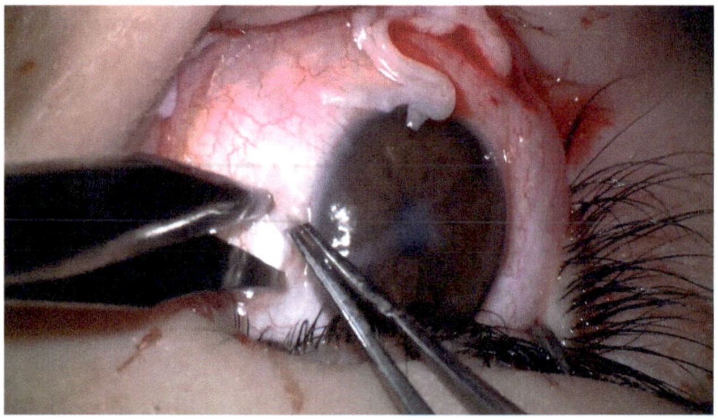

Fig. 58.4 A 5 mm conjunctival and Tenon's incision is made parallel to and 5 mm from the superonasal corneal limbus

5. A 5 mm conjunctival and Tenon's incision is made parallel to and 5 mm posterior to the superonasal corneal limbus (Fig. 58.4). Another incision is created in the superior and medial upper fornix, through which a Wright fascia needle is directed, to create a tunnel from the conjunctival incision to the ipsilateral skin incision below the brow. The nerve graft is loaded into the eyelet and gently passed through the tunnel and under the Tenon's fascia towards the first incision. Now the graft fascicles are separated via epineurectomy of the distal 3–4 cm of the nerve graft. Three to four corneoscleral insertion points are mapped out such that they are evenly distributed around the limbus to create a homogenous reinnervation pattern. A sub-Tenon tunnel is created using blunt dissection with Westcott scissors, extending in a constant 5 mm distance to the corneoscleral junction. Subsequently, the individual fascicles are tunneled to their predefined insertion points.

A short, partial-thickness corneoscleral tunnel (2.0 mm wide, 1.5 mm from the limbus) is established with a 1.25 mm crescent blade at each individual nerve graft insertion point, extending 0.5 mm into the clear cornea (Fig. 58.5). The end of the fascicles is trimmed with Vannas scissors, and the fascicle is carefully inserted into the corneoscleral tunnel (Fig. 58.6). Right proximal to the corneoscleral tunnel, the fascicle is fixated to the sclera using a single perineural stitch with 10-0 absorbable monofilament suture or fibrin glue (Fig. 58.7). After inserting all fascicles in an analogous manner, the conjunctival incisions are closed with 10-0 absorbable, monofilament suture.

6. Fibrin glue or epineural sutures can be used to connect the distal end of the harvested nerve graft to the donor nerve. The donor nerve is transected, and the end of the nerve graft is trimmed and gently apposed to the distal end of the donor nerve(s) with thorough epineural alignment in an end-to-end fashion. Then the coaptation site is covered with fibrin glue, and fibrin aggregation is awaited before skin incisions are closed.
7. The operated eye is irrigated with sterile saline, and corticoid-antibiotic ointment (e.g., Tobradex, Novartis AG, Switzerland) is applied to control postsurgical swelling and inflammation. A temporary tarsorrhaphy protects the operated eye (Fig. 58.8) and is typically left for a week. The tarsorrhaphy of the unaffected eye can be removed at the end of the procedure.

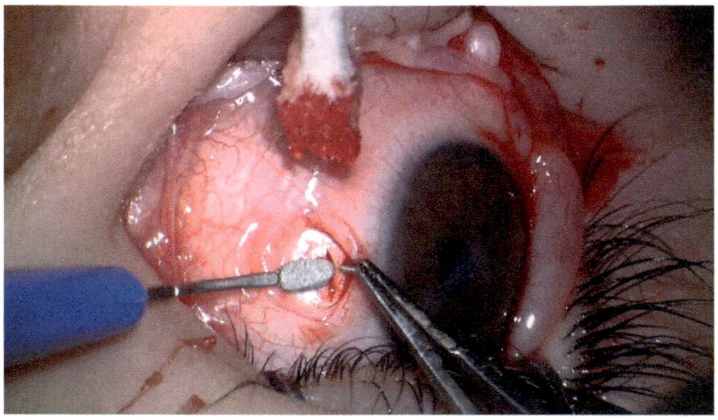

Fig. 58.5 Using a crescent blade, a partial-thickness corneoscleral tunnel is established at each individual nerve graft insertion point, extending 0.5 mm into clear cornea

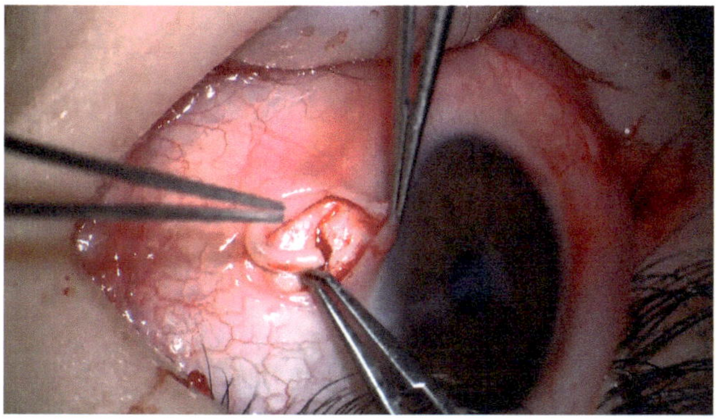

Fig. 58.6 After trimming the fascicle, its end is carefully inserted into the corneoscleral tunnel

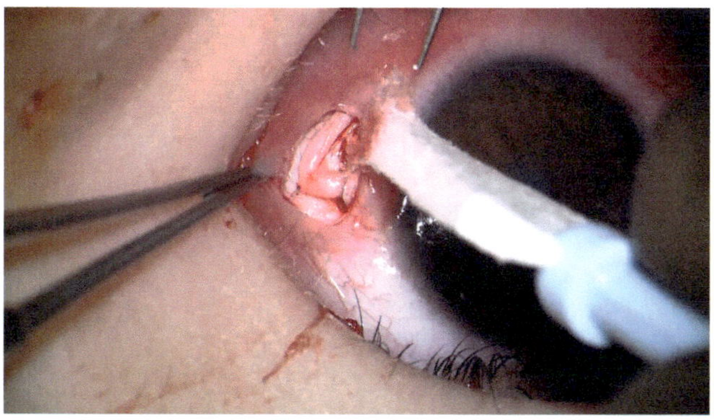

Fig. 58.7 Proximal to the corneoscleral tunnel, the fascicle is fixated on the sclera using a single perineural stitch with 10-0 absorbable monofilament suture

Potential Complications

Potential complications of corneal neurotization include general postsurgical complications such as bleeding, hematoma, surgical site infection, and wound healing deficit, as well as the accidental lesion of functionally relevant structures such as nerves or blood vessels.

Specific complications of corneal neurotization may include temporary paresthesia or pain at the donor site, extrusion or displacement of the nerve graft, as well as neuroma development at the nerve coaptation site or the corneoscleral insertion sites. In theory, neuroma formation may also occur along the course of the graft (neuroma in continuity) due to intraneural scarring as a result of rough nerve graft handling, but we have not observed this complication in practice.

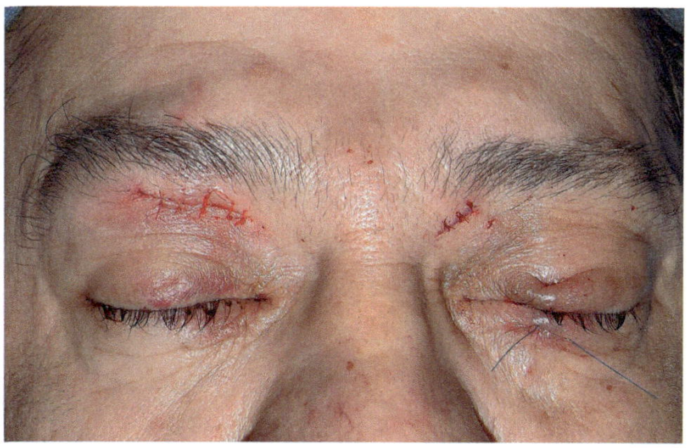

Fig. 58.8 Closed skin incisions post-surgery. A temporary tarsorrhaphy protects the operated eye

References

1. Dua HS, Said DG, Messmer EM, Rolando M, Benitez-Del-Castillo JM, Hossain PN et al (2018) Neurotrophic keratopathy. Prog Retin Eye Res 66:107–131. https://doi.org/10.1016/j.preteyeres.2018.04.003
2. Terzis JK, Dryer MM, Bodner BI (2009) Corneal neurotization: a novel solution to neurotrophic keratopathy. Plast Reconstr Surg 123(1):112–120. https://doi.org/10.1097/PRS.0b013e3181904d3a
3. Catapano J, Fung SSM, Halliday W, Jobst C, Cheyne D, Ho ES et al (2019) Treatment of neurotrophic keratopathy with minimally invasive corneal neurotisation: long-term clinical outcomes and evidence of corneal reinnervation. Br J Ophthalmol 103(12):1724–1731. https://doi.org/10.1136/bjophthalmol-2018-313042
4. Bains RD, Elbaz U, Zuker RM, Ali A, Borschel GH (2015) Corneal neurotization from the supratrochlear nerve with sural nerve grafts: a minimally invasive approach. Plast Reconstr Surg 135(2):397e–400e. https://doi.org/10.1097/prs.0000000000000994

Penile Reinnervation

59

Fausto Viterbo, Balduino F. M. Neto, and Lucas V. Magnani

Indication

Erectile dysfunction (ED) is a multifactorial disease that has had a great evolution in treatment with the arrival of phosphodiesterase inhibitors, but it continues with high rates of therapeutic failure. For cases that are refractory to traditional measures, a somatic-autonomic end-to-side neurorrhaphy technique to improve erections in ED patients after radical prostatectomy was created [1]. We present the surgical technique that can be performed in patients with different causes of ED.

Surgical Technique (Video)

The surgery is divided into three stages: harvest of two nerve grafts (preferably sural), dissection of the femoral nerves and dorsal nerves of the penis, and neurorrhaphies. Bilateral sural nerve graft harvest [2] is essential due to the need for long nerves to be divided into four grafts of about 15 cm each.

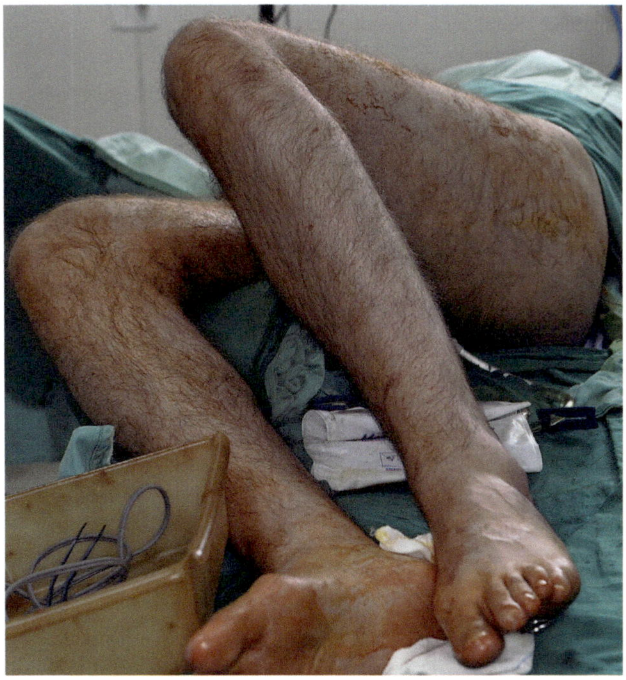

Fig. 59.1 Orthostatic position with hip flexion and internal rotation

1. Position: The harvest is easier with the patient in the prone position; however, to save surgical time, we chose the orthostatic position with hip flexion and internal rotation to expose the posterolateral region of the legs at the same time (Fig. 59.1).
2. A transverse incision is made at the midpoint between the lateral malleolus and the Achilles tendon, measuring approximately 1–1.5 cm, identifying the sural nerve. It is important to try to make the smallest number of incisions, but at least three are needed.
3. Harvest: Through detachment, using the Viterbo blunt dissector (Doctus, Curitiba-Brazil) [3], and performing nerve traction distally, the sural nerve path is superiorly identified, and transverse incisions similar to the first are made up to the popliteal fossa region (Fig. 59.2). The nerve is sectioned distally to avoid accidental sectioning of the fibular nerve. A mild to moderate traction helps in the nerve harvest. Once harvested, the nerve is divided in half.

Supplementary Information The online version contains supplementary material available at https://doi.org/10.1007/978-3-031-73931-6_59.

F. Viterbo (✉)
Fausto Viterbo's Plastic Clinic, School of Medicine of Botucatu, São Paulo, Brazil
e-mail: fv@faustoviterbo.com.br

B. F. M. Neto
Botucatu School of Medicine, HC-FMB, UNESP, São Paulo, Brazil

L. V. Magnani
School of Medicine of Botucatu, São Paulo State University, UNESP, São Paulo, Brazil
e-mail: lucas.v.magnani@unesp.br

A. S. Hanna (ed.), *Nerves: Anatomy, Exposures, and Techniques*, https://doi.org/10.1007/978-3-031-73931-6_59

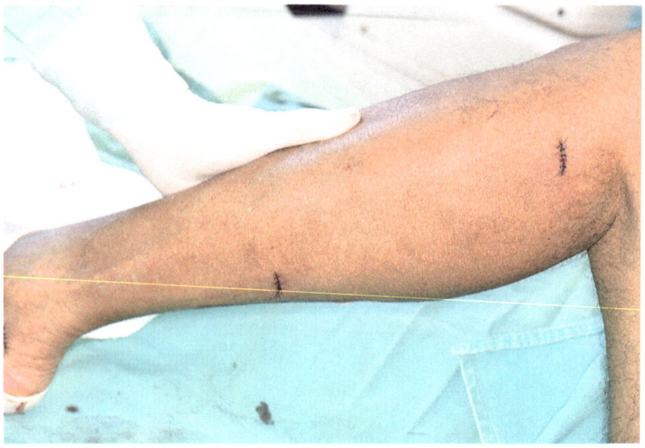

Fig. 59.2 Sural nerve harvest in three incisions

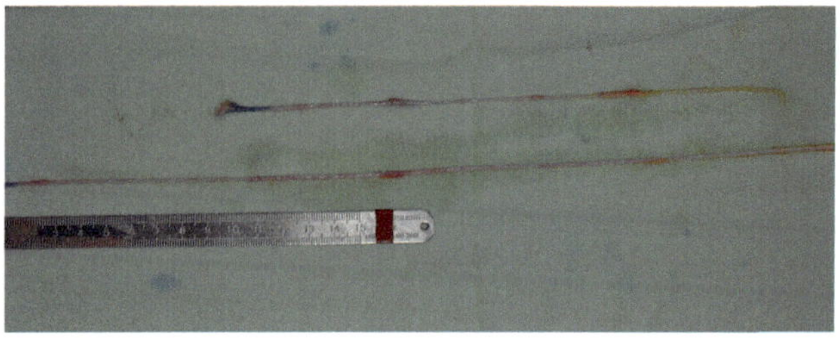

Fig. 59.3 Harvested sural nerve graft from both legs. The distal stumps are always marked

4. Prevention of neuromas: It is essential that the stumps are sutured with two transfixing stitches with non-absorbable monofilament threads, such as nylon 4-0.
5. The harvested sural nerves are measured, marked on their distal ends, and placed in saline solution (Fig. 59.3).

In parallel to this step, it is better if a second team prepares the donor and recipient sites. The procedure is done bilaterally.

1. An incision in each inguinal crease of about 4 cm and another incision at the base of the penis, slightly curved downwards, are made to expose the femoral nerves and the base of the penis, respectively. Through palpation of the femoral artery, a dissection is performed lateral to it to find the femoral nerve, which is prepared to perform neurorrhaphy. In the incision at the base of the penis, the suspensory ligament of the penis is released, which, in addition to having the potential to lengthen the penis, allows better access to the most basal portion of the male organ, where Buck's fascia is released to expose the dorsal nerves of the penis (lateral to the dorsal arteries of the penis) and the corpora cavernosa.
2. Using a cylindrical nerve passer with 2 mm in diameter, the nerve grafts are taken from the inguinal incisions to the base of the penis by a subcutaneous path.

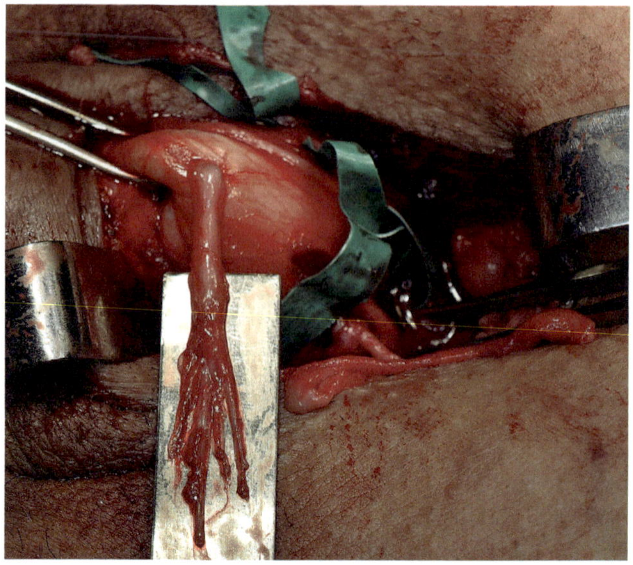

Fig. 59.4 Corpora cavernosa neurotization

3. The distal end of the two sural nerves harvested is sutured with end-to-side neurorrhaphies to the femoral nerve after identifying this nerve using a nerve stimulator, with at least 6–12 stitches using 8-0 nylon sutures after the removal of an epi-perineurium window [4]. It is essential that the stitches create good coaptation with positive pressure, which allows for better axonal sprouting.
4. Two nerves are used for the corpora cavernosa neurotization. Two Allis forceps (Rhosse, Ribeirão Preto, Brazil) grasp the tunica albuginea, one proximally and one distally, and both are pulled in opposite directions. Two 3 mm incisions with an 11-blade scalpel are made in the tunica albuginea on the lateral side of the penis. One proximal, at the base, and another 2–3 cm distally, and must be deep enough to allow the opening of the cavernous bodies, causing bleeding. A Mixter forceps (Rhosse, Ribeirão Preto, Brazil) is then introduced into the distal incision, emerging at the proximal one where it grasps the nerve graft and pulls it, causing its externalization through the distal incision. The "fraying" maneuver is performed to allow a greater chance of contact between the axons of the nerve graft and the corpora cavernosa (Fig. 59.4). The nerve graft is then pulled back through the proximal incision so that the nerve endings are in the corpora cavernosa. The incision sites in the corpora cavernosa are then sutured with 4-0 nylon to prevent bleeding.
5. The penile dorsal nerves are dissected using loupe magnification, and one graft on each side is sutured in an end-to-side fashion to this nerve without any epineural window (Figs. 59.5 and 59.6).
6. Finally, all skin incisions are closed in at least two layers.

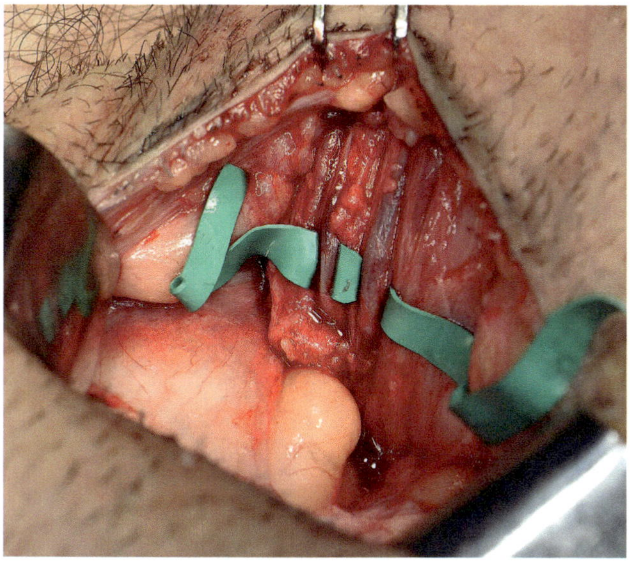

Fig. 59.5 The two dorsal nerves of the penis

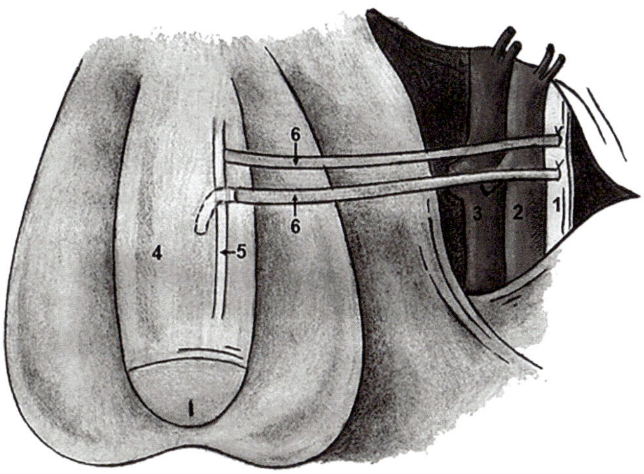

Fig. 59.6 Overview figure showing the sural nerve grafts (*6*) connecting the femoral nerve (*1*) to the dorsal nerve of the penis (*5*) and neurotizing the corpora cavernosa (*4*). The procedure is done bilaterally. *2* femoral artery; *3* femoral vein

Postoperative Care

The patient is allowed to walk on the first postoperative day and is released home, with a return for the removal of stitches in 7–10 days.

All patients are instructed to purchase a portable electrostimulator to perform electrostimulation of the inguinal region towards the base of the penis at least five times a day, for 10 min, for at least 6 months. After 8 weeks, they are released and encouraged to seek various penile stimulations, including masturbation, and attempting sexual intercourse.

References

1. Souza Trindade JC, Viterbo F, Petean Trindade A, Fávaro WJ, Trindade-Filho JCS (2017) Long-term follow-up of treatment of erectile dysfunction after radical prostatectomy using nerve grafts and end-to-side somatic-autonomic neurorraphy: a new technique. BJU Int 119(6):948–954. https://doi.org/10.1111/bju.13772. Epub 2017 Mar 10
2. de Menezes Neto BF, Viterbo F, Secanho MS, Moragas WR, Carvalho LB (2022) Bilateral sural nerve harvest in adult patients: a plastic surgery medical residency experience in Brazil. Eur J Plast Surg 45:327–332. https://doi.org/10.1007/s00238-021-01867-5
3. Viterbo F (2013) Improved blunt dissectors for greater safety in face lift surgery. Plast Reconstr Surg 131(5):858e–859e. https://doi.org/10.1097/PRS.0b013e318287a1bc
4. Viterbo F, Trindade JC, Hoshino K, Mazzoni NA (1992) Latero-terminal neurorrhaphy without removal of the epineural sheath. Experimental study in rats. Rev Paul Med 110(6):267–275

Nerve Transfers for Cervical Spinal Cord Injury

60

Stanley F. Bazarek, Margaret S. Sten, Jasmine A. Thum, Benjamin R. Johnston, and Justin M. Brown

Abbreviations

AIN	Anterior interosseous nerve
APL	Abductor pollicis longus
BB	Biceps brachii
BR	Brachioradialis
BRA	Brachialis branch of musculocutaneous nerve
ECRB	Extensor carpi radialis brevis
ECRL	Extensor carpi radialis longus
ECU	Extensor carpi ulnaris
ED	Extensor digitorum
EDM	Extensor digiti minimi
EI	Extensor indicis
EMG	Electromyogram
EPB	Extensor pollicis brevis
EPL	Extensor pollicis longus
FCU	Flexor carpi ulnaris
FDP	Flexor digitorum profundus
FPL	Flexor pollicis longus
LABC	Lateral antebrachial cutaneous nerve
LAT	Latissimus dorsi
LHT	Long head triceps branch of radial nerve
MCN	Musculocutaneous nerve
MRC	Medical Research Council
PIN	Posterior interosseous nerve
PQ	Pronator quadratus
SCI	Spinal cord injury
SSRN	Superficial sensory radial nerve
SUP	Supinator branch of radial nerve
TMi	Teres minor branch of axillary nerve

Stanley F. Bazarek and Margaret S. Sten contributed equally to this work.

Supplementary Information The online version contains supplementary material available at https://doi.org/10.1007/978-3-031-73931-6_60.

S. F. Bazarek
Department of Neurological Surgery, Case Western Reserve University School of Medicine, Cleveland, OH, USA
e-mail: stanley.bazarek@uhhospitals.org

M. S. Sten
Georgetown University School of Medicine, Washington, DC, USA
e-mail: msten@mgh.harvard.edu

J. A. Thum
Department of Neurosurgery, Massachusetts General Hospital, Harvard Medical School, Boston, MA, USA

Department of Neurosurgery, University of Alabama at Brimingham, Birmingham, AL, USA

B. R. Johnston
Department of Neurological Surgery, Brigham and Women's, Boston Children's Hospital, Harvard Medical School, Boston, MA, USA
e-mail: bjohnston2@bwh.harvard.edu

J. M. Brown (✉)
Department of Neurosurgery, Massachusetts General Hospital, Harvard Medical School, Boston, MA, USA
e-mail: jmbrown@mgh.harvard.edu

Indications

A C5 spinal cord injury (SCI) typically preserves function at the shoulder along with elbow flexion and supination. A subset of these predominant C5 innervated targets may be redistributed via nerve transfers to provide volitional control of elbow extension, finger flexion, and finger extension, resulting in a significant gain of function and independence [1, 2]. These reconstructive procedures are typically delayed 6–9 months following injury to allow for spontaneous recovery. Pre-operative assessment includes both physical examination and neurophysiology to determine the quality of the donor nerve (and recipient nerve in chronic cases). It is critical that donor sacrifice does not induce further functional deficit; therefore, another redundant muscle function must be available to back up the original donor function. Function should be confirmed by electromyography (EMG), as it is

A. S. Hanna (ed.), *Nerves: Anatomy, Exposures, and Techniques*, https://doi.org/10.1007/978-3-031-73931-6_60

often difficult to distinguish by clinical examination alone. The donor must demonstrate sufficient strength against resistance (at least an MRC Grade 4 and more than 3 motor units on EMG). The recipient nerve must be evaluated for signs of denervation from lower motor neuron injury, which would limit the time window for intervention due to irreversible fibrosis and atrophy (preferably within a year). This can be determined by direct muscular stimulation, with no activation of the target muscles indicating extensive lower motor neuron injury and thus a time limit for reconstruction.

Surgical Techniques

General anesthesia without the use of muscle relaxants is used for all procedures. Bipolar stimulation is used to limit the current spread and activation of unintended neighboring targets.

Teres Minor Branch of the Axillary Nerve to the Long Head of Triceps Branch of the Radial Nerve (Fig. 60.1)

Surgical Anatomy

The posterior cord of the brachial plexus first gives rise to the axillary nerve (AN) and continues as the radial nerve (RN). The AN typically contains an anterior division that supplies the anterior/middle deltoid, the posterior division that supplies the posterior deltoid and a cutaneous branch to the overlying skin of the deltoid, and a branch to the teres minor muscle (TMi). The first branch of the RN supplies the long head of the triceps (LHT). In the anterior approach, the latissimus dorsi (LAT) tendon can be used to identify the overlying proximal RN and the medially located quadrangular space containing the AN.

Clinical Significance

Elbow extension (C7, 8) is critical for expanding an individual's workspace to reach for objects in addition to elbow stabilization, particularly when the patient is in the recumbent position. It also allows the subject with SCI to do transfers to and from the wheelchair. Nerve transfer of the TMi to the LHT (largest triceps head) has been shown to restore adequate elbow extension for this purpose [3]. The TMi contributes to external rotation of the shoulder, which is also supported by the infraspinatus muscle; thus, external rotation is preserved following harvesting of TMi.

Exposure

1. The patient is placed supine with an arm board to position the arm in shoulder abduction and elbow extension to expose the axilla.
2. The incision is designed to anteriorly circumvent the glandular axillary skin to decrease infection risk and extends distally into the medial brachial neurovascular region.
3. A table-mounted retractor system may be used to facilitate the exposure. The brachial fascia is divided to expose the underlying neuro-vascular bundle. The brachial plexus branches are carefully dissected, working proximally to identify the major nerves and follow them to their origins at the level of the cords.

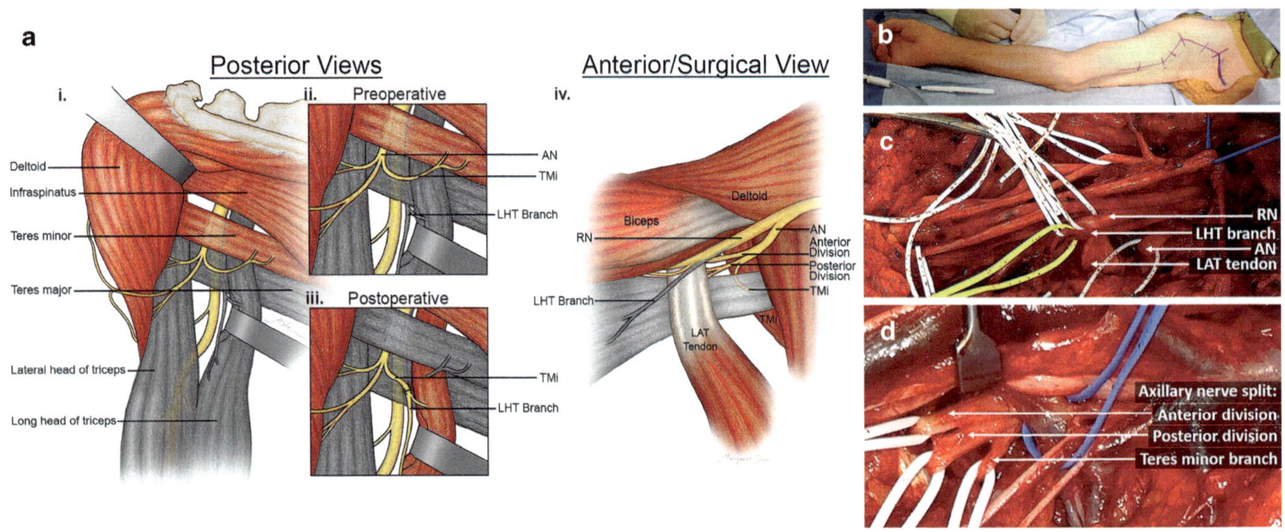

Fig. 60.1 TMi branch of the RN to the LHT for elbow extension. (**a**) The posterior view is shown to demonstrate the target muscles of the nerves with the coaptation (*i–iii*). (Denervated muscles are depicted in gray and innervated in red.) The surgery is performed through an anterior approach (*iv*). The LAT tendon insertion to the humerus serves as an initial landmark to identify the AN passing through the quadrangular space (just proximal to the LAT tendon) and the RN overlying the LAT tendon. (**b**) The incision is designed to access the axilla and avoid the glandular skin. (**c**) Operative view as depicted in the graphic. The LHT (*yellow loop*) is identified by following the RN proximally. (**d**) The AN is subsequently neurolyzed into its three main branches: anterior division to the bulk of the deltoid muscle, the posterior division to the posterior deltoid and cutaneous sensation overlying the deltoid, and the teres minor branch

4. The LAT tendon is identified at its insertion into the humerus and completely exposed to facilitate identification of the quadrangular space (borders: LHT, humerus, TMi, and teres major). The AN can be palpated just proximal to the LAT insertion on the humerus and further exposed. AN stimulation should demonstrate robust shoulder abduction and external rotation.
5. The RN lies on the surface of the LAT tendon and is just posterior to the median and ulnar nerves. The RN is traced proximally to identify the branch to the LHT, which is the first branch of the RN. The nerve should be followed to confirm insertion into the LHT muscle belly. RN stimulation will be variable depending on the extent of lower motor neuron injury but should activate at least the brachioradialis and supinator muscles in most cases (typically C5–6).
6. The microscope is utilized to further separate the AN from the circumflex arteries and to neurolyze the branch to the TMi from the anterior and posterior axillary divisions. The posterior deltoid can be preserved as a backup tendon transfer option for elbow extension. Strong external rotation should be definitively demonstrated upon stimulation of the teres minor branch (this is facilitated by bringing the arm into slight adduction and internal rotation before stimulating).
7. The teres minor branch is sharply transected as distally as possible and the branch to the long head of the triceps should be neurolyzed away from the main radial nerve to gain as much additional length as possible before it is transected proximally. The nerves are coapted by 9-0 nylon epineurial sutures. A collagen tube is used to relieve tension and reinforce the repair site, secured with 8-0 nylon sutures, and covered with fibrin glue.
8. Closure is performed with intra-dermal 3–0 braided Vicryl sutures and skin glue. An abdominal pad is placed in the axillary fold to absorb moisture. A sling is used to minimize shoulder movement in the early post-operative period to protect the repair site. Typically, abduction is limited to 45° for 3 weeks, then 90° for 3 weeks, then full range. This restriction depends upon the available range of motion following the completion of the repair.

Brachialis Branch of the Musculocutaneous Nerve to Anterior Interosseous Nerve (Fig. 60.2)

Surgical Anatomy

The musculocutaneous nerve (MCN) supplies the most powerful elbow flexors (biceps brachii (BB) and brachialis (BRA) muscles) and terminates as the lateral antebrachial cutaneous nerve (LABC) to provide cutaneous innervation to the lateral forearm. The anterior interosseous nerve (AIN) is a branch of the median nerve (MN) that supplies the flexor pollicis longus (FPL), the flexor digitorum profundus (FDP) to digits 2 and 3, and the pronator quadratus (PQ).

Clinical Significance

Hand function is critical for independence and requires the ability to both grasp and release objects. The AIN is a desired target, particularly as it controls the ability to flex the thumb, index, and middle fingers. Distal donors in the forearm, such as the pronator teres and the nerve to the extensor carpi radialis brevis (ECRB) (C6, 7), are unavailable in a C5 injury, but the nerve to the brachialis is typically available as a donor [4]. Elbow flexion is preserved by the BB and brachioradialis following harvesting of the BRA. While there are multiple methods for implementing this transfer, we will describe the direct transfer.

Exposure

1. The patient is supine with the arm extended on the hand table.
2. A Bruner's incision (zigzag to limit skin contractures) is drawn across the antecubital fossa and extended proximally into the medial brachial region.
3. Subcutaneous dissection is performed on the forearm and brachial fascia. In the forearm, the lacertus fibrosus (bicipital aponeurosis) is released, and the forearm fascia is divided to develop the plain between the flexor-pronator mass and the brachioradialis to expose the MN and the AIN as it branches from the main MN trunk.
4. The AIN is identified distally and neurolyzed proximally. NOTE: There are typically several interconnecting fascicles between the proximal AIN and MN as we progress proximally beyond the antecubital fossa. It is critical to include only AIN fibers to avoid dispersion of axons to non-desired targets. This will ultimately limit the extent of proximal neurolysis.
5. The MCN can then be identified between the BB and BRA muscles, with the BB branch arising proximal to the mid-humeral level. The incision should be extended proximally to identify the branch to the BB and verify its stimulation in isolation will provide sufficient elbow flexion. The MCN continues until a branch arises to innervate the BRA. The BRA branch splits and enters the muscle in 2 or 3 final branches. Following this, only the LABC branch should continue distally. Stimulation of the BRA nerve should elicit strong elbow flexion. The BRA nerve can be followed into the muscle to harvest maximal length, but it becomes larger in caliber the further distally it is followed.
6. The AIN should be sharply transected at its most proximal point, where only pure AIN fibers remain. It is then rerouted superficially to gain length. If this is insufficient,

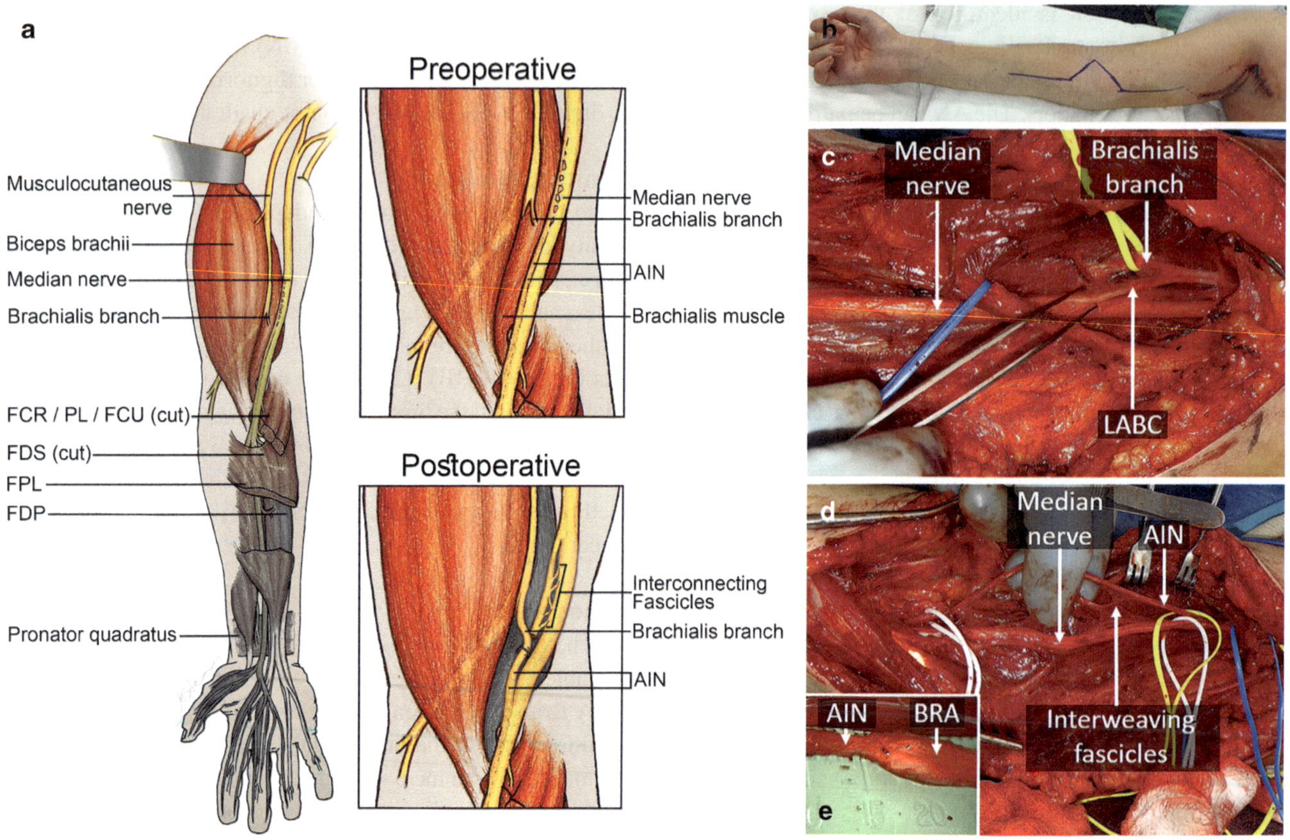

Fig. 60.2 BRA branch of the MCN to the AIN. (**a**) The AIN branches of the MN innervate the FPL, FDP (Digits 2 and 3), and the PQ. The proximal neurolysis of the AIN is limited by interweaving fascicles with the MN (inset). The dissection is continued proximally until the AIN can no longer be separated from the MN. The BRA nerve is identified under the BB and the inset demonstrates the BRA coapted to the AIN just distal to any remaining interweaving AIN-MN fascicles. (Denervated muscles are depicted in gray and innervated in red.) (**b**) A Bruner type incision is marked across the antecubital fossa and into the intermuscular plane of the arm. (**c**) The proximal aspect of the surgical field is shown with the BRA branch (*yellow loop*) of the MCN and the continuing LABC in addition to the pre-neurolyzed MN. (**d**) The AIN is shown with the interweaving fascicles between the AIN and MN. (**e**) The BRA-AIN coaptation is shown

the elbow may require flexion to enable tensionless repair. The table-mounted retractor may be used to maintain elbow flexion, and the rest of the operation would then proceed with the elbow held in a flexed position.

7. The nerves are coapted by 9-0 nylon epineurial sutures under the microscope. A collagen tube is used to relieve tension and reinforce the repair site, secured with 8-0 nylon sutures, and covered with fibrin glue.
8. Closure is performed with intradermal 3-0 braided Vicryl sutures and skin glue. An adjustable immobilizing brace is used to gradually extend the elbow following a 3-week period of immobilization at 90°. Depending on the tightness of the repair, the gradual extension could last 6 weeks or more. (Of note, when time is not of the essence, our team now frequently bypasses this lengthy dissection and immobilization by using a nerve graft in a 2-part operation: brachialis to graft tunneled distally, followed in 6 months by connection of the distal graft to the AIN within the forearm).

Supinator Branches of the Radial Nerve to the Posterior Interosseous Nerve for Finger Extension (Fig. 60.3)

Surgical Anatomy

The RN innervates the posterior compartment of the arm and forearm. Following innervation of the triceps, there are branches to the brachioradialis (BR), radial wrist extensors (ECRL and ECRB), and supinator (SUP) muscles. The nerve then continues as the superficial sensory radial nerve (SSRN) to provide cutaneous innervation to the radial dorsum of the hand and as the posterior interosseus nerve (PIN), which provides innervation to all finger extensors and extensor carpi ulnaris. The SUP branches arise just proximal to the PIN, diving deep to the SUP muscle. The SUP branches are innervated primarily by the C5–6 nerve roots, while PIN contains fibers primarily from C7 to C8.

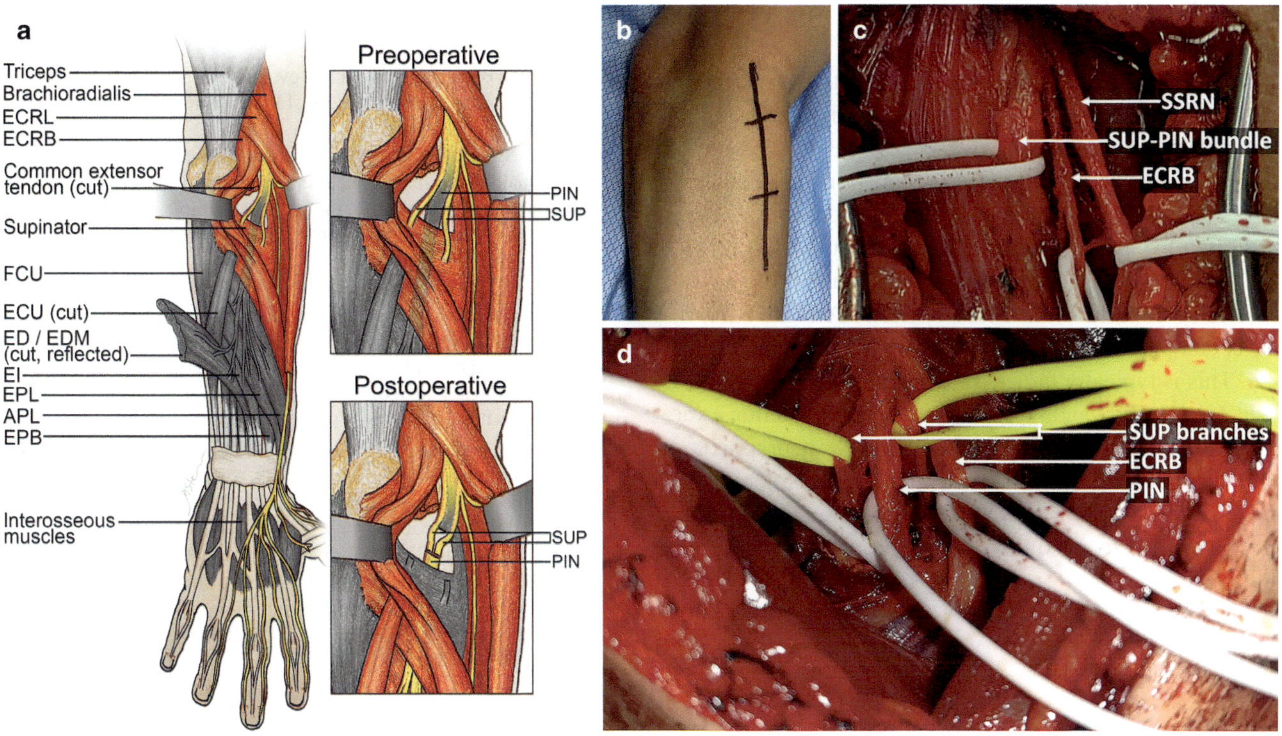

Fig. 60.3 SUP branches of RN to the PIN. (**a**) The SUP branches off the deep RN with the PIN continuing to innervate the posterior compartment of the forearm. The insets show the SUP branches (often two to four branches) combined as multiple fascicles and coapted to the PIN. (Denervated muscles are depicted in gray and innervated in red.) (**b**) The incision is made in the proximal forearm posterior to the brachioradialis muscle (between BR and ECRL). (**c**) The SSRN and ECRB are typically first identified and neurolyzed from the deep RN containing the PIN and SUP branches. (**d**) The SUP branches (*yellow loops*) are neurolyzed from the PIN

Clinical Significance

Finger extension is critical to create an aperture by which to get the hand around objects to grasp them and then to release them. This function has been achieved in tetraplegics with the transfer of the SUP branches of the RN to the PIN [5, 6]. Supination of the forearm is preserved by the BB, which supinates in addition to providing elbow flexion.

Exposure

1. The patient is positioned supine with arm extended on hand table. A Penrose drain secured to the hand table may be used to maintain the wrist in pronation for exposure of the posterior compartment of the forearm. We avoid a tourniquet in these cases so as to not diminish the response to stimulation.
2. The incision is drawn in the proximal forearm along the plane between the BR and the extensor muscles (palpate the border of the BR).
3. Care must be taken during the superficial dissection to avoid injury to the LABC, which would create a sensory deficit in the lateral forearm (often the best preserved distal sensation in these patients).
4. A color distinction is observed between the thicker white ECRL and red BR muscle fascia. This fascial interval is sharply divided, and the intermuscular plane leads directly to the fat pad containing the radial nerve. A cerebellar retractor is used to maintain this exposure.
5. The SSRN is first encountered and can be proximally neurolyzed to the main radial trunk to identify branches to ECRB and the PIN. The vascular leash of Henry (recurrent radial artery branch) can be divided to enhance exposure.
6. The PIN and the SUP branches typically form a trifurcation, with the largest branch being the PIN. The PIN is neurolyzed proximally and separated from the supinator branches. Once they are safely separated from the main trunk of the PIN, it is divided as proximally as possible, just distal to their origin. The SUP branches are all followed distally and divided as well. Note: There is often an additional SUP branch posterior to the PIN. Typically, between 2 and 4 SUP branches are found. It is important to incorporate all the SUP branches, as failure to include all branches may lead to persistent coactivation of supination and finger extension. This will limit the utility of the transfer.
7. The nerves are coapted by 9-0 nylon epineurial sutures under the microscope. A collagen tube is used to relieve tension and reinforce the repair site, secured to the more proximal epineurium with 8-0 nylon sutures, and covered with fibrin glue.
8. Closure is performed with intra-dermal 3-0 braided Vicryl sutures and skin glue. This repair is typically free from the risk of tension from positioning.

Complications

Infections and hematoma are rare but potential post-operative complications. Transient weakness of wrist extension following retraction of wrist extensor muscles for this transfer is not uncommon. Weakness of the function provided by the nerve being cut and transferred is always a concern, but these are often avoidable with careful preoperative evaluation of the backup agonist. Separation at the coaptation site is of particular concern with the direct BRA-AIN transfer, and strict compliance to wearing the immobilizing brace is critical. This is typically far less of a concern with the SUP-PIN transfer. Careful handling of the nerves and retraction awareness is important to prevent post-operative neurapraxia, as any loss of function, even transient, is poorly tolerated in a patient who already has an SCI. Rigorous occupational therapy is critical to maximize the functional benefit of these transfers.

References

1. Bazarek S, Brown JM (2020) The evolution of nerve transfers for spinal cord injury. Exp Neurol 333:113426. https://doi.org/10.1016/j.expneurol.2020.113426
2. van Zyl N, Hill B, Cooper C, Hahn J, Galea MP (2019) Expanding traditional tendon-based techniques with nerve transfers for the restoration of upper limb function in tetraplegia: a prospective case series. Lancet 394(10198):565–575. https://doi.org/10.1016/s0140-6736(19)31143-2
3. Bertelli JA, Ghizoni MF, Tacca CP (2011) Transfer of the teres minor motor branch for triceps reinnervation in tetraplegia. J Neurosurg 114(5):1457–1460. https://doi.org/10.3171/2010.12.JNS101519
4. Bertelli JA, Ghizoni MF (2017) Nerve transfers for restoration of finger flexion in patients with tetraplegia. J Neurosurg Spine 26(1):55–61. https://doi.org/10.3171/2016.5.SPINE151544
5. Bazarek S, Sten M, Nin D, Brown JM (2021) Supinator to posterior interosseous nerve transfer for restoration of finger extension. Oper Neurosurg (Hagerstown) 21(5):E408–EE13. https://doi.org/10.1093/ons/opab263
6. Bertelli JA, Tacca CP, Ghizoni MF, Kechele PR, Santos MA (2010) Transfer of supinator motor branches to the posterior interosseous nerve to reconstruct thumb and finger extension in tetraplegia: case report. J Hand Surg Am 35(10):1647–1651. https://doi.org/10.1016/j.jhsa.2010.07.012

61 Selective Neurectomies and Myectomies for Cervical Dystonia

Robert J. Spinner and Brandon W. Smith

Indications

The indications for selective denervation for cervical dystonia include refractory pain and deformity that have not improved with physical therapy, medications, and injections of neuromuscular blockers. Surgical indications include idiopathic cases of rotational torticollis, laterocollis, and retrocollis.

Surgical Anatomy

The main targets of denervation procedures for cervical dystonia are the dorsal rami of the cervical spinal nerves and the spinal accessory nerve in the neck. Neurosurgeons may be unfamiliar with the nuances of this anatomy. A detailed understanding of the surgical anatomy of the posterior cervical paraspinal muscles (including the dorsal rami of the cervical spinal nerves) and the sternocleidomastoid (SCM) (and the spinal accessory nerve) is necessary to perform selective denervation procedures for cervical dystonia.

While most posterior cervical surgery is directed in the midline towards the spinous processes and laminae, the paramedian plane deep to the trapezius and splenius capitis muscles allows identification of the dorsal rami of the cervical spinal nerves between the semispinalis capitis and cervicis muscles. Knowledge of the course of the spinal accessory nerve from the skull base through the posterior triangle is needed. The spinal accessory nerve exits the jugular foramen and runs through or deep to the SCM. It then passes obliquely towards the trapezius muscle. The identification of the branching pattern of the accessory nerve is needed to perform safe selective denervation and avoid injury to the trapezius branch. Dysfunction of the trapezius would produce scapular instability.

Surgical Techniques

The surgical procedure targeting the most affected muscles on the more affected side of the posterior cervical paraspinal muscles and the SCM is evolving. Decision-making is based on the clinical phenotype and findings of overactive muscle contraction on special movement disorders electromyography (EMG). Most commonly, procedures are done on both sides. Our surgical approach and results have been reported [1, 2]. In general, for rotational torticollis, the ipsilateral cervical paraspinals and the contralateral SCM are targeted. For laterocollis, the ipsilateral cervical paraspinals, SCM, and levator scapulae muscles are targeted. For retrocollis, bilateral cervical paraspinal muscles are denervated.

Supplementary Information The online version contains supplementary material available at https://doi.org/10.1007/978-3-031-73931-6_61.

R. J. Spinner (✉)
Department of Neurologic Surgery, Mayo Clinic, Rochester, MN, USA
e-mail: Spinner.robert@mayo.edu

B. W. Smith
Cone Health Neurosurgery, Burlington, NC, USA
e-mail: Brandon.Smith2@conehealth.com

A. S. Hanna (ed.), *Nerves: Anatomy, Exposures, and Techniques*, https://doi.org/10.1007/978-3-031-73931-6_61

Selective Denervation of Cervical Paraspinal Muscles (C2–6 Dorsal Rami)

1. Surgery is performed in a seated position. The occiput and neck are prepped and draped widely for good exposure.
2. A posterior midline incision is used exposing the occiput to C7. A hockey stick type incision with a transverse curved limb (Bertrand incision) may be used to flap the side of the exposure but is not necessary in our experience.
3. The midline fascia is opened. The dissection is not taken to bone. At the deepest muscle layer (deep to the trapezius and splenius capitis muscles), the interval between the semispinalis capitis and cervicis muscles is developed where the medial branches of the C2–6 dorsal rami of the cervical spinal nerves are identified (Fig. 61.1a). They are traced proximally to the respective foramina where they are divided. Ligaclips are placed.
4. For the C2 nerve (and C1), the rectus capitis posterior major (Fig. 61.1b) and inferior oblique are divided (Fig. 61.1c).
5. The gutter lateral to the foramina is then accessed by dividing the origin of semispinalis capitis. In the plane beneath it, the lateral branches of the C3–6 dorsal rami can be found, which are also divided (Fig. 61.1d).
6. Muscle resection either of semispinalis capitis or splenius capitis can be performed (Fig. 61.1e). Limbs of the levator scapulae muscle may be divided (Fig. 61.1f).

Division of Sternocleidomastoid Muscle and Neurectomy of the Accessory Nerve Branch to the SCM

1. A separate 3–4 cm incision is made halfway between the turn of the trapezius and the pinna of the ear in one of the neck creases (Fig. 61.2a).
2. The incision is deepened, and the great auricular nerve is identified on the SCM and mobilized (Fig. 61.2b). The posterior belly of the SCM is identified and reflected.
3. About 2 cm posterior to the great auricular nerve, the SCM is then divided in a controlled manner, taking care to identify the accessory nerve and its branches to the SCM trapezius. The accessory nerve can be identified after the SCM has been partially or near completely divided from superficially to deep; it can also be identified prior to the myectomy; however, the SCM is often hypertrophied, making this option not easy.
4. The terminal branches are identified (Fig. 61.2c and d). A nerve stimulator is used to confirm the anatomy by producing muscle contractions from the individual branch(es). The branch to the trapezius (which is more transverse) is maintained, and to the SCM (which is more vertical) is divided (Fig. 61.2e).
5. Remaining deep muscle fibers of the SCM are divided.

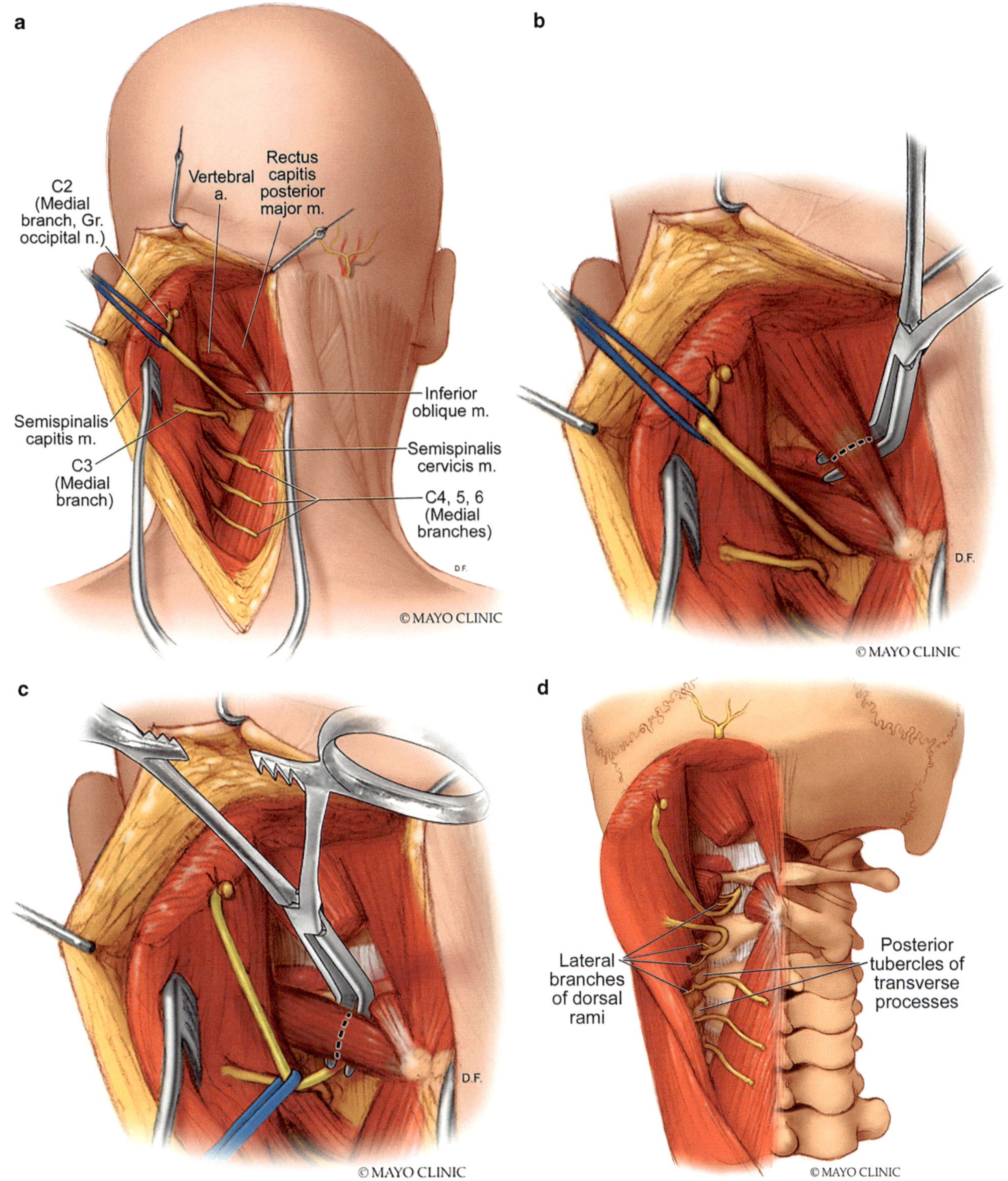

Fig. 61.1 Selective denervation of cervical paraspinal muscles (C2–6 dorsal rami). (**a**) Dorsal rami of C2–6 are identified in the interval between the semispinal capitis and cervicis muscles. C2,3 are typically found deep to semispinalis capitis while C4-6 superficial to semispinalis cervicis. C5,6 are the smallest in diameter. (**b**) For proximal dissection of C2 nerve and exposure of C1, rectus capitis posterior major is divided. (**c**) Inferior oblique muscle is also divided. (**d**) Ligaclips are placed proximally at the level of the foramina, and the medial branches are divided. The lateral branches are identified near the Ligaclips in the gutter after the semispinalis capitis muscle is divided. (**e**) The splenius capitis or the semispinalis capitis is resected. (**f**) The levator scapulae muscle may be divided. (Used with permission of Mayo Foundation for Medical Education and Research. All rights reserved [2])

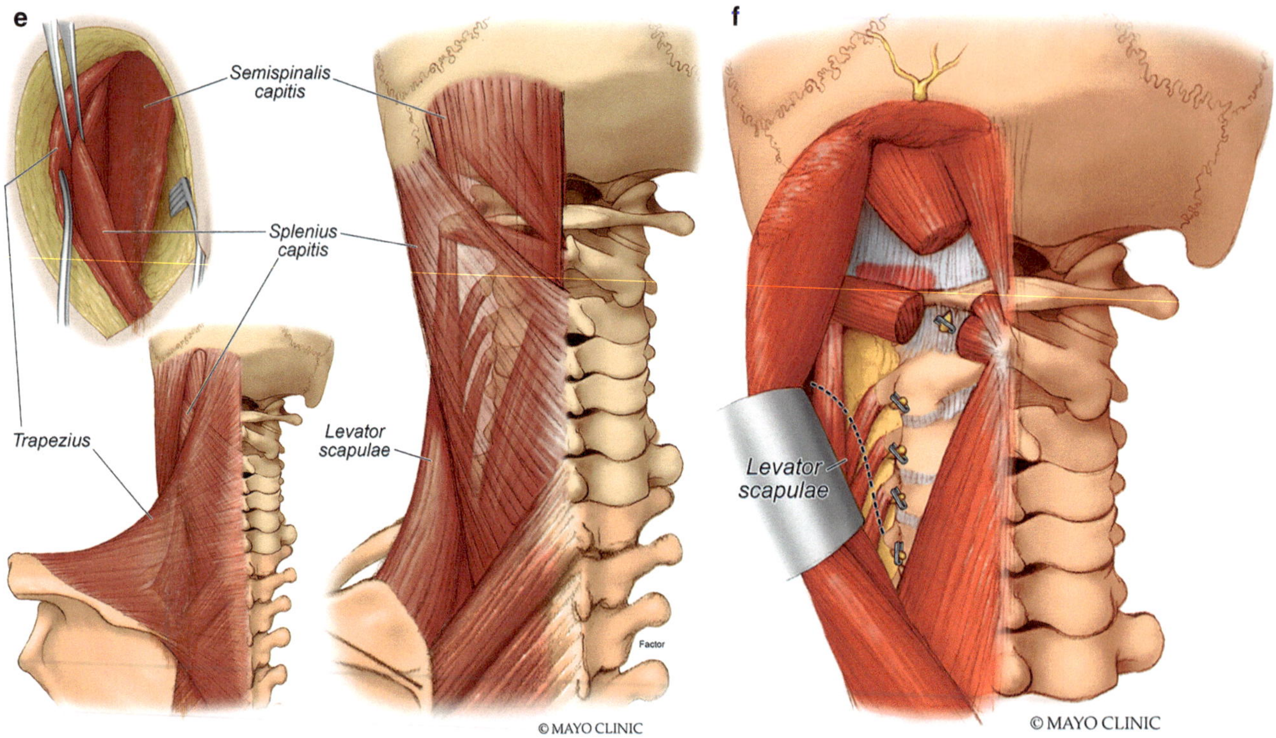

Fig. 61.1 (continued)

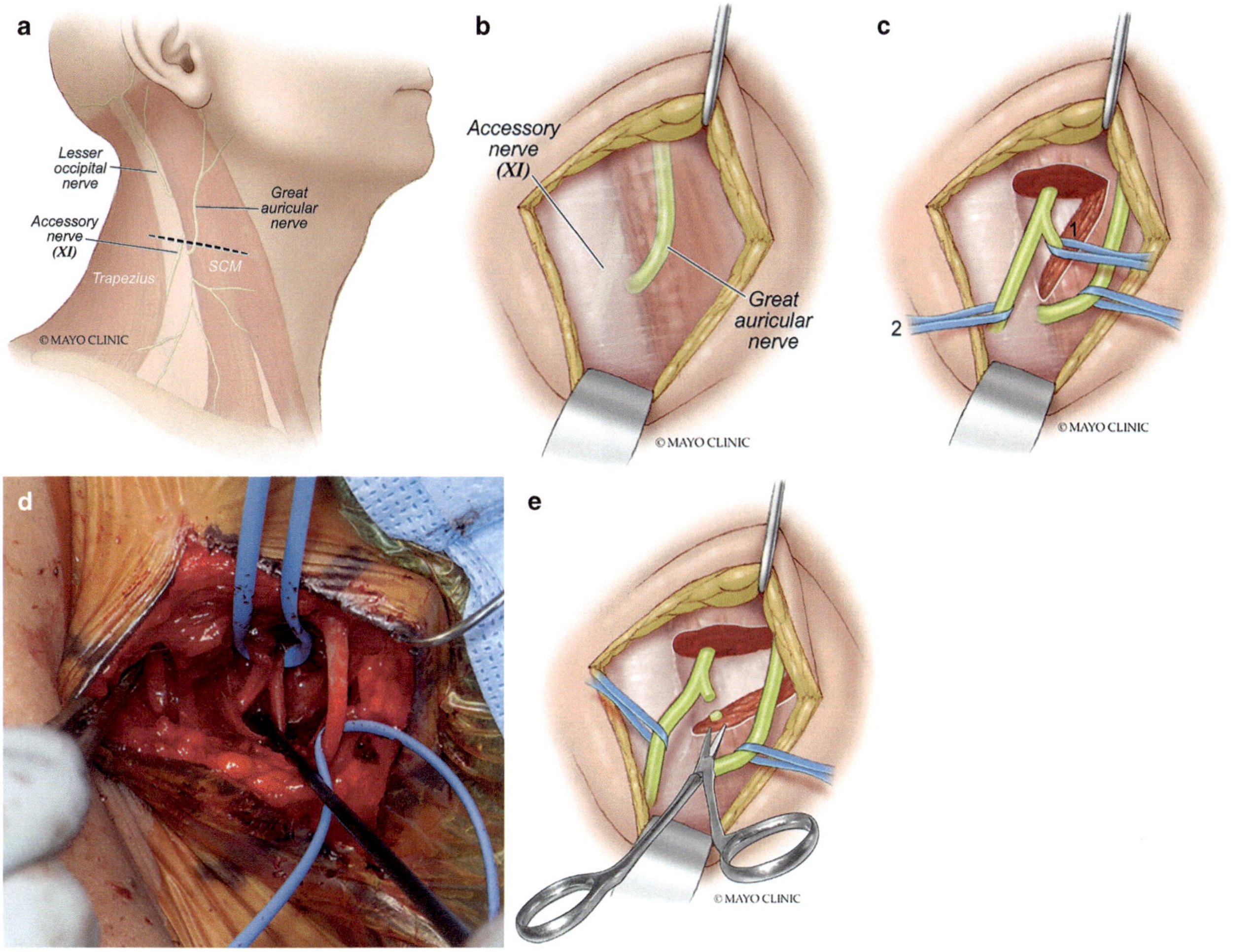

Fig. 61.2 Division of the SCM and neurectomy of the accessory nerve branch to the SCM. (**a**) An oblique incision in the mid-neck is planned at the posterior border of the SCM. (**b**) The great auricular nerve is identified and mobilized. (**c**) The SCM is divided approximately 2 cm posterior to the great auricular nerve. The accessory nerve and its branches to the SCM (1) and the trapezius (2) muscles are identified. (**d**) The great auricular nerve is seen in a vasoloop to the right of the photograph. The accessory nerve has been identified in a vasoloop just proximal to its branching point. The spatula shows the SCM branch. (**e**) After stimulation of the nerve branches is done and confirms the anatomy, the accessory branch to the SCM is divided. (Used with permission of Mayo Foundation for Medical Education and Research. All rights reserved)

Outcomes

Selective denervation is a safe and highly effective procedure for dystonia. Still, realistic goals need to be set for patients with this disabling condition. While the surgery can dramatically straighten the abnormal head position and decrease the pulling sensation and spasm, it does not cure the dystonia; the tendency to pull with stress or fatigue will likely remain to some degree. Improvement in the head position is achieved in about 80% of patients (Fig. 61.3). Neck pain, while multifactorial in nature, can be improved in about 50%. Patients with post-traumatic cervical dystonia do not respond as favorably to selective denervation. The surgery, however, is not aimed at tremor, which may coexist in the initial presentation of the patient with dystonia.

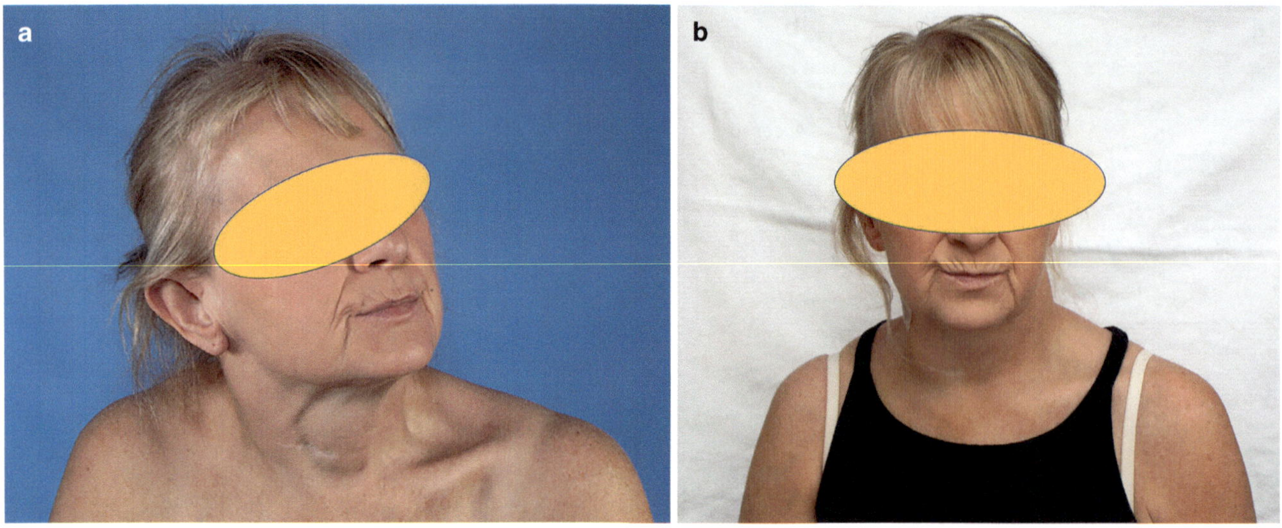

Fig. 61.3 A 58-year-old woman with a 5-year history of severe left rotational torticollis underwent selective denervation of her left cervical paraspinals and right SCM. She had a previous anterior cervical discectomy and fusion without benefit. (**a**) Preoperative photograph shows severe left rotational torticollis and the prominent right SCM. (**b**) Clinical photograph shows improvement in the abnormal head position immediately after the surgery

Complications

Complications are usually minor or temporary.

1. Hypesthesia in a portion of the scalp is expected, but the denervation may rarely result in dysesthesias.
2. Numbness in the earlobe may also occur from the mobilization of the great auricular nerve.
3. Shoulder weakness from the dissection of the accessory nerve may occur.
4. There is a small risk of air emboli related to the seated position.
5. Vertebral artery injury has been reported but is minimized by the current technique which does not address the C1 nerve directly and instead includes myectomy of the semispinalis capitis, rectus capitis posterior major, and inferior oblique.

References

1. Cohen-Gadol AA, Ahlskog JE, Matsumoto JY, Swenson MA, McClelland RL, Davis DH (2003) Selective peripheral denervation for spasmodic torticollis: experience with 168 patients at the Mayo Clinic. J Neurosurg 98:1247–1254. https://doi.org/10.3171/jns.2003.98.6.1247
2. Wilson TJ, Spinner RJ (2018) Selective cervical denervation for cervical dystonia: modification of the Bertrand procedure. Neurosurgery 14:546–555. https://doi.org/10.1093/ons/opx147

62 Selective Neurectomies for Treatment of Limb Spasticity

Forrest A. Hamrick and Mark A. Mahan

Indications

Patients who continue to experience refractory focal limb spasticity may be candidates for HSN. Refractory spasticity is often diagnosed after serial botulinum toxin injections and antispasmodic medication trials [1]. Individuals who remain severely and stably spastic for greater than 12 months despite these therapies are more likely to benefit from HSN [2, 3]. Some patients will have also received intrathecal baclofen therapy or tendon surgeries without relief.

Preoperative assessment includes evaluating factors that may guide the extent of neurectomy, such as the degree of residual motor control, the use of spasticity for function, and the identity of the affected muscle(s). Those suffering from only moderate spasticity with preserved motor control and functional use of the affected limb may benefit from a partial neurectomy approximating 50% of the cross-sectional area of the target nerve branch. Individuals with severe spasticity, minimal motor control, and limited limb functionality will likely benefit from a more aggressive partial neurectomy, approximating 75–80% of the cross-sectional area of the nerve branch [1, 2].

Identifying contraindications to HSN requires an assessment of the predominant motor pathology. Patients with progressive disorders such as multiple sclerosis, fixed contracture, or an overriding movement disorder like dystonia or athetosis are considered noncandidates [2, 3]. Generalized spasticity, such as spastic tetraplegia, is a relative contraindication, as well as impaired cognition that would limit the ability to meaningfully engage in physical therapy. Typical surgical contraindications such as continuous anticoagulation should also be strongly considered during preoperative evaluation.

Physiological Basis

Spasticity arising from central nervous system injuries, most commonly stroke, traumatic brain injury, and spinal cord injury, results from a complex response to the loss of descending motor control. While reduction in descending inhibition has previously been attributed as the primary pathologic lesion [4], further studies have shown that the reflex arc is amplified by pathologic filling of denervated synapses on motor neurons by sensory afferents. In essence, the loss of motor control is replaced by sensory input from the periphery, leading to a dysregulated, amplified sensory reflex [5].

Surgical Techniques

1. An incision is made superficial to the innervating nerve of the targeted spastic muscle(s).
2. Identify the branch(es) of the targeted nerve that innervate the spastic muscle(s).
   (a) Additionally, the surface of the muscle is stimulated with a monopolar stimulator to detect branch variation and avoid missing occult, sub-millimeter nerves.
   (b) We typically use 1 mA stimulation to "inspect" the region for localization of occult branches, which are branches of the primary nerve to the muscle of interest.
3. Open the epineurium longitudinally to identify fascicles within the branch.

Supplementary Information The online version contains supplementary material available at https://doi.org/10.1007/978-3-031-73931-6_62.

F. A. Hamrick
School of Medicine, University of Utah, Salt Lake City, UT, USA
e-mail: Forrest.Hamrick@hsc.utah.edu

M. A. Mahan (✉)
Division of Nerve and Pain Surgery, Department of Neurosurgery, University of Utah, Salt Lake City, UT, USA
e-mail: mark.mahan@hsc.utah.edu

A. S. Hanna (ed.), *Nerves: Anatomy, Exposures, and Techniques*, https://doi.org/10.1007/978-3-031-73931-6_62

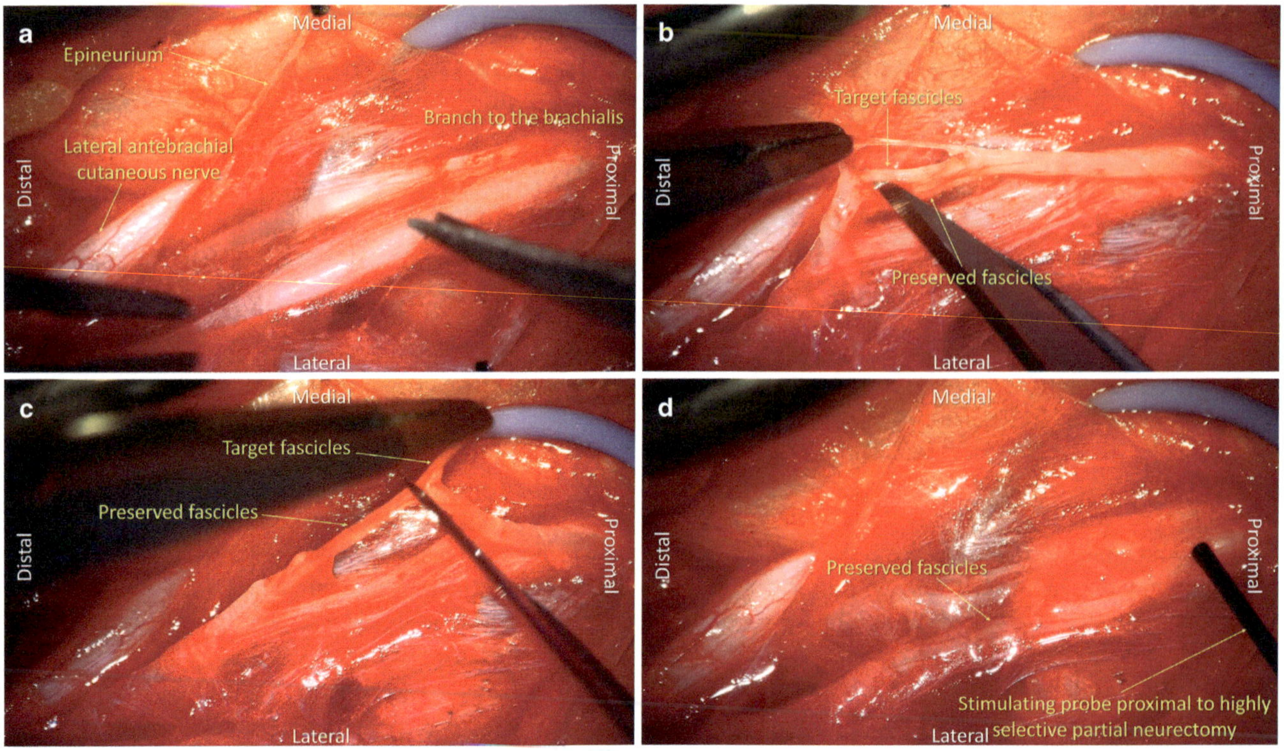

Fig. 62.1 Intraoperative still images of the selective fascicle sectioning of the branch to the brachialis. (**a**) Opening of the epineurium of the nerve to the brachialis with visualization of two fascicles. The nerve to the brachialis is often inferior/posterior to the lateral antebrachial cutaneous nerve in origin from the distal musculocutaneous nerve. (**b**) Once a fascicle is selected for sectioning, often in response to electrical stimulation, the fascicle is divided through a longitudinal cut with a #11 scalpel blade. Fascicles that are desired to be preserved are not touched. (**c**) Approximately 10 mm of sectioned fascicle is removed to reduce regeneration. (**d**) Muscle response to stimulation is compared between stimulation proximal to the highly selective partial neurectomy and distal to the lesion. We expect minimal response to stimulation proximal to the iatrogenic lesion, despite continuity of the intact fascicles. While electrical stimulation at low amperage is abrogated, the patient typically (>90%) awakes with retained motor control, if it was present prior to the surgery

4. Place a 4-0 suture in the epineurium on either side of the nerve to elevate the nerve from the field to enhance visualization (Fig. 62.1a).
5. Stimulate the fascicles within the nerve branch to assess for exaggerated responses.
   (a) Apply low-amperage electrical stimulation to each nerve branch to low-threshold activation, exaggerated reflex, or pathological spread within the spastic muscle. More reactive/lower threshold branch(es) are noted for more substantial nerve reduction.
   (b) We use current amperages of 0.1–0.5 mA, based on clinical context (such as prior phenol injection, etc.) once the epineurium has been opened.
6. Open the perineurium longitudinally.
7. Section fascicles preferentially based on exaggerated response, with the goal of achieving the preoperatively planned percentage (50–80%) of cross-sectional area of the nerve or fascicle (Fig. 62.1b).
   (a) If a target nerve branch contains only a single fascicle, open the perineurium and separate the endoneurial tissue lengthwise before sectioning a portion of the endoneurium to achieve partial neurectomy.
   (b) Remove a 1-cm segment of the sectioned fascicle(s) (Fig. 62.1c).
8. Stimulate the proximal parent nerve to assess the resultant reduction in excitability, either confirming achieving the desired result or the need for further sectioning [6] (Fig. 62.1d). Loss of stimulation is common, especially once the perineurium is opened; however, this does not reflect a postoperative palsy. The degree of sectioning determines the amount of weakness postoperatively, not the electrical response after opening the perineurium.
9. Variations: Numerous variations have been published on the surgical technique, including sectioning some fascicles while leaving other fascicles untreated [7] as well as sectioning branches of nerve further distally, i.e., within the muscle. To date, there have been no head-to-head comparisons of different surgical techniques. While such a study would be worthwhile, there is substantial variation in patient spasticity pathophysiology, retained motor control, tendon and/or joint contracture,

and other confounding variables that would make it challenging to draw definitive conclusions between surgical techniques.

Complications

The most common complication after HSN procedures is re-emergent spasticity or insufficient reduction in spasticity. In our experience, patients at the highest risk of this outcome were those with a history of deep cerebral hemorrhages. Neurectomy is unlikely to result in sensitive neuroma formation since cutaneous afferents are avoided. There is a low risk of paresis, paresthesia, and dysesthesia. Other operative complications common to all surgical procedures are possible, including hematoma and wound infection.

References

1. Leclercq C (2018) Selective neurectomy for the spastic upper extremity. Hand Clin 34(4):537–545. https://doi.org/10.1016/j.hcl.2018.06.010
2. Mahan MA, Eli I, Hamrick F, Abou-Al-Shaar H, Shingleton R, Tucker Balun K et al (2021) Highly selective partial neurectomies for spasticity: a single-center experience. Neurosurgery 89(5):827–835. https://doi.org/10.1093/neuros/nyab303
3. Leclercq C, Perruisseau-Carrier A, Gras M, Panciera P, Fulchignoni C, Fulchignoni M (2021) Hyperselective neurectomy for the treatment of upper limb spasticity in adults and children: a prospective study. J Hand Surg Eur Vol 46(7):708–716. https://doi.org/10.1177/17531934211027499
4. Nagel SJ, Wilson S, Johnson MD, Machado A, Frizon L, Chardon MK et al (2017) Spinal cord stimulation for spasticity: historical approaches, current status, and future directions. Neuromodulation 20(4):307–321. https://doi.org/10.1111/ner.12591
5. Sindou M, Duraffourg M, Georgoulis G (2022) Neurosurgery for spasticity, a practical guide for treating children and adults, 2nd edn. Springer, Switzerland. https://doi.org/10.1007/978-3-030-92717-2
6. Abou-Al-Shaar H, Mahan MA (2021) Highly selective partial neurectomy for lower-extremity spasticity: 2-dimensional operative video. Oper Neurosurg (Hagerstown) 20(6):E442–E443. https://doi.org/10.1093/ons/opab020
7. Sitthinamsuwan B, Chanvanitkulchai K, Phonwijit L, Nunta-Aree S, Kumthornthip W, Ploypetch T (2013) Surgical outcomes of microsurgical selective peripheral neurotomy for intractable limb spasticity. Stereotact Funct Neurosurg 91(4):248–257. https://doi.org/10.1159/000345504. Epub 2013 Mar 26.

63 Neuroma

Amgad S. Hanna

Indications

The main indication for surgery is a painful neuroma intractable to medical management. These can be very challenging. There are numerous methods to treat neuromas; below are some examples. The main risks are failure to improve the pain and recurrent neuroma. A painful neuroma should be resected unless on a major motor nerve with residual function. In the latter case, extensive release should be performed with the opening of the epineurium or consider neuromodulation.

Surgical Techniques (Fig. 63.1)

Resection and Grafting (Fig. 63.2)

- For a neuroma in continuity where there is a proximal and distal nerve accessible, assuming that the nerve is not functional.
- The neuroma is resected down to normal-appearing nerve proximally and distally.
- A bridge graft can be used to bridge the gap between the proximal and distal nerve stumps.
- Autografts can be used but have the risk of developing a neuroma on the donor nerve causing a new source of pain. Allografts are preferred.

Supplementary Information The online version contains supplementary material available at https://doi.org/10.1007/978-3-031-73931-6_63.

A. S. Hanna (✉)
Department of Neurosurgery, University of Wisconsin School of Medicine and Public Health, Madison, WI, USA

Resection and Tube Repair

- As an alternative to grafting, after neuroma resection, a connecting tube can be used to bridge the gap.
- The proximal and distal nerve stumps are sutured to the ends of the tube.

Resection and Diversion (Fig. 63.3)

- When a distal stump is not available for repair.
- The neuroma is resected down to normal-appearing nerve.
- The new stump needs to be diverted away from the skin incision and the neighboring joints to avoid recurrence of a painful neuroma.
- To achieve this goal, the proximal stump can be buried deep in a muscle [1], another nerve (end-to-side) [2], a vein, a bone, or a vascularized fascial flap [3]. The distal stump can also be placed in a dead-end tube or connected to a very long nerve graft with the hope that the axons will not make it to the other end of the graft.

Resection and Dispersion (Fig. 63.4)

- After resecting a neuroma from a large mixed nerve, when there is not enough length to bury the proximal stump deep in muscle. This is usually the case in amputation stumps after multiple surgical resections.
- The neuroma is first resected.
- The proximal stump is divided into multiple fascicles.
- Several grafts are used to suture to different groups of fascicles.
- The distal ends of the grafts are sutured to different locations deep in a neighboring muscle/tissue.
- Allografts are preferred.

A. S. Hanna (ed.), *Nerves: Anatomy, Exposures, and Techniques*, https://doi.org/10.1007/978-3-031-73931-6_63

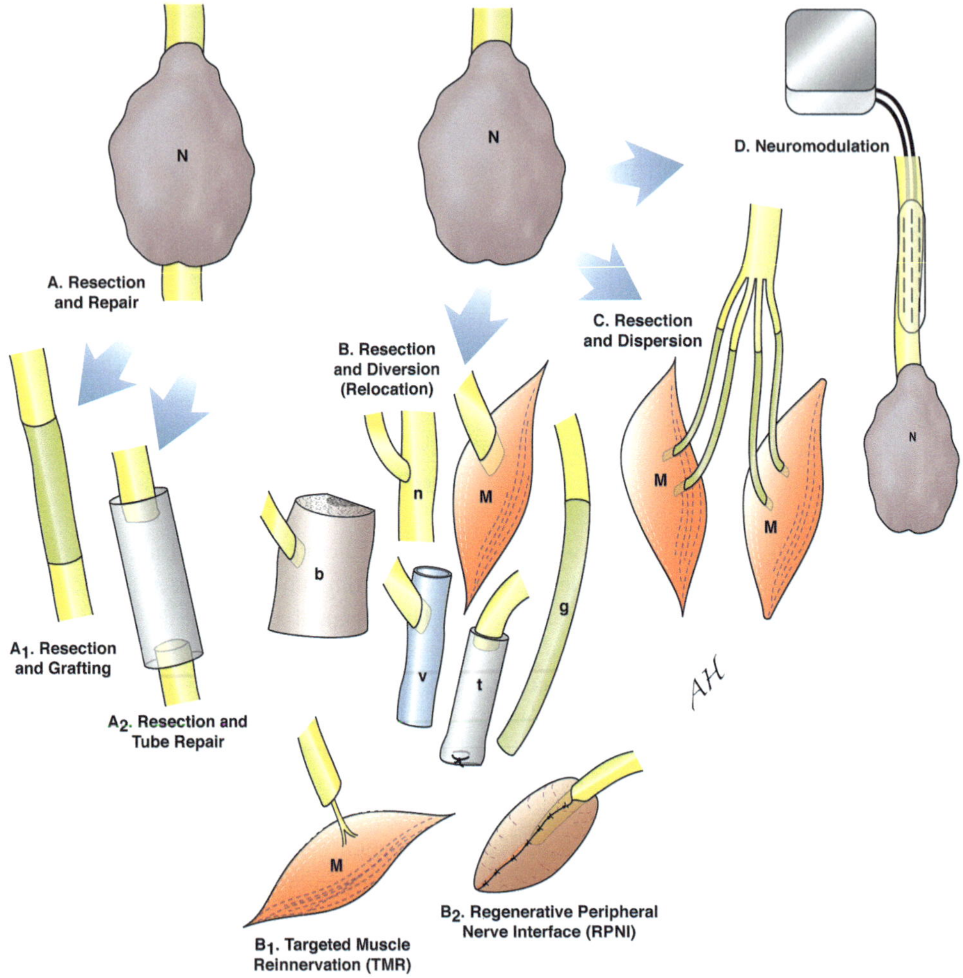

Fig. 63.1 Diagrammatic representation of different techniques to treat a painful neuroma (*N*). The painful neuroma should be resected, and the nerve stump should be directed to a target. **A.** Repair: If distal normal nerve is available, one may attempt repair with a nerve graft (**A$_1$**) (allograft vs. autograft) or a tube (**A$_2$**). **B.** Diversion: If no distal nerve is available, the nerve stump can be relocated into muscle (*M*), bone (*b*), another nerve (*n*)—end-to-side, a vein (*v*), a dead-end tube (*t*), or a long graft (*g*). **B$_1$**. Targeted Muscle Reinnervation (TMR): A neighboring motor nerve is cut, and the neuroma stump is coapted to the distal motor nerve stump. **B$_2$**. Regenerative Peripheral Nerve Interface (RPNI): A piece of muscle is cut and wrapped around the nerve ending. **C.** Dispersion: For a large neuroma on a mixed nerve with a short stump, the nerve can be divided into several fascicles, grafts can be used to gain length and bury the distal end in different targets as in B. **D.** Neuromodulation: Placing a nerve stimulator, a dorsal root ganglion (DRG) stimulator, or a spinal cord stimulator. Copyright Amgad Hanna. Published with permission

Targeted Muscle Reinnervation (TMR) [4, 5]

This technique entails using a nerve stimulator to find neighboring motor nerves. If it can be sacrificed without functional deficits, the motor nerve branch is cut and the distal stump connecting to the muscle is sutured to the free nerve ending after cutting out the neuroma (Fig. 63.1B$_1$).

Regenerative Peripheral Nerve Interface (RPNI) [6]

A piece of muscle is cut and brought in to wrap around the nerve endings after cutting out the neuroma (Figs. 63.1B$_2$ and 63.5).

The latter two techniques are also used for myoelectric control of advanced prostheses, as the signal obtained from the muscle is much more robust compared to the one from the nerve.

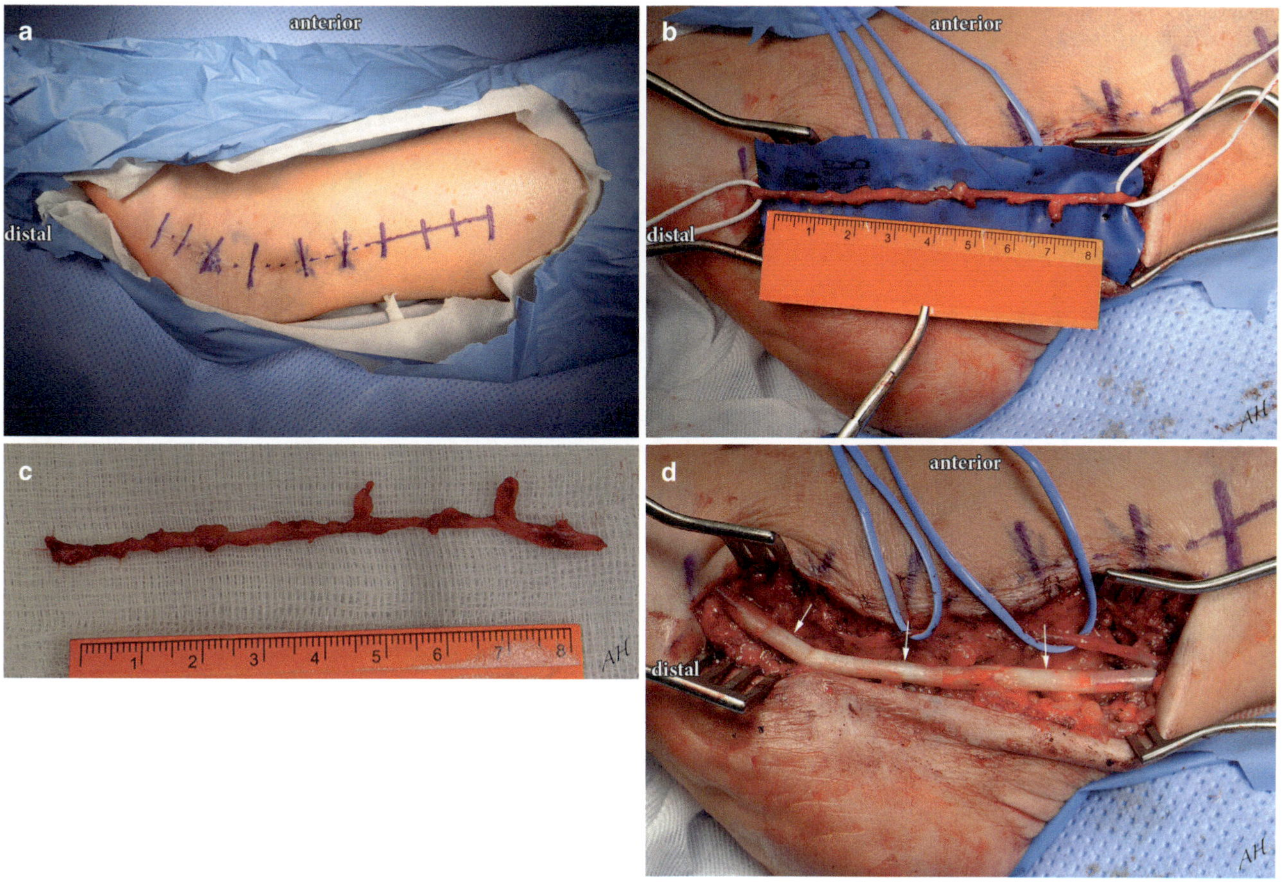

Fig. 63.2 This patient had a painful scarred left sural nerve after ankle surgery, treated by resection and grafting. (**a**) The patient is positioned lateral on a beanbag. (**b**) About 9 cm of sural nerve is exposed, with evidence of scarring and nerve damage. (**c**) The damaged nerve is first resected. (**d**) Allograft repair (*arrows*) with stitching to both proximal and distal nerve stumps. The suture sites are covered with wrap tubes; glue is then applied. Note the short saphenous vein in blue loops. The goal is to avoid pain recurrence, restoring sensation would be a bonus

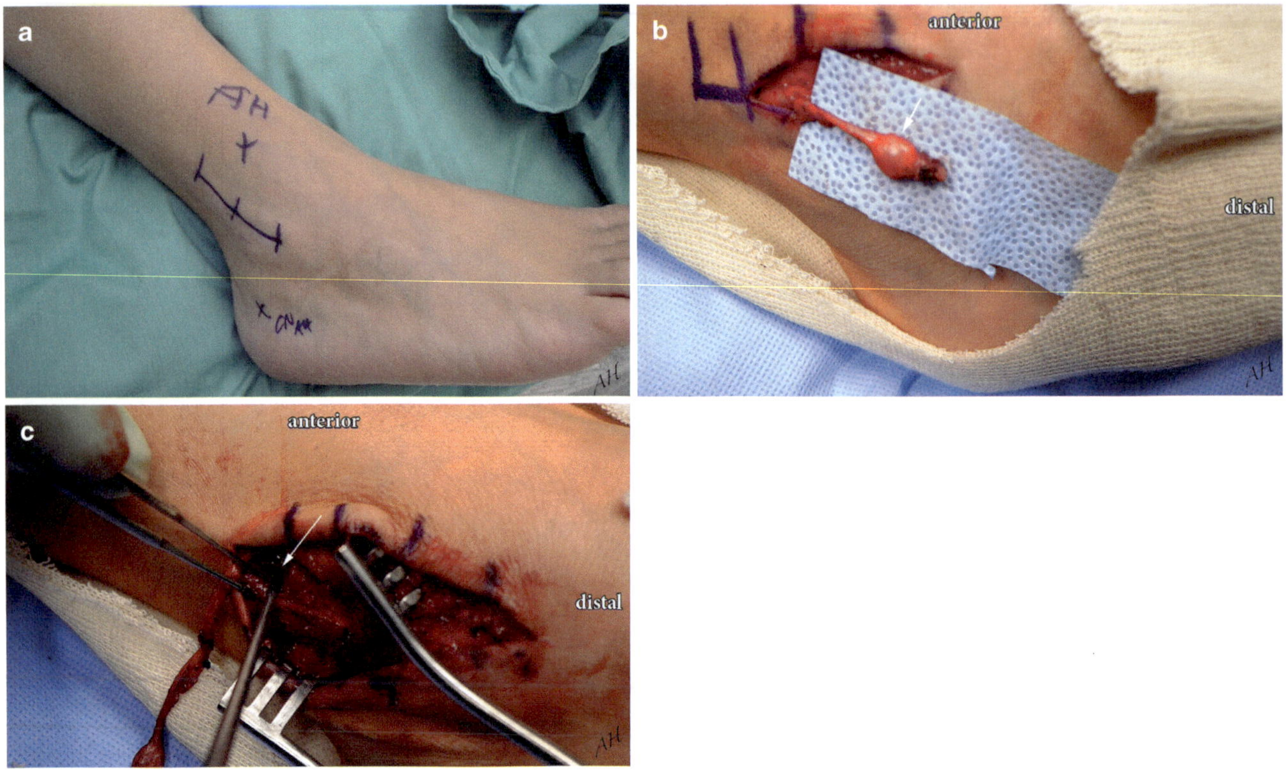

Fig. 63.3 This patient had a painful neuroma along the intermediate dorsal cutaneous nerve. (**a**) She is positioned supine with a bump. (**b**) The neuroma is exposed (*arrow*), but no distal stump is found. (**c**) A bed is created in a neighboring muscle (*arrow*). The neuroma is then resected, and the nerve ending is diverted into the muscle bed

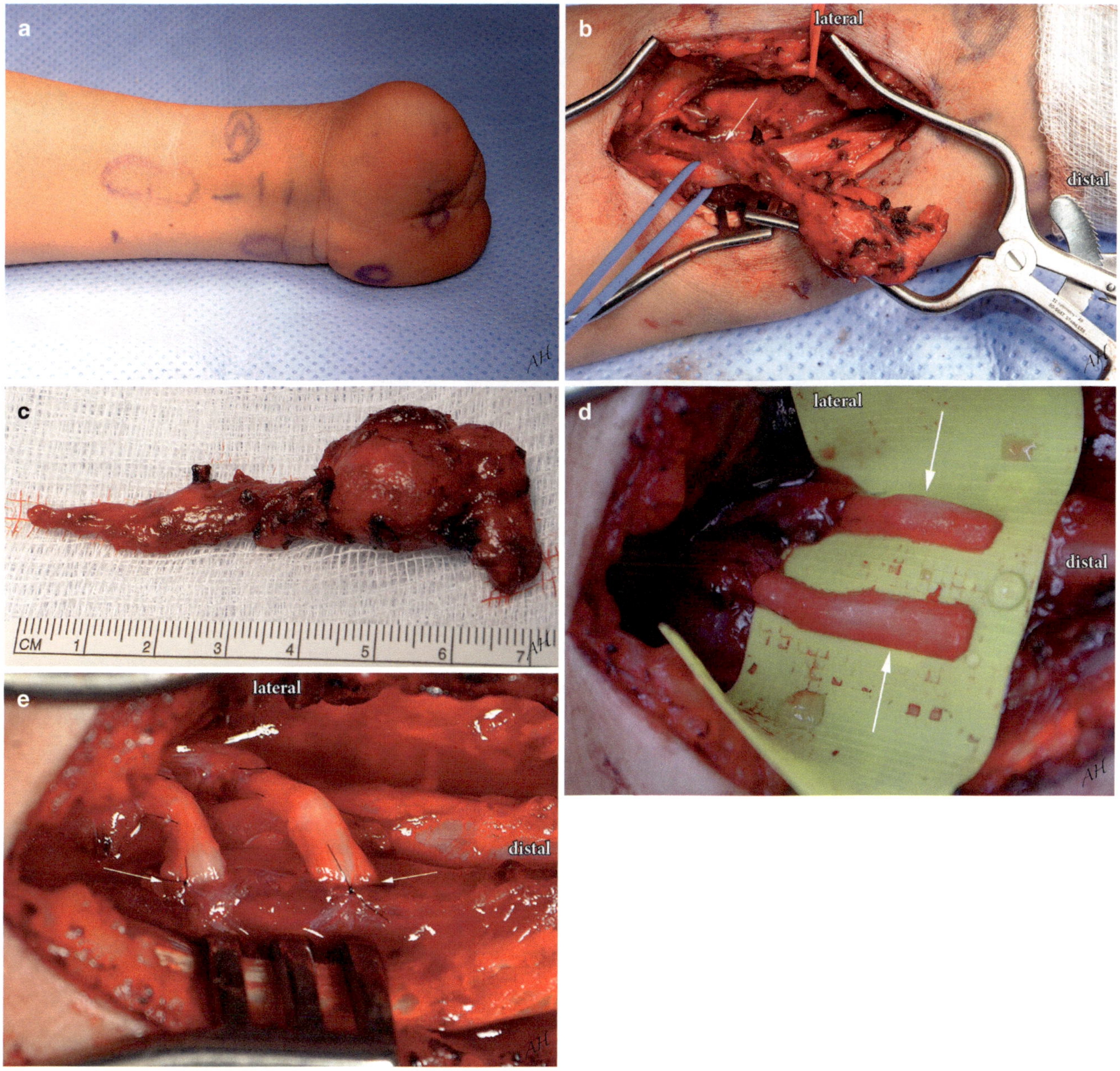

Fig. 63.4 This patient suffered from a severely painful left amputation stump. (**a**) Neuroma sites are mapped with ultrasound. (**b**) A neuroma is found at the end of the anterior interosseous nerve (AIN) (*arrow*). Note the median nerve in a blue loop and the radial artery in a red loop. (**c**) The neuroma is resected. (**d**) The nerve stump is divided into two, and each part received a piece of allograft (*arrows*). (**e**) The distal ends of the allografts are buried separately in a muscle (*arrows*)

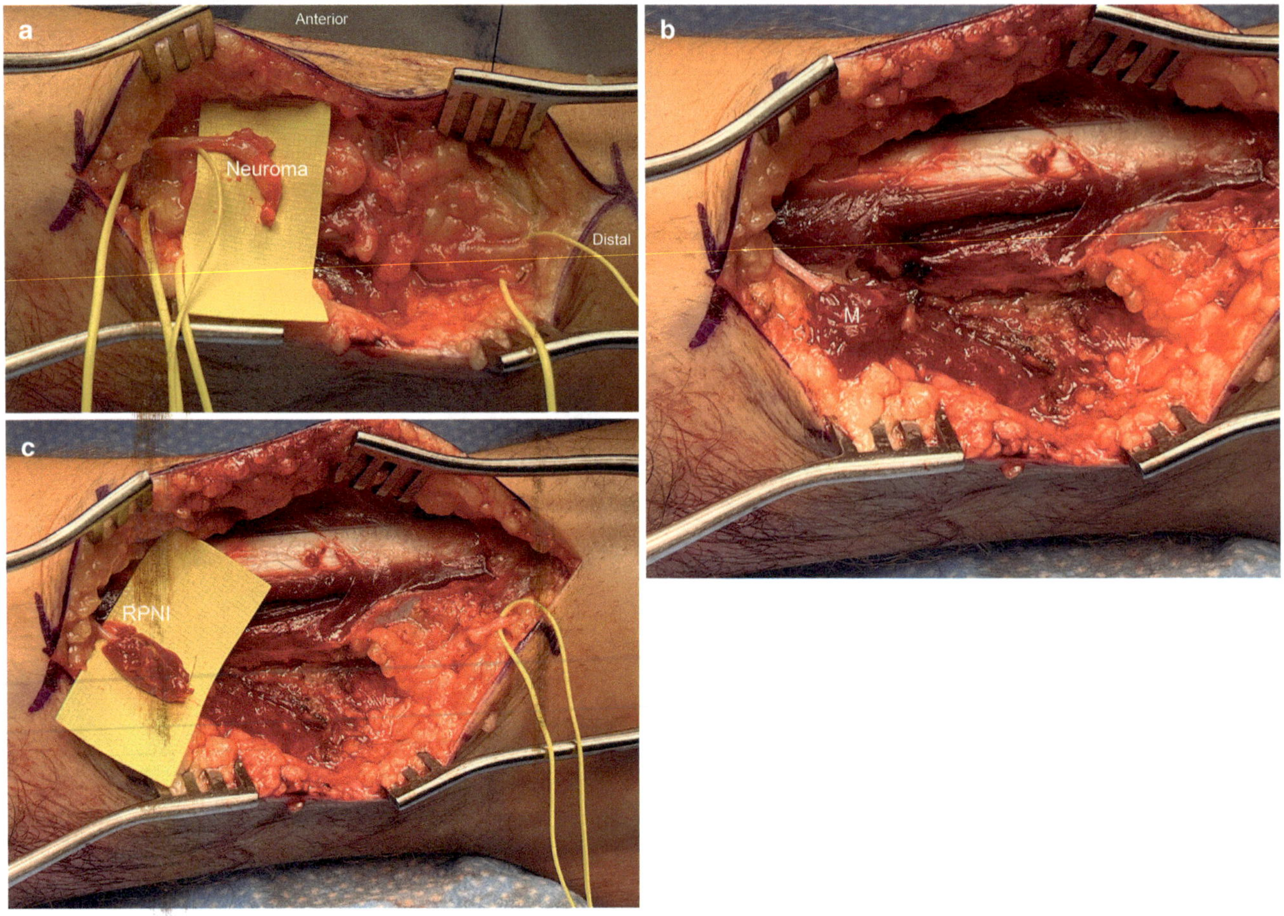

Fig. 63.5 Regenerative peripheral nerve interface (RPNI). (**a**) Right superficial peroneal nerve neuroma. (**b**) The neuroma is resected, and a free piece of muscle is harvested. The nerve is sutured to the center of the muscle (*M*). (**c**) The free muscle is then wrapped around the nerve ending and closed with sutures, thus forming the *RPNI*

References

1. Mackinnon SE, Dellon AL, Hudson AR, Hunter DA (1985) Alteration of neuroma formation by manipulation of its microenvironment. Plast Reconstr Surg 76(3):345–353. https://doi.org/10.1097/00006534-198509000-00001
2. Aszmann OC, Moser V, Frey M (2010) Treatment of painful neuromas via end-to-side neurorraphy. Handchir Mikrochir Plast Chir 42(4):225–232. https://doi.org/10.1055/s-0030-1255053. Epub 2010 Aug 3
3. Elliot D (2014) Surgical management of painful peripheral nerves. Clin Plast Surg 41(3):589–613. https://doi.org/10.1016/j.cps.2014.03.004
4. Dumanian GA, Potter BK, Mioton LM, Ko JH, Cheesborough JE, Souza JM et al (2019) Targeted muscle reinnervation treats neuroma and phantom pain in major limb amputees: a randomized clinical trial. Ann Surg 270(2):238–246. https://doi.org/10.1097/SLA.0000000000003088
5. Janes LE, Fracol ME, Dumanian GA, Ko JH (2021) Targeted muscle reinnervation for the treatment of neuroma. Hand Clin 37(3):345–359. https://doi.org/10.1016/j.hcl.2021.05.002
6. Santosa KB, Oliver JD, Cederna PS, Kung TA (2020) Regenerative peripheral nerve interfaces for prevention and management of neuromas. Clin Plast Surg 47(2):311–321. https://doi.org/10.1016/j.cps.2020.01.004. Epub 2020 Feb 1

Open Nerve Stimulation

64

Amgad S. Hanna

Indication

It is used for intractable pain in a nerve distribution, refractory to medical management, especially with complex regional pain syndrome (CRPS) [1, 2].

Surgical Technique

1. Most upper limb implants can be placed in the supine position (Fig. 64.1), sciatic nerve implants are placed in the prone position.
2. The target nerve is exposed as described in previous chapters addressing approaches to different nerves (Fig. 64.2).
3. A subcutaneous pocket is created for the implantable pulse generator (IPG) placement either in the infraclavicular area for the upper limb or in the buttock for the lower limb.
4. An extension cable is tunneled between the two incisions using a shunt passer (Fig. 64.3).
5. Different electrodes can be used. The electrode with a mesh allows suturing to surrounding tissues to prevent migration. The electrode is placed under the nerve, and 2-0 Ethibond is usually used to secure it in place (Fig. 64.4). If an electrode without a mesh is being used, the suture can be placed through the silicone part of the lead, making sure not to damage the wire itself.
6. The electrode is connected to the extension cable and secured using a screwdriver, the provided sleeve, a suture, and glue. If the electrode is long enough, no extension cable is needed.

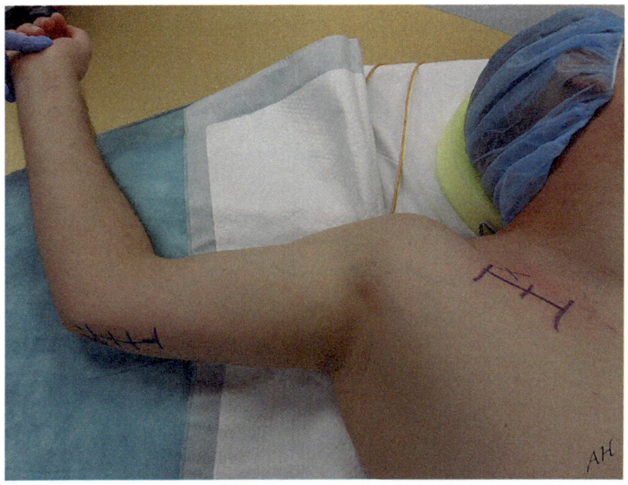

Fig. 64.1 This patient had intractable pain in the ulnar nerve distribution from previous nerve injury. He is positioned supine with the arm abducted for open placement of a nerve stimulator

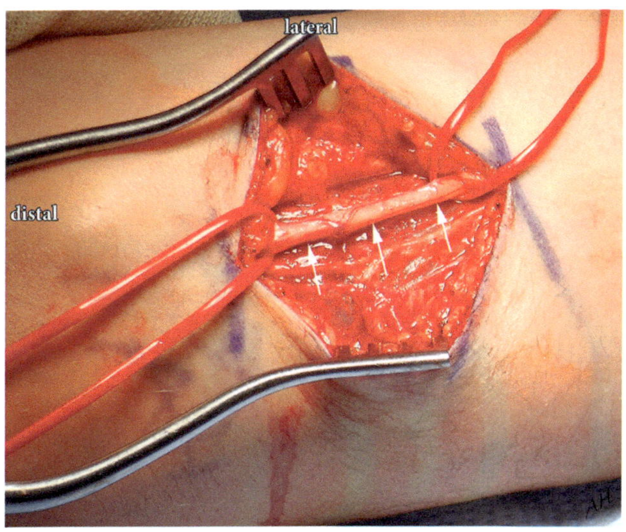

Fig. 64.2 The right ulnar nerve (*arrows*) is exposed in the lower arm

Supplementary Information The online version contains supplementary material available at https://doi.org/10.1007/978-3-031-73931-6_64.

A. S. Hanna (✉)
Department of Neurosurgery, University of Wisconsin School of Medicine and Public Health, Madison, WI, USA

A. S. Hanna (ed.), *Nerves: Anatomy, Exposures, and Techniques*, https://doi.org/10.1007/978-3-031-73931-6_64

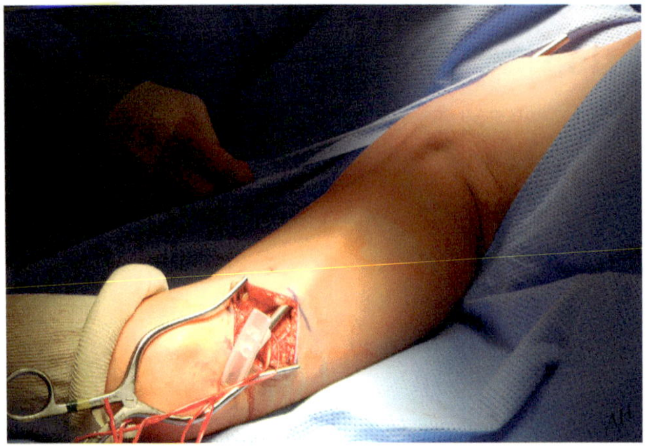

Fig. 64.3 A shunt passer is used to tunnel the extension cable between the two incisions

7. The cable is then connected to the IPG, and impedance is checked before final placement of the IPG.
8. The IPG is placed in the subcutaneous pocket created (1–2 cm deep to the skin surface) and secured with sutures; we use 2-0 Ethibond (Fig. 64.5).
9. At the proximal and distal sites, extra loops of cable are fashioned to allow for limb mobility without disconnecting the system (Fig. 64.6).

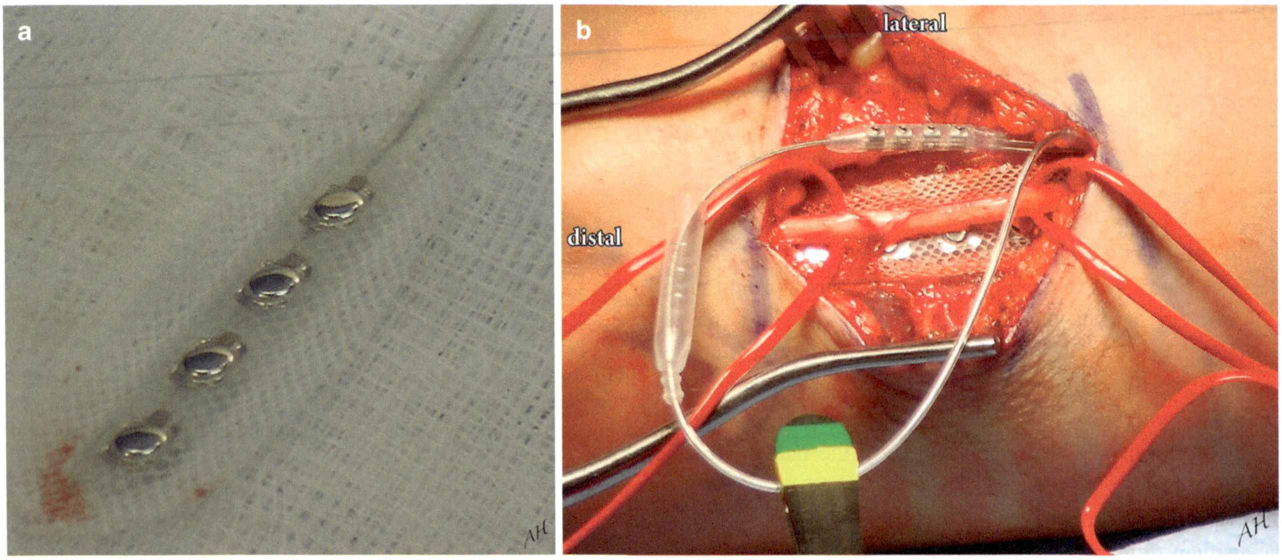

Fig. 64.4 (a) An electrode with a mesh is used. (b) It is placed under the ulnar nerve, sutured to the underlying tissues, then connected to the extension cable

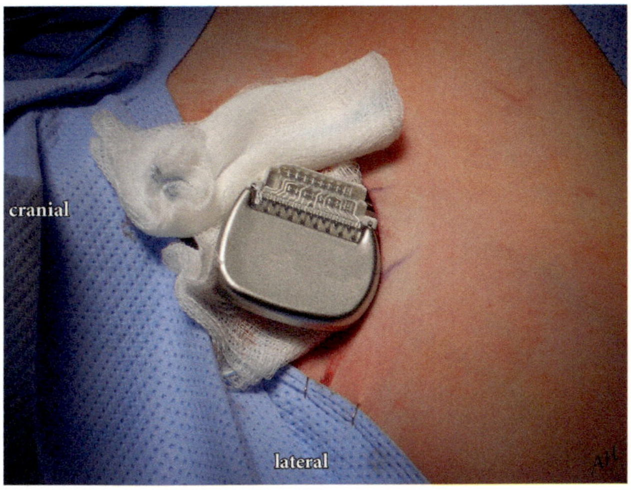

Fig. 64.5 An implantable pulse generator (IPG) is connected to the other end of the connection cable, and once impedance is tested and acceptable, it can be placed in a pocket created in the infraclavicular area

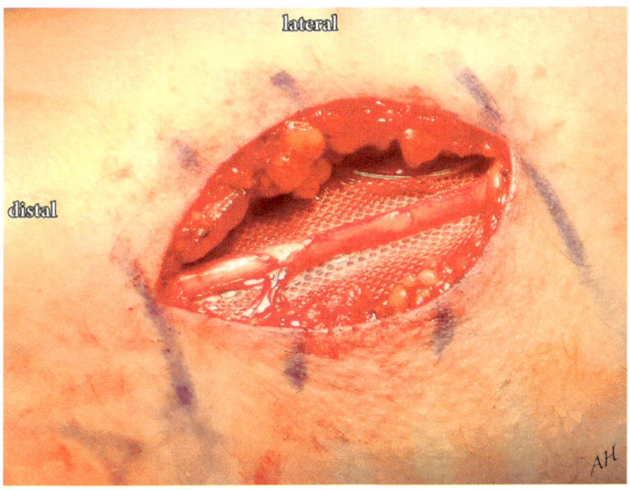

Fig. 64.6 Final position of the electrode under the ulnar nerve, with a loop of cable secured with sutures. Loops made of extra wire should be fashioned at both incision sites to allow for limb movement without disruption of the system

References

1. Nashold BS Jr, Goldner JL, Mullen JB, Bright DS (1982) Long-term pain control by direct peripheral-nerve stimulation. J Bone Joint Surg Am 64(1):1–10
2. Reverberi C, Dario A, Barolat G, Zuccon G (2014) Using peripheral nerve stimulation (PNS) to treat neuropathic pain: a clinical series. Neuromodulation 17(8):777–783; discussion 783. https://doi.org/10.1111/ner.12157

Percutaneous Nerve Stimulation for Pain

65

Caroline A. Varlotta and David A. Spinner

Introduction

The modern origins of nerve stimulation to treat pain date to 1965 when Dr. Wall and Dr. Sweet implanted a pair of silastic ring platinum electrodes around the ulnar and median nerves, providing an electrical stimulus along the median nerve that resulted in a pleasant tingling in the lateral three fingers of the hand and stopped pain in the medial three fingers [1]. Since then, nerve stimulation has evolved significantly due to new technologies and ultrasound/fluoroscopic-guided procedures. These advances have led to the ability to treat a variety of conditions, including but not limited to hemiplegic shoulder pain, complex regional pain syndrome (CRPS), and phantom pain [2].

Treatment with percutaneous nerve stimulation (PNS) involves the temporary placement of a percutaneous electrode along the nerve supplying the region or origin of pain. The objective of PNS is to trigger action potentials in axons of the targeted nerve fascicles to evoke nonpainful signals instead of painful ones (neuromodulation). Selectively stimulating Aβ fibers results in nonpainful sensations such as vibration and tingling (Table 65.1) [3, 4]. Other proposed mechanisms of PNS include cortical reorganization by spinothalamic inhibition and central neurochemical mechanisms. PNS may also provide dermatomal, myotomal, and sympathetic stimulation, local blood flow alteration, and peripheral neurochemical mechanisms to aid in pain relief.

The components of the PNS system include an external pulse transmitter (EPT), a gel electrode patch, a patient programmer, and the implanted lead. The lead described here is 15 cm in length and contains three electrodes and an integrated receiver (Fig. 65.1). The electrodes have an anchoring system to prevent migration. The EPT transmits an electrical field stimulation to the receiving end of the lead implanted under the skin (Fig. 65.2). Gel electrode patches are used to adhere to the EPT device and to the skin. The EPT can operate for about 6 h to 2 days based on the usage. The gel electrode patches may be replaced every 2–4 days. The patient controls the type and intensity of stimulation from the EPT with the wireless patient programmer. Data from the patient programmer also include compliance and usage information.

Understanding fascicular anatomy is essential to effective PNS. A large nerve is a bundle of its smaller branches held together by a connective tissue framework. The component fascicles may retain their identity and relative positions as the nerve courses distally. However, the proximal larger

Table 65.1 Classification and physiologic characteristics of nerve fibers [3, 4]

Nerve fiber class	Function	Myelination
Aα	Motor	Yes
Aβ	Touch, pressure, vibration	Yes
Aγ	Muscle spindle	Yes
Aδ	Temperature, sharp pain	Yes
B	Sympathetic (preganglionic)	Yes
C	Temperature, dull pain, burning pain	No

C. A. Varlotta · D. A. Spinner (✉)
Department of Rehabilitation and Human Performance, Mount Sinai Hospital, New York, NY, USA

A. S. Hanna (ed.), *Nerves: Anatomy, Exposures, and Techniques*, https://doi.org/10.1007/978-3-031-73931-6_65

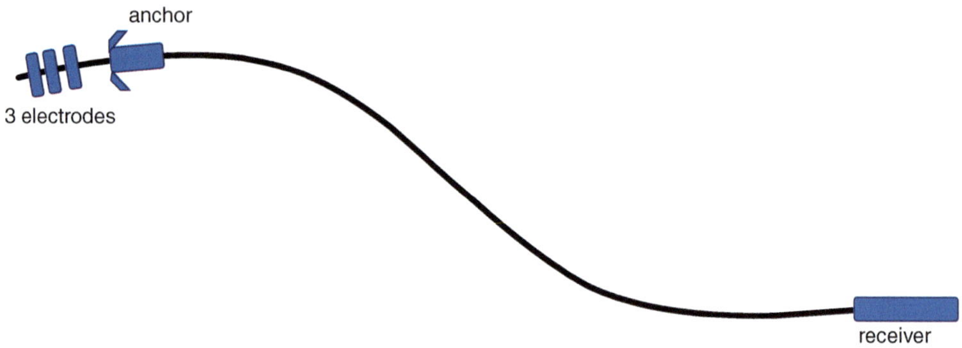

Fig. 65.1 Implantable lead components

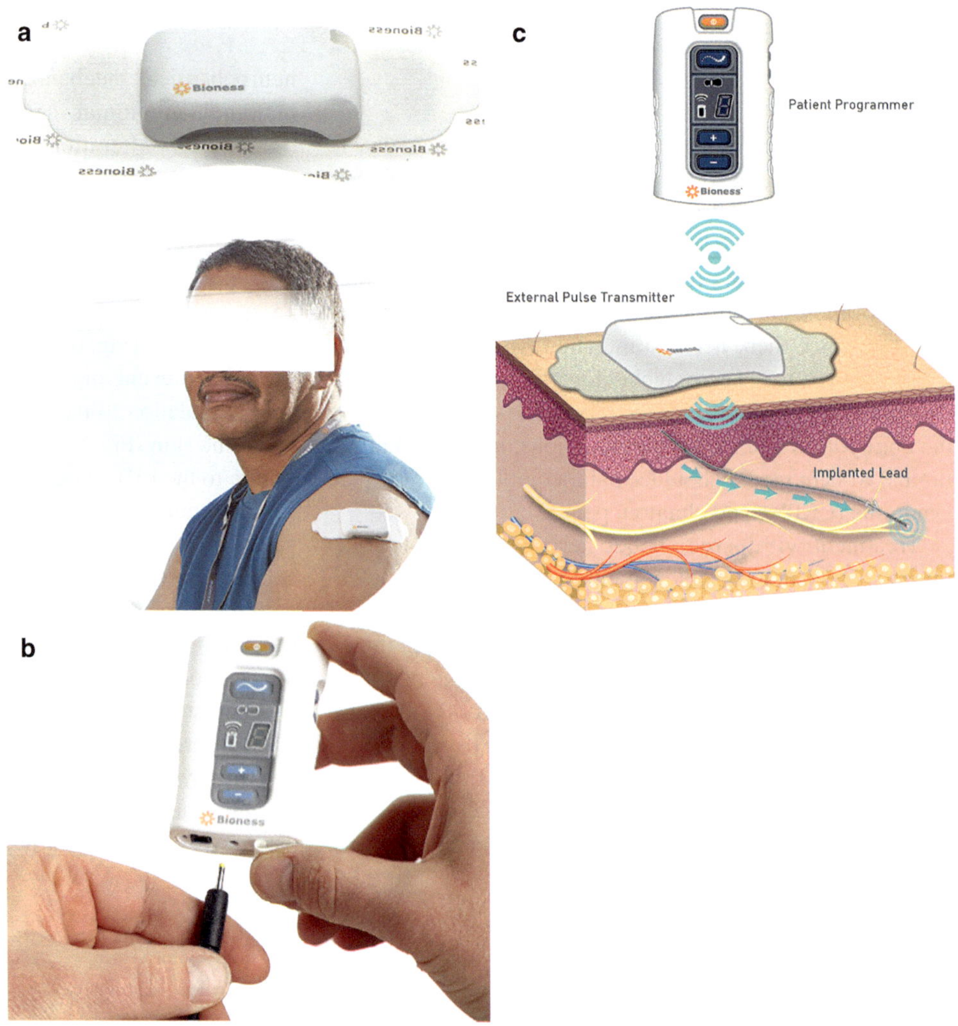

Fig. 65.2 System components for PNS. (**a**) The external pulse transmitter (EPT). (**b**) Patient programmer. (**c**) Photo of entire system components. (Used with permission from Bioventus LLC)

nerves will have cross-over between their nerve fibers, so individual fascicles may contain components from nearby fibers. As large nerves course distally, the fibers may have a more distinct distribution [5]. A fascicular map of a compound nerve relates each fascicle to the distal nerve branch it gives origin to, therefore to specific muscles or dermatomes innervated by that distal nerve branch [6]. Available techniques allow us to selectively stimulate individual fascicles or areas within a compound nerve.

Contraindications (3Cs)

- Cancerous lesions near the target area of stimulation or electrode patch, as PNS contains diathermy and therapeutic ultrasound, which can cause potential spread of malignant cells
- Cardiac pacemaker, defibrillator, and metallic implant in the immediate area of the proposed PNS implant
- Central pain syndromes

General Principles of PNS

- Plan for final active lead position.
- Plan for final position of receiver.
- Use color doppler to avoid vascular injury.
- Avoid lead placement at the injured segment of the nerve.
- Generally, viewing nerves in the short axis is preferred because nerves are easier to identify (honeycomb appearance with ultrasound; see also Chap. 5).
- Ensure there is sufficient distance between the target and needle entry point to assure parallel placement of electrodes onto the nerve.
- Most procedures are completed under local anesthesia or light-monitored anesthesia care (MAC). Pediatric cases are typically completed with moderate sedation.

Knowledge of the anatomy and the above principles apply to any nerve in the body. This chapter will focus on common lower and upper extremity nerve targets for PNS: femoral, sciatic, and radial nerves.

Equipment (Figs. 65.1, 65.2, and 65.3)

- Stimulation probe with a blunt tip
  - Has markings in white and black with an isolated longer black marking.
- Tunneling needle and stylet
- Introducer sheath and dilator
  - To unscrew, hold the wings and then remove the dilator from the sheath.
- Small lead adaptor
  - Used to test stimulation with the lead itself.
  - There is a lever or hook to secure the receiver end of the lead.
- Lead
  - Will be inside a lead loader when removed from the PNS kit.
  - Remove the rubber band if present.
  - Has electrodes on one end with a small anchor to maintain the lead in its position and a receiver on the other end.
  - Only component of the system that is implanted in the patient.
- Stimulation cable to provide electrical current in stimulation testing of the nerve
- Scalpel (#11 blade)
- Local anesthetic (Lidocaine 1% or 2%)
- Echogenic 18-gauge 3.5-inch spinal needle
  - Used to move through fascial planes (as the other items are blunt tips).
- External pulse transmitter (EPT)
  - Part of the PNS kit.
  - Can be programmed to various stimulation patterns and intensities.
  - Patient needs to charge every day or every other day.
  - Attaches to the body by a gel electrode patch, which adheres to the skin overlying the receiver end of the lead.
- Gel electrode patch
  - Part of the PNS kit.
  - Should be placed on the area of the skin overlying receiver end of the lead.
  - Can be disposed of and replaced when no longer adhesive or every 2–5 days.
- Patient programmer
  - Wireless remote to control the EPT.
  - Can turn on/off and adjust intensity.
  - Allows for patient-controlled stimulation by selecting programs and intensity.
  - Tracks patient's compliance and usage.
  - Patients need to charge every day or every other day.

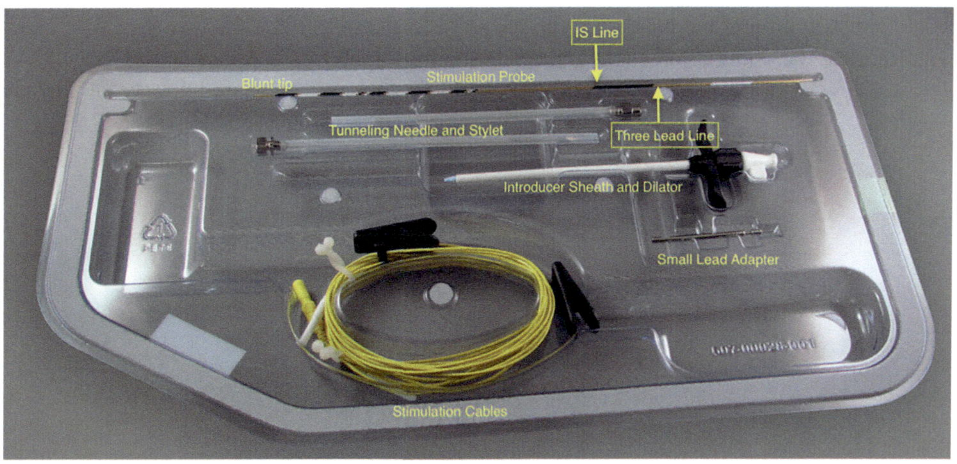

Fig. 65.3 Labeled procedure kit for implant. *IS Line* Introducer sheath line. Three lead line is the line on the stimulation probe to be lined up with the black portion of the introducer sheath, indicating the three leads are in place

Femoral Nerve

Key Facts

- Supplied by L2–L4 nerves.
- Innervates the muscles of the anterior thigh.
- Femoral nerve at the site of lead placement will usually be about 2 cm deep.

Position

- Supine

Procedure (Fig. 65.4)

1. Identify the femoral head, then the femoral nerve, artery, and vein (from lateral to medial, respectively) with the ultrasound probe in short axis.
2. Turn on color flow to confirm location of vasculature.
3. Using the ultrasound, take note of the depth of the target nerve and plan the needle trajectory.
4. Administer local anesthetic to the targeted area of incision, avoiding excess that can track to the target nerve.
5. Using the scalpel, make a stab incision a few centimeters in-line and distal to the US probe.
6. Insert the 18-gauge spinal needle with the bevel facing the nerve. The tip will be hyperechoic.
7. Adjust placement of the spinal needle until the bevel is facing down in an acceptable position for lead placement. The tip of the needle should be overlying the nerve.
8. Remove the ultrasound probe.
9. Pass the stimulation probe through the spinal needle.
10. Remove the spinal needle over the stimulation probe.
11. Use the provided cable to stimulate in the location of the stimulation needle. Ensure the area of stimulation covers the distribution of the patient's pain.
12. Remove the stimulation cable and guide the introducer over the stimulation needle. Stop once the distal longer black line of the stimulation probe meets the white part of the introducer.
13. Stimulate again to make sure the area of the patient's pain is still covered.
14. Remove the stimulation probe while keeping the introducer in place. The "wings" of the introducer can be used to assist in this.
15. Feed the lead and lead loader into the introducer.
16. Once the beginning of the black line on the lead loader is reached, the first lead is on top of the nerve. When most of the black line is covered, then the third lead is on the nerve.
17. Stimulate with the stimulation cable again to ensure electrode placement, covering fascicles that supply coverage to the painful area.
18. Once there is an appropriate stimulation response, remove the stimulation cable while holding the lead loader in place so the electrodes are not displaced.
19. Start to remove the introducer. This deploys the anchor on the lead.
20. Apply pressure while continuing to remove the lead loader and introducer.
21. Place the lead adaptor onto the receiver end of the lead and stimulate one last time to ensure proper placement.
22. Decide where to tunnel the receiver end of the lead.
    (a) Avoid crossing a joint line, this would provide too much mobility around the lead.
    (b) Ideal placement is lateral thigh.
    (c) By using a sterile marker, the distance can be measured, and ideal placement marked.
23. Pass the tunneling needle and stylet through the stab incision to the marked target for the intended receiver placement.
24. Once you pass back through, then advance the receiver end into the loader, pull through to the marked target. The lead and receiver should be in the subcutaneous tissue.
25. Close with Dermabond (Ethicon, Johnson & Johnson), small gauze, and Tegaderm (3M).

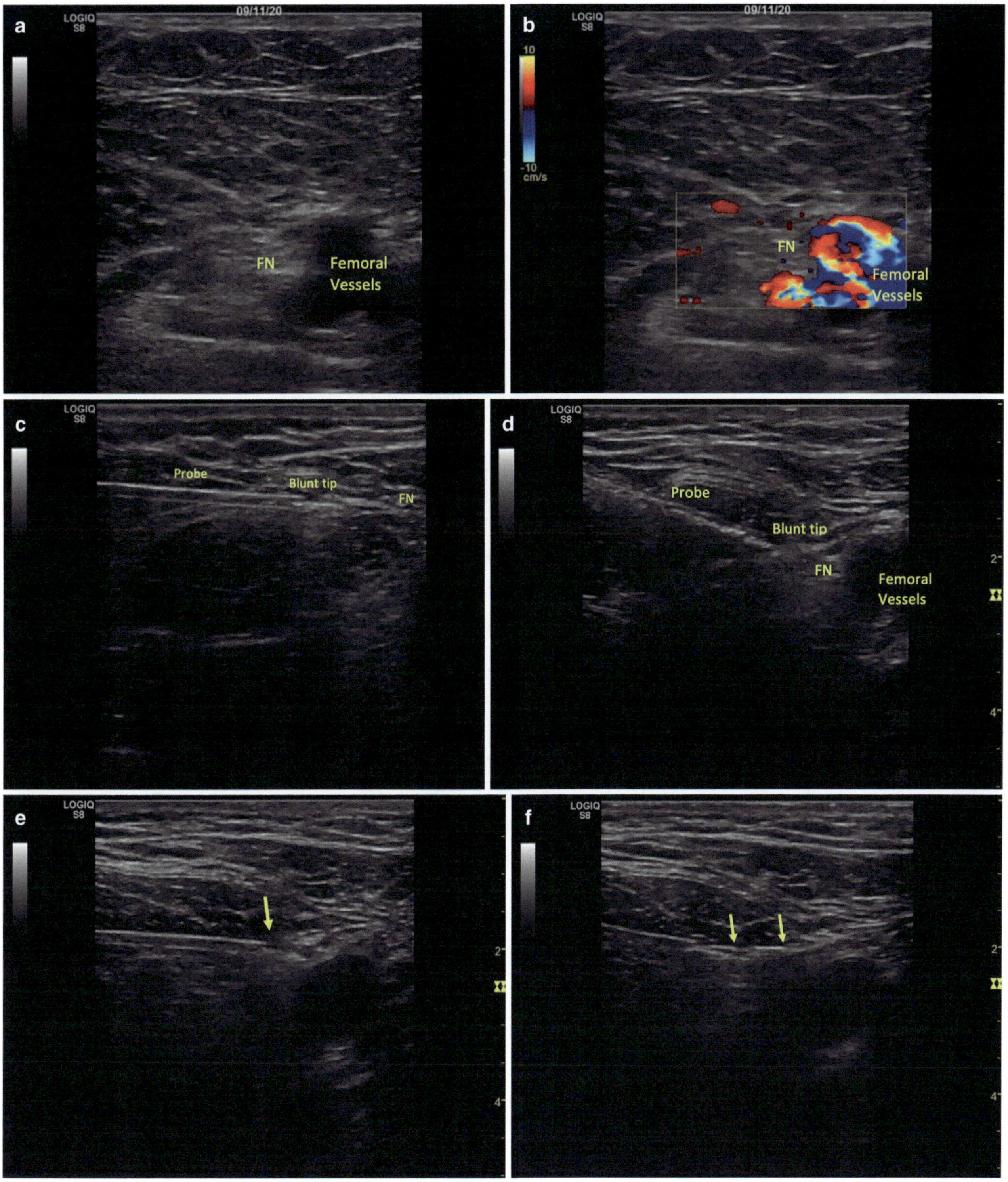

Fig. 65.4 Femoral nerve out of plane approach. (**a**) Identification of femoral neurovascular bundle. (**b**) Color flow neurovascular bundle. (**c** and **d**) Needle approach to the femoral nerve. (**e**) First contact of nerve stimulator (*arrow*). (**f**) Multiple contacts of nerve stimulator (*arrows*)

Sciatic Nerve

Key Facts

- Supplied by L4–S3 nerves.
- Courses down the buttock, then posterior thigh.
- Composed of the tibial nerve medially and common fibular (peroneal) nerve laterally, surrounded by a common sheath. The terminal branches start to separate distally towards the popliteal fossa.
- The common fibular nerve travels laterally towards the fibular head, while the tibial nerve will stay deep and midline in the leg.
- Sciatic nerve at the site of lead placement will usually be about 2.0–2.5 cm deep.

Position

- Prone

Procedure (Fig. 65.5)

1. Start by scanning with the ultrasound on the distal posterior thigh, just cephalad to the knee. The goal is to visualize the tibial and the common fibular portions of the sciatic nerve. Trace proximally up the posterior thigh. The target is identified once the two nerves are visualized under one sheath as a large nerve (approximately at the lower buttock). The target can also be identified below the piriformis muscle.

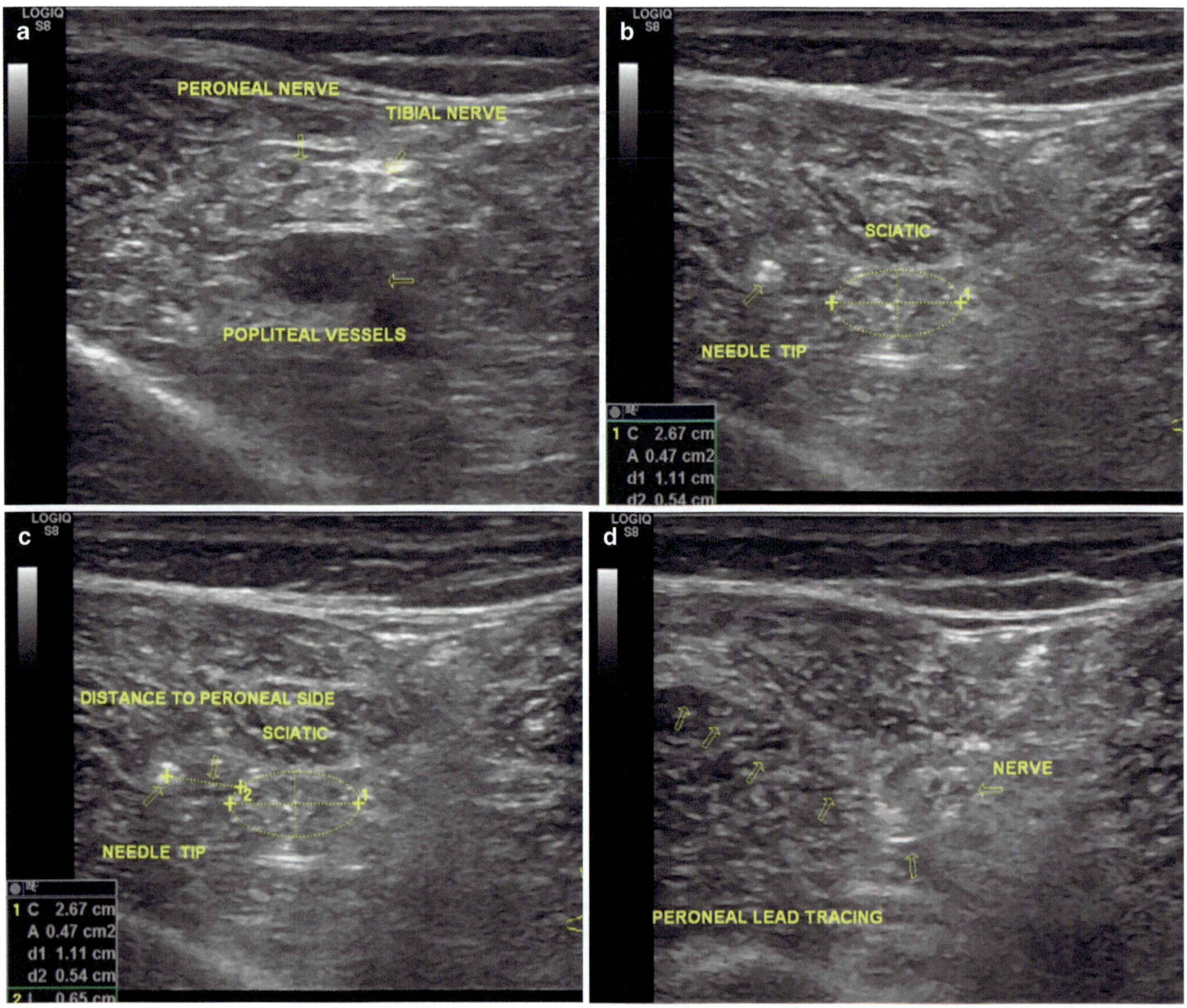

Fig. 65.5 Sciatic nerve out of plane approach. (**a**) Identification of the popliteal vessels, adjacent peroneal nerve, and adjacent tibial nerve. (**b**) Needle tip approaching the sciatic nerve. (**c**) Needle tip progresses and identification of the peroneal side of the sciatic bundle. (**d**) Lead placed on peroneal side of sciatic nerve. (**e**) Identification of the tibial portion of the sciatic nerve

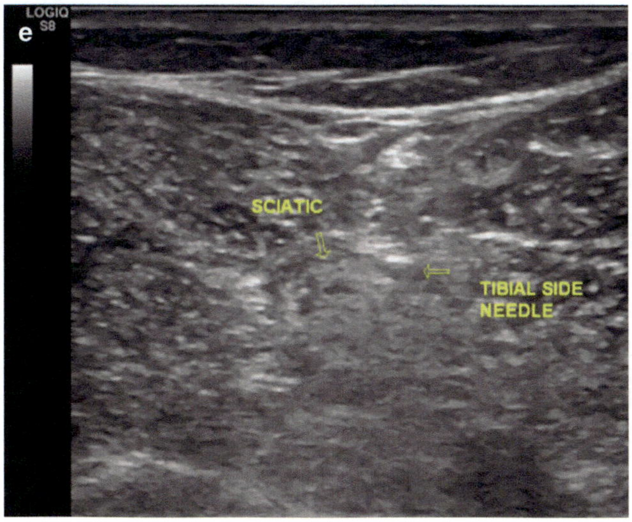

Fig. 65.5 (continued)

2. The remaining steps follow the procedure described above for the femoral nerve. Make sure that the tip of the spinal needle is overlying the center of the sciatic nerve in order to "split the difference" between its tibial and common fibular components.

Radial Nerve

Key Facts

- Supplied by the posterior cord of the brachial plexus from C5 to T1 nerves.
- Courses posterior to the axillary artery in the axilla and will enter the posterior compartment of the arm distal to the teres major, continuing through the spiral groove of the humerus along with the profunda brachii artery towards the elbow joint.
- Divides into superficial and deep radial nerves and gives off the posterior interosseous nerve.
- Radial nerve at the site of lead placement will usually be about 1.0 cm deep.

Position

- Supine with the lateral aspect of the upper arm exposed.

Procedure (Fig. 65.6)

1. Start scanning just below the elbow. Identify the radial nerve and identify the superficial and deep portions as they branch distally. Scan proximally at the elbow and above the elbow.
2. Center the radial nerve when scanning to visualize the humerus and radial nerve in the spiral groove at approximately 1 cm deep. The goal is to target the radial nerve in this area. The needle approach will be from a few centimeters distal or proximal to the probe.
3. The remaining steps follow the general scheme described above under the femoral nerve, with the following nuances:
   (a) When inserting the 18-gauge spinal needle, start with the needle more superficial at first until you see the hyperechoic dot. Pull back, steepen the course, and drop down until the needle tip is placed just superficial to the radial nerve.
   (b) Ideal placement of the receiver is the lateral arm.

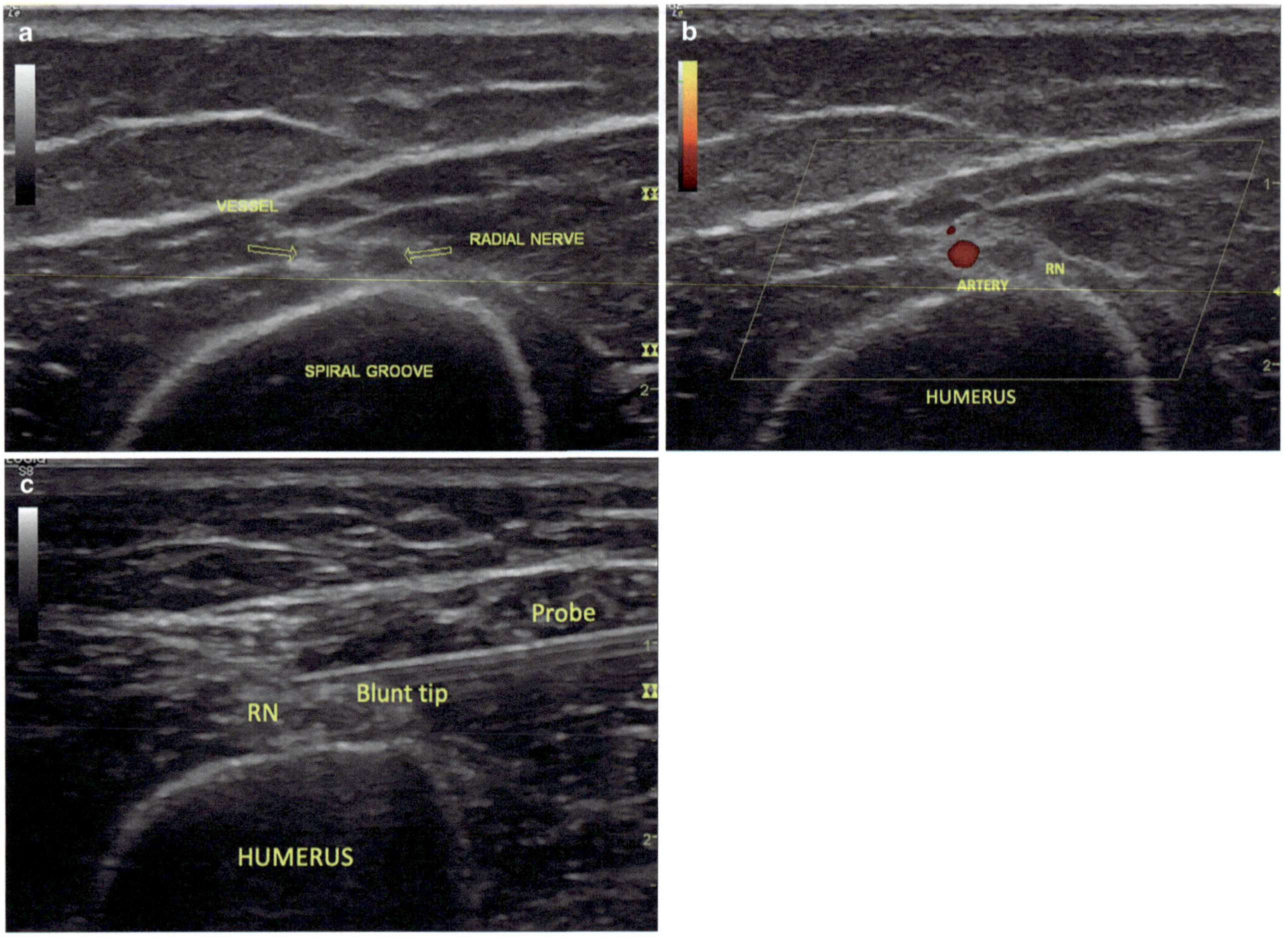

Fig. 65.6 Radial nerve out of plane approach. (**a**) Identification of radial nerve (*RN*) and adjacent neurovascular in spiral groove of humerus. (**b**) Identification of vessels adjacent to the radial nerve with color flow. (**c**) Needle overlying radial nerve

Complications

Adverse effects from PNS are minimal and include complications universal to any surgical procedure. The risks of the implantation procedure and afterwards include pain, discomfort, bleeding, skin discoloration, infection, and other generalized skin changes. Pain may resolve or persist after the procedure. During the procedure, damage to the nerve is possible, but rare. When using the stimulation device, the patient may experience discomfort, pain, or an undesired motor response, such as muscle spasm. If these occur, the patient should turn off the device and remove the gel electrode pad. Once the device is implanted, the patient should avoid therapeutic ultrasound and diathermy. The leads are not compatible with direct magnetic resonance imaging (MRI) over that region and would require removal prior to an MRI. However, for imaging distant from the system, the leads are compatible with MRI at a certain distance from the coil [7].

Illustrative videos [8].

References

1. White JC, Sweet WH (1969) Pain and the neurosurgeon: a forty-year experience. Charles C Thomas, Springfield
2. Wilson R, Bennett M, Nguyen V, Bock W, O'Dell M, Watanabe T et al (2018) Fully implantable peripheral nerve stimulation for hemiplegic shoulder pain: a multi-site case series with two-year follow-up. Neuromodulation 21(3):290–295. https://doi.org/10.1111/ner.12726
3. Cousins MJ, Bridenbaugh PO (1980) Absorption and disposition of local anesthetics: pharmacokinetics. In: Neural blockade in clinical anesthesia and management of pain. JB Lippincott, Philadelphia, p 54
4. Yam M, Loh Y, Tan C, Adam SK, Abdul Manan N, Basir R (2018) General pathways of pain sensation and the major neurotransmitters involved in pain regulation. Int J Mol Sci 19(8):2164. https://doi.org/10.3390/ijms19082164
5. Sunderland S (1945) The intraneural topography of the radial, median, and ulnar nerves. Brain 68(4):243–299. https://doi.org/10.1093/brain/68.4.243
6. Gustafson KJ, Pinault GCJ, Neville JJ, Syed I, Davis JA Jr, Jean-Claude J, Triolo RJ (2009) Fascicular anatomy of human femoral nerve: implications for neural prostheses using nerve cuff electrodes. J Rehabil Res Dev 46(7):973. https://doi.org/10.1682/jrrd.2008.08.0097
7. https://stimrouter.com/physicians/mri-safety-following-stimrouter-implant/
8. https://www.wapmu.org/training-videos-1. Used with permission from Bioventus LLC

Dorsal Root Entry Zone (DREZ) Lesion

66

Amgad S. Hanna

Indication

This chapter describes dorsal root entry zone (DREZ) lesion as indicated in brachial plexus avulsion. Deafferentation pain is difficult to treat and can sometimes be intractable to medical management. DREZ lesion has an 85% success rate at 2 years in treating neuropathic pain following brachial plexus avulsion (Fig. 66.1) [1].

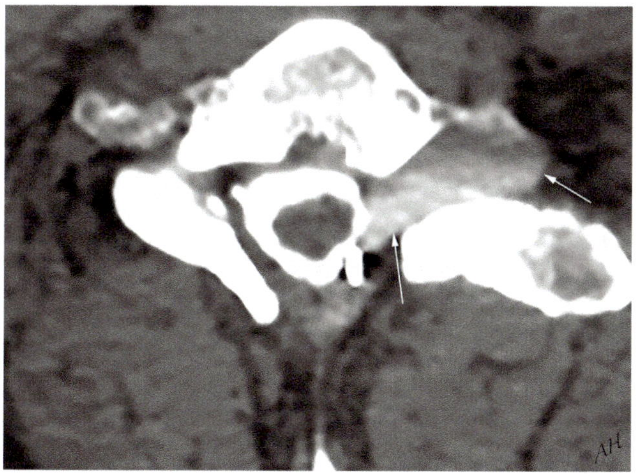

Fig. 66.1 Axial CT-myelogram revealing left pseudomeningocele (*arrows*) from brachial plexus avulsion

Supplementary Information The online version contains supplementary material available at https://doi.org/10.1007/978-3-031-73931-6_66.

A. S. Hanna (✉)
Department of Neurosurgery, University of Wisconsin School of Medicine and Public Health, Madison, WI, USA

Technique

1. Position prone on chest rolls (or Wilson frame) in head pins.
2. Neuromonitoring with somatosensory evoked potentials (SSEPs) and motor evoked potentials (MEPs).
3. The skin is opened in the midline. The paraspinal muscles can be dissected unilaterally for a hemilaminectomy or bilaterally for laminectomy or laminoplasty.
4. We use the harmonic bone scalpel (Fig. 66.2) to perform bilateral laminectomy and a plate/screw system for laminoplasty.
5. The dura mater is opened using an 11-blade scalpel in the midline or paramedian on the side of the injury. The opening is enlarged using a Woodson tool and a scalpel. The dura is tacked up using 4-0 braided Nylon sutures.
6. The arachnoid mater is opened with a nerve hook and micro scissors and tacked to the dura using hemoclips.
7. The operative microscope is brought into the field.
8. Identification of the DREZ:
   - The DREZ lines up with an imaginary line joining the last normal rootlet cranially to the first normal rootlet caudal to the injury (Fig. 66.3).
   - The distance from the DREZ on the avulsed side to the dorsal median sulcus of the cord should be the same as from the latter to the normal dorsal rootlets on the other side. However, the cord can be shifted or rotated due to the injury.
   - Pits (the most reliable): These are the sites of avulsion of the dorsal rootlets from the spinal cord (Fig. 66.4). They are defects in the pia mater with scarring and are darker in color (greyish).
9. The lesion can be done mechanically (Fig. 66.5) [2] or using radiofrequency [3]. Here we describe the mechanical lesion. The lesion should include the avulsed segment with or without a few normal rootlets cranially and caudally.
10. Bipolar coagulation with fine tips is used to coagulate the vessels and pia in the DREZ.

A. S. Hanna (ed.), *Nerves: Anatomy, Exposures, and Techniques*, https://doi.org/10.1007/978-3-031-73931-6_66

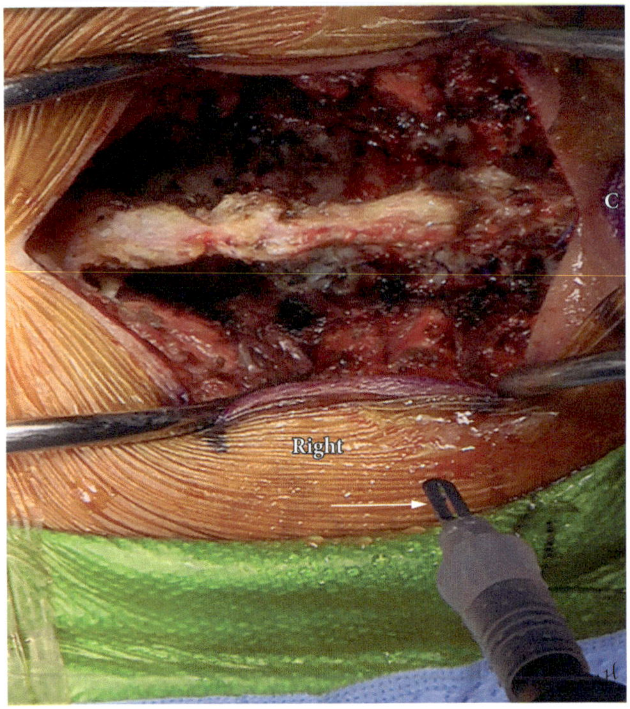

Fig. 66.2 A harmonic bone scalpel (*arrow*) is used to perform a laminectomy at the target levels. *C* cranial

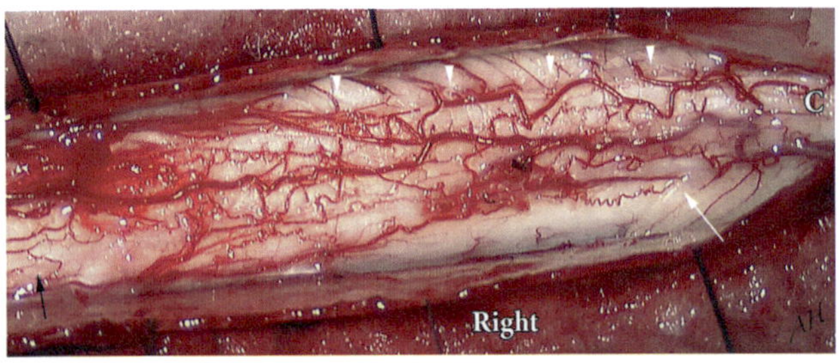

Fig. 66.3 After opening the dura and arachnoid, normal rootlets were observed on the left side (*arrowheads*). The DREZ on the avulsion side is identified by a line joining the last normal rootlet cranial to the injury (*white arrow*) to the first normal rootlet caudal to the injury (*black arrow*). *C* cranial

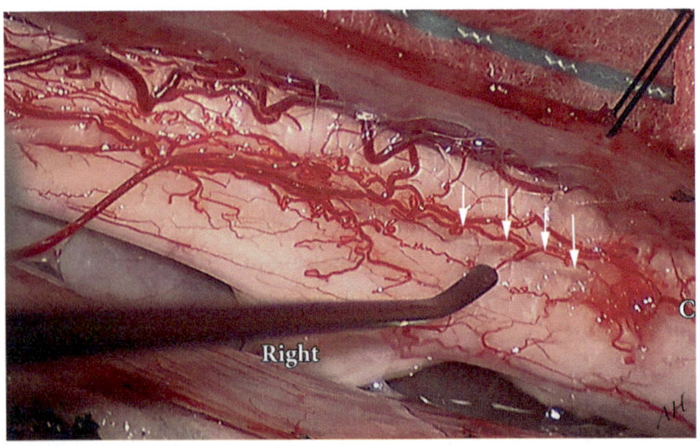

Fig. 66.4 The sites of nerve root avulsion are identified by pits (*arrows*) that look darker (greyish) in color compared to the surrounding pia. *C* cranial

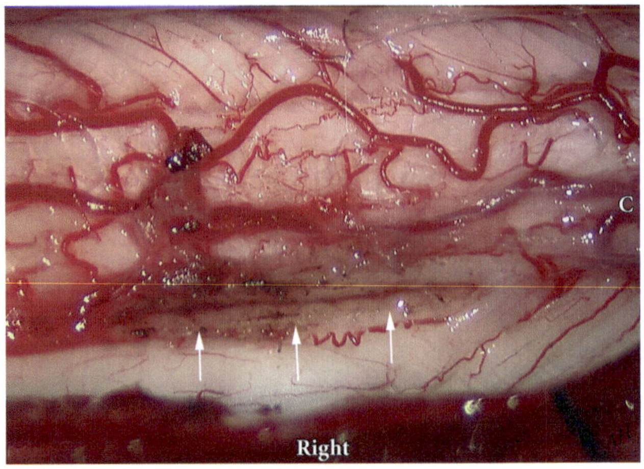

Fig. 66.5 Under the operative microscope, the DREZ lesion is performed (*arrows*) using a myelotomy knife and bipolar coagulation: angle, 30–45° medially with the spinal cord; depth, 2–3 mm. The lesion could also be performed using radiofrequency (RF). *C* cranial

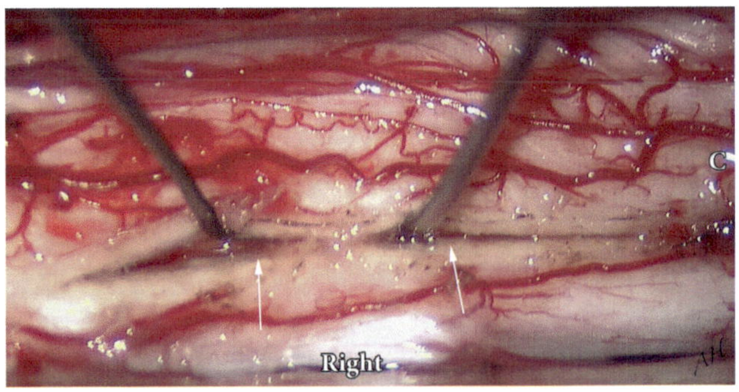

Fig. 66.6 Skip lesions of 1.5–2 cm in length are performed (*arrows*), leaving 1–2 mm of intact pia in-between. The latter is then coagulated. *C* cranial

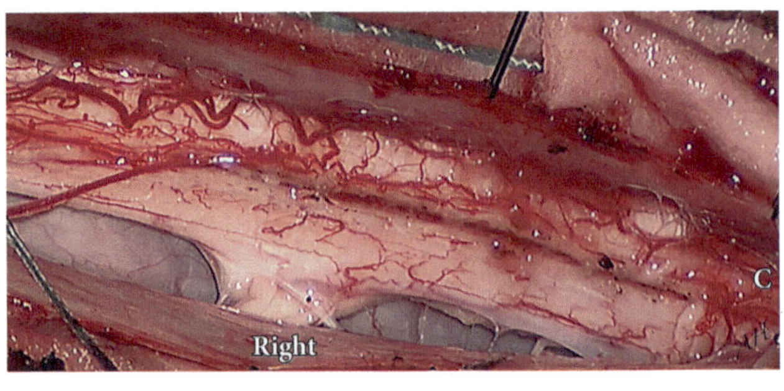

Fig. 66.7 Overview of the end of the procedure showing the entire extent of a right DREZ lesion. *C* cranial

11. A myelotomy knife is used to create skip lesions in the DREZ, at about 30–45° to the spinal cord surface, to a depth of 2–3 mm. The lesions are 1.5–2 cm in length, leaving 1–2 mm of intact pia in between (Fig. 66.6).
12. Bipolar coagulation is used again to coagulate the walls of the lesion and the skip areas (Fig. 66.7).

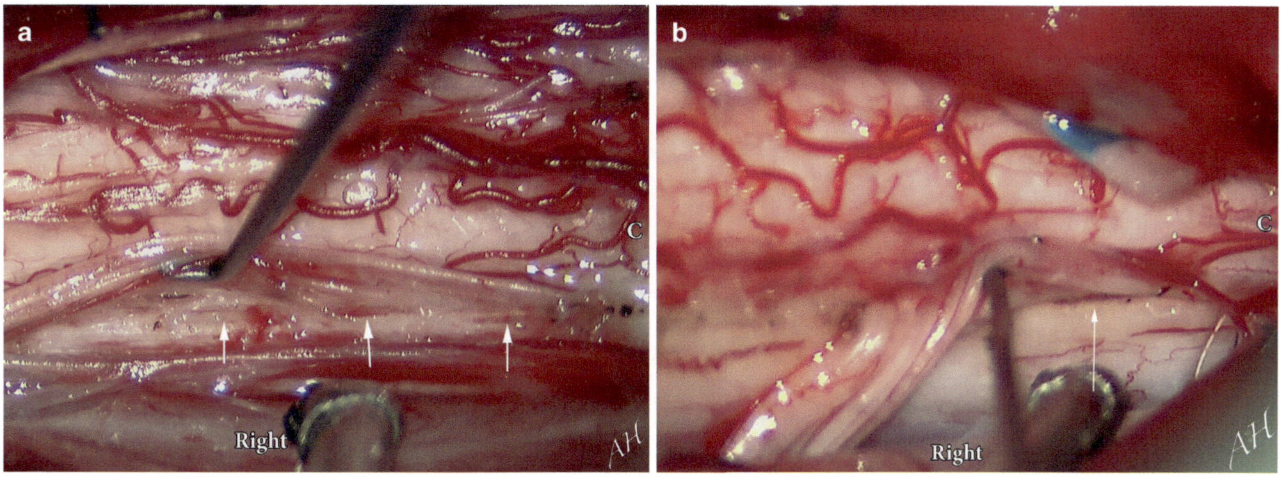

Fig. 66.8 The DREZ (*arrows*) could also include the nerve rootlets caudal (**a**) and cranial (**b**) to the avulsion. *C* cranial

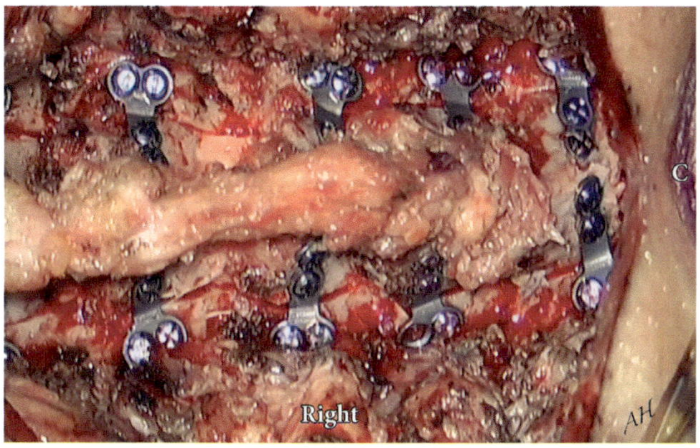

Fig. 66.9 The laminae are replaced with laminoplasty plates and screws. *C* cranial

13. If normal rootlets above and below are to be included, these are lifted up by an assistant using a nerve hook, and the lesion is created as above (Fig. 66.8).
14. Hemostasis is performed, and then copious irrigation is used to wash out any blood and replenish the cerebrospinal fluid (CSF).
15. The dura is closed using 6-0 GoreTex, 5-0 Prolene, or 4-0 Nylon.
16. This is secured by fibrin or hydrogel glue.
17. The laminae are replaced with miniplates and screws if laminoplasty is the goal (Fig. 66.9).
18. Careful hemostasis of the muscle. No drain is left. Vancomycin powder can be used in the muscle and subcutaneous layer. Long acting anesthetic could be injected in the muscle and subcutaneous layers.
19. The fascia is closed tightly with 0 Vicryl sutures.
20. The subcutaneous tissue is approximated with 2-0 Vicryl.
21. The skin is closed with running 3-0 Nylon.

Complications

1. Failure to treat the pain.
2. Recurrent pain.
3. Loss of SSEPs and/or MEPs. Troubleshoot: check the connections, raise the blood pressure, warm irrigation to the spinal cord, and wait a few minutes. If significant changes persist, a wake-up test may be performed or the procedure aborted.
4. Spinal cord injury.
5. CSF leak. This can be treated by elevating the head of the bed, over-sewing the incision, or inserting a lumbar drain. If unsuccessful, it will require wound revision.
6. Wound infection.
7. Postoperative hematoma.

References

1. Cetas JS, Saedi T, Burchiel KJ (2008) Destructive procedures for the treatment of nonmalignant pain: a structured literature review. J Neurosurg 109(3):389–404. https://doi.org/10.3171/JNS/2008/109/9/0389
2. Sindou M, Mifsud JJ, Boisson D, Goutelle A (1986) Selective posterior rhizotomy in the dorsal root entry zone for treatment of hyperspasticity and pain in the hemiplegic upper limb. Neurosurgery 18(5):587–595. https://doi.org/10.1227/00006123-198605000-00013
3. Friedman AH, Nashold BS Jr, Bronec PR (1988) Dorsal root entry zone lesions for the treatment of brachial plexus avulsion injuries: a follow-up study. Neurosurgery 22(2):369–373. https://doi.org/10.1227/00006123-198802000-00016

Part VI

Axial Cuts

Upper Limb Axial Cuts

67

Amgad S. Hanna, Natalia Guevara-Moriones, and Luis Rafael Moscote-Salazar

Cadaveric axial cuts matched with axial MRI images of the upper limb Figs. 67.1, 67.2, 67.3, 67.4, 67.5, 67.6, and 67.7.

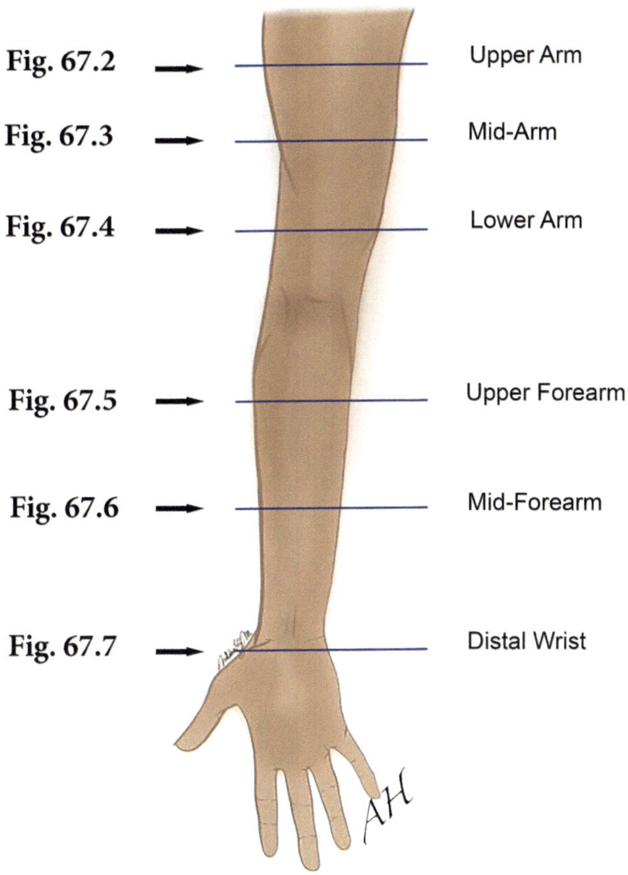

Fig. 67.1 Overview of the right upper limb showing the location of the axial cuts depicted in the following figures. In all the following figures: *A* anterior, *P* posterior, *M* medial, *L* lateral

A. S. Hanna (✉) · L. R. Moscote-Salazar
Department of Neurosurgery, University of Wisconsin School of Medicine and Public Health, Madison, WI, USA

N. Guevara-Moriones
Faculty of Medicine, Universidad Juan N. Corpas, Bogotá, Colombia
e-mail: nataliam-guevara@juanncorpas.edu.co

A. S. Hanna (ed.), *Nerves: Anatomy, Exposures, and Techniques*, https://doi.org/10.1007/978-3-031-73931-6_67

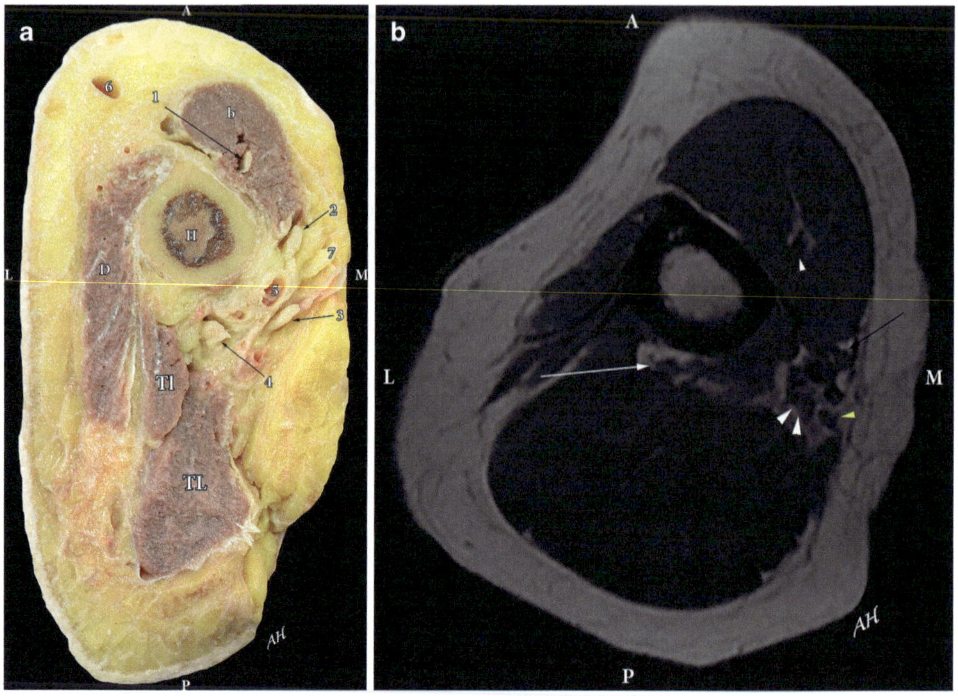

Fig. 67.2 Upper arm. (**a**) Axial cut. *H* humerus, *D* deltoid, *b* biceps brachii, *Tl* triceps, lateral head, *TL* triceps, long head, *1* musculocutaneous nerve, *2* median nerve, *3* ulnar nerve, *4* radial nerve, *5* brachial artery and veins, *6* cephalic vein, *7* medial antebrachial cutaneous nerve. (**b**) Axial T1-weighted MRI. *White arrow* radial nerve, *white arrowhead* musculocutaneous nerve, *black arrow* median nerve, *yellow arrowhead* medial antebrachial cutaneous nerve, *double white arrowheads* ulnar nerve

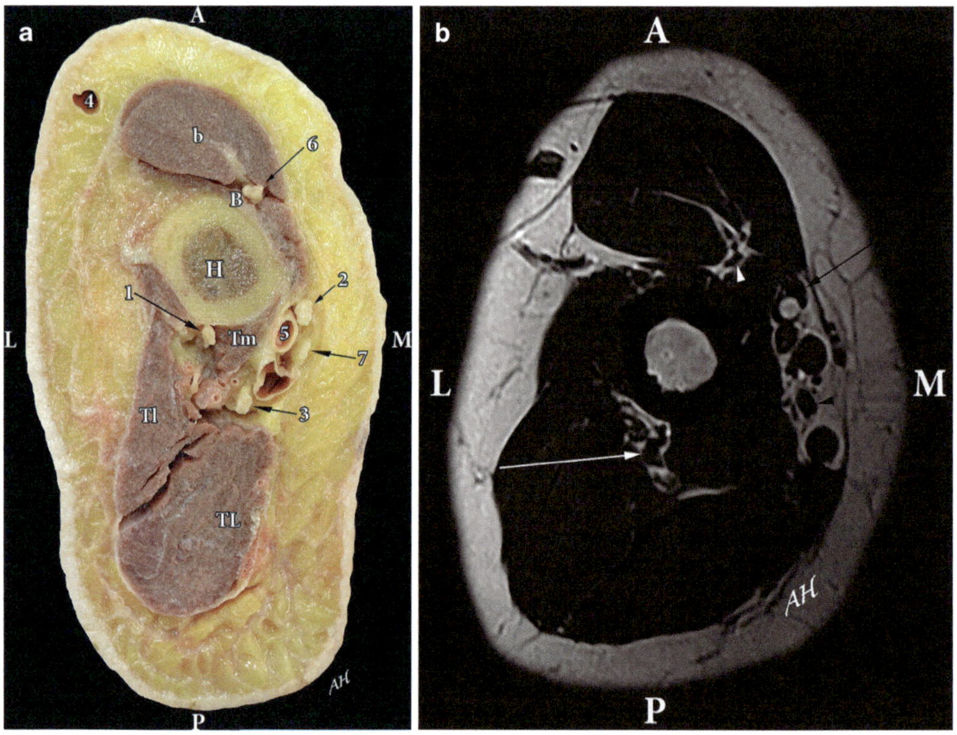

Fig. 67.3 Mid-arm. (**a**) Axial cut. *H* humerus, *B* brachialis, *b* biceps brachii, *Tm* triceps, medial head, *Tl* triceps, lateral head, *TL* triceps, long head, *1* radial nerve in the spiral groove, *2* median nerve, *3* ulnar nerve, *4* cephalic vein, *5* brachial artery, *6* musculocutaneous nerve, *7* medial antebrachial cutaneous nerve. (**b**) Axial T1-weighted MRI. *White arrow* radial nerve in the spiral groove, *white arrowhead* musculocutaneous nerve, *black arrow* median nerve, *black arrowhead* ulnar nerve

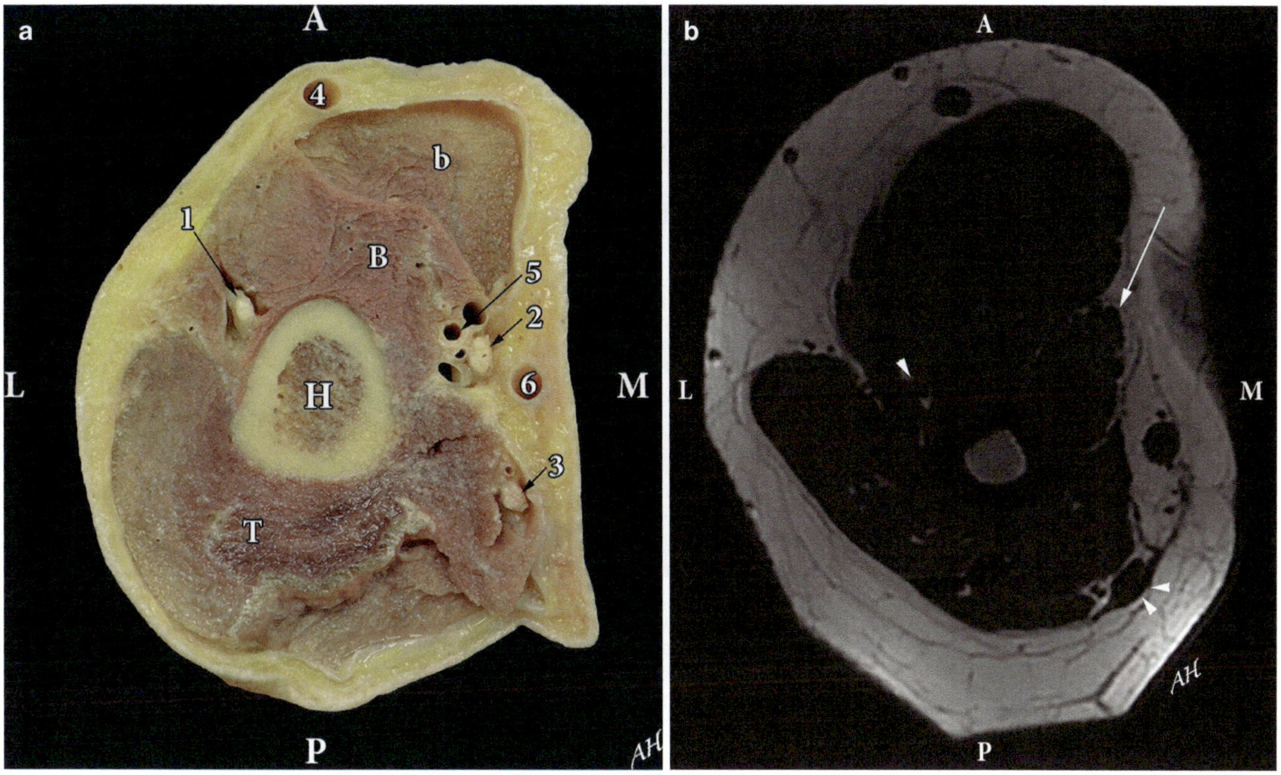

Fig. 67.4 Lower arm. (**a**) Axial cut. *H* humerus, *B* brachialis, *b* biceps brachii, *T* triceps, *1* radial nerve, *2* median nerve, *3* ulnar nerve, *4* cephalic vein, *5* brachial vessels, *6* basilic vein. (**b**) Axial T1-weighted MRI. *Arrow* median nerve, *double arrowheads* ulnar nerve (swollen), *arrowhead* radial nerve

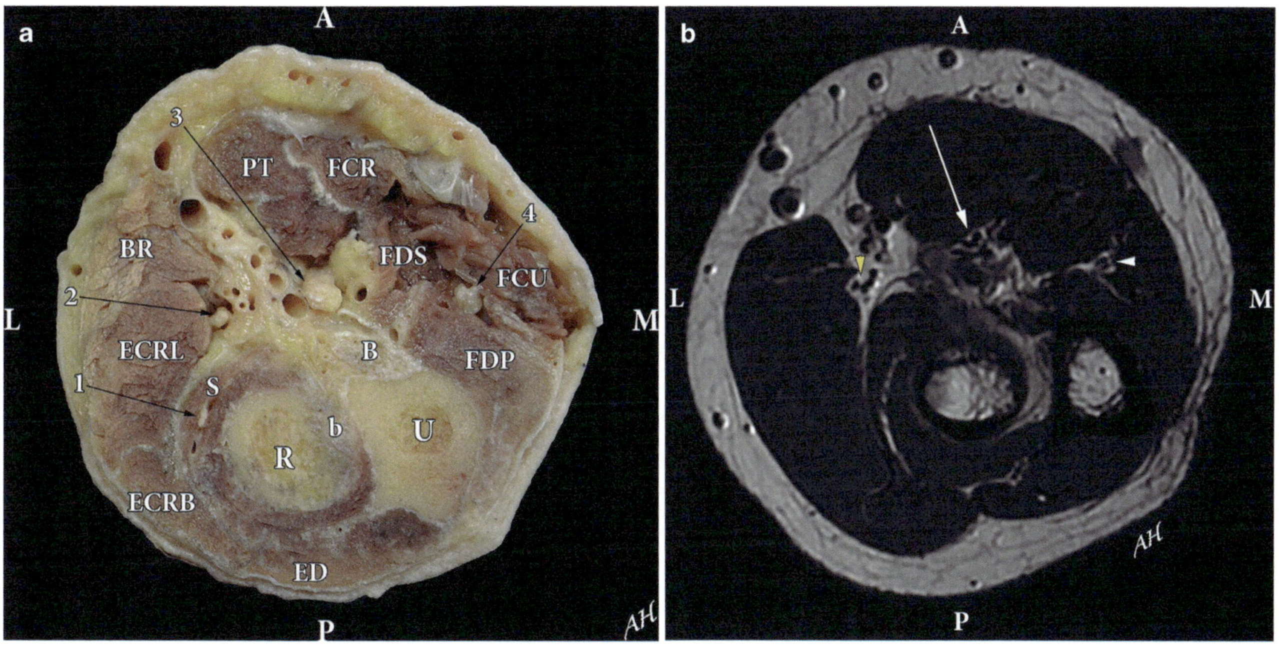

Fig. 67.5 Upper forearm. (**a**) Axial cut. *R* radius, *U* ulna, *BR* brachioradialis, *ECRL* extensor carpi radialis longus, *ECRB* extensor carpi radialis brevis, *ED* extensor digitorum, *S* supinator, *PT* pronator teres, *FCR* flexor carpi radialis, *FDS* flexor digitorum superficialis (sublimis), *FCU* flexor carpi ulnaris, *FDP* flexor digitorum profundus, *B* brachialis, *b* biceps brachii, *1* posterior interosseous nerve (PIN), *2* superficial radial nerve, *3* median nerve, *4* ulnar nerve. (**b**) Axial T1-weighted MRI. *White arrow* median nerve, *white arrowhead* ulnar nerve, *yellow arrowhead* radial nerve

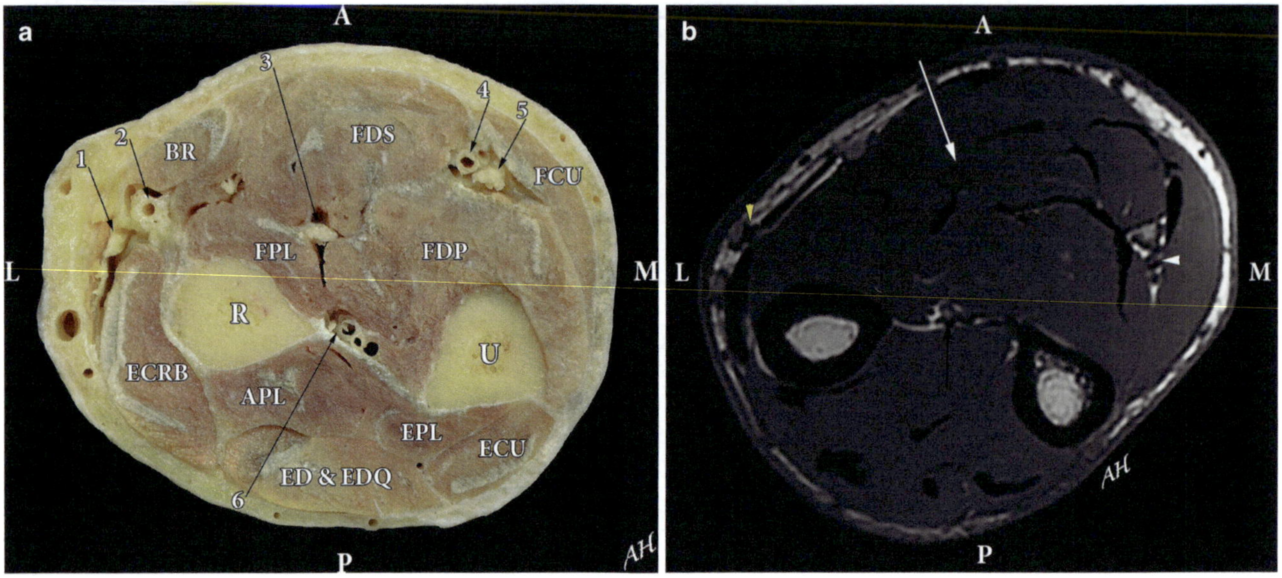

Fig. 67.6 Mid-forearm. (**a**) Axial cut. *R* radius, *U* ulna, *BR* brachioradialis, *FDS* flexor digitorum superficialis (sublimis), *FCU* flexor carpi ulnaris, *FPL* flexor pollicis longus, *FDP* flexor digitorum profundus, *ECRB* extensor carpi radialis brevis, *APL* abductor pollicis longus, *EPL* extensor pollicis longus, *ECU* extensor carpi ulnaris, *ED and EDQ* extensor digitorum and extensor digiti quinti (minimi), respectively, *1* superficial radial nerve, *2* radial artery, *3* median nerve, *4* ulnar artery, *5* ulnar nerve, *6* anterior interosseous nerve (AIN) and vessels. (**b**) Axial T1-weighted MRI. *White arrow* median nerve, *white arrowhead* ulnar nerve, *black arrow* anterior interosseous nerve and vessels, *yellow arrowhead* superficial radial nerve

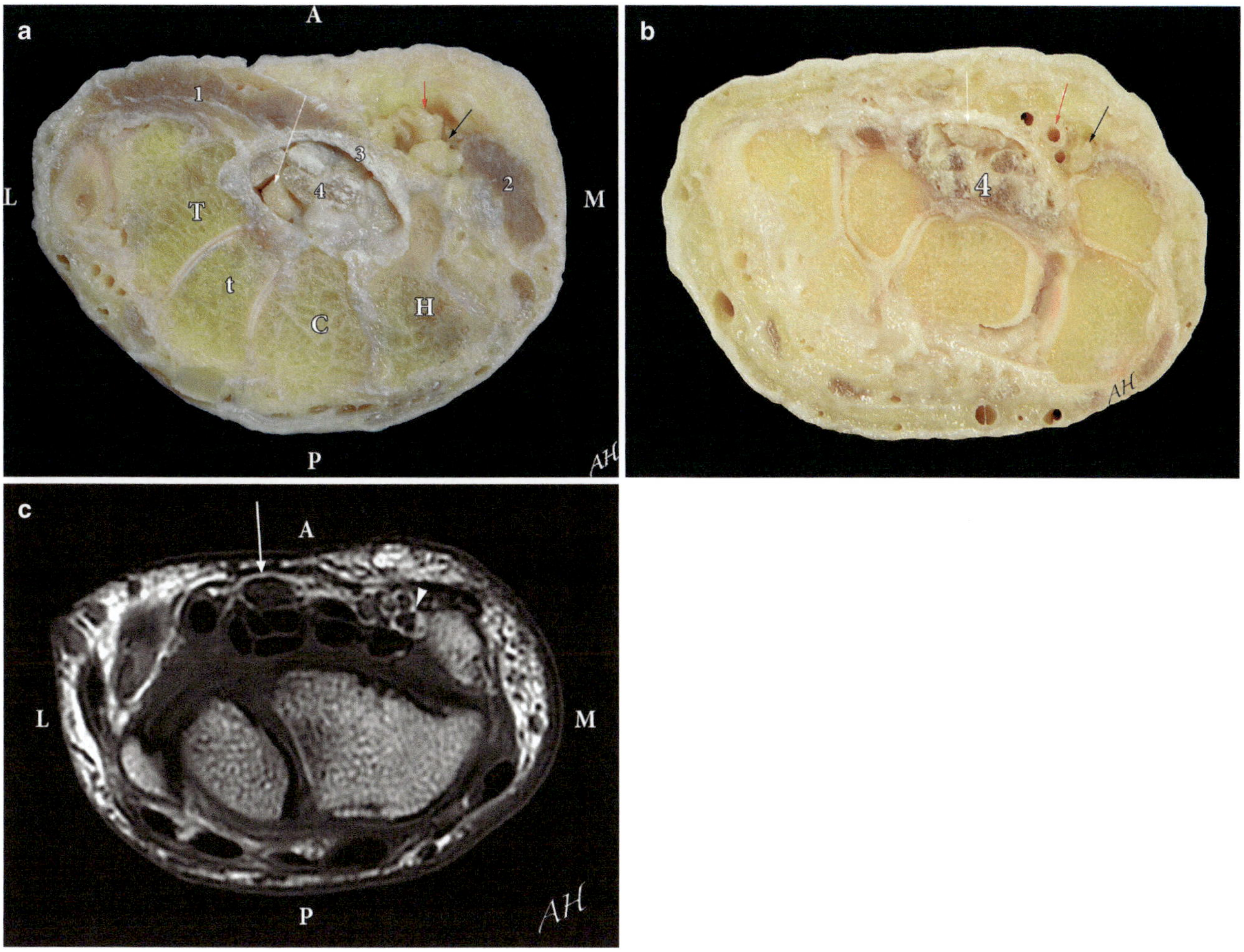

Fig. 67.7 Distal wrist. (**a**) Axial cut. *T* trapezium, *t* trapezoid, *C* capitate, *H* hamate, *1* thenar muscles, *2* hypothenar muscles, *3* transverse carpal ligament, *4* flexor tendons, *white arrow* median nerve, in this specimen abnormally located deep to the flexor tendons, *black arrow* ulnar nerve, *red arrow* ulnar artery. (**b**) Axial cut through a different specimen; here, the median nerve (*white arrow*) is in its normal anatomical location superficial to the flexor tendons (*4*). *Black arrow* ulnar nerve, *red arrow* ulnar artery. (**c**) Axial T1-weighted MRI. *Arrow* median nerve in carpal tunnel, *arrowhead* ulnar nerve in Guyon's canal

68 Lower Limb Axial Cuts

Amgad S. Hanna, Natalia Guevara-Moriones, and Luis Rafael Moscote-Salazar

Cadaveric axial cuts matched with axial MRI images of the lower limb. Figs. 68.1, 68.2, 68.3, 68.4, 68.5, 68.6, and 68.7.

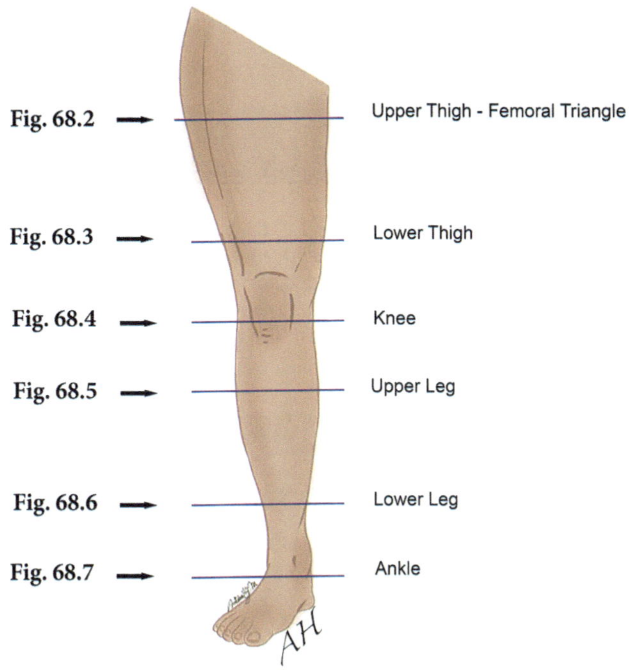

Fig. 68.1 Overview of the right lower limb showing the location of the axial cuts depicted in the following figures. In all the following figures: *A* anterior, *P* posterior, *M* medial, *L* lateral

A. S. Hanna (✉) · L. R. Moscote-Salazar
Department of Neurosurgery, University of Wisconsin School of Medicine and Public Health, Madison, WI, USA

N. Guevara-Moriones
Faculty of Medicine, Universidad Juan N. Corpas, Bogotá, Colombia
e-mail: nataliam-guevara@juanncorpas.edu.co

A. S. Hanna (ed.), *Nerves: Anatomy, Exposures, and Techniques*, https://doi.org/10.1007/978-3-031-73931-6_68

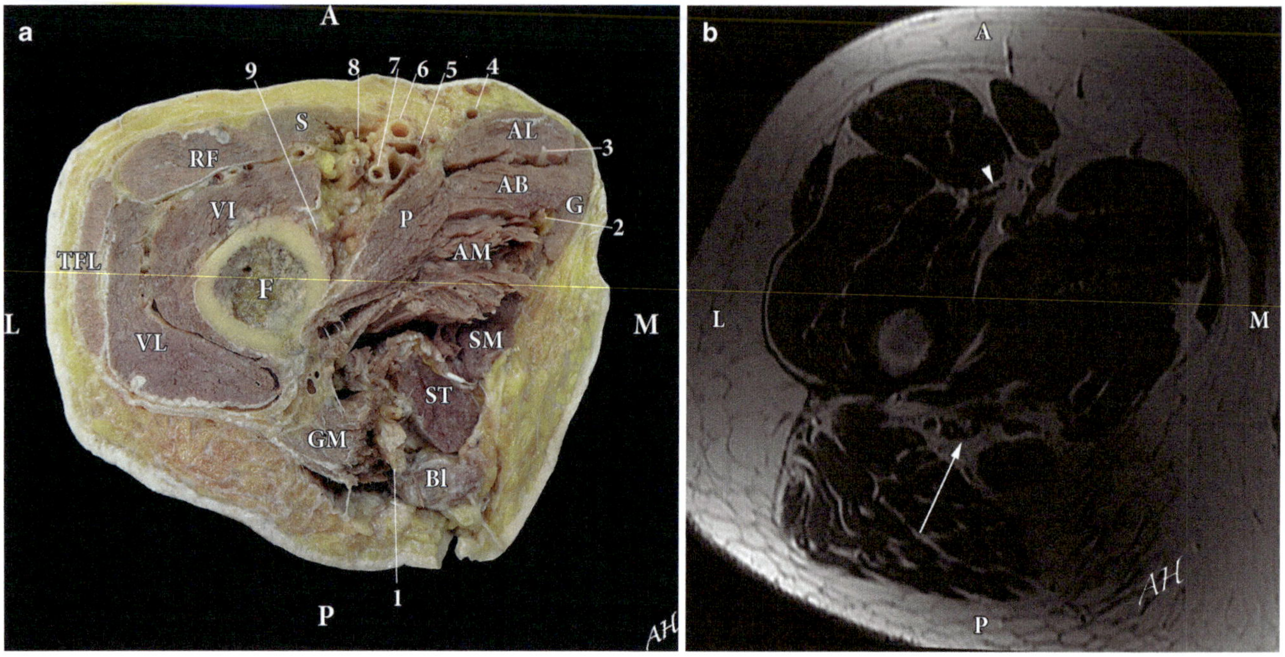

Fig. 68.2 Right upper thigh—femoral triangle. (**a**) Axial cut. *S* sartorius, *RF* rectus femoris, *VI* vastus intermedius, *VL* vastus lateralis, *TFL* tensor fasciae latae, *G* gracilis, *AL* adductor longus, *AB* adductor brevis, *AM* adductor magnus, *P* pectineus, *SM* semimembranosus, *ST* semitendinosus, *Bl* biceps femoris, long head, *GM* gluteus maximus, *1* sciatic nerve, *2* obturator nerve, posterior division, *3* obturator nerve, anterior division, *4* long saphenous vein, *5* femoral vein, *6* femoral artery, *7* profunda femoris artery, *8* femoral nerve, *9* vastus medialis. (**b**) Axial T1-weighted MRI. *Arrow* sciatic nerve, *arrowhead* femoral nerve branches

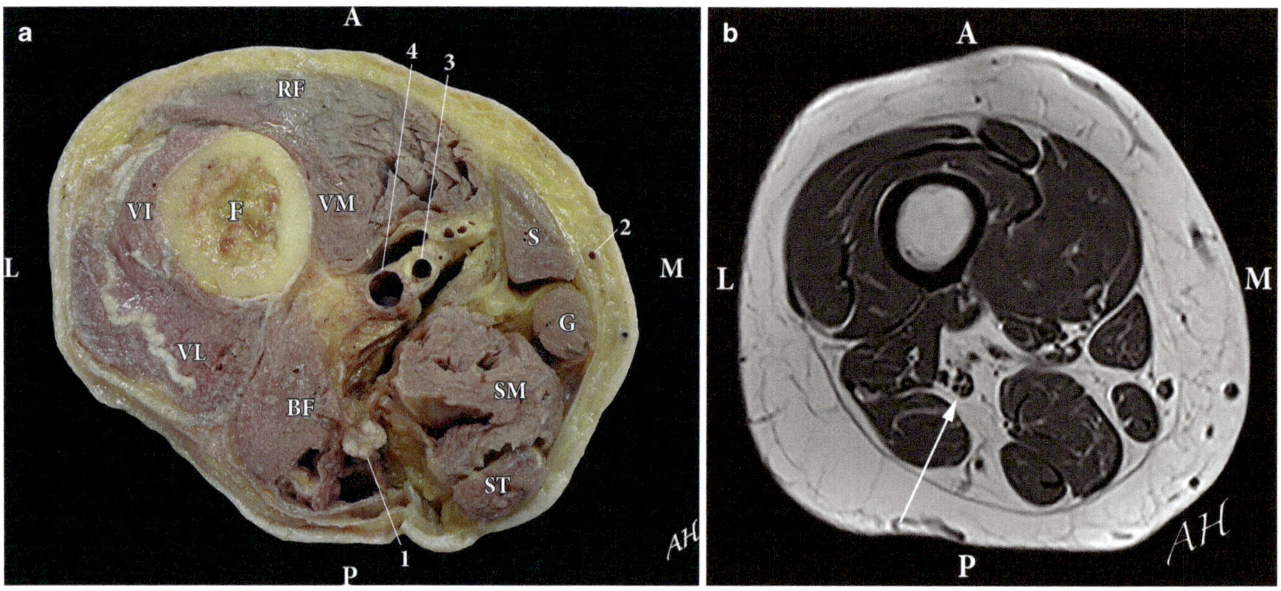

Fig. 68.3 Lower thigh. (**a**) Axial cut. *S* Sartorius, *G* gracilis, *SM* semimembranosus, *ST* semitendinosus, *BF* biceps femoris, *VL* vastus lateralis, *VI* vastus intermedius, *VM* vastus medialis, *RF* rectus femoris, *1* sciatic nerve, *2* long saphenous vein, *3* popliteal artery, *4* popliteal vein. (**b**) Axial T1-weighted MRI. *Arrow* sciatic nerve

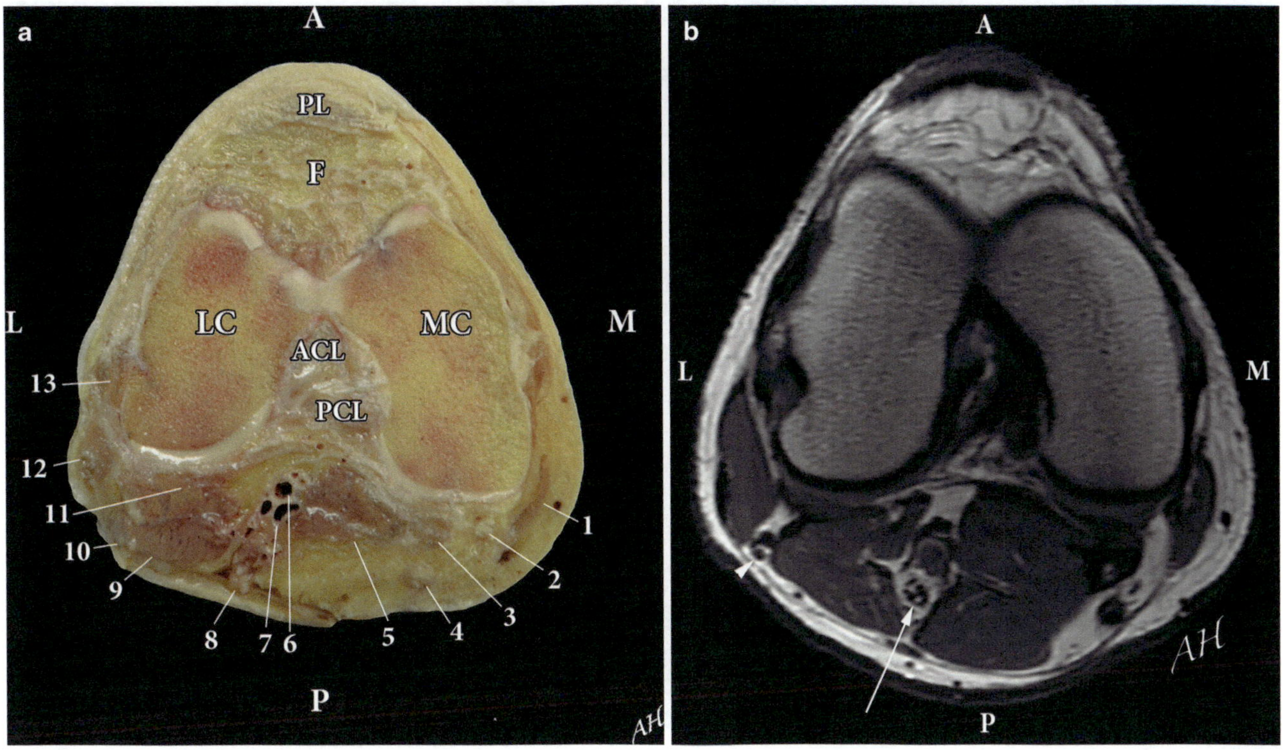

Fig. 68.4 Knee. (**a**) Axial cut. *MC* medial femoral condyle, *LC* lateral femoral condyle, *ACL* anterior cruciate ligament, *PCL* posterior cruciate ligament, *F* infrapatellar pad of fat, *PL* patellar ligament, *1* sartorius, *2* gracilis, *3* semimembranosus, *4* semitendinosus, *5* gastrocnemius, medial head, *6* popliteal artery, *7* popliteal vein, *8* tibial nerve, *9* gastrocnemius, lateral head, *10* common peroneal (fibular) nerve, *11* plantaris, *12* biceps femoris, *13* popliteus. (**b**) Axial T1-weighted MRI. *Arrow* tibial nerve, *arrowhead* common peroneal (fibular) nerve

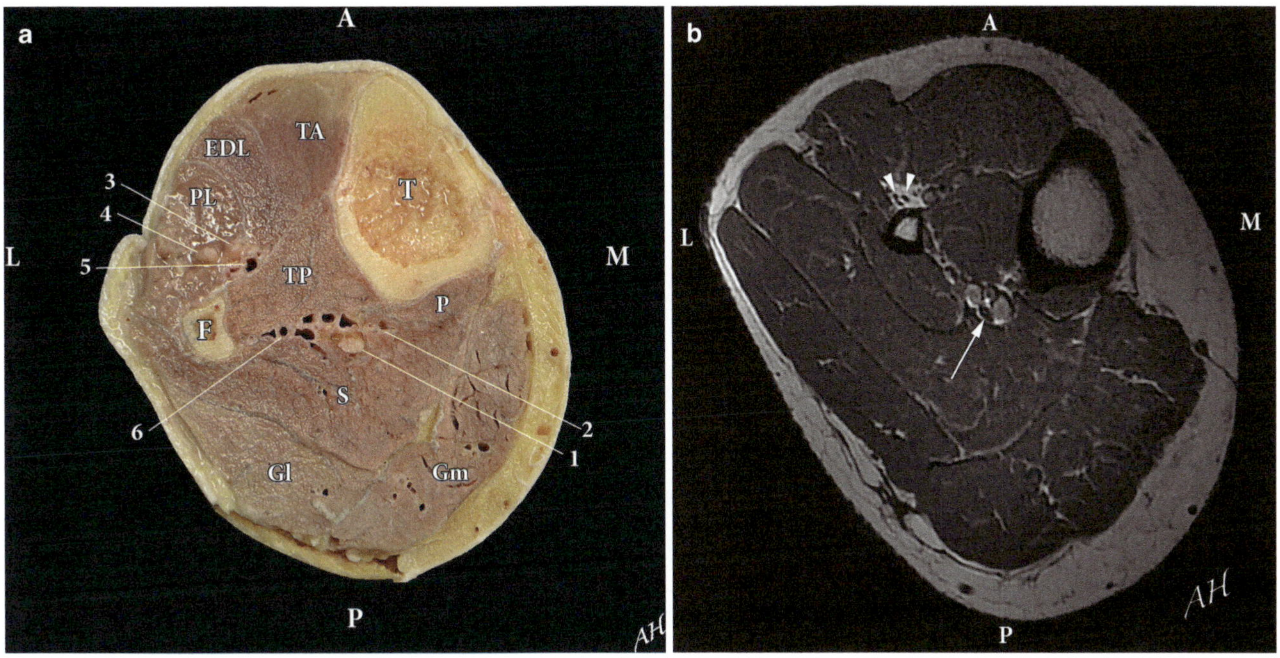

Fig. 68.5 Upper leg—just distal to tibial tuberosity. (**a**) Axial cut. *T* tibia, *F* fibula, *TA* tibialis anterior, *EDL* extensor digitorum longus, *PL* peroneus longus, *TP* tibialis posterior, *P* popliteus, *S* soleus, *Gl* gastrocnemius, lateral head, *Gm* gastrocnemius, medial head, *1* tibial nerve, *2* posterior tibial vessels, *3* deep peroneal (fibular) nerve, *4* superficial peroneal (fibular) nerve, *5* anterior tibial vessels, *6* peroneal vessels. (**b**) Axial T1-weighted MRI. *Arrow* tibial nerve, *arrowheads* superficial and deep peroneal nerves (from lateral to medial)

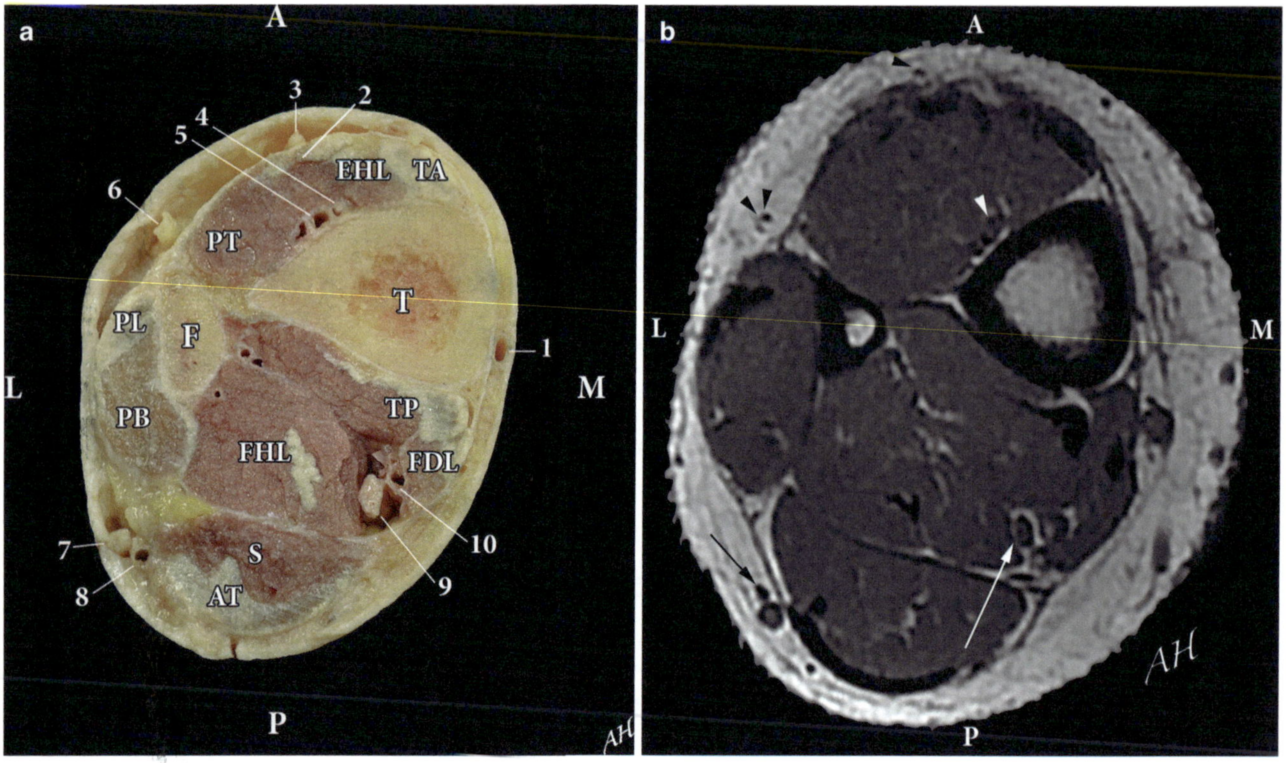

Fig. 68.6 Lower leg, above the ankle. (**a**) Axial cut. *T* tibia, *F* fibula, *TA* tibialis anterior, *EHL* extensor hallucis longus, *PT* peroneus tertius, *TP* tibialis posterior, *FDL* flexor digitorum longus, *FHL* flexor hallucis longus, *S* soleus, *AT* Achilles tendon, *PL* peroneus longus, *PB* peroneus brevis, *1* long saphenous vein, *2* extensor digitorum longus, *3* medial dorsal cutaneous nerve, *4* deep peroneal nerve, *5* anterior tibial vessels, *6* intermediate dorsal cutaneous nerve, *7* sural nerve, *8* short saphenous vein, *9* tibial nerve, *10* posterior tibial artery. *3 and 6* are branches of the superficial peroneal nerve. (**b**) Axial T1-weighted MRI. *White arrow* tibial nerve, *white arrowhead* deep peroneal nerve, *black arrow* sural nerve, anterior to the short saphenous vein, *black arrowhead* medial dorsal cutaneous nerve, *double black arrowheads* intermediate dorsal cutaneous nerve. The latter two are branches of the superficial peroneal nerve

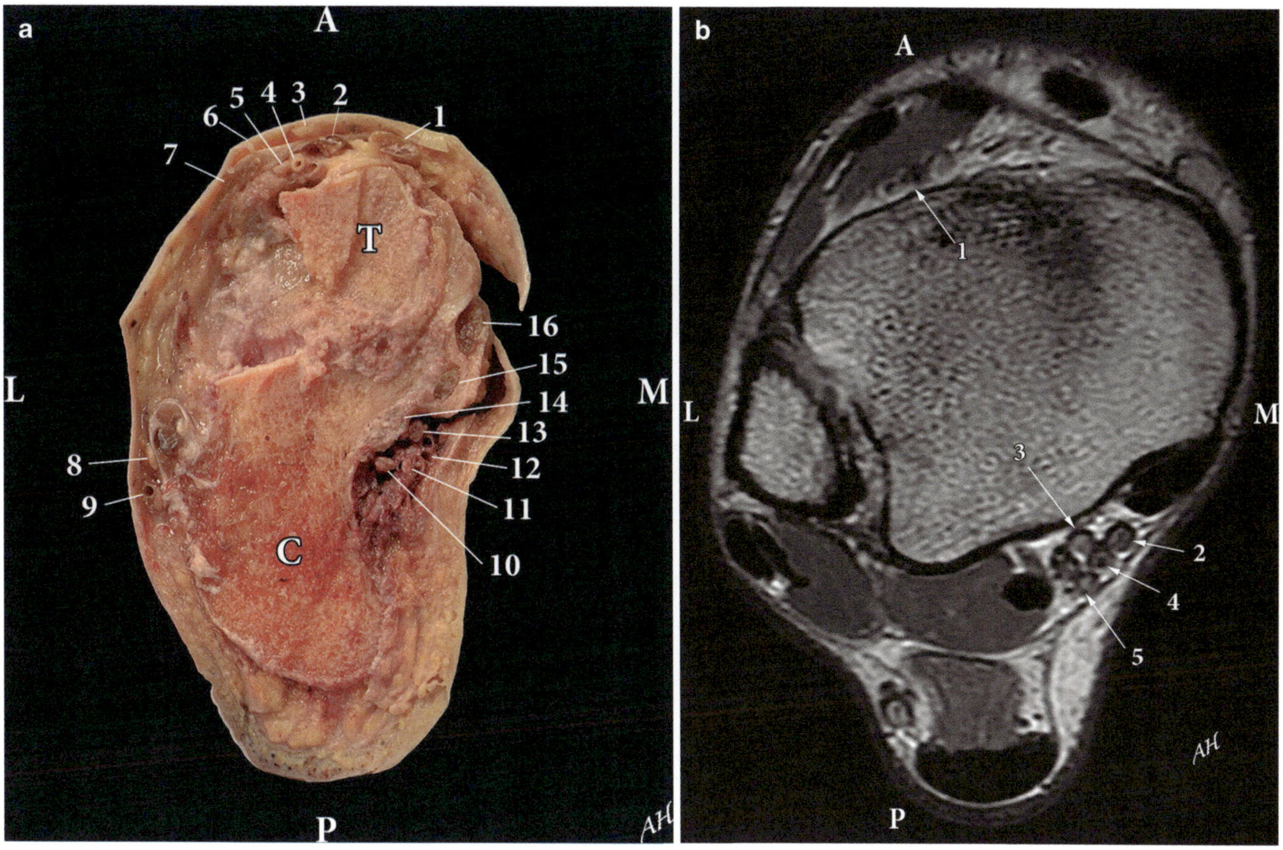

Fig. 68.7 Right ankle. (**a**) Axial cut at the level of the ankle joint and tarsal tunnel. *C* calcaneus, *T* talus, *1* tibialis anterior, *2* extensor hallucis longus, *3* medial dorsal cutaneous nerve, *4* anterior tibial artery and veins, *5* deep peroneal nerve, *6* intermediate dorsal cutaneous nerve, *7* extensor digitorum longus, *8* sural nerve, *9* short saphenous vein, *10* lateral plantar nerve, *11* calcaneal branch, *12* posterior tibial vessels, *13* medial plantar nerve, *14* flexor hallucis longus, *15* flexor digitorum longus, *16* tibialis posterior. (**b**) Axial proton density MRI, just proximal to the ankle joint. *1* deep peroneal nerve and anterior tibial vessels, *2* medial plantar nerve, *3* lateral plantar nerve, *4* posterior tibial vessels, *5* calcaneal branch

Part VII

The Future of Nerve Surgery

Bionic Reconstruction After Severe Neural Loss

69

Udo Maierhofer and Oskar C. Aszmann

Indications

- Targeted muscle reinnervation (TMR) in bionic reconstruction is best suited for patients who experienced above-elbow or glenohumeral amputation, as these patients lack sufficient electromyography (EMG) signals to control myoelectric prostheses. In patients with transcarpal or transradial amputation, sufficient muscle signals may be present, TMR may be used for neuroma treatment [1].
- The ideal patient for bionic reconstruction has a history of sharp amputation without significant soft tissue or plexus damage. Extensive preoperative assessment of the brachial plexus, including magnetic resonance neurography, is necessary to ensure healthy nerve fascicles and intact residual muscles are present [2]. Neuroma can be addressed during the same surgery [3].
- Patients should be capable and motivated to undergo a long rehabilitation process, including extensive physical therapy, to achieve intuitive prosthesis control [4].
- In above-elbow amputees, optimal prosthetic fitting requires 50–70% of the original humerus length.
- Patients with insufficient bone length or lack of viable muscle for TMR may require bone lengthening or free tissue transfer.

Supplementary Information The online version contains supplementary material available at https://doi.org/10.1007/978-3-031-73931-6_69.

U. Maierhofer · O. C. Aszmann (✉)
Clinical Laboratory for Bionic Extremity Reconstruction, Department of Plastic, Reconstructive and Aesthetic Surgery, Medical University of Vienna, Vienna, Austria
e-mail: udo.maierhofer@meduniwien.ac.at; oskar.aszmann@meduniwien.ac.at

Surgical Techniques

This surgery is performed under general anesthesia. The use of muscle relaxers should be avoided, as identifying motor nerves and evaluating function by stimulation are essential.

The patient is positioned supine with the head turned to the opposite side at a 30° angle. The shoulder is slightly elevated to facilitate access to the posterior shoulder and axilla. The entire extremity, the shoulder, the axilla, and the neck are surgically prepared (Fig. 69.1).

Exploration of the supraclavicular brachial plexus can be performed at the beginning of surgery to evaluate and simultaneously treat proximal nerve damage. The surgical concept is adapted based on available recipient motor nerves (Table 69.1).

Above Elbow Amputation

1. The remaining stump is placed on a hand table in an abducted position.
2. A medial incision reaching from the axilla is made to access the median, the ulnar, and the musculocutaneous nerves.
3. The musculocutaneous nerve is identified and its motor branches to the brachialis (BR), and the biceps' short (SB) and long heads are dissected (Fig. 69.2).
4. The short head of the biceps is detached from its origin at the coracoid process (Fig. 69.2).
5. Overlaying subcutaneous adipose tissue is removed to improve subsequent EMG signal recording, and an adipose tissue flap is mobilized to separate the biceps heads. Nerve transfers of the median nerve to the BR and the ulnar nerve to the SB.
6. An incision is made in the lateral aspect of the arm to access the radial nerve.
7. The heads of the triceps brachii are dissected, and the motor branches of the radial nerve are identified (Fig. 69.3).

A. S. Hanna (ed.), *Nerves: Anatomy, Exposures, and Techniques*, https://doi.org/10.1007/978-3-031-73931-6_69

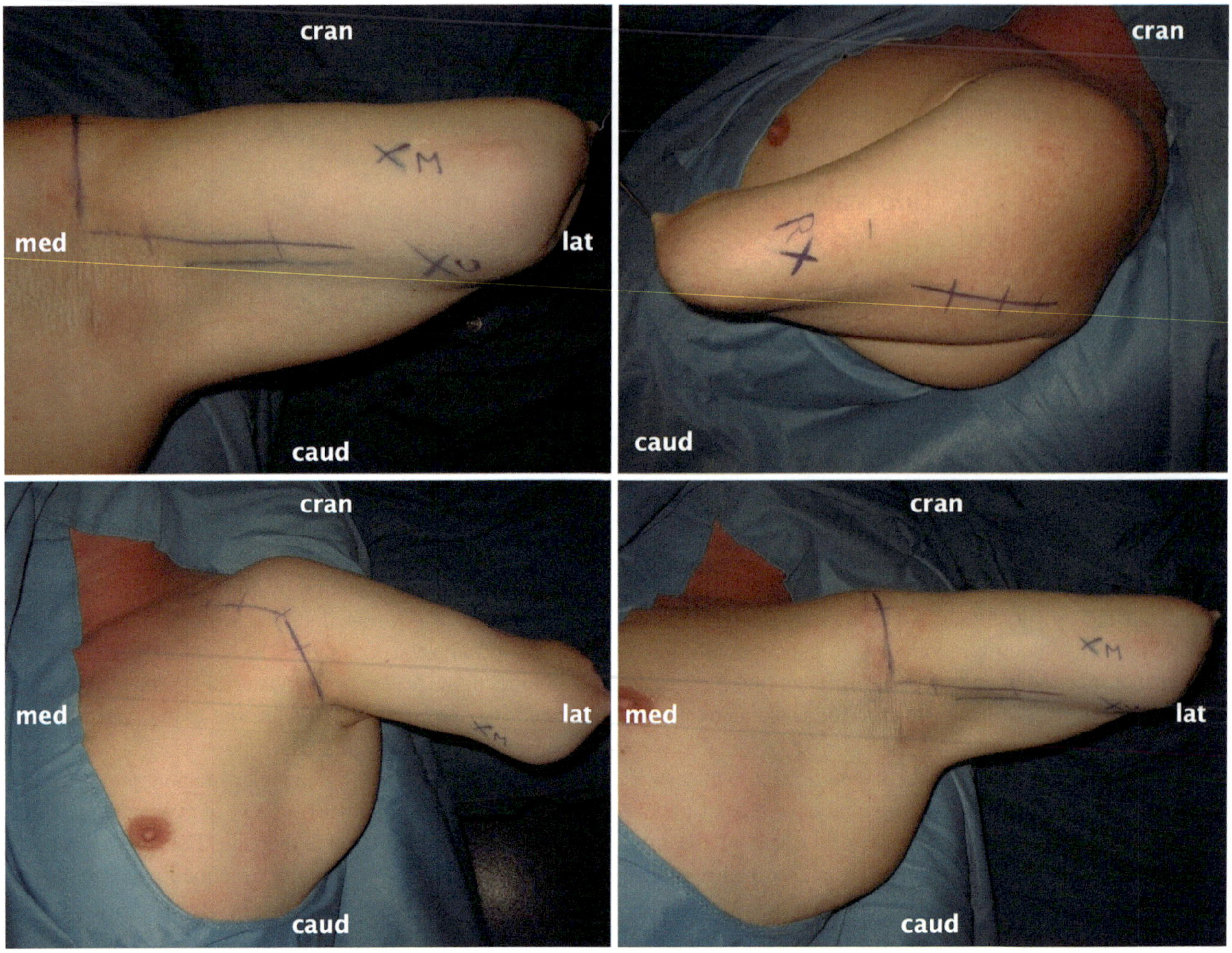

Fig. 69.1 Surgical site marking for a transhumeral amputee. *M* distal end of the median nerve, *U* distal end of the ulnar nerve, *R* distal end of the radial nerve, *cran* cranial, *caud* caudal, *med* medial, *lat* lateral

Table 69.1 Nerve transfer scheme for above-elbow amputees and glenohumeral amputees [5]

Amputation level	Nerves	Target muscles	Prosthetic function	Innervation
Above-elbow	Musculocutaneous	Biceps long head	Elbow flexion	Native
	Ulnar	Biceps short head	Hand close	Transferred
	Median	Brachialis	Pronation	Transferred
	Radial	Triceps long and medial head	Elbow extension	Native
	Split radial	Triceps lateral head	Hand open	Transferred
	Split radial	Brachioradialis	Supination	Transferred
Glenohumeral	Musculocutaneous	Pectoralis major clavicular part	Elbow flexion	Transferred
	Ulnar	Pectoralis minor	Hand close	Transferred
	Median	Pectoralis major sternocostal part	Hand close/wrist rotation	Transferred
	Median	Pectoralis major abdominal part	Wrist rotation	Transferred
	Radial	Latissimus dorsi	Elbow extension	Transferred
	Deep radial branch	Infraspinatus	Hand open	Transferred

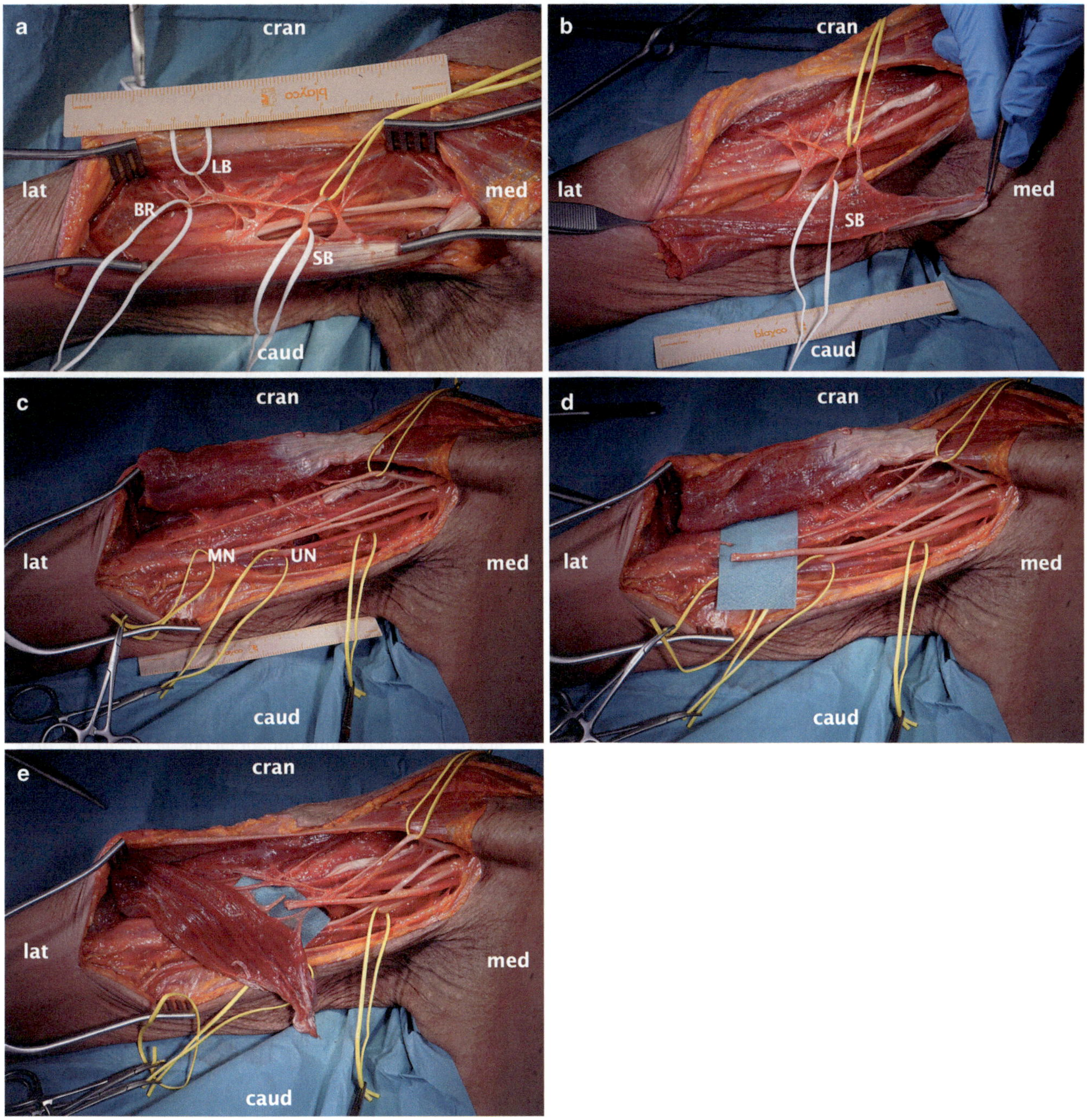

Fig. 69.2 (**a**) Motor branches innervating the brachialis (*BR*), the long head of the biceps (*LB*), and the short head of the biceps (*SB*) are identified and dissected. (**b**) The short head of the biceps (*SB*) is released from its origin at the coracoid process and relocated medially. (**c**) The ulnar nerve (*UN*) and median nerve (*MN*) are identified and dissected free. (**d**) Nerve transfer of the median nerve to the brachialis motor branch. (**e**) Nerve transfer of the ulnar nerve to the short head of the biceps motor branch. *cran* cranial, *caud* caudal, *med* medial, *lat* lateral

8. The motor branch to the lateral head of the triceps brachii (LT) is dissected toward its origin at the radial nerve (Fig. 69.3).
9. If the brachioradialis muscle is preserved, intraneural dissection of the distal radial nerve is performed to identify its motor branch (BRA) and separate supination from hand opening after coaptations.
10. Amputated donor nerves are released from scar tissue and dissected free proximally to prevent neuroma formation.
11. Recipient motor branches are tested by stimulation and transected. Proximal stumps are shortened and buried deep in the tissue.

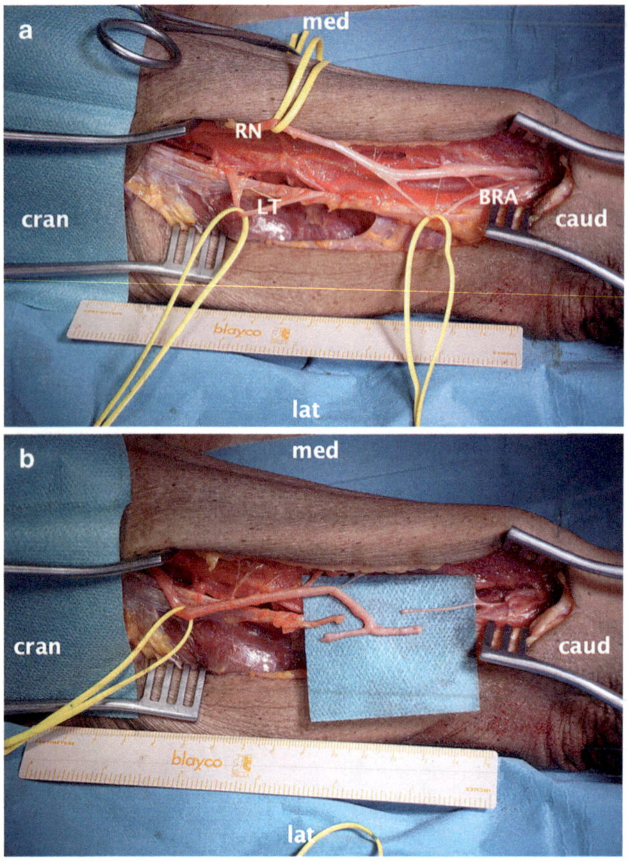

Fig. 69.3 (**a**) The radial nerve (*RN*), the motor branch to the lateral head of the triceps (*LT*), and the motor branch to the brachioradialis (*BRA*) are identified. (**b**) Subsequently, the deep radial nerve is split. The fascicular group responsible for hand opening is transferred to the LT, and the fascicular group responsible for supination is transferred to the BRA. *cran* cranial, *caud* caudal, *med* medial, *lat* lateral

12. The deep radial nerve is split. Nerve transfers are performed in a tension-free manner using 9-0 monofilament sutures and fibrin glue: the fascicular group responsible for hand opening is transferred to the LT, and the fascicular group responsible for supination is transferred to the BRA (Fig. 69.3).
13. Wound closure is performed.

Glenohumeral Amputation

1. The amputation scar is reopened, and the incision is extended infraclavicularly to expose the pectoralis major muscle.
2. Deflection of the pectoralis major (PM) medially and dissection of its motor branches after division of the clavipectoral fascia from proximal to distal (Fig. 69.4).
3. The motor branches to the clavicular, sternocostal, and abdominal portions of the pectoralis major muscle are identified and confirmed by stimulation. Similarly, pectoralis minor (Pm) branch is identified.
4. The ulnar, median, musculocutaneous, and radial nerves are identified in the scar tissue and dissected free proximally. Topography of the axillary artery can be useful in nerve identification (Fig. 69.4).
5. The suprascapular and thoracodorsal (TD) nerves are identified.
6. The clavicular, sternocostal, and abdominal parts of the pectoralis major are mobilized and divided to separate EMG signals.
7. Recipient motor branches are tested by stimulation and transected; proximal stumps are shortened and buried deep in the tissue.
8. Nerve transfers are performed in a tension-free manner using 9-0 monofilament sutures and fibrin glue: ulnar nerve to the Pm, musculocutaneous nerve to the upper PM, median nerve to the lower PM, and radial nerve to TD.
9. Wound closure is performed.

Complications

1. Pneumothorax
2. Iatrogenic vascular injuries
3. Iatrogenic injuries to the brachial plexus or its branches
4. Neuroma formation
5. Wound infection

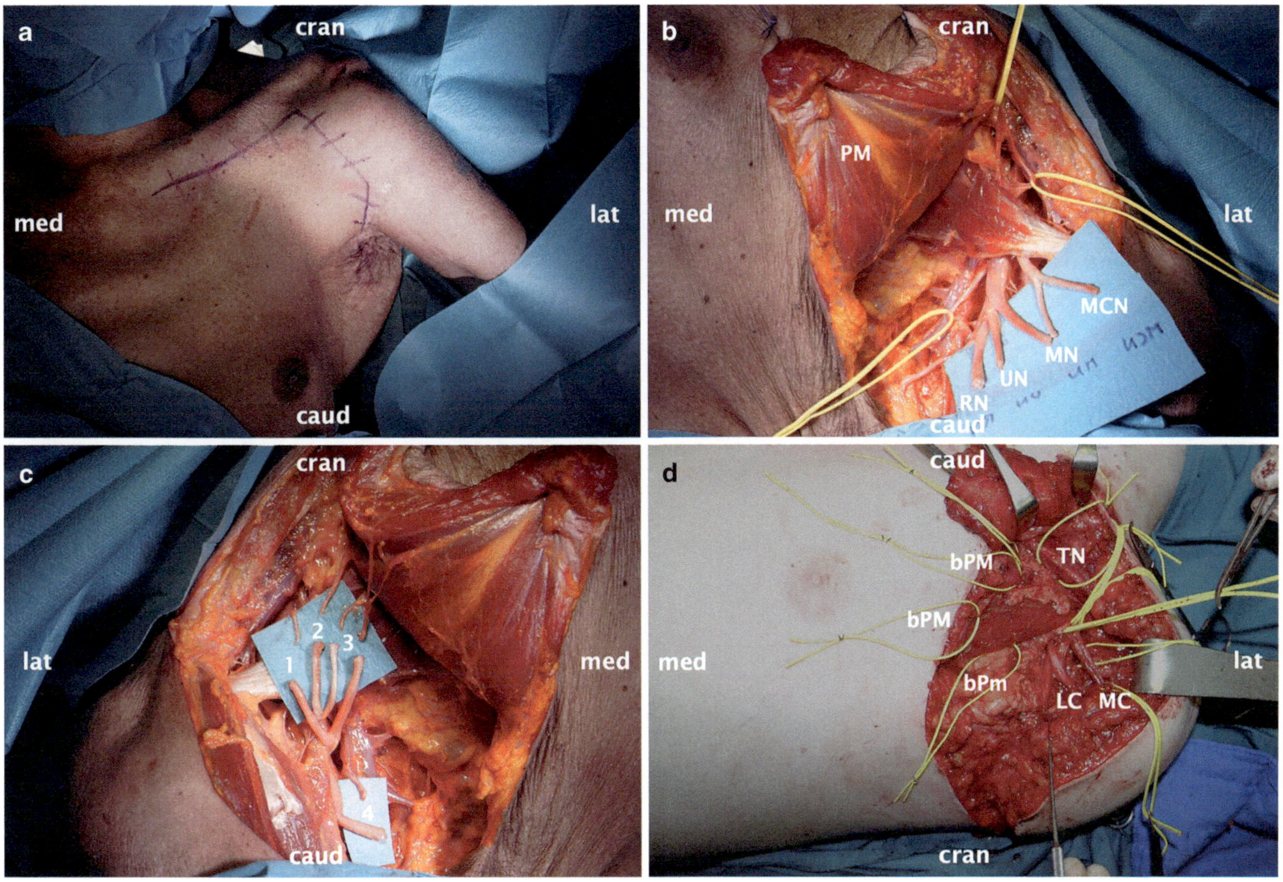

Fig. 69.4 (**a**–**c**) Cadaveric illustration. (**a**) Surgical site marking for a glenohumeral amputee. (**b**) The pectoralis motor branches are identified at the deep surface of the pectoralis major muscle (*PM*). The ulnar nerve (*UN*), median nerve with its two components (*MN*), musculocutaneous nerve (*MCN*), and radial nerve (*RN*) are identified and dissected from scar tissue. (**c**) Nerve transfers of the ulnar nerve to the pectoralis minor motor branch (*1*); the musculocutaneous to the upper pectoralis major motor branches (*2*); the median nerve to the lower pectoralis major motor branches (*3*); and the radial nerve to the latissimus dorsi motor branch (*4*). (**d**) Intraoperative view after nerve identification. *bPM* motor branch to the pectoralis major, *bPm* motor branch to the pectoralis minor, *TN* thoracodorsal nerve, *LC* lateral cord, *MC* medial cord, *cran* cranial, *caud* caudal, *med* medial, *lat* lateral

References

1. Kuiken TA, Dumanian GA, Lipschutz RD, Miller LA, Stubblefield KA (2004) Targeted muscle reinnervation for improved myoelectric prosthesis control in a bilateral shoulder disarticulation amputee. Prosthet Orthot Int 28(3):245–253. https://doi.org/10.3109/03093640409167756
2. Farina D, Aszmann O (2014) Bionic limbs: clinical reality and academic promises. Sci Transl Med 6(257):257ps12. https://doi.org/10.1126/scitranslmed.3010453
3. Dumanian GA, Potter BK, Mioton LM, Ko JH, Cheesborough JE, Souza JM et al (2019) Targeted muscle reinnervation treats neuroma and phantom pain in major limb amputees: a randomized clinical trial. Ann Surg 270(2):238–246. https://doi.org/10.1097/SLA.0000000000003088
4. Ortiz-Catalan M, Mastinu E, Sassu P, Aszmann O, Brånemark R (2020) Self-contained neuromusculoskeletal arm prostheses. N Engl J Med 382(18):1732–1738. https://doi.org/10.1056/NEJMoa1917537
5. Salminger S, Sturma A, Roche AD, Mayer JA, Gstoettner C, Aszmann OC (2019) Outcomes, challenges, and pitfalls after targeted muscle reinnervation in high-level amputees: is it worth the effort? Plast Reconstr Surg 144(6):1037e–1043e. https://doi.org/10.1097/PRS.0000000000006277

Between Stimulation and Biologics

70

Stephen P. Miranda, Emily Xu, Maya Alexis, and Zarina S. Ali

Introduction

The field of nerve surgery has witnessed exciting advances in recent years. Current research seeks to identify technologies and therapeutics that may accelerate nerve regeneration and improve function after surgical repair. Promising avenues for future clinical application can be broadly categorized by their aims: improving the substrates used for nerve repair (e.g., Schwann cell transplantation, stem cell-based tissue-engineered grafts, olfactory ensheathing cells), accelerating the nerve regeneration process (e.g., administration of biologic growth factors, electrical stimulation), and augmenting recovery of function (e.g., myoelectric prosthetics). In this chapter, we provide an overview of select topics as a primer for the practicing nerve surgeon and for surgical trainees. This is a rapidly evolving field, and newer discoveries may build on, confirm, or negate what's written here at this point in time.

Schwann Cells

Given the physiologic role of Schwann cells in nerve regeneration [1, 2], it is not surprising that much research has focused on whether their presence or activity could be modulated to support nerve repair [3]. Schwann cell transplantation via nerve conduits has been proposed for long-gap nerve injuries, for which there are limited reconstruction options [2]. In animal models, Schwann cell grafts have demonstrated significant potential in augmenting myelinated axon regrowth within repairs. For example, immunostaining and light microscopy revealed enhanced numbers of myelinated axons within nerve grafts containing Schwann cells as opposed to acellular grafts alone, as early as 4 weeks post-transplant [4–6]. There is also evidence that the addition of Schwann cells to a graft conduit increases the microvessel density around the repair site [7]. Motor functional recovery, as assessed by compound muscle action potentials (CMAP), has also been enhanced with the use of Schwann cell grafts in rodent models [7–9]. Several materials have successfully been trialed as potential conduits for autologous Schwann cell transplantation, including chitosan, cellulose, hydrogel, and polycaprolactone [5, 9–13].

In humans, autologous Schwann cells can be harvested either from a donor nerve or from a traumatized nerve stump during an initial exploration, at least 3–4 weeks prior to definitive nerve repair [2, 12, 13]. Over this time, the cell population is cultured and expanded, before being infused into a conduit used for neurorrhaphy [2, 12]. There are some drawbacks to this approach. If sacrificing a donor nerve is necessary to obtain Schwann cells, the patient could potentially have a better functional outcome if the donor nerve were used as autograft instead, especially if it takes several weeks to culture enough Schwann cells for implantation, or if Schwann cells at the repair site potentially contribute to scar formation [3]. Nevertheless, early in-human case reports have shown success with long-gap sciatic nerve injuries. Autologous Schwann cells harvested both from sural nerve and from traumatized sciatic nerve ends were cultured and used to supplement sural nerve graft repairs, with excellent outcomes as patients regained near-complete or complete motor function in some muscle groups as well as partial sensation [13, 14]. While these promising reports suggest that this technique is both safe and feasible, further clinical stud-

S. P. Miranda
Neurosurgery Department, University of Pennsylvania, Philadelphia, PA, USA
e-mail: stephen.miranda@pennmedicine.upenn.edu

E. Xu · M. Alexis
Perelman School of Medicine, University of Pennsylvania, Philadelphia, PA, USA
e-mail: emily.xu1@pennmedicine.upenn.edu; maya.alexis@pennmedicine.upenn.edu

Z. S. Ali (✉)
Department of Neurosurgery, Penn Presbyterian Medical Center, University of Pennsylvania, Philadelphia, PA, USA
e-mail: Zarina.Ali@pennmedicine.upenn.edu

A. S. Hanna (ed.), *Nerves: Anatomy, Exposures, and Techniques*, https://doi.org/10.1007/978-3-031-73931-6_70

ies with long-term follow-up will be needed to elucidate the indications, risks, and benefits of Schwann cell transplantation.

Stem Cells

While autologous nerve graft remains the ideal substrate for the surgical repair of injured nerves, this approach is limited by some disadvantages, including donor-site morbidity, donor nerve mismatch, and limited length and availability of the donor nerve, all of which may limit the potential for functional recovery [15]. Stem cell-based, tissue-engineered nerve grafts represent a promising alternative. These artificial grafts consist of a biomaterial-based scaffold containing seed cells and neurotrophic factors, which can ultimately be sutured in place to bridge nerve defects. Stem cells from a variety of sources have been used to develop tissue-engineered nerve grafts, including embryonic stem cells [16], neural stem cells [17, 18], bone marrow-derived stem cells (BMSCs) [19, 20], adipose-derived stem cells (ADSCs) [21, 22], skin-derived precursor stem cells [23–25], and induced pluripotent stem cells [26, 27]. After nerve graft transplantation, these stem cells can differentiate into Schwann-like cells that secrete neurotrophic factors and extracellular matrix components to promote axonal regeneration and myelination [28, 29].

Mesenchymal stem cells, including BMSCs and ADSCs, have received the most research interest because of their relative ease of collection and ability to differentiate into neurons, astrocytes, and Schwann-like cells [30–35]. Animal models of sciatic nerve injuries have demonstrated that BMSCs led to superior recovery as measured by motor nerve conduction velocity and amplitude when compared with autologous nerve graft alone [36]. Rats treated with BMSCs grew thicker axons, had a greater extent of myelination, and developed thicker myelin in a dose-dependent fashion [37]. Similarly, ADSCs improved regeneration of atrophied muscle and motor recovery in rodent models of sciatic nerve injuries [38, 39].

Despite such promise in animal models, there are only a few reported clinical case series supporting the translational potential of stem cell-based grafts. One group developed a collagen tube graft filled with autologous skin-derived stem cells and used these grafts to supplement sural nerve transplantation in a patient with long-gap nerve injuries in the arm (8–10 cm). After 3 years, some motor and sensory recovery was documented on pinch gauge test, two-point discrimination, monofilament testing, and electromyography (EMG) in the median and ulnar nerves [25]. In another study, 22 patients who presented in delayed fashion with median or ulnar nerve transection injuries underwent resection of neuroma and reconstruction using silicon tubes with autologous BMSCs. These patients were reported to have superior motor and sensory outcomes compared to a historical control group of 22 patients who received only empty silicone tubes [40]. More rigorous clinical studies will be needed to evaluate whether stem-cell-based grafts can eventually be incorporated into surgical strategies for nerve reconstruction.

Biologics and Therapeutics

Supplementation of nerve repair sites with biologics or immunosuppressants is an emerging technique to enhance nerve regeneration. While damaged nerve stumps have been shown to increase growth factor expression, such endogenous upregulation is not always sufficient to support the regenerating axon or myelination [41–43]. However, exogenous administration may aid the recovery process. Compounds that have shown promise include brain-derived neurotrophic factor (BDNF), nerve growth factor (NGF), fibroblast growth factor (FGF), insulin-like growth factor (IGF), and glial-derived neurotrophic factor (GDNF) [41]. For example, in rodent models, exogenous BDNF increased the survival and differentiation of human neural precursor cells after auditory nerve damage [44]. FGF administration led to enhanced nerve regeneration and ambulatory function after sciatic nerve injury [45].

Combining growth factors with grafted biomaterial or nerve conduits allows for extended growth factor activity, better targeting of growth factors to the repair site, potential control over spatiotemporal release, and enhancement of the regenerative microenvironment [41]. Various biomaterials have demonstrated success for this purpose, including chitosan and polycaprolactone [46, 47]. The delivery of multiple growth factors also appears to offer advantages, as infusion of a single growth factor may insufficiently support the different neuronal subpopulations that are required for successful regeneration. Madduri et al. demonstrated that co-delivery of GDNF and NGF via a cross-linked collagen conduit led to enhanced early nerve regeneration in nerve gaps as compared to GDNF alone [48]. Similarly, Hellenbrand et al. delivered NGF and GDNF in a sustained-release fashion through mineral-coated microparticles with promising results [49].

Beyond growth factors, therapeutics with immunosuppressant properties have also been regarded as a potential tool for improving nerve repair. For example, FK506, an FDA-approved immunosuppressant also known as tacrolimus, has demonstrated the ability to enhance nerve regeneration in rat models at lower doses than required for immunosuppression [50–52]. In human cases, early reports suggested that recovery of sensory and motor function could be attributed to the use of FK506 [53, 54], but a later case series found no long-term benefit to the administration of

FK506 after surgical repair of median, ulnar, and sciatic nerve transections [55]. Routine clinical use of FK506 is limited by its known systemic side effects [51]. Vehicles for local delivery of FK506 are under study, including hydrogels and micropatterned films [50, 56]. It is possible that enhanced local delivery may mitigate these side effects and create the incentive for more widespread use of FK506 for nerve recovery in the future.

Electrical Stimulation

Brief electrical stimulation (BES) is a regeneration technique that can be applied after surgical repair, in which low-frequency electrical current (typically 20 Hz) is used to stimulate injured motor and sensory nerves [57]. Animal models have demonstrated that BES can promote nerve regeneration by accelerating axonal outgrowth and preventing growth cone collapse [58]. Although the mechanisms are incompletely understood, it is hypothesized that BES promotes upregulation of regeneration-associated genes and drives production of neurotrophic factors in neurons and Schwann cells, including BDNF, neurotrophin-4/5 (NT-4/5) and tropomyosin-related kinase B (trkB) receptors [59–61].

Stimulation has been shown to be safe and efficacious for different types of nerve injury [62], and clinical trials have begun to demonstrate the translational potential of BES in nerve repair, both intraoperatively and postoperatively [63]. One trial conducted in 2010 recruited patients with severe carpal tunnel syndrome, defined as thenar atrophy on clinical examination with at least 50% axonal loss on motor unit number estimation (MUNE), and randomized them to carpal tunnel release with or without BES immediately after surgery. After BES, patients achieved thenar muscle reinnervation sooner, although there were no significant differences in functional outcomes [64]. However, in a similar randomized study for patients with severe cubital tunnel syndrome, BES was associated with accelerated axonal regeneration by MUNE, and patients demonstrated greater improvement in grip and key pinch strength after BES, with significantly improved CMAP amplitudes compared to sham stimulation [65].

BES has also shown potential to improve regeneration after nerve transection. A 2015 randomized, double-blind placebo-controlled trial investigated the impact of postoperative BES on digital tip sensation and functional outcomes after digital nerve transection. Compared to the surgery-only group, patients who received BES recovered greater temperature, tactile discrimination, and pressure detection sense by 5–6 months [66]. Finally, BES has also been used in head and neck cancer patients who suffered spinal accessory nerve damage during neck dissection. Intraoperative BES was shown to increase objective and subjective measures of shoulder function at 12 months postoperatively [67].

Future work is ongoing to determine optimal stimulation parameters, the efficacy of BES on cranial nerve injury, and the utility of preoperative BES [68–70]. Furthermore, ongoing development of implantable nerve stimulators [71, 72] including biodegradable ones and surface electrode stimulators [73] could broaden the applicability of BES to other clinical settings.

Myoelectric Prosthesis

Some forms of nerve injury pose major reconstructive challenges. For instance, brachial plexus injuries with lower nerve root avulsions often leave patients with permanently disabled hands, despite optimal surgical management [74]. However, recent technological advances have made it possible to leverage surviving nerves and residual muscle activity to control a prosthetic limb. Such myoelectric prostheses detect EMG signals generated by skeletal muscles and translate them into movement of an orthosis [75]. Surgical techniques have been used to amplify these EMG signals. Targeted muscle reinnervation (TMR) is a strategy by which surviving nerves are rerouted to remnant muscles to allow for more intuitive control of the prosthesis and improved functional outcomes [76, 77].

Myoelectric prosthetics and TMR have been studied for several clinical applications, including nerve injury and reconstruction after amputation. The MyoPro (Myomo, Inc., Cambridge, MA, USA) is a commercially available upper limb myoelectric device that can be used after nerve injury/reconstruction, stroke, and traumatic brain injury (Fig. 70.1) [79, 80]. The use of TMR has enabled restoration of distal function among upper- and lower-limb amputees with these devices [77, 81]. In recent case series, this approach has also been applied to patients with traumatic brachial plexus injuries who failed to regain antigravity function in the affected arm after primary reconstruction [78, 82]. Use of the myoelectric orthosis provided significant improvement in muscle strength, overall physical functioning, and pain scores [78, 82].

One of the major challenges with myoelectric prosthetics is precise and accurate EMG signal sensing. To address this issue, there have been several developments in novel electrode designs [83, 84], wireless implantable EMG sensors [85–88], and sensor placement [89]. Beyond the detection of the EMG signals, there have also been advances in signal processing algorithms that allow for improved EMG pattern recognition [90–92]. Instead of relying on precise detection of an EMG signal to directly control the prosthetic, devices that use pattern recognition can identify user-specific EMG signatures and predict the intended movement pattern.

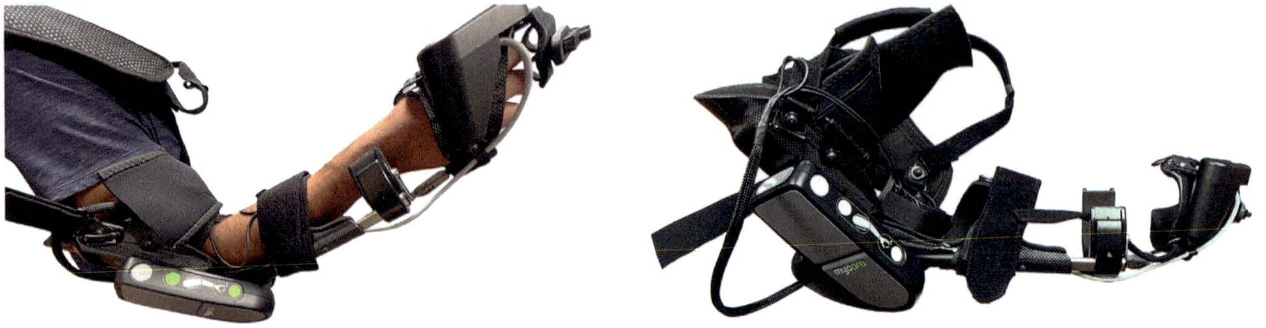

Fig. 70.1 MyoPro G device (Myomo, Inc., Cambridge, MA, USA) is a commercially available upper extremity myoelectric powered wearable orthosis, which has been used to improve elbow flexion strength and function after brachial plexus reconstruction [78]

Advances in machine learning and computation could potentially overcome current mechanical barriers and propel this technology to new heights. Sensory feedback has been a great challenge and a subject of big research interest [93]. Preventing Wallerian Degeneration And why not? Polyethylene glycol (PEG)-fusion has shown promising results in preventing Wallerian degeneration and enhancing nerve recovery after injury [94].

Conclusion

The past two decades have seen considerable innovation in the domain of nerve repair and regeneration, but many of these novel therapies require further study and testing in humans before widespread clinical adoption can be considered. So far, Schwann cell transplantation, stem cell-based tissue-engineered grafts, growth factor administration, and electrical stimulation have shown significant promise in animal models and in some clinical case series. Similarly, myoelectric prosthetics offer vital support for patients who plateau in their recovery, and this technology will only improve with ongoing advances in computing and robotics. Moving forward, the development of systems for trial enrollment and long-term follow-up of patients with nerve injuries will be essential for testing and scaling these therapies and their successors.

References

1. Hood B, Levene HB, Levi AD (2009) Transplantation of autologous Schwann cells for the repair of segmental peripheral nerve defects. Neurosurg Focus 26(2):E4. https://doi.org/10.3171/FOC.2009.26.2.E4
2. Vallejo FA, Diaz A, Errante EL, Smartz T, Khan A, Silvera R et al (2022) Systematic review of the therapeutic use of Schwann cells in the repair of peripheral nerve injuries: advancements from animal studies to clinical trials. Front Cell Neurosci 16:929593. https://doi.org/10.3389/fncel.2022.929593
3. Fowler JR, Lavasani M, Huard J, Goitz RJ (2015) Biologic strategies to improve nerve regeneration after peripheral nerve repair. J Reconstr Microsurg 31(4):243–248. https://doi.org/10.1055/s-0034-1394091
4. Berrocal YA, Almeida VW, Gupta R, Levi AD (2013) Transplantation of Schwann cells in a collagen tube for the repair of large, segmental peripheral nerve defects in rats. J Neurosurg 119(3):720–732. https://doi.org/10.3171/2013.4.JNS121189
5. Gonzalez-Perez F, Hernandez J, Heimann C, Phillips JB, Udina E, Navarro X (2018) Schwann cells and mesenchymal stem cells in laminin- or fibronectin-aligned matrices and regeneration across a critical size defect of 15 mm in the rat sciatic nerve. J Neurosurg Spine 28(1):109–118. https://doi.org/10.3171/2017.5.SPINE161100
6. Morrissey TK, Kleitman N, Bunge RP (1991) Isolation and functional characterization of Schwann cells derived from adult peripheral nerve. J Neurosci 11(8):2433–2442. https://doi.org/10.1523/JNEUROSCI.11-08-02433.1991
7. Ma T, Zhu L, Yang Y, Quan X, Huang L, Liu Z et al (2018) Enhanced in vivo survival of Schwann cells by a synthetic oxygen carrier promotes sciatic nerve regeneration and functional recovery. J Tissue Eng Regen Med 12(1):e177–e189. https://doi.org/10.1002/term.2284
8. Das S, Sharma M, Saharia D, Sarma KK, Muir EM, Bora U (2017) Electrospun silk-polyaniline conduits for functional nerve regeneration in rat sciatic nerve injury model. Biomed Mater 12(4):045025. https://doi.org/10.1088/1748-605X/aa7802
9. Wang Y, Li WY, Jia H, Zhai FG, Qu WR, Cheng YX et al (2017) KLF7-transfected Schwann cell graft transplantation promotes sciatic nerve regeneration. Neuroscience 340:319–332. https://doi.org/10.1016/j.neuroscience.2016.10.069
10. McGrath AM, Novikova LN, Novikov LN, Wiberg M (2010) BD PuraMatrix peptide hydrogel seeded with Schwann cells for peripheral nerve regeneration. Brain Res Bull 83(5):207–213. https://doi.org/10.1016/j.brainresbull.2010.07.001
11. Chang CJ (2009) The effect of pulse-released nerve growth factor from genipin-crosslinked gelatin in schwann cell-seeded polycaprolactone conduits on large-gap peripheral nerve regeneration. Tissue Eng Part A 15(3):547–557. https://doi.org/10.1089/ten.tea.2007.0342
12. Errante EL, Diaz A, Smartz T, Khan A, Silvera R, Brooks AE et al (2022) Optimal technique for introducing Schwann cells into peripheral nerve repair sites. Front Cell Neurosci 16:929494. https://doi.org/10.3389/fncel.2022.929494
13. Levi AD, Burks SS, Anderson KD, Dididze M, Khan A, Dietrich WD (2016) The use of autologous Schwann cells to supplement sciatic nerve repair with a large gap: first in human experience. Cell Transplant 25(7):1395–1403. https://doi.org/10.3727/096368915X690198
14. Gersey ZC, Burks SS, Anderson KD, Dididze M, Khan A, Dietrich WD et al (2017) First human experience with autologous Schwann cells to supplement sciatic nerve repair: report of 2 cases with

long-term follow-up. Neurosurg Focus 42(3):E2. https://doi.org/10.3171/2016.12.FOCUS16474
15. Evans GR (2001) Peripheral nerve injury: a review and approach to tissue engineered constructs. Anat Rec 263(4):396–404. https://doi.org/10.1002/ar.1120
16. Jones I, Novikova LN, Novikov LN, Renardy M, Ullrich A, Wiberg M et al (2018) Regenerative effects of human embryonic stem cell-derived neural crest cells for treatment of peripheral nerve injury. J Tissue Eng Regen Med 12(4):e2099–e2109. https://doi.org/10.1002/term.2642
17. Zhang H, Wei YT, Tsang KS, Sun CR, Li J, Huang H et al (2008) Implantation of neural stem cells embedded in hyaluronic acid and collagen composite conduit promotes regeneration in a rabbit facial nerve injury model. J Transl Med 6:67. https://doi.org/10.1186/1479-5876-6-67
18. Guo BF, Dong MM (2009) Application of neural stem cells in tissue-engineered artificial nerve. Otolaryngol Head Neck Surg 140(2):159–164. https://doi.org/10.1016/j.otohns.2008.10.039
19. Yang Y, Yuan X, Ding F, Yao D, Gu Y, Liu J et al (2011) Repair of rat sciatic nerve gap by a silk fibroin-based scaffold added with bone marrow mesenchymal stem cells. Tissue Eng Part A 17(17–18):2231–2244. https://doi.org/10.1089/ten.TEA.2010.0633
20. Hu N, Wu H, Xue C, Gong Y, Wu J, Xiao Z et al (2013) Long-term outcome of the repair of 50 mm long median nerve defects in rhesus monkeys with marrow mesenchymal stem cells-containing, chitosan-based tissue engineered nerve grafts. Biomaterials 34(1):100–111. https://doi.org/10.1016/j.biomaterials.2012.09.020
21. Watanabe Y, Sasaki R, Matsumine H, Yamato M, Okano T (2017) Undifferentiated and differentiated adipose-derived stem cells improve nerve regeneration in a rat model of facial nerve defect. J Tissue Eng Regen Med 11(2):362–374. https://doi.org/10.1002/term.1919
22. di Summa PG, Kalbermatten DF, Pralong E, Raffoul W, Kingham PJ, Terenghi G (2011) Long-term in vivo regeneration of peripheral nerves through bioengineered nerve grafts. Neuroscience 181:278–291. https://doi.org/10.1016/j.neuroscience.2011.02.052
23. McKenzie IA, Biernaskie J, Toma JG, Midha R, Miller FD (2006) Skin-derived precursors generate myelinating Schwann cells for the injured and dysmyelinated nervous system. J Neurosci 26(24):6651–6660. https://doi.org/10.1523/jneurosci.1007-06.2006
24. Khuong HT, Kumar R, Senjaya F, Grochmal J, Ivanovic A, Shakhbazau A et al (2014) Skin derived precursor Schwann cells improve behavioral recovery for acute and delayed nerve repair. Exp Neurol 254:168–179. https://doi.org/10.1016/j.expneurol.2014.01.002
25. Grimoldi N, Colleoni F, Tiberio F, Vetrano IG, Cappellari A, Costa A et al (2015) Stem cell salvage of injured peripheral nerve. Cell Transplant 24(2):213–222. https://doi.org/10.3727/096368913x675700
26. Uemura T, Takamatsu K, Ikeda M, Okada M, Kazuki K, Ikada Y et al (2012) Transplantation of induced pluripotent stem cell-derived neurospheres for peripheral nerve repair. Biochem Biophys Res Commun 419(1):130–135. https://doi.org/10.1016/j.bbrc.2012.01.154
27. Kimura H, Ouchi T, Shibata S, Amemiya T, Nagoshi N, Nakagawa T et al (2018) Stem cells purified from human induced pluripotent stem cell-derived neural crest-like cells promote peripheral nerve regeneration. Sci Rep 8(1):10071. https://doi.org/10.1038/s41598-018-27952-7
28. Cui L, Jiang J, Wei L, Zhou X, Fraser JL, Snider BJ et al (2008) Transplantation of embryonic stem cells improves nerve repair and functional recovery after severe sciatic nerve axotomy in rats. Stem Cells 26(5):1356–1365. https://doi.org/10.1634/stemcells.2007-0333
29. Ziegler L, Grigoryan S, Yang IH, Thakor NV, Goldstein RS (2011) Efficient generation of Schwann cells from human embryonic stem cell-derived neurospheres. Stem Cell Rev Rep 7(2):394–403. https://doi.org/10.1007/s12015-010-9198-2
30. Mathot F, Shin AY, Van Wijnen AJ (2019) Targeted stimulation of MSCs in peripheral nerve repair. Gene 710:17–23. https://doi.org/10.1016/j.gene.2019.02.078
31. Brohlin M, Mahay D, Novikov LN, Terenghi G, Wiberg M, Shawcross SG et al (2009) Characterisation of human mesenchymal stem cells following differentiation into Schwann cell-like cells. Neurosci Res 64(1):41–49. https://doi.org/10.1016/j.neures.2009.01.010
32. Yu Z, Xu N, Zhang N, Xiong Y, Wang Z, Liang S et al (2019) Repair of peripheral nerve sensory impairments via the transplantation of bone marrow neural tissue-committed stem cell-derived sensory neurons. Cell Mol Neurobiol 39(3):341–353. https://doi.org/10.1007/s10571-019-00650-2
33. Reichenberger MA, Mueller W, Hartmann J, Diehm Y, Lass U, Koellensperger E et al (2016) ADSCs in a fibrin matrix enhance nerve regeneration after epineural suturing in a rat model. Microsurgery 36(6):491–500. https://doi.org/10.1002/micr.30018
34. Wei Y, Gong K, Zheng Z, Liu L, Wang A, Zhang L et al (2010) Schwann-like cell differentiation of rat adipose-derived stem cells by indirect co-culture with Schwann cells in vitro. Cell Prolif 43(6):606–616. https://doi.org/10.1111/j.1365-2184.2010.00710.x
35. Jiang L, Mee T, Zhou X, Jia X (2022) Augmenting peripheral nerve regeneration with adipose-derived stem cells. Stem Cell Rev Rep 18(2):544–558. https://doi.org/10.1007/s12015-021-10236-5
36. Wang Y, Li ZW, Luo M, Li YJ, Zhang KQ (2015) Biological conduits combining bone marrow mesenchymal stem cells and extracellular matrix to treat long-segment sciatic nerve defects. Neural Regen Res 10(6):965–971. https://doi.org/10.4103/1673-5374.158362
37. Raheja A, Suri V, Suri A, Sarkar C, Srivastava A, Mohanty S et al (2012) Dose-dependent facilitation of peripheral nerve regeneration by bone marrow-derived mononuclear cells: a randomized controlled study: laboratory investigation. J Neurosurg 117(6):1170–1181. https://doi.org/10.3171/2012.8.Jns111446
38. Park JU, Kwon ST (2017) Potential of autologous adipose-derived stem cells to regenerate atrophied muscle in a rat model. Wound Repair Regen 25(6):944–955. https://doi.org/10.1111/wrr.12598
39. Rodríguez Sánchez DN, de Lima Resende LA, Boff Araujo Pinto G, de Carvalho Bovolato AL, Possebon FS, Deffune E et al (2019) Canine adipose-derived mesenchymal stromal cells enhance neuroregeneration in a rat model of sciatic nerve crush injury. Cell Transplant 28(1):47–54. https://doi.org/10.1177/0963689718809045
40. Braga-Silva J, Gehlen D, Padoin AV, Machado DC, Garicochea B, Costa da Costa J (2008) Can local supply of bone marrow mononuclear cells improve the outcome from late tubular repair of human median and ulnar nerves? J Hand Surg Eur Vol 33(4):488–493. https://doi.org/10.1177/1753193408090401
41. Li R, Li DH, Zhang HY, Wang J, Li XK, Xiao J (2020) Growth factors-based therapeutic strategies and their underlying signaling mechanisms for peripheral nerve regeneration. Acta Pharmacol Sin 41(10):1289–1300. https://doi.org/10.1038/s41401-019-0338-1
42. Hoke A, Redett R, Hameed H, Jari R, Zhou C, Li ZB et al (2006) Schwann cells express motor and sensory phenotypes that regulate axon regeneration. J Neurosci 26(38):9646–9655. https://doi.org/10.1523/JNEUROSCI.1620-06.2006
43. Cui Q (2006) Actions of neurotrophic factors and their signaling pathways in neuronal survival and axonal regeneration. Mol Neurobiol 33(2):155–179. https://doi.org/10.1385/MN:33:2:155
44. Jiao Y, Palmgren B, Novozhilova E, Englund Johansson U, Spieles-Engemann AL, Kale A et al (2014) BDNF increases survival and neuronal differentiation of human neural precursor cells cotransplanted with a nanofiber gel to the auditory nerve in a rat model of neuronal damage. Biomed Res Int 2014:356415. https://doi.org/10.1155/2014/356415

45. Ma F, Xiao Z, Chen B, Hou X, Dai J, Xu R (2014) Linear ordered collagen scaffolds loaded with collagen-binding basic fibroblast growth factor facilitate recovery of sciatic nerve injury in rats. Tissue Eng Part A 20(7–8):1253–1262. https://doi.org/10.1089/ten.TEA.2013.0158
46. Chung TW, Yang MC, Tseng CC, Sheu SH, Wang SS, Huang YY et al (2011) Promoting regeneration of peripheral nerves in-vivo using new PCL-NGF/Tirofiban nerve conduits. Biomaterials 32(3):734–743. https://doi.org/10.1016/j.biomaterials.2010.09.023
47. Xu H, Yan Y, Li S (2011) PDLLA/chondroitin sulfate/chitosan/NGF conduits for peripheral nerve regeneration. Biomaterials 32(20):4506–4516. https://doi.org/10.1016/j.biomaterials.2011.02.023
48. Madduri S, di Summa P, Papaloizos M, Kalbermatten D, Gander B (2010) Effect of controlled co-delivery of synergistic neurotrophic factors on early nerve regeneration in rats. Biomaterials 31(32):8402–8409. https://doi.org/10.1016/j.biomaterials.2010.07.052
49. Hellenbrand DJ, Haldeman CL, Lee JS, Gableman AG, Dai EK, Ortmann SD et al (2021) Functional recovery after peripheral nerve injury via sustained growth factor delivery from mineral-coated microparticles. Neural Regen Res 16(5):871–877. https://doi.org/10.4103/1673-5374.297786
50. Tajdaran K, Chan K, Shoichet MS, Gordon T, Borschel GH (2019) Local delivery of FK506 to injured peripheral nerve enhances axon regeneration after surgical nerve repair in rats. Acta Biomater 96:211–221. https://doi.org/10.1016/j.actbio.2019.05.058
51. Zuo KJ, Saffari TM, Chan K, Shin AY, Borschel GH (2020) Systemic and local FK506 (tacrolimus) and its application in peripheral nerve surgery. J Hand Surg Am 45(8):759–765. https://doi.org/10.1016/j.jhsa.2020.03.018
52. Yang RK, Lowe JB 3rd, Sobol JB, Sen SK, Hunter DA, Mackinnon SE (2003) Dose-dependent effects of FK506 on neuroregeneration in a rat model. Plast Reconstr Surg 112(7):1832–1840. https://doi.org/10.1097/01.PRS.0000091167.27303.18
53. Martin D, Pinsolle V, Merville P, Moreau K, Pelissier P, Baudet J (2005) [First case in the world of autoreplantation of a limb associated with oral administration of an immunosuppressant agent (FK 506-tacrolimus)]. Ann Chir Plast Esthet 50(4):257–263. https://doi.org/10.1016/j.anplas.2005.02.001
54. Owen ER, Dubernard JM, Lanzetta M, Kapila H, Martin X, Dawahra M et al (2001) Peripheral nerve regeneration in human hand transplantation. Transplant Proc 33(1–2):1720–1721. https://doi.org/10.1016/s0041-1345(00)02656-7
55. Phan DQ, Schuind F (2012) Tolerance and effects of FK506 (tacrolimus) on nerve regeneration: a pilot study. J Hand Surg Eur Vol 37(6):537–543. https://doi.org/10.1177/1753193411427826
56. Davis B, Wojtalewicz S, Labroo P, Shea J, Sant H, Gale B et al (2018) Controlled release of FK506 from micropatterned PLGA films: potential for application in peripheral nerve repair. Neural Regen Res 13(7):1247–1252. https://doi.org/10.4103/1673-5374.235063
57. Gordon T (2020) Peripheral nerve regeneration and muscle reinnervation. Int J Mol Sci 21(22):8652. https://doi.org/10.3390/ijms21228652
58. Zuo KJ, Gordon T, Chan KM, Borschel GH (2020) Electrical stimulation to enhance peripheral nerve regeneration: update in molecular investigations and clinical translation. Exp Neurol 332:113397. https://doi.org/10.1016/j.expneurol.2020.113397
59. Al-Majed AA, Brushart TM, Gordon T (2000) Electrical stimulation accelerates and increases expression of BDNF and trkB mRNA in regenerating rat femoral motoneurons. Eur J Neurosci 12(12):4381–4390
60. Al-Majed AA, Tam SL, Gordon T (2004) Electrical stimulation accelerates and enhances expression of regeneration-associated genes in regenerating rat femoral motoneurons. Cell Mol Neurobiol 24(3):379–402. https://doi.org/10.1023/b:cemn.0000022770.66463.f7
61. Geremia NM, Gordon T, Brushart TM, Al-Majed AA, Verge VMK (2007) Electrical stimulation promotes sensory neuron regeneration and growth-associated gene expression. Exp Neurol 205(2):347–359. https://doi.org/10.1016/j.expneurol.2007.01.040. Epub 2007 Feb 21
62. Günter C, Delbeke J, Ortiz-Catalan M (2019) Safety of long-term electrical peripheral nerve stimulation: review of the state of the art. J Neuroeng Rehabil 16(1):13. https://doi.org/10.1186/s12984-018-0474-8
63. Willand MP, Nguyen MA, Borschel GH, Gordon T (2016) Electrical stimulation to promote peripheral nerve regeneration. Neurorehabil Neural Repair 30(5):490–496. https://doi.org/10.1177/1545968315604399
64. Gordon T, Amirjani N, Edwards DC, Chan KM (2010) Brief post-surgical electrical stimulation accelerates axon regeneration and muscle reinnervation without affecting the functional measures in carpal tunnel syndrome patients. Exp Neurol 223(1):192–202. https://doi.org/10.1016/j.expneurol.2009.09.020
65. Power HA, Morhart MJ, Olson JL, Chan KM (2020) Postsurgical electrical stimulation enhances recovery following surgery for severe cubital tunnel syndrome: a double-blind randomized controlled trial. Neurosurgery 86(6):769–777. https://doi.org/10.1093/neuros/nyz322
66. Wong JN, Olson JL, Morhart MJ, Chan KM (2015) Electrical stimulation enhances sensory recovery: a randomized controlled trial. Ann Neurol 77(6):996–1006. https://doi.org/10.1002/ana.24397
67. Barber B, Seikaly H, Ming Chan K, Beaudry R, Rychlik S, Olson J et al (2018) Intraoperative brief electrical stimulation of the spinal accessory nerve (BEST SPIN) for prevention of shoulder dysfunction after oncologic neck dissection: a double-blinded, randomized controlled trial. J Otolaryngol Head Neck Surg 47(1):7. https://doi.org/10.1186/s40463-017-0244-9
68. Senger J-L, Chan KM, Macandili H, Chan AWM, Verge VMK, Jones KE et al (2019) Conditioning electrical stimulation promotes functional nerve regeneration. Exp Neurol 315:60–71. https://doi.org/10.1016/j.expneurol.2019.02.001
69. Senger J-LB, Chan KM, Webber CA (2020) Conditioning electrical stimulation is superior to postoperative electrical stimulation, resulting in enhanced nerve regeneration and functional recovery. Exp Neurol 325:113147. https://doi.org/10.1016/j.expneurol.2019.113147
70. Mendez A, Hopkins A, Biron VL, Seikaly H, Zhu LF, Côté DWJ (2018) Brief electrical stimulation and synkinesis after facial nerve crush injury: a randomized prospective animal study. J Otolaryngol Head Neck Surg 47(1):20. https://doi.org/10.1186/s40463-018-0264-0
71. Koo J, MacEwan MR, Kang S-K, Won SM, Stephen M, Gamble P et al (2018) Wireless bioresorbable electronic system enables sustained nonpharmacological neuroregenerative therapy. Nat Med 24(12):1830–1836. https://doi.org/10.1038/s41591-018-0196-2. Epub 2018 Oct 8
72. Chu XL, Song XZ, Li YR, Wu ZR, Li Q, Li QW et al (2023) An ultrasound-guided percutaneous electrical nerve stimulation regimen devised using finite element modeling promotes functional recovery after median nerve transection. Neural Regen Res 18(3):683–688. https://doi.org/10.4103/1673-5374.350215
73. Chan I, Brown AR, Park K, Winfree CJ (2010) Ultrasound-guided, percutaneous peripheral nerve stimulation. Neurosurgery 67(3 Suppl Operative):ons136–ons139. https://doi.org/10.1227/01.NEU.0000383137.33503.EB
74. Bertelli JA, Ghizoni MF (2011) Results and current approach for brachial plexus reconstruction. J Brachial Plex Peripher Nerve Inj 6(1):2. https://doi.org/10.1186/1749-7221-6-2

75. Geethanjali P (2016) Myoelectric control of prosthetic hands: state-of-the-art review. Med Devices (Auckl) 9:247–255. https://doi.org/10.2147/mder.S91102
76. Gart MS, Souza JM, Dumanian GA (2015) Targeted muscle reinnervation in the upper extremity amputee: a technical roadmap. J Hand Surg Am 40(9):1877–1888. https://doi.org/10.1016/j.jhsa.2015.06.119
77. Dumanian GA, Ko JH, O'Shaughnessy KD, Kim PS, Wilson CJ, Kuiken TA (2009) Targeted reinnervation for transhumeral amputees: current surgical technique and update on results. Plast Reconstr Surg 124(3):863–869. https://doi.org/10.1097/PRS.0b013e3181b038c9
78. Pulos N, van den Berg C, Kaufman KR, Shin AY (2021) Application of myoelectric elbow flexion assist orthosis in adult traumatic brachial plexus injury: a retrospective clinical study. Prosthet Orthot Int 45(6):521–525. https://doi.org/10.1097/pxr.0000000000000046
79. Pundik S, McCabe J, Skelly M, Salameh A, Naft J, Chen Z et al (2022) Myoelectric arm orthosis in motor learning-based therapy for chronic deficits after stroke and traumatic brain injury. Front Neurol 13:791144. https://doi.org/10.3389/fneur.2022.791144
80. McCabe JP, Henniger D, Perkins J, Skelly M, Tatsuoka C, Pundik S (2019) Feasibility and clinical experience of implementing a myoelectric upper limb orthosis in the rehabilitation of chronic stroke patients: a clinical case series report. PLoS One 14(4):e0215311. https://doi.org/10.1371/journal.pone.0215311
81. Kuiken TA, Barlow AK, Hargrove L, Dumanian GA (2017) Targeted muscle reinnervation for the upper and lower extremity. Tech Orthop 32(2):109–116. https://doi.org/10.1097/bto.0000000000000194
82. Aszmann OC, Roche AD, Salminger S, Paternostro-Sluga T, Herceg M, Sturma A et al (2015) Bionic reconstruction to restore hand function after brachial plexus injury: a case series of three patients. Lancet 385(9983):2183–2189. https://doi.org/10.1016/s0140-6736(14)61776-1
83. Schlink BR, Nordin AD, Ferris DP (2020) Comparison of signal processing methods for reducing motion artifacts in high-density electromyography during human locomotion. IEEE Open J Eng Med Biol 1:156–165. https://doi.org/10.1109/OJEMB.2020.2999782. eCollection
84. Welle EJ, Patel PR, Woods JE, Petrossians A, Della Valle E, Vega-Medina A et al (2020) Ultra-small carbon fiber electrode recording site optimization and improved in vivo chronic recording yield. J Neural Eng 17(2):026037. https://doi.org/10.1088/1741-2552/ab8343
85. Dewald HA, Lukyanenko P, Lambrecht JM, Anderson JR, Tyler DJ, Kirsch RF et al (2019) Stable, three degree-of-freedom myoelectric prosthetic control via chronic bipolar intramuscular electrodes: a case study. J Neuroeng Rehabil 16(1):147. https://doi.org/10.1186/s12984-019-0607-8
86. Vaskov AK, Vu PP, North N, Davis AJ, Kung TA, Gates DH et al (2022) Surgically implanted electrodes enable real-time finger and grasp pattern recognition for prosthetic hands. IEEE Trans Robot 38(5):2841–2857. https://doi.org/10.1109/tro.2022.3170720. Epub 2022 Jun 1
87. Salminger S, Sturma A, Hofer C, Evangelista M, Perrin M, Bergmeister KD et al (2019) Long-term implant of intramuscular sensors and nerve transfers for wireless control of robotic arms in above-elbow amputees. Sci Robot 4(32):eaaw6306. https://doi.org/10.1126/scirobotics.aaw6306
88. Vu PP, Vaskov AK, Irwin ZT, Henning PT, Lueders DR, Laidlaw AT et al (2020) A regenerative peripheral nerve interface allows real-time control of an artificial hand in upper limb amputees. Sci Transl Med 12(533):eaay2857. https://doi.org/10.1126/scitranslmed.aay2857
89. Mastinu E, Clemente F, Sassu P, Aszmann O, Brånemark R, Håkansson B et al (2019) Grip control and motor coordination with implanted and surface electrodes while grasping with an osseointegrated prosthetic hand. J Neuroeng Rehabil 16(1):49. https://doi.org/10.1186/s12984-019-0511-2
90. Spanias JA, Simon AM, Finucane SB, Perreault EJ, Hargrove LJ (2018) Online adaptive neural control of a robotic lower limb prosthesis. J Neural Eng 15(1):016015. https://doi.org/10.1088/1741-2552/aa92a8
91. Jiang N, Rehbaum H, Vujaklija I, Graimann B, Farina D (2014) Intuitive, online, simultaneous, and proportional myoelectric control over two degrees-of-freedom in upper limb amputees. IEEE Trans Neural Syst Rehabil Eng 22(3):501–510. https://doi.org/10.1109/tnsre.2013.2278411
92. Young AJ, Simon AM, Fey NP, Hargrove LJ (2014) Intent recognition in a powered lower limb prosthesis using time history information. Ann Biomed Eng 42(3):631–641. https://doi.org/10.1007/s10439-013-0909-0
93. Antfolk C, D'Alonzo M, Rosén B, Lundborg G, Sebelius F, Ciprian (2013) Sensory feedback in upper limb prosthetics. Expert Rev Med Devices 10(1):45–54. https://doi.org/10.1586/erd.12.68
94. Bittner GD, Tuffaha S, Shores JT (2024) Polyethylene glycol-fusion repair of peripheral nerve injuries. Hand Clin 40(3):389–397. https://doi.org/10.1016/j.hcl.2024.05.001

Index

A. S. Hanna (ed.), *Nerves: Anatomy, Exposures, and Techniques*, https://doi.org/10.1007/978-3-031-73931-6

GPSR Compliance

The European Union's (EU) General Product Safety Regulation (GPSR) is a set of rules that requires consumer products to be safe and our obligations to ensure this.

If you have any concerns about our products, you can contact us on ProductSafety@springernature.com

In case Publisher is established outside the EU, the EU authorized representative is:

Springer Nature Customer Service Center GmbH
Europaplatz 3
69115 Heidelberg, Germany

Batch number: 10731661

Printed by Printforce, the Netherlands